Medical Imaging:
Essentials for Physicians

Medical Imaging: Essentials for Physicians

Anthony B. Wolbarst, PhD

Associate Professor
Department of Radiology, College of Medicine
Department of Radiation Science, College of Health Sciences
University of Kentucky
Lexington, KY, USA

Patrizio Capasso, MD, DSc

Professor of Radiology and Surgery
Vice Chair, Department of Radiology
University of Kentucky
Lexington, KY, USA

Andrew R. Wyant, MD

Assistant Professor
Department of Clinical Sciences
College of Health Sciences
University of Kentucky
Lexington, KY, USA

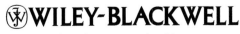

A John Wiley & Sons, Ltd., Publication

Library of Congress Cataloging-in-Publication Data

Wolbarst, Anthony B.
  Medical imaging : essentials for physicians / Anthony B. Wolbarst, Andrew R. Wyant, Patrizio Capasso.
    p. ; cm.
  ISBN 978-0-470-50570-0 (cloth : alk. paper) – ISBN 978-1-118-48024-3 (ebook) – ISBN 978-1-118-48027-4 (emobi) – ISBN 978-1-118-48028-1 (epdf) – ISBN 978-1-118-48026-7 (obook)
  I. Wyant, Andrew R.   II. Capasso, Patrizio.   III. Title.
  [DNLM: 1. Diagnostic Imaging – methods.   2. Image Enhancement – methods. WN 180]
  616.07′54–dc23   2012047813

Front cover image: Photo kindly provided by Charles Smith, MSEE, MD, and David Powell, PhD, of the Magnetic Resonance Imaging and Spectroscopy Center (MRISC), University of Kentucky, Lexington

Back cover image: Courtesy of Brian Gold, PhD, University of Kentucky

Cover design: Michael Rutkowski

Illustrations by Anthony Wolbarst and Gordon Cook

Set in 9.5/12pt Minion by Aptara® Inc., New Delhi, India

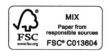

We dedicate this effort to

    Ling and Zea, who mean everything (ABW),

    Tara, Pier Andrea, and Melanie, who have all of my love (PC),

    My amazing wife Krystal and our six wonderful children (AW),

and to the patients and healthcare-providers it may serve.

"Everything should be made as simple as possible, but no simpler."

On educating, attributed to Albert Einstein

Contents

Preface

Recall how, after several years of college French, or Spanish, or Urdu, you ventured abroad and discovered that you could actually get by? You could order more or less what you wanted for dinner, you began to find your way around town. And when people asked you, slowly and clearly, where you were from and what you were doing there, you could both make out much of what they were saying and respond reasonably coherently. It might take you another year or so before you began sounding like a native, but you definitely could survive.

The objective of this book is to help and encourage you to acquire survival-level medical imaging. As such, it is designed to provide a technically solid, clear, largely non-mathematical understanding of the most significant ideas underlying the field, and yet be as short as possible (but no shorter). We include references to several much longer texts that provide reams of factual details, which are important for those who wish to go farther. The idea here, however, is to get you up and going, with a reasonable degree of competence and confidence, and to do so quickly.

Medical Imaging: Essentials for Physicians is a survival-level introduction to the extraordinary instruments and processes that create medical images, and to the ways in which radiologists, cardiologists, orthopedists, neurosurgeons, and most other physicians employ them to assist in resolving medical problems. While intended primarily for attending physicians, radiology and other residents, and medical students with limited direct familiarity with imaging, it should also be accessible to other senior medical professionals, and to biological and physical scientists as well.

This is not a textbook, nor is it written in a formal style. Hopefully you will find the manner to be relaxed and engaging, more or less like the way people speak. (We sometimes even split infinitives and end sentences with prepositions, if there's reason to.) But it is nonetheless a very serious and nontrivial book written for professionals who wish to acquire enough command of the imaging tools of their trade to be able to explain the general ideas accurately to students, nurses and technologists, to discuss them self-confidently with medical and technical colleagues and vendors, and to describe them effectively to concerned patients and loved ones. While there are no prerequisites, the read will be much more pleasurable if you happen to be the curious type. You will come to grasp a good deal about *what* and *how* imaging things happen, in any case, but it should be a more rewarding experience if you, like the authors, tend to frequently ask yourself *why*, as well. We like to explain things, not just describe them.

The reward for your perseverance will be a firm and technically rigorous qualitative understanding of the basic ideas of how computed tomography (CT), magnetic resonance imaging (MRI), digital subtraction angiography (DSA), and the other principal modalities really work – along with the strengths and risks of each, and the reasons that the knowledgeable physician finds one technology to be preferable to the others in a particular clinical situation. You will come to see the reasons that digital radiography (DR) and single photon emission computed tomography (SPECT) may be able to detect hairline bone fractures, say (although nuclear medicine is only rarely employed for that purpose), while ultrasound and fluoroscopy cannot. And why positron emission tomography (PET) is so adept at seeking out and searching out neoplasms, while few of the other modalities are.

You will also learn the essential role that quality assurance and safety programs play in determining that devices are delivering images with clinically optimal contrast and resolution, and at the same time with as little risk as possible from radiation or other hazards. Distressingly large numbers of physicians misread images and overdose patients with radiation, in part because they do not realize that their equipment is producing less than adequate pictures, or how to check on that routinely. Nor are they aware of just how great, or not, are the risks and benefits from routine screening mammograms, or from CT of a neonate – or that it may be possible to reduce the doses to kids considerably without compromising clinical efficacy.

In most situations, the issue of greatest importance in a diagnostic image is the visual *contrast* that allows the viewer to distinguish among and examine organs and other tissues, both normal and pathological. For X-ray technologies, including screen-film and digital radiography, digital subtraction angiography, and CT, contrast arises because X-ray probes collide with the atoms of different tissues in different ways and by different amounts; the shadows of bone emerge in a radiograph because that material is much more adept at absorbing and scattering away X-rays than are the surrounding soft tissues, so fewer of them make it through to expose the film or digital image receptor. There is contrast in nuclear medicine images, including SPECT and PET, because various radiopharmaceuticals concentrate preferentially in certain specific biological compartments, resulting in the differential emission of high-energy photons that can be detected and imaged from outside the body. High-frequency vibrational waves of ultrasound radiation reflect at boundaries between tissues that differ in density or elasticity, and processing the echoes can give rise to those cute pre-baby pictures of such extraordinary clarity and detail. And with MRI, in all its glory, one can generate contrast among tissues in multiple ways, based on differences in their proton density; the proton spin relaxation times T1 and T2; the flow of blood through vessels; the diffusion of water along the tracts of neural axons in the brain; the motion of relatively well-oxygenated blood to parts of the brain that require it; the list goes on.

These approaches give rise to contrast among the tissues in remarkably dissimilar ways. The resulting various kinds of contrast naturally accentuate different aspects of anatomy or physiology, and one

of them may provide exceptionally valuable kinds of clinical information in a given medical situation. Much of the discussion herein will therefore focus on the ways in which the diverse methods of imaging exploit distinct biophysical processes to create contrast, on how the operator can draw it out and enhance it most effectively, on the relative risks, costs, and availability of the technologies, and ultimately on the medical reasons that a particular modality may be especially diagnostically useful in a given case.

The authorship of the book reflects its intent. The first draft was prepared by a medical physicist who has written a widely used text for radiology residents on imaging science and technology. It was then edited by a practicing interventional radiologist, who cut out some of the stuff unnecessary or uninteresting for most doctors; translated the rest into proper medicalese; and added a large number of cases to illustrate important points. Then an emergency-room physician with much experience but no special training in imaging went through it carefully to ensure the clarity of presentation and its intelligibility to non-radiologists, and to add further cases. Finally, each completed chapter on a modality was sent for review to radiologists, medical physicists, and other radiological specialists. As in the Acknowledgments section, the authors wish to express here again their great and sincere sense of indebtedness to these extremely busy professionals who took time out of their packed schedules to critique the chapters and to offer ideas for improvements.

A challenge to the authors has been, of course, to determine what topics to discuss, and in how much depth and breadth. We have attempted to cover enough to satisfy readers searching for a rapid, practical understanding of the whole field, yet also to whet the appetites of others to pursue more. Some will brush through the central topics quickly, just to pick up the main points, at least on the first pass, while others will wish to dig in a bit deeper. The presentation is therefore on two levels: the main story line appears in normal type, but paragraphs containing more detail or explanation than might be needed for a first encounter will be presented in this manner. We welcome suggestions from readers on what should be added in future editions of the book, or cut back or deleted, or changed, bearing in mind that we are making a conscious effort to keep it as short as possible while it can still do its job.

A comment on equations: in some places it clarifies ideas to express them in the language of elementary algebra. Nothing is more mathematically demanding in the text than linear equations ($y = mx + b$), or sine waves ($\sin x$), or the occasional exponential ($e^{-\mu x}$). The equations will serve to summarize and elucidate notions by re-phrasing them in another form, not to complicate them, and they are guaranteed not to cause tachycardia or severe gastric distress.

Another comment, about repetition: we use it, very intentionally so, because it is well known to aid in learning the central points in an extensive and sometimes challenging new subject. We feel that it will be helpful for many readers – but if you got the idea the first time around, please be patient if it comes up again. In any case, additional information is almost always added each time a topic is revisited – material that might have seemed less relevant or confusing earlier.

One good thing you might consider doing, after completing a chapter, is to wander into an imaging clinic, talk with both the physicians and the technologists there, perhaps even learn to drive their machines a little. And before long, you yourself will start sounding somewhat like an imaging native.

Bon voyage, and bring back lots of good pictures!

Acknowledgments

A number of friends and colleagues have helped us, in some cases a great deal, with the preparation of this book, and also with reviewing the chapters. The following may look like just a list of names, but in reality we dealt with each of these people, sometimes closely, and every one of those interactions was important to us and hopefully pleasant for them. It is with heartfelt appreciation that we thank the following for their time, efforts, and good ideas:

Mathew Maxwell, Chief Resident in the Department of Radiology at UK, for his heroic efforts in scrounging up a number of excellent clinical case images, and collaboration in their interpretation.

Nathan Yanasek, who kindly went through the two MRI chapters carefully and made a number of thoughtful, detailed suggestions that have improved them significantly. Likewise, Fred Fahey helped us regarding nuclear medicine.

Two medical physics graduate students of one of us (A.B.W.), Xin Xie, PhD, and Thomas Baker, MS, went through the whole thing, caught many typos, and provided numerous ideas for making the presentation clearer.

In addition, Bruce Curran, Peter Hardy, Joseph Hornak, Yang Jiang, Phil Judy, Kevin F. King, Baojun Li, Christine Luerman, Walter Miller, David Powell, Gerald Schlenker, Partha Sinha, Charles Smith, Michael Steckner, Margaret Szabunio, Lifeng Yu, Charles Willis, Robert Zamenhof, and Jie Zhang all provided considerable help and guidance. Again, thank you all.

And finally, an especial thanks to Mel Clouse for his encouragement and support on this project. They have meant a great deal.

We are greatly indebted to Thom Moore, Gill Whitley, Jane Kerr of Castlecrab, Wales, wherever that may be, and the other folks at Wiley who have been supportive, accommodating, and wise in guiding us through this process; one couldn't ask for a better team of publishers.

And finally, our profoundest thanks to our three wives, without whom this effort would never have gotten beyond the dream stage. They have been unfailingly encouraging, patient, and understanding throughout, and they have helped to turn an arduous burden into a labor of love.

Dr. Doe's Headaches

An Imaging Case Study

Jane Doe, for several decades the sole physician in a small town in rural eastern Kentucky, began having mild but disruptive headaches that responded completely to Advil or Tylenol. After they continued for two months, she referred herself to the small community clinic 30 miles away.

The patient presented to the clinic's internist as a healthy 52-year-old woman in no apparent distress, apart from mild hypertension that was controlled by medication. Other aspects of her physical examination were unremarkable. In particular, neurologic examination revealed no focal deficits. She followed a good diet and exercised moderately several times a week. She claimed to be happily married to her best friend, and reported no major stresses or anxieties, apart from those arising from a daughter fortunately emerging from teenagehood.

Computed tomography

Uncomfortable with the duration of the problem, the internist ordered an immediate *unenhanced computed tomography* (CT) scan of the brain.

A CT machine is a highly specialized X-ray instrument. Like an ordinary radiographic or fluoroscopic device, it produces X-rays, which can be thought of as minute, particle-like bundles of energy that can flow through matter unimpeded – until, that is, they collide with atoms. X-rays tend to interact more frequently with bone or pieces of metal, and thereby be removed from the X-ray beam, than with soft tissues, which are less dense and are composed of lighter elements like hydrogen, carbon and oxygen; for this reason, the beam creates a *shadowgram* that reveals such differences.

Suppose a child may have swallowed some dangerous objects lying on a desk, possibly including tacks and razor blades within paper wrappers. You take an antero-posterior (AP) radiograph in the region of interest, but cannot tell for sure, from that image alone, what he ingested. You are very concerned about radiation exposure, especially in one so young, but feel it is necessary to have a better idea about what you are dealing with before proceeding. You take a lateral radiograph, and hope to make sense of the pair of images together (Figure 0.1). What entities (and in what configuration) could possibly give rise to this particular set of radiographs?

A CT carries out this program to extremes, in effect obtaining shadowgrams from hundreds of angles around the patient; its computer's mathematical *reconstruction algorithm* then calculates how much X-ray attenuation must be occurring at every point within the body to result in this particular *set* of many such planar shadowgrams. That is, from a vast amount of measured data, CT *reconstructs* and displays maps of the local rates of interaction of the X-rays with matter throughout one or more adjacent transverse slices of tissue, all at the same time. And that, in turn, provides separate two-dimensional maps of the various tissue types within

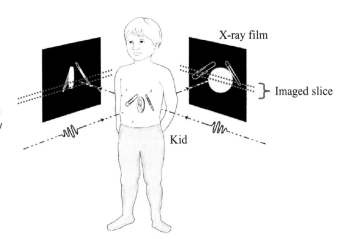

X-ray film

Imaged slice

Figure 0.1 While a single radiograph of a child's stomach taken from one angle may not reveal much with certainty, a few pictures together may allow you to determine what he had swallowed – or rather, the spatial distribution of attenuating materials within the body that could give rise to this *set* of X-ray images, obtained from multiple vantage points.

Kid

every slice, with good *contrast* between materials that differ significantly in composition, and with no visual patterns from over- or underlying tissues to obscure what is of interest.

For technical reasons, older CT machines did not examine a tall block of the body, but only a pan-cake transverse slice of tissues a centimeter or so high; modern devices can capture 10 cm or more of body in 64, or even hundreds, of slices with a single rotation of the gantry.

The computer is not clever enough to reveal anything medical about what it finds; all it can do, rather, is to determine how readily the material at any point can soak up or scatter X-rays, a purely physical measurement and computation. Making sense of it all is up to the physician.

For Dr. Doe, sixteen transverse CT slices of the brain were obtained on a rather antiquated machine. Nearly all the scans were normal, apart from a probable right posterior temporo-occipital irregularity adjacent to the occipital horn of the right lateral ventricle, appearing in two adjacent slices. There was no radiologist on-site, and the internist arranged for Dr. Doe to undergo a magnetic resonance imaging (MRI) examination right away at a large, tertiary hospital center. He copied the CT images onto a DVD, to take with her.

Picture archiving and communication system

The next day her husband drove her the three hours to the University of Kentucky (UK) Medical Cen-ter in Lexington. But, in his haste, he misplaced the DVD of the CT study, so we cannot display it here.

Unlike her rural clinic, modern imaging centers tend now to be fully digital, and they rely heavily on a computer-based *picture archiving and communications system* (PACS), rather than on film, for nearly all of their activities (Figure 0.2). A PACS is a data management network that interconnects the various digital image acquisition and processing devices, local workstations, short-term image storage, and long-term archiving. It allows live viewing and image manipulation at any workstation, and can rapidly call up from storage images obtained earlier. Its *teleradiology* capabilities allow it to send and receive images instantaneously for examination by colleagues down the hall or across the country. It can even transfer them to a *computer-assisted detection* (CAD) artificial intelligence program to aid in detecting and perhaps identifying irregularities in images – acting, in effect, as a second pair of trained eyes.

A state-of-the-art PACS and associated radiology information system (RIS) also welcome input of pathology slides, colonoscopy photographs, and other diagnostic image information, including digitized versions of prior X-rays for comparison, and links to similar systems in other departments. After she arrived at the UK Medical Center, all of Dr. Doe's subsequent images, along with lab results and other medical records, were stored safely and kept available for immediate retrieval on the Department of Radiology's PACS and RIS.

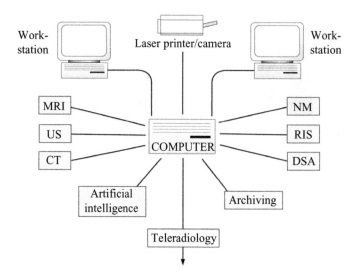

Figure 0.2 A picture archiving and communications system (PACS) links together the various devices and activities of a modern imaging center.

The CT had already performed an essential service by drawing attention to the possible irregularity, and in any case, the MRI studies would be far more revealing of soft-tissue lesions. MRI can create contrast between normal background tissues and abnormalities in a number of related but dissimilar ways, and these can yield somewhat different but complementary kinds of clinical information. She began with three standard, distinct image techniques known as T1-weighted, T2-*w*, and FLAIR.

T1, T2, and FLAIR MRI

For an MRI study, a patient is placed within the bore of an extremely powerful *superconducting* magnet: the magnetic field of a standard 1.5 tesla (1.5 T) device is 30 000 times that of the earth.

The nuclei of the hydrogen atoms of the water, lipid, and other molecules in her tissues are just isolated protons. But they act like *spinning* charged bodies, and since any moving charge produces its own magnetic field, they behave somewhat like submicroscopic compass needles. The protons tend to align along the strong external field of the magnet, but carefully sculpted short pulses of radio waves can drive their spin axes briefly away from the direction of the field, which is when the interesting things begin to happen.

Most of MR involves the imaging of inter- and intracellular water, so we'll stick with that for now.

Various biophysical interactions between the water and the other cellular constituents encourage the water protons to *relax* back toward their original preferred orientation along the main field. There are several friction-like mechanisms that affect such proton spin relaxation, each with its own characteristic rate of relaxation or, equivalently, its own *proton relaxation time.* Every cell type creates a unique internal physico-chemical environment, moreover, and the values of the several proton relaxation times for it depend on the kind of tissue found there, and even on its state of health or the presence of disease. It is the mapped spatial variations in the relaxation times of various tissues that give rise to the sometimes remarkable degree of contrast appearing in most MR images.

The two clinically dominant relaxation processes, in particular, take place with relaxation times called T1 and T2. An MR image that emphasizes the variations in the value of T1 at the different points throughout a slice of tissues is said to be *T1-weighted.* So, too, for a *T2-weighted* image. A FLAIR (*FLuid Attenuation Inversion Recovery*) image is similar to these but provides the advantage of suppressing signals from aqueous fluids; in the brain, for example, it can eliminate the appearance of cerebrospinal fluid, thereby enhancing periventricular lesions like some gliomas and multiple sclerosis plaques.

Dr. Doe's T1 and T2 images supported the CT report, noting additionally the extension of the well-circumscribed 1.7 × 1.1 cm lesion to the ependymal lining of the ventricle (Figure 0.3a). There was a significant mass effect, but no midline shift or hydrocephalus. The T1 scan was then repeated following the injection of 20 ml of gadolinium contrast agent, and there was little change. Higher-grade neoplasms in the brain are more likely to disrupt the blood–brain barrier, and are thus associated with more avid contrast enhancement. The failure of the region to take up the agent suggested that there was no breach of the blood–brain barrier, which implied that the lesion was probably not a high-grade neoplasm, a hopeful sign.

The FLAIR study proved to be clinically even more revealing, and the reading radiologist felt that it indicated a lower-grade glioma protruding into the ventricle, with consideration (although less likely) of a tumefactive demyelinating lesion in the differential (Figure 0.3b). There were also several small punctuate T2 signal abnormalities scattered throughout the subcortical white matter of the cerebral hemispheres, possibly representing chronic small-vessel ischemic changes or conceivably further areas of demyelation.

MR spectroscopy and a virtual biopsy

The gold standard in identifying a tumor is a physical biopsy, of course, but an MRI *virtual biopsy* can provide excellent preliminary information quickly and non-invasively. This advanced procedure, known also as *MR spectroscopy* (*MRS*), exploits the other most fundamental process that, in addition to proton relaxation, underlies MRI.

One way to view protons in an external field is that they behave like sub-microscopic spinning gyroscopes that are precessing in a gravitational field. A top precesses one sixth as fast in the weaker field of the Moon as when on Earth; similarly, the precession of proton spins is highly sensitive to the exact strength of the local magnetic field. Now, the uneven circulation of electrons (again, moving charges) throughout a biomolecule will affect the local magnetic fields at the various points within it. This results in parts-per-million shifts in the rates of precession of protons in different local molecular environments. These changes are usually far too small to show up with MRI images, but an MRS

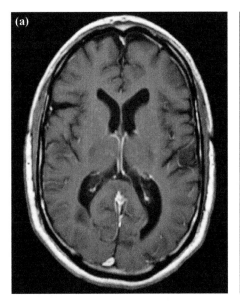 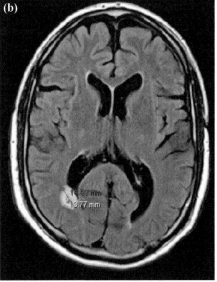

Figure 0.3 Two MRI images of the same thin (1 mm), transverse slice. (**a**) T1-weighting reveals a hypointense right posterior temporo-occipital lesion, adjacent to occipital horn of the right lateral ventricle. (**b**) A FLAIR sequence, in which signals from CSF and other fluids are suppressed, yields a somewhat different type of MRI contrast, better demonstrating the lesion, which is now hyperintense. Courtesy of Charles Smith, Peter Hardy, David Powell, University of Kentucky, MR Imaging and Spectroscopy Center (MRISC).

machine is more refined, and exquisitely responsive to these slight *chemical shifts.*

The proton resonance spectrum of acetic acid (CH_3COOH), for example, appears as two peaks, close in local magnetic field and therefore in proton precession frequency, but clearly distinct, whose amplitudes are in the ratio 3:1 (Figure 0.4a). The three protons within the methyl (CH_3-) group all experience the same swirl of electrons and identical local environments. The electron flow within the $-COOH$ group is a bit different, however, and its single proton resides in a slightly lower local field. Hence the two lines in the spectrum are separated in frequency, indicating the different local magnetic fields and rates of precession.

For brain tissue away from the lesion, the proton spectra for *N*-acetylaspartate (NAA), creatine and phospho-creatine (Cr), and choline (Cho) appeared normal (Figure 0.4b). The lesion itself, however, reveals a statistically significant irregularity in the relative concentrations (areas under the peaks) of Cr and Cho (Figure 0.4c). The spectral signatures for numerous normal and abnormal tissues have been studied, and the pattern seen here is indicative of a glioma, but of indeterminate stage.

Functional MRI

Treatment of a tumor depends on its type, grade, stage, and anatomical location. In this case, its position is such that therapy such as surgery or radiation might result in the loss of one of her two fields of vision. While Dr. Doe could accept that, she made it unambiguously clear that she would not agree to any action that would seriously jeopardize her ability to read; she would prefer to leave the disease untreated, and take her chances. So before proceeding to a needle biopsy, which itself could impose a risk to reading vision, she underwent two non-invasive MRI-based studies that would help to determine the distance of optically active regions from the apparent tumor. The first was *functional MRI (fMRI).*

While oxyhemoglobin is magnetically practically neutral (diamagnetic), deoxyhemoglobin is paramagnetic, producing a small additional magnetic presence when the molecule happens to be sitting in a strong magnetic field. When brain tissues are active, they consume extra oxygen and transform oxyhemoglobin into deoxyhemoglobin, and *f*MRI can detect where such changes are occurring; this provides an altogether different type of MRI contrast.

In an *f*MRI study, a subject is made to experience a periodic mental process of some sort, such as by repeatedly tapping her finger, and variations in the MR signal are monitored (Figure 0.5a). Resulting deviations in the balance of the two kinds of hemoglobin may produce detectable tissue contrast where associated parts of the brain are being triggered. What may not be expected is that neurons are *not* simply burning more oxygen there; as will be seen later, the brain is much more clever than that, and the process is actually more subtle and interesting.

Dr. Doe underwent *f*MRI with two separate stimuli, self-directed finger tapping and visual images. From the scale to the left, it is evident that the temporal *variations* (which is what is of interest here) in the MR signal are much smaller than the average value of the signal itself, so effective noise-rejection and statistical information-processing programs must be invoked. The finger-tapping task demonstrated robust activation within the expected region of the motor cortex of the cerebral hemispheres. Her response to an intermittent visual stimulus, shown here in a 1 mm thin sagittal *f*MRI slice through the lesion, indicates that one optically active region of the brain lies nearly adjacent to it (Figure 0.5b).

Diffusion tensor MR imaging

In view of the discouraging *f*MRI results, it was felt to be important to carry out a *diffusion tensor image (DTI)* study for her. With DTI, contrast arises from the uni-directional *diffusion* of water molecules along the axons of a nerve trunk, against a background of other water molecules that are diffusing isotropically, in all directions. A sagittal, thin-slice DTI corroborated the earlier *f*MRI finding that Dr. Doe's probable glioma lies directly adjacent to, and possibly infiltrating, superior portions of the optic radiation (Figure 0.6).

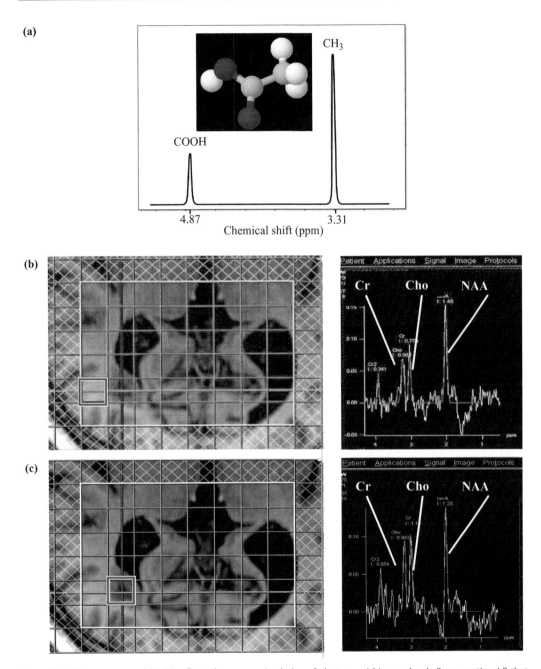

Figure 0.4 MR spectroscopy. (a) MRS reflects the uneven circulation of electrons within a molecule (here, acetic acid) that give rise to small differences in *local* magnetic field, hence in parts per million (ppm) shifts in proton Larmor frequency of precession. (b) MRS is performed here on two adjacent small volumes of tissue in the right posterior temporo-occipital region, adjacent to occipital horn of the right lateral ventricle. The measured spectra are adjusted so that the amplitudes of the *N*-acetylaspartate (NAA) peaks are the same. The spectrum from this region of healthy tissue appears normal. (c) That from the region of the abnormality, however, displays differences in the heights of the creatine plus phospho-creatine (Cr) and the choline (Cho) peaks that are suggestive of a glioma. This "virtual biopsy" was subsequently confirmed through examination of a tissue sample.

(a)

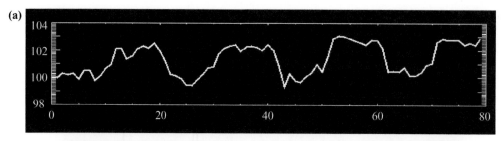

(b)

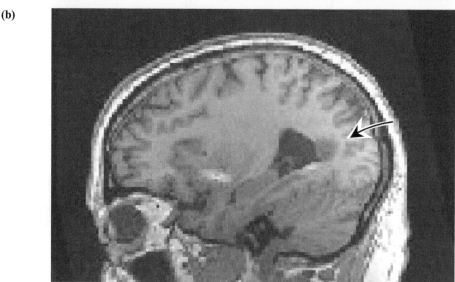

Figure 0.5 Contrast in functional MRI (*f*MRI) comes from the detection of changes, induced by certain stimuli, in the consumption of oxygen and in the patterns of blood flow in specific parts of the brain. **(a)** The periodic change in MRI signal strength from a small region of the brain results from a stimulus of the same periodicity. **(b)** The image of a 1 mm thin sagittal slice of Dr. Doe's brain that indicates that one area activated by a visual stimulus, in green, lies close to her lesion (arrow).

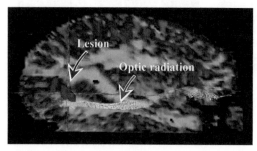

Figure 0.6 With diffusion tensor imaging (DTI) of the optic radiation, contrast arises between the water molecules that happen to be diffusing along trunks of axons and the others that are diffusing isotropically.

MR guided biopsy

After viewing all the evidence, and particularly the DTI, a neurosurgeon felt that with MRI guidance of the needle, she could very probably obtain a tissue biopsy sample at little risk to the optic radiations, and Dr. Doe agreed to the two-step process. First, under local anesthesia, a rigid, non-magnetic head-frame was screwed firmly into the skull providing a fixed coordinate system within which to localize the lesion (Figure 0.7a). A sub-assembly was attached to the frame that could provide positional markers visible to the MRI device, and so any point within the head can be expressed as a set of *x*-, *y*-, and *z*-coordinates relative to the frame, to within one millimeter. MR images were now taken with the technique known as MP RAGE, and from the

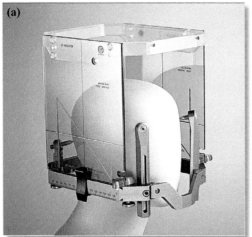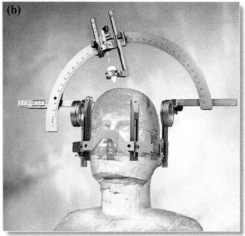

Figure 0.7 A stereotactic thin-needle biopsy device consists of a frame screwed rigidly into the skull plus two separate attachments. **(a)** The first attachment consists of an array of slightly magnetic "rulers" embedded in plastic planes, which can be read precisely by the MRI device during the study. These make possible precise localization of a target point within the lesion. **(b)** With the frame still in place, the first assembly was removed and the second attached. This one can guide insertion, within the OR, of a needle along any direction such that its tip will end up within 1 mm of the target point. Courtesy of Elekta.

resulting images the surgeon decided exactly where she would obtain the sample, and the path she would follow in getting there.

Then, with the MRI-imaging sub-assembly removed but the frame still fixed to the skull, the stereotactic biopsy needle assembly was attached in the operating room (Figure 0.7b). A medical physicist experienced in the use of the equipment made the necessary calculations, based on the images just obtained, and he and the surgeon set the required angles and distance limiters on the mechanical needle-control assembly. Soon thereafter, the surgeon obtained the sample without incident.

Pathology

The biopsy provided only minute fragments of tissue (Figure 0.8). A few showed an increase in cellularity, and were characterized by small to medium-sized nuclei lying in an eosinophilic (pink-staining) background. Other fragments were paucicellular but contained large pleomorphic cells with hyperchromatic nuclei. The nuclei of the commonly seen multinucleated cells were more densely staining and atypical, and some appeared to be undergoing degeneration. No mitoses were found, and neither endothelial proliferation nor necrosis was

seen. There was increased reactivity of the GFAP immunostain in most fragments, most prominently in the more densely cellular foci. The MIB-1 immunostain labeled only a few cells, and the GMS stain revealed nothing abnormal.

Initially there was no certain consensus among the pathologists on a tissue diagnosis. Their final report was that while grading this type of lesion is difficult, since most low-grade gliomas usually do not have this degree of cellular pleomorphisms and nuclear atypia, it was most likely a grade 1, or possibly grade 2, astrocytoma.

Positron emission tomography?

A final diagnostic test was considered, but rejected. Tumors commonly oxidize glucose at a faster rate than do healthy tissues of the same type, and *positron emission tomography* (PET) is a nuclear medicine modality highly sensitive at detecting excessive cellular uptake of it. The sugar is labeled with radioactive fluorine-18, and injected fluorodeoxyglucose (^{18}FDG) concentrates preferentially in fast-metabolizing neoplasms. The fluorine nucleus decays with the emission of a positron, which immediately collides with an electron, its anti-particle; the two self-annihilate, giving birth

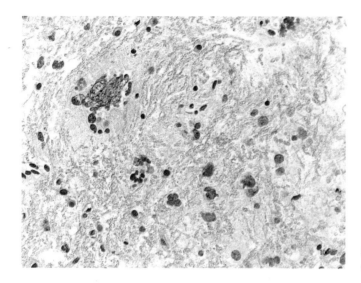

Figure 0.8 Photomicrograph from one of Dr. Doe's biopsy slides.

to a pair of X-ray-like *annihilation photons*, which fly away from the site of the interaction in opposite directions. If the two are detected simultaneously by a PET imager, they will contribute to the formation of a PET image of the region that had taken in the radiopharmaceutical. Another source of tissue contrast!

PET findings would probably have little or no effect on the patient's treatment, however, and Dr. Doe and her physicians decided against pursuing it.

Treatment and follow-up

What to do? There evolved general agreement that a reasonable strategy would be to do nothing for now, to wait and see. Surgery, radiation therapy, and chemotherapy could all have serious deleterious effects even if she retained her ability to read and, after all, there was a good chance that the tumor might grow extremely slowly.

Dr. Doe followed that advice. She has had follow-up MRI examinations twice annually for the past 3 years, during which time the images have not changed appreciably. She did learn, upon returning home, that a number of other people in her building were also experiencing headaches. The epidemic ended, as did Dr. Doe's own headaches, when the large construction project next door, which occasionally produced noxious fumes, came to an end. So the ultimate cause of Dr. Doe's initial problem was never fully confirmed.

＊　＊　＊

Hopefully, this actual medical case will encourage you to delve into what follows. The rest of the book will explore in greater depth the workings of the various extraordinary imaging devices that inform so much of medical care, and will display their diagnostic power by considering many examples of clinical applications. It should be a good read, since there are few things as fascinating, or as significant, as the cutting edge tools of modern high-technology medicine.

CHAPTER 1

Sketches of the Standard Imaging Modalities

Different Ways of Creating Visible Contrast Among Tissues

The principal job of a medical imaging modality is to provide clear maps of anatomy, or to make it possible to identify irregularities in physiology, or both (Figure 1.1). It does so by creating contrast among tissues, and the various modalities do this in biophysically diverse ways.

This chapter provides brief sketches of the major imaging technologies that are employed routinely in modern diagnostic clinics to examine the structure and functioning of the body. It begins with modalities slowly developed over the first three quarters of the twentieth century, like screen-film

Medical Imaging: Essentials for Physicians, First Edition. Anthony B. Wolbarst, Patrizio Capasso and Andrew R. Wyant.
© 2013 John Wiley & Sons, Inc. Published 2013 by John Wiley & Sons, Inc.

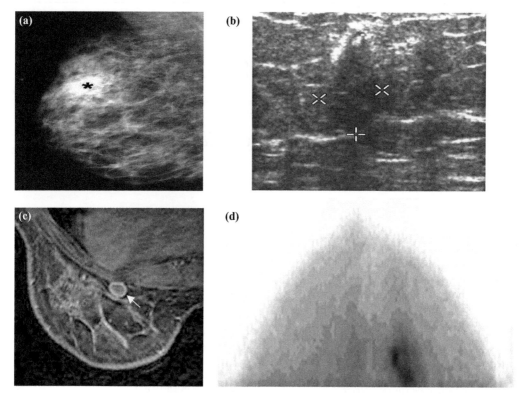

Figure 1.1 Breast imaging for a patient with a biopsy-proven lobular carcinoma. **(a)** When a woman has her routine annual digital mammographic examination after the age of 40, two nearly orthogonal views are obtained of each breast. Mammography demands high soft-tissue contrast to detect neoplasms and fine resolution to examine microcalcifications but, at the same time, very low dose deposition. **(b)** B-mode ultrasound is often able to distinguish quickly, reliably, and inexpensively between a fluid-filled cyst and a solid tumor detected earlier with mammography. Here, the acoustic attenuation confirms the presence of a suspicious solid lesion. **(c)** MRI is often the screening tool of choice for patients at high risk for breast cancer. **(d)** PET with its standard radiopharmaceutical fluorine-18 deoxyglucose (^{18}FDG) is highly sensitive to tissues that, like many tumors, consume an excessive amount of glucose. These modalities produce contrast through radically different biophysical mechanisms, and provide complementary kinds of medical information.

radiography and mammography, image-intensifier tube fluoroscopy, and analog nuclear medicine (NM) and ultrasound (US) imaging. Then came twenty-first century technologies that have flourished only with the advent of high-speed and powerful, but small and affordable, computers – digital planar imaging like computed radiography (CR); digital radiography (DR); digital mammography (DM); digital fluoroscopy (DF), including digital subtraction angiography (DSA); computed tomography (CT), culminating in helical, multi-detector ring CT (MDCT); single photon emission computed tomography (SPECT) and positron emission tomography (PET); advanced forms of B-mode and Doppler US; and magnetic resonance imaging (MRI) in all its glory, with T1-, T2-, and proton density-weighted imaging, functional MRI (*f*MRI), MR angiography (MRA), diffusion tensor imaging (DTI), and many other variants. All of these modalities will be discussed further in the forthcoming chapters.

"Roentgen has surely gone crazy!"

Although no one realized it at the time, the discovery of X-rays in 1895 foreshadowed the quantum upheavals that would turn the physical sciences upside down in the first quarter of the twentieth century. More immediately and spectacularly, however, it flung open a door that led into a new and

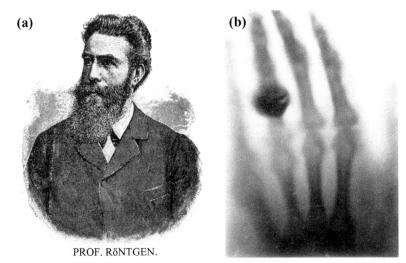

(a)

PROF. RöNTGEN.

(b)

Figure 1.2 In the beginning ... **(a)** An engraving of Wilhelm Conrad Roentgen, from *Something About X-rays for Everyone*, which was published in 1896, less than a year after his discovery. Reproduced from Trevert E, *Something about X-rays for Everyone*, 1896. Reprinted by Medical Physics Publishing Company, Madison, WI, 1988. Soon thereafter, one visitor described him as "a very tall man, with a scholarly stoop, his face somewhat pockmarked, stern but kindly, and very modest in his remarks upon his achievements" (Mould RE, *A Century of X-Rays and Radioactivity in Medicine*, Institute of Physics Publishing, London, 1993). **(b)** The earliest extant X-ray record, of Roentgen's wife Bertha's hand and signet ring, taken by her husband on December 22, 1895. Courtesy of the Deutsches Roentgen-Museum, Remscheid-Lennep, Germany.

completely unanticipated dimension in the practice of medicine – the ability to look non-invasively within a patient's body, without having to cut into it.

A century ago, medical diagnosis was as much art as science. The doctor could measure body temperature, blood pressure, pulse rate, and a few simple chemical attributes of blood and urine, but not much else. Odors and subtle aspects of a patient's appearance during a physical examination often provided equally important clues. But medicine lacked any means to view the interior of the body directly, apart from surgery, to reach critically important diagnoses.

That abiding problem ceased to exist, literally overnight, on the evening of November 8, 1895, when the German physicist Wilhelm Conrad Roentgen chanced upon X-rays (Figure 1.2a). Roentgen, a respectable but little known professor at the University of Würzburg, had been experimenting with an apparatus of widespread scientific interest at the time that is now called a *cathode ray tube* – a partially evacuated glass tube containing two metal electrodes at its opposite ends that were attached to the outside world by means of a pair of

wires passing through the glass. Scientists had been intrigued by what happens when a high voltage is applied between the electrodes: the thin gas within would glow, as would the glass itself in the area near the anode (the electrode attached to the positive pole of the voltage source). It was argued that the agent responsible for this phenomenon was some sort of wave or particle, perhaps negatively charged, that emerged from the cathode (the negative electrode) and that was attracted toward the anode. These so-called "cathode rays" presumably excited the gas and, on striking glass, caused it to fluoresce as well. The nature of cathode rays themselves, now understood to be ordinary electrons, remained obscure for several more years after Roentgen's discovery.

It is not clear what Roentgen was attempting on November 8, since his will stipulated that all of his laboratory notes be burned unread upon his death. In any case, as he worked in a darkened room late in the evening, something unusual caught his eye: when an electric discharge occurred in his tube, a nearby piece of paper that happened to be coated with a chemical compound of barium, platinum, and cyanide produced a glow. With his glass tube completely enveloped in black cardboard, there was no way that visible light from the tube could be reaching the coated paper. So something invisible had to be passing through the cardboard and reaching the barium platinum cyanide, inducing it to give off light. Roentgen had, in fact, discovered X-ray radiation by observing X-ray fluorescence (the emission of light caused by an X-ray stimulus) in a nearby material that was fluorescent. (Patton [1–3] provides a fascinating and detailed accounting of Roentgen's discovery.)

Roentgen was aware that he might have stumbled onto something altogether new, and he was excited and shaken by the remarkable thing he was seeing. But as he explored this totally unexpected phenomenon, he worried that perhaps there might be a simple, obvious explanation that he was overlooking. Far more disturbing was the possibility that perhaps he could not trust his own senses – after all, this appeared to be a physical process that was trivially easy to produce, and undeniably of extraordinary significance, so why had no-one else already seen it and reported it? He knew the physics literature well, and was quite certain that nothing like this had been described before. But were his observations genuine, or might they possibly be the creation of his own mind?

"I believed," he later recalled, "that I was the victim of deception when I observed the phenomenon of the ray" [4]. He wrote to his longtime friend, physicist Ludwig Zehnder: "I had spoken to no one about my work. To my wife I merely mentioned that I was working on something about which people would say, when they found out about it, 'Roentgen has surely gone crazy.'"

But Roentgen persevered. Placing various objects between the tube and the fluorescent screen, he learned that they affected the brightness of the emitted light by different amounts. A few pieces of paper or cardboard had little impact, but a thick sheet of metal quenched the light completely. And when he held his hand in the path of the beam, he could make out the bones of his fingers projected in silhouette upon the screen. A short while later, Roentgen produced the first X-ray record, permanently capturing his wife Bertha's hand and signet ring on a glass photographic plate (Figure 1.2b). Bertha, regrettably, was not overly impressed by the medical significance of the discovery – she had long harbored a terrifying premonition of an early death, and seeing the resemblance of her hand to a skeleton gave her a most unpleasant shock. She ran screaming from her husband's laboratory and never went near it again.

On December 28, Roentgen submitted a paper describing his findings, "On a new kind of ray," to a local scientific journal. Within days, news of the discovery was excitedly picked up by the press and spread like wildfire throughout the world, along with the instantly famous picture of Bertha's hand. People found the experiment easy to reproduce, and within months physicians everywhere were using the pictures it produced to set broken bones and to remove bullets and shrapnel. Over the single year following the discovery, more than a thousand technical and medical papers were published on the subject. With his new kind of rays, Roentgen had discovered a splendid window for looking within the living body and painlessly examining organs and bones.

For his work, Roentgen was offered a title, which he refused, and received numerous awards, including the first Nobel Prize in Physics in 1901. Soon after unveiling his discovery, Roentgen returned to his former research interests, and wrote only seven more papers. In October of 1914, he joined 92 other professors in issuing a manifesto in support of German militarism, an action that he later regretted. His family lost their wealth and suffered considerable hardship during the First World War and the depression that followed. After a short illness, during which he kept careful records of his own symptoms, Roentgen died in Munich on February 20, 1923.

Different imaging probes interact with different tissues in different ways and yield different kinds of medical information

Much of the information content of a medical image will invariably be irrelevant, or tend to detract from or obscure the diagnostically critical features – or worst of all, appear to be real but not be so. When confronted with the results of an X-ray, CT, NM, US, or MRI study, the viewer must detect any significant anomaly in it, regardless of how slight

Figure 1.3 Creation of a transmission image of the body with a beam of X-ray probes, by keeping track of the fate of those that enter it and do, or do not, interact with it. An (ideally) uniform X-ray beam is directed at the chest; some of the X-rays incident on it are either absorbed or scattered through interactions with its atoms and molecules, predominantly in the dense bones. The differential attenuation of X-rays by the various body tissues is revealed in the (no longer uniform) residual beam emerging from its far side, and captured by the image receptor. This process is the basis for all X-ray imaging, including CT.

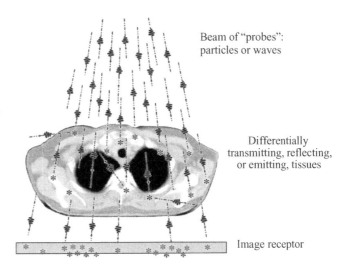

Beam of "probes": particles or waves

Differentially transmitting, reflecting, or emitting, tissues

Image receptor

or well hidden it may be, and correctly identify a corresponding irregularity in the patient's body. She must then interpret this in terms of a deviation from normal anatomy or physiology — the what, how, and why of what has actually gone wrong with the cells, tissues, and organs. After determining the pathophysiology, she will hopefully be able to arrive at a reasonable differential diagnosis that ultimately enables selection of the best treatment.

A medical image will be considered good enough if it helps to achieve any or all of this — efficiently, reliably, safely, and, preferably, inexpensively. A diagnostic imaging system must therefore be able to display the specific, distinctive aspects of the patient's anatomy or physiology that are the cause of the problem, and be sensitive enough to pick up even very subtle early signs of the disease process. It may seem ironic that a "good enough" image is good enough, incidentally, especially since we so often strive for the "best." But there are likely to be hidden real costs from "better than good enough," especially *unnecessary* radiation dose, and the quality of the image itself is only part of the overall picture.

The specificities, sensitivities, and other characteristics of the various imaging tools, in turn, are determined by how they work — and they work in remarkably disparate ways. But while the imaging technologies make use of quite different physical processes in carrying out their appointed tasks, they do share a central, fundamental commonality of approach: they all gather information by creating,

following, and recording, by some means or other, the transmission or reflections of suitable *probes* as they attempt to pass through a patient's body, or by monitoring the emission of signals coming from within it.

For transmission X-ray imaging, such as radiography, fluoroscopy, and CT, the body must be *partially*, but only partially, transparent to the probes (Figure 1.3). If the X-rays all slip through bones and organs without interacting with them, like light through a pane of clear glass, then no differences among the tissues can be visualized. Similarly, if their passage is completely blocked, nothing shows up. But if the probes are only somewhat affected – absorbed, scattered, reflected, delayed, whatever – we may be able to detect small differences in how they interact with the molecular constituents of diverse biological materials. And these small differences can then serve as the raw material for the creation of diagnostically useful images.

A beam of X-rays consists of such probes. X-rays are a form of electromagnetic (EM) radiation, as are gamma- and ultraviolet rays, visible light of all colors, infrared radiation, and radio waves. Physicists discovered a century ago that all of these display both wave-like and particle-like characteristics, if you know how to look for them; in the next chapter, we shall return briefly to this and other cases of what is sometimes called "quantum weirdness."

In the production of radiographs, however, only the particle-like attributes of EM radiation are relevant. You can think of an X-ray beam as consisting of a stream of vast numbers of small, discrete, compact particle-like bundles of EM energy, called *photons*. X-ray photons travel in straight lines at the speed of light and, unless something absorbs or scatters them, they just keep on going. Most importantly when considering formation of an image, however, they can collide with atoms within the body, and in this way be removed from the beam.

When a fairly uniform beam of X-ray photons enters a chest, say, the skin, muscles, and bones attenuate it (i.e., thereby removing X-ray photons from it, and reducing its intensity) by different amounts, and in so doing cast a distinctive spatial pattern of X-ray shadows in it. The no-longer-uniform beam that emerges from the far side of the chest then falls upon and exposes an *image receptor*. In Roentgen's case, the first image receptor happened to be a sheet of cardboard covered with fluorescent material that glowed when his cathode ray tube was activated. Later he used a glass plate coated with a photographic emulsion that contained microscopic, transparent silver halide crystals; if sensitized by an X-ray photon, a crystal would transform into a minute speck of black pure silver when the plate was subsequently developed. The more X-ray photons that reached a part of the plate, the more silver halide crystals were altered, and the blacker, more visually opaque, that part of it became. Where absorption and scattering are relatively low, such as in the lung or the edge of the breast, more photons make it through to expose the image receptor, and the corresponding area on developed film appears darker. Conversely, the image of a bone, with its high beam attenuation, is much clearer, showing up brightly on a view box.

What is of interest in radiography (and fluoroscopy), and what is ultimately responsible for the patterns of clear and dark in a radiograph, is the three-dimensional (3D) distribution of the tissues within the body. What is recorded on film and available for diagnostic purposes is a 2D representation of the spatially varying X-ray intensity that was transmitted through the body. The radiographic process is thus a mapping, or condensation, if you prefer, of the patient's anatomy in three dimensions onto a two-dimensional visual map.

In *emission imaging*, the body itself may produce diagnostic signals naturally (thermography, electroencephalography, magnetocardiography), and image irregularities may indicate related health issues. Alternatively, a signal-emitting substance may be introduced into it intentionally (radiopharmaceuticals in PET, fluorescent dyes in infrared imaging); the tracer is designed to be taken up nonuniformly by the various tissues, and their spatial distribution is subsequently revealed by differential emission captured in the resultant images.

Ultrasound employs another approach, namely the *reflection* of the probes. A *transducer* generates high-frequency (1–10 MHz) mechanical vibrations and, when it is pressed against the skin, these initiate US waves that propagate through tissue. When the US energy comes to a boundary between tissues of different mechanical properties, however, it bounces back, like a tennis ball from a wall; the transducer senses these echoes upon their return to it, and transforms them into electrical signals that the computer untangles to create an echo-image.

MR imaging is something of an amalgam. It directs probes, radiofrequency (RF) electromagnetic waves, into the body which, under special conditions (including the application of a strong, constant magnetic field), will be absorbed by the hydrogen nuclei (protons) of tissue water and lipids. This interaction of EM waves with the protons leads to the emission immediately thereafter by the body of other RF radiation that is modulated by the behavior of these protons. The newer RF signal induces voltages in a wire pickup-coil, which are sent to the MRI's computer for image reconstruction.

In any case, regardless of whether these "probes" or "signals" are transmitted through, reflected in, or are emitted from the body or behave in some more subtle fashion, they go on to activate a probe-specific *image receptor* (IR) to create a medical picture. Older IRs, such as radiographic film and fluoroscopic image intensifiers, are said to be *analog* devices because they produce images that are continuous and smooth, like a photograph. A *digital* image, by contrast, can exist only in a computer system and monitor, and is comprised of a matrix of thousands or millions of tiny, distinct, square *pixels* of a discrete set of shades of gray or color. A digital system must be designed, incidentally, to ensure that these squares are small and numerous enough not to be individually noticeable, and that

Table 1.1 Typical values of the general characteristics of the principal imaging modalities: analog and digital radiography and fluoroscopy (R/F), and CT; nuclear medicine, including SPECT and PET; US; and MRI. These create images from probes such as X-rays transmitted through the body, gamma-rays emitted from within it, high-frequency sound waves reflected at tissue boundaries, and MRI radiofrequency waves that behave in more subtle ways. The different probes interact with tissues and image receptors by way of different physical mechanisms, and are influenced by different attributes of them. They are all effective at presenting some aspects of anatomy or tissue physiology or both, but they differ in the extent to which they can reveal either contrast among tissues or fine detail.

Modality	Probe/signal	Detector	Source of contrast: Δ ...	Anatomy/ physiology
Analog R/F	X-rays through body	Screen + film; II + CCD	x, ρ, Z, (kVp)	A
Digital R/F; CT	X-rays through body	AMFPI; CsI array	x, ρ, Z, (kVp)	A
Nuclear medicine, SPECT; PET	Gamma-rays from body; 511 keV	NaI single crystal; BGO array	Radiopharmaceutical uptake	P
US	MHz sound	Piezoelectric transducer	ρ, κ	A
MRI	RF, magnet	AM radio receiver	Proton spin relaxation	A, P

Δ ... , "differences in ... "; x, tissue thickness; ρ, density; Z, atomic number; kVp, tube potential; II, image intensifier; CCD, charge coupled device; AMFPI, active matrix flat panel imager; κ, tissue elasticity; RF, radiofrequency EM.

the gray-scale levels are close enough together to appear smoothly graded.

Whether point-by-point on film or pixel-by-pixel for CT, the image receptor transforms the pattern of probes or signals that actually reach it into a visual image. The resultant image can be highly informative about healthy or diseased patient anatomy (radiography; CT), or about functional pathophysiology (nuclear medicine, including SPECT and PET; US), or both (MRI).

Some characteristics of the major imaging modalities are summarized in Table 1.1.

Twentieth-century (analog) radiography and fluoroscopy: contrast from differential attenuation of X-rays by tissues

When a patient shows up at her door today, a physician will perform a history and physical examination, and perhaps order and evaluate pertinent laboratory data. From her interpretation of the results, she can develop a tentative differential diagnosis. Medical imaging may now step in to play a decisive role in confirming or refuting a challenging differential diagnosis, and it may lead directly to a refinement of the final diagnosis. Imaging may also

be invaluable in guiding treatment and in following disease progression or response.

X-ray film of a cracked phalange

The easiest of the modalities to describe, and still the most widely used around the world (away from modern medical centers) is conventional screen-film radiography.

Zea W. is a slender, elegant 18-year-old accomplished scholar and figure skater, and also the only daughter of one of the authors (A.B.W.). She's also tougher than she looks: several years ago, she was one of only two girls on her high school's JV ice hockey team. In a collision, however, a misplaced skate blade crushed the left hand, causing a great deal of pain, rapid swelling, and a brief and highly embarrassing burst of tears. After carefully inspecting the hand, the emergency room physician at the local clinic sent the patient to the radiology suite for an X-ray. If no bones were damaged, then Zea could get by with conservative management such as the elevation of her hand, intermittent application of a cold pack, and medications to reduce the swelling and discomfort. If the radiologist found a hairline fracture, the hand might need a cast to counteract any stresses on the injury during healing. If a bone had been broken into separate pieces, it might even necessitate wiring them together surgically for proper setting. Before there were X-ray images, a physician would have to place a limb in a cast without being able to see clearly how to position the bones, and that could result in weakness and deformity after healing.

The clinic's digital X-ray system was under repair, so it was necessary to revert to an old film unit. The entire procedure took less than five minutes. The radiologic technologist (also known as a radiographer) protected Zea's entire body and neck with a lead-lined apron, which strongly absorbs any stray X-rays. He positioned her hand on a light-tight cassette, within which resided a sheet of specialized photographic film (Figure 1.4a). He then adjusted the height of the X-ray tube above it, and reduced the dimensions of the rectangular X-ray field (indicated by a coincident light field) until it barely covered the hand. He stepped behind a shielding wall, set the controls of the X-ray machine, and kept watch on his patient through a lead-glass window as he shot the film. He then replaced the exposed film with a fresh one, repositioned the hand, and made a second image.

The films were developed, ready for inspection. Both were of adequate quality for the radiologist to identify the problem, and so to guide the patient's treatment. As with nearly all radiographic studies, the contrast between bone and soft tissue was very good. High attenuation by a bone leads to a pale area on film, giving a "negative" appearance of the skeletal structures, with the surrounding, more radiolucent, soft tissues showing up darker. There was no visual noise in either film, and they had sufficient sharpness and resolution of detail to reveal a clean, simple break in one of the bones into two separate pieces, indicated by the arrows in Figure 1.4b and c. The radiolucent line corresponds to the fracture, with an interruption of the dense cortex that enabled X-rays to cross without as much absorption. These pieces had not been significantly displaced relative to one another, but the treatment required a cast to immobilize the bone, allowing it time to heal by consolidation with callous formation.

A month later, Zea was back on the ice.

Meanwhile, a lot was going on behind the scenes. In creating a radiograph, the real action occurs in three places – the anode of the *X-ray tube*, the *patient's body*, and the *image receptor*. In that order...

Generating the beam at the anode of the X-ray tube

A typical modern X-ray tube is a highly-evacuated container, made of glass or metal, within which reside two metal *electrodes*, a *cathode* and an *anode* (Figure 1.5a). The cathode consists of a thin tungsten metal filament housed within a focusing cup; a dedicated, low-voltage power supply drives current through the filament and heats it white-hot, so that it "boils" off electrons.

Almost all of the time, the *exposure* or *"beam-on" switch* is *open*, so that there is no electrical current from cathode to anode, in which case that's the end of the story. During the brief fraction of a second that the exposure switch is held *closed*, the cathode and anode become attached to the negative and positive poles, respectively, of a *generator* of very high, constant electric potential, which acts somewhat like a high-voltage battery (Figure 1.5b). For historical reasons, the potential applied across the tube is known also as the *peak kiloVoltage* (*kVp*), and most X-ray images are produced in the 60−120 kVp range.

The electrons boiling off the negatively charged cathode are accelerated to great velocity toward the positive anode. When they crash into it, something like $\frac{1}{2}$% of their collective energy is transformed into highly energetic X-ray photons; the rest becomes non-productive and potentially destructive heat that must somehow be removed rapidly from the anode and tube.

The result of all this is that a nearly uniform, rectangular beam of X-rays exits the tube via its *window* and heads off toward, say, a patient's hand.

The process brings to mind the time Fluffy curled up a little too close to your favorite Ming treasure (Figure 1.5c). As the vase accelerated downward, its gravitational potential energy transformed smoothly into kinetic energy of motion; when it crashed, most of its kinetic energy was expended abruptly in shattering it into tiny pieces, heating them, and scattering them in all directions – but a small amount was radiated away as sound energy. Same sort of thing happens here with the electrons at the anode.

Contrast from differential attenuation of the beam within the body

Contrast is the principal measure of the extent to which tissues that are anatomically or

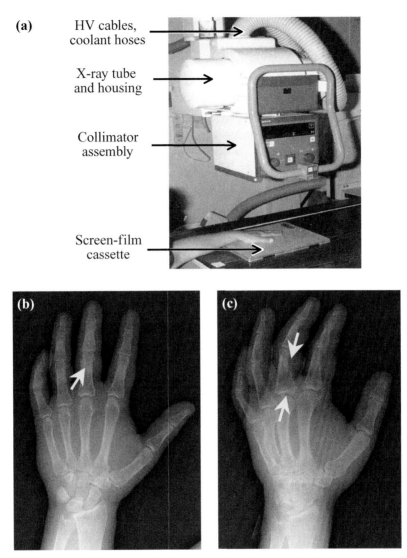

(a) HV cables, coolant hoses

X-ray tube and housing

Collimator assembly

Screen-film cassette

Figure 1.4 X-ray study of a hand. (**a**) A screen-film X-ray unit, with the X-ray tube (inside the horizontal, white cylindrical housing) pointing its beam downward at the hand, which is resting on a film-cassette image receptor. Apart from the X-ray window, the tube is surrounded with lead for radiation protection. The corrugated white tubing carries the *high-voltage cables* from the *generator*, which is outside the room, and hoses for circulating *coolant oil* around the tube. The two knobs on the front of the *collimator assembly* allow adjustment of the beam size, to minimize the volume of tissue that has to be directly irradiated; this also cuts down on the amount of *scatter radiation* produced, which would otherwise both degrade image quality and contribute additional non-productive dose to the hand. Only some of the X-ray photons pass through to darken the film and create a shadowgram; the rest are scattered or absorbed, predominantly in the bones. (**b**) The developed film displayed sufficient image *contrast* and *resolution*, and low enough visual *noise*, to reveal clearly a slightly displaced, oblique fracture of the proximal phalanx of the third finger of the left hand (arrow). (**c**) The same fracture line is better demonstrated in the oblique projection, showing how it extends proximally to the proximal metaphysis of the proximal phalanx to the level of the articular cartilage of the metacarpo-phalyngeal joint (arrows). This has therapeutic implications and demonstrates how one must obtain several views (preferably orthogonal) of the target region, since a 3D structure will project on the film only in 2D.

(a)

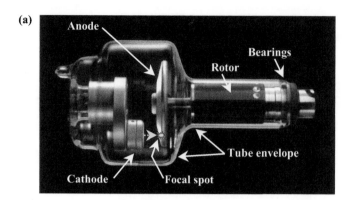

(b)

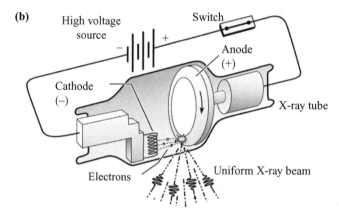

(c)

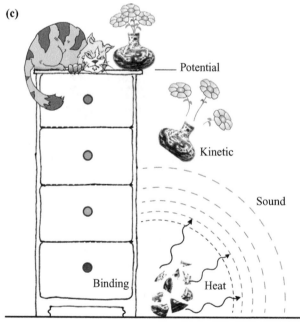

Figure 1.5 Creation of an X-ray beam. (a) A typical radiographic/fluoroscopic (R/F) X-ray tube. (b) For a fraction of a second, electrons from the cathode are accelerated to very high velocity and smash into the anode. Only about $\frac{1}{2}$% of their energy is converted into X-ray energy there, the rest being wasted as heat – an extremely inefficient process! To spread out the heat deposited in the anode and prevent overheating in any one spot, the anode is made to spin rapidly. (c) Production of another form of radiation.

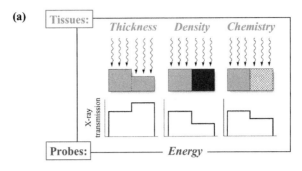

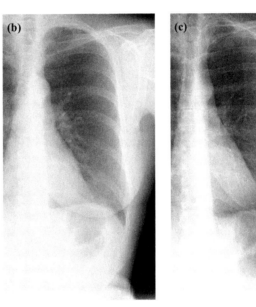

Figure 1.6 X-ray contrast. (**a**) For X-rays, three primary determinants of contrast are *differences* in the thicknesses of tissues, in their densities, such as between lung, muscle, and bone, and in their chemical makeup. (**b**) A fourth important influence on subject contrast is the effective energy of the X-ray beam, as determined by the setting the adjustable *kVp*. This PA image of the left lung of a patient presenting with chest pain was taken at 110 kVp. (**c**) When more detail of the ribs is needed (as in the search of fractures following trauma), then a lower applied voltage, such as 70 kVp, is selected. (b) and (c) modified from the Teaching File images of the American College of Radiology (ACR).

physiologically different appear as such in an image. While other aspects, like resolution or noise level, can be especially important in certain studies, usually it is the visual contrast in a diagnostic image that allows the viewer to distinguish among and examine organs and other tissues, both normal and pathological.

With X-rays, various types of soft tissue and bone absorb and scatter a beam's photons at different rates, which is responsible for the contrast. The amount of attenuation of the beam along any geometric "ray-path" through the body, in turn, depends on the thicknesses and densities of the materials it traverses, and on their chemical compositions (Figure 1.6a). The consequent *differential attenuation* of the beam imprints an X-ray shadow in it, and it is the two-dimensional pattern of X-ray intensity emerging from the far side of the patient, the *primary X-ray image*, that is subsequently captured by the image receptor (IR).

The amount of X-ray contrast among tissues in an image is thus governed primarily by the *differences* in attenuation along the countless ray-paths, hence by the relative *differences* in tissue thicknesses, densities, and chemical makeup of the tissues.

Rates of attenuation, hence amounts of contrast, can be affected strongly also by the setting of the kVp applied to the tube. It may be possible to improve subject contrast for a specific clinical task by selecting a more appropriate kVp (Figures 1.6b and c), but probably at the price of greater radiation dose to the patient.

Radiography can provide excellent contrast for locating and viewing objects that have densities

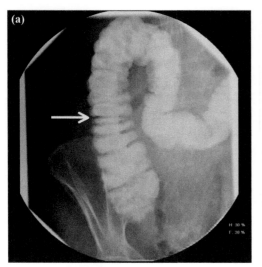
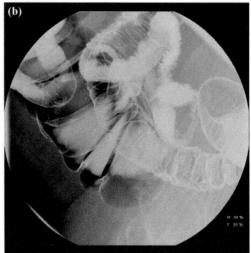

Figure 1.7 Fluoroscopic examination of the GI tract with contrast agent. **(a)** In a barium enema study, a suspension of barium, which is unusually effective at absorbing X-rays, will opacify the lumen of the colon after being administered per rectum, enabling the examination of its diameter and contours. In this image centered at the level of the cecum, one can see areas of normal narrowing of the colon called *haustrae* (arrow), along with abnormal projections from the lumen such as diverticula or filling defects such as polyps. **(b)** A radiolucent material such as insufflated air can then be introduced to fill the lumen of the colon. The remaining barium coats the colonic wall, which is now distended, giving a *double contrast* study, enabling viewing of the partially translucent bowel *en face*.

or chemical makeup significantly different from those of the surrounding tissues – as with bullets, bones, or fluid or masses in lungs. Subject contrast among similar soft tissues, however, can sometimes be barely discernible. Because its density and other properties may be close to those of nearby healthy tissues, a cancerous growth also may give rise to little radiographic contrast. Still, a lesion may reveal its presence through a *mass effect*, displacing or otherwise altering the appearance of an adjacent structure (such as the wall of a bowel coated with barium contrast agent) that *can* be visualized.

The contrast for some tissues can be enhanced artificially by altering their physical properties with a *contrast agent*. Because iodine atoms happen to absorb X-rays especially strongly, blood vessels containing intravenously injected iodine compounds tend to stand out clearly from the surrounding soft tissues. Barium has similar application for fluoroscopy of the esophagus, stomach, and intestine (Figure 1.7a). Following a barium enema, moreover, air can be infused into the colon and function as a second kind of contrast agent because air does *not* soak up X-rays (Figure 1.7b).

Alternatively, it may well be appropriate to turn to another modality. Even when almost nothing shows up on film or DR, for example, CT may adequately depict the organs of interest. Likewise, US may quickly and inexpensively distinguish between a cyst and a solid lesion and, in addition, it poses no radiation risk. And in many situations MRI can create soft-tissue contrast far better than that of CT, also with no dose of ionizing radiation. But however you do it, the critical objective is normally to generate enough relevant image contrast to allow a good clinical diagnosis.

The usefulness of an image may depend not only on the degree of contrast it displays among tissues, but also on its *resolution* or *sharpness*, and on the level of interfering *visual noise* or *artifacts* that might be present. Some of these will be of greater importance than others in a given medical situation. The search for tumors requires the high contrast offered by SPECT and PET, for example, but these deliver poor resolution – which, however, is not a problem for this application. The inherently high resolution of X-ray films and digital radiography, on the other hand, enables them to provide critical details of fine structure, revealing hairline cracks in bone, microcalcifications in breast, and irregularities in narrow blood vessels made visible with iodine contrast agent. And while visual random noise plays almost no role in radiography, it can be a dominant factor in CT, nuclear medicine, US, and MRI.

Exposure of a screen-film image receptor

The third step in creating a radiograph is to transform the *subject contrast* in the primary X-ray image emerging from the patient into visible *image contrast* in a permanent record in the IR.

Not many X-ray photons manage to pass completely through the body, as it happens, but a good fraction of those that do are captured by the image receptor. In traditional analog radiography, the IR is a sheet of photographic film sandwiched between the two flat *fluorescent screens* of a light-tight *radiographic cassette* (Figure 1.8a). When an X-ray photon strikes an atom in a transparent microcrystal of fluorescent material in a screen, its energy is converted into a pinpoint flash of thousands of visible light photons (Figure 1.8b).

Many of the light photons created this way head into the adjacent sheet of film. The two surfaces of standard film are coated with thin layers of *emulsion*, which contains a suspension of translucent microcrystals composed of a mix of *silver bromide* and *iodide* plus trace amounts of other goodies (Figure 1.9a). If a half dozen or more light photons from a screen happen to strike a particular silver halide microcrystal, then it will become *sensitized* and, during the subsequent chemical *development* of the film, it will be transformed into a minute black fleck of nearly pure silver (Figure 1.9b). Crystals in the emulsion that are *not* sensitized in this fashion will be dissolved and removed from the film during fixation and washing.

In this fashion, a single X-ray photon striking a fluorescent screen typically results in a microscopic black cluster of hundreds of minute specks of silver. Where more radiation passes through the patient and reaches the cassette, there arises a higher spatial density of these opaque dots. Here, the developed film is darker, with a higher *optical density* (OD). The pattern of X-ray photons emerging from the patient is thus distilled into a permanent visible record, to be placed on a view box for inspection.

The reason for the fluorescent screen is that the indirect two-step process, X-ray-to-light and then light-to-film, is greatly more efficient than direct X-ray-to-film. With screens, the IR requires one or two orders of magnitude less radiation to achieve a usable average OD, with a correspondingly lower *dose* to the patient. There is, however, a significant trade-off: thicker and therefore more sensitive screens may reduce patient dose, but they also lower resolving capability, and the solution to this dilemma must rely on clinical considerations.

To summarize: transmission X-ray imaging involves the *differential attenuation* of a previously flat X-ray beam through interaction with the various tissues, followed by *differential exposure* of the image receptor. This is true for all X-ray imaging, whether screen-film or digital planar, or CT, or fluoroscopy.

Image intensifier-based fluoroscopy with a CCD/CMOS electronic optical camera

Fluoroscopy is radiography's first cousin, the clever one that lets the physician watch continuously changing processes live in real time as they take place, rather than as one or a few radiographic snapshots developed later. To achieve this, it employs a more complex image receptor (Figure 1.10).

The X-rays that pass through and emerge from the patient do not expose a film cassette but rather, in most fluoro systems, they project directly onto the front face of an *image intensifier* (II) tube. An II is an electronic vacuum tube device that can transform a life-sized, very faint pattern of X-ray energy into a small, bright corresponding pattern of visible light. The output of the II tube used to be photographed directly with a still or cine film camera or viewed with a TV camera. These days, a solid state electronic *charge-coupled device* (*CCD*) or a *complementary metal oxide semiconductor* (*CMOS*) optical camera does the job.

As with X-ray filming, fluoroscopy is most adept at distinguishing objects that differ significantly from soft tissue in either density or chemical constitution — such as the passage of intravenously injected iodine-based contrast agent to or through constrictions in blood vessels, or the movement of barium past partial obstructions in the GI tract.

(a)

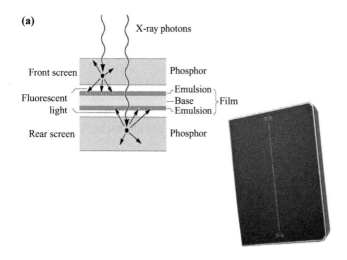

(b)

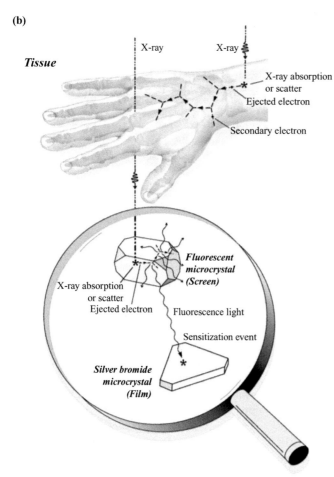

Figure 1.8 A screen-film X-ray image receptor. **(a)** The cassette consists normally of a pair of fluorescent screens in a light-tight, mechanically rigid housing; it can be opened in a darkroom to insert or remove film from between the screens. This cassette contains an embedded anti-scatter grid for easier and quicker imaging. Photograph courtesy of Reina Imaging. **(b)** An X-ray photon that happens to pass through the body and then strike a fluorescent microcrystal in the screen will excite it; the crystal relaxes immediately thereafter with the emission of thousands of visible light photons that will expose the film.

Figure 1.9 What makes photographic film dark? (**a**) A dispersion in the emulsion of tiny translucent microcrystals of silver iodobromide, seen here with the aid of an electron microscope. Several light photons striking a silver halide microcrystal will activate, or sensitize, it such that (**b**) upon chemical development, it transforms into a microscopic, opaque speck of silver metal, one of which is shown here. Courtesy of Arthur Haus, Eastman Kodak Company.

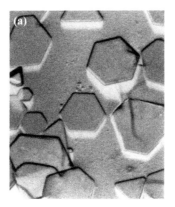
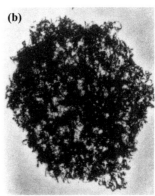

Fluoroscopy can also guide the removal of a radiopaque body from within the body, such as a bullet or urolith, or the insertion of one into it (e.g., a catheter or stent).

With most systems, the X-ray tube points upward from beneath the patient table (Figure 1.10a). It may be possible to tilt the whole assembly upward, including the table, for imaging the patient in the vertical orientation. Alternatively, as is standard in modern angiography suites, the X-ray tube and image receptor are held at opposite ends of a rigid *C-*

arm support, as in Figure 1.10b, that can be rotated about one or more axes.

Modern angiography units are replacing the bulky, unwieldy II tube plus camera combination with a much thinner, lighter, and more maneuverable solid-state *active matrix flat-panel image* (AMFPI) receptor. A flat panel IR, the technology of which evolved from that of liquid crystal and plasma display monitors, makes things digital from the outset but currently at considerably greater cost. The most advanced interventional/angiographic

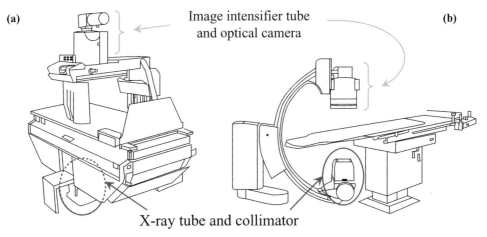

Figure 1.10 With fluoroscopy, the X-ray image receptor is an image intensifier (II) plus electronic optical camera combination, rather than screens and film. The X-ray beam is pulsed rapidly, but each pulse is of much lower intensity than for radiography. (**a**) With a standard radiography/fluoroscopy (R/F) system, the X-ray tube lies below the patient table, so that the lead-lined curtains surrounding it will cut down on scatter dose to the operators near the machine. The image receptor views the patient from above. The signal from the camera may be digitized and fed into a computer, making possible quasi-digital fluoroscopy and digital subtraction angiography. (**b**) An angiography device is mechanically more flexible and complex. The X-ray tube and image receptor (where, in the more advanced and totally digital systems, a solid-state *active matrix flat-panel imager* replaces the II tube and CCD pair) reside on opposite ends of a *C-arm* support that can be rotated about up to three axes. Modified from Bushberg JT, Seibert JA, Leidholdt, Jr. EM, Boone JM, *The Essential Physics of Medical Imaging*, 2nd edn, Philadelphia, Lippincott, Williams, and Wilkins (2002), fig. 9-15.

(a)   **(b)**

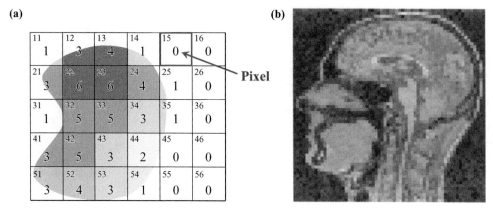

Figure 1.11 Two-dimensional digital image. **(a)** The number in the upper left corner of each pixel, or picture element, is its *pixel address*. The larger, central number represents the *pixel value* – that is, the degree of brightness, averaged over the entire pixel, where (in this example) the number 0 refers to the lightest and 6 is the darkest. The image can then be presented as a single string (i.e., a *one*-dimensional representation) of pixel addresses coupled with the corresponding pixel values. **(b)** The importance of many, small pixels and enough shades of gray. This MRI image of a head utilizes 256 shades of gray, which is OK, but only a 64 × 64 pixel matrix, which does not provide sufficient resolution. Courtesy of WS Kiger, III, Massachusetts Institute of Technology.

biplanar systems support two X-ray tubes and two flat panels, a configuration that allows simultaneous antero-posterior and lateral observation of the patient (or with other pairs of angles); such orthogonal imaging is often helpful in making visual sense of three-dimensional, tortuously complex vascular, biliary, and renal structures.

Twenty-first century (digital) images and digital planar imaging: computer-based images and solid-state image receptors

Conventional X-ray radiography is still the most common, and least expensive, way of obtaining diagnostic medical and dental images, and often it is perfectly adequate. But modern imaging departments have other options from which to choose – and just about all are built around computers.

Computers are invaluable for image enhancement with II-based fluoro, planar NM, and US. They are absolutely essential, moreover, for image generation with CT, MRI, CR, DR, SPECT, and PET. But either way, for computers to work their wonders, an image must be present in digital form.

Digital images

Creating a digital image is like the converse of painting by numbers. In simplest two-dimensional form,

the computer partitions an image, obtained somehow with an image acquisition device, into an imaginary 2D array or *matrix* of many small square *pixels* (*pic*ture *el*ements), each corresponding to a tissue *voxel* (*vo*lume *el*ement) within the patient's body. Every pixel is assigned a unique *pixel address*, or numerical spatial location; the associated *pixel value* is the number that corresponds to the value of the biophysical parameter being assessed in the voxel. The matrix addresses for the 30-pixel matrix of Figure 1.11a, for example, consist of pairs of integer indices, where the first and second label the five rows and six columns of the matrix, respectively, such as 11, 12, 13, 14, 15, 16, 21, 22, . . . , 55, 56. The range of degrees of brightness on a black-and-white monitor is referred to as the *gray scale*; each pixel's gray scale level is set to correspond to a specific pixel value, in this case with a range from 0 to 6; the same general approach would apply to a color display. The entire image can then be represented as a long *one*-dimensional string of the addresses and corresponding pixel value numbers, such as: 11-1; 12-3; 13-4; 14-1; 15-0; 16-0; 21-3; 22-6, . . . , 55-0, 56-0. Perhaps a very simple form of *image compression* comes to mind that greatly reduces the amount of data that must be retained in such a string.

There are two digital imaging technologies that have been rapidly displacing screen-film radiography. Computed radiography (CR) is relatively simple and inexpensive, and employs an IR that is similar to a screen-film combination, but one in which the active element is developed electronically, rather than chemically. Digital radiography (DR) is more advanced and much faster. A DR image receptor is built around an active matrix flat panel imager, which consists of several million independent sensors, each capable of determining the local X-ray intensity. With the sensors arranged as a 1024 × 2048 matrix, for example, there would be about two million pixels, and two million numbers would be required to represent the shades of gray of those two million pixels in a complete digital encoding of an image.

There are great advantages of both DR and CR over film, such as the capacity for image processing, rapid storage, and instantaneous communications, and Chapters 6 and 7 will cover these extensively. The same is true for digital fluoroscopy and digital subtraction angiography, which can capture events changing in real time far better than systems based on II tubes.

For MRI, the pixel matrix is most likely to be 512 × 512, requiring less computer memory to store an image, but considerably more calculational power to generate it in the first place. Troubles can arise, as with any other digital modality, if the pixel size is not handled properly: Figure 1.11b was reconstructed, for example, with a 64 × 64 grid, instead, an example that exaggerates the difficulty, but the pixelation would likely still be noticeable even at 256 × 256. Other problems arise if there are not enough distinct shades of gray, or if all the pixels are all shown somewhat too dark or too light – that is, if improperly *windowed*.

Computed tomography: three-dimensional mapping of X-ray attenuation by tissues

Conventional radiographic and fluoroscopic images are relatively easy to produce. But the superimposed shadows from overlapping tissues may obscure the critical details that the physician needs to see — the shadows from an intricate three-dimensional structure can project into hopeless two-dimensional disarray on film or with CR and DR.

The idea behind CT is straightforward, and was described in connection with Figure 0.1. CT creates, digitizes, and stores in a computer the radiologic images from a large number of different perspectives.

Imagine a patient as comprised of many thin transverse slices. In the early days, CT generated an image of the tissues within only a single slice 1 cm or so thick, for technical reasons, but now it is most common to scan the patient with 64 slices each 0.5 mm or so thick, all at the same time (Figure 1.12a).

It is perhaps easiest to visualize the operation of a CT by considering the first commercial head scanner, produced by the British company EMI (Figure 1.12b). It swept a very narrow "pencil" beam of X-rays across the head, in a direction perpendicular to the beam orientation, while monitoring the amount of energy transmitted through it, at 160 points along the way, with a small, co-linear X-ray detector, also being shifted sideways (Figure 1.12c). It then rotated the tube plus detector assembly rigidly 1° around the patient, and repeated. This set of motions is known as "translate/rotate" data acquisition, and the first and 60th such scans are shown. After the accumulation of data from 180 angles, the computer then worked backward through vast numbers of complex calculations to *reconstruct* and display the spatial distribution of the materials (or, more precisely, of the X-ray attenuation properties of the materials) that must have been responsible for this particular set of images. Obtaining the data and reconstructing a single slice of the head took over four minutes.

The patient table was then advanced 1 cm or so, and the entire procedure carried out again to produce the next, adjacent slice. The resulting information was shown as a sequence of images of individual thin transverse slices of tissue (Figure 1.12d). This slice happens to display a *star artifact* caused by the inability of the CT's computational *reconstruction algorithm* to deal with the abrupt change in rate of attenuation that occurs at a small metal aneurysm clip.

By eliminating the interfering patterns that come from over- and underlying bones and organs, CT provides ample contrast among the various soft tissues, far better than standard radiography or fluoroscopy can do. So CT is routinely used for detailed studies of abdominal and pelvic organs, the lungs,

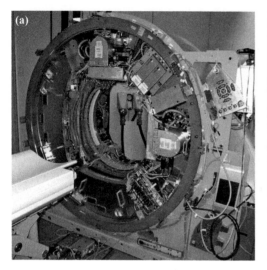
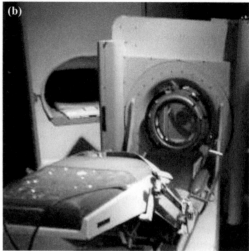

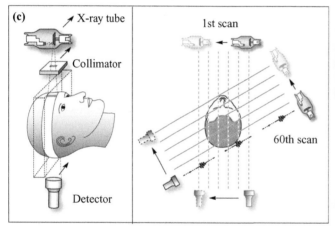
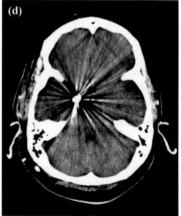

Figure 1.12 CT data acquisition. **(a)** An immodest view of a modern dual-source, multi-slice CT scanner, with a pair of X-ray tubes at right angles and a corresponding pair of multi-slice detector assemblies. **(b)** The first commercial scanner, manufactured by the British company EMI, Ltd, with development funds provided largely by the Fab Four, also an EMI product. **(c)** The geometry of data acquisition by a first-generation CT device, such as the EMI machine, known as "translate-rotate." The tube and its narrow pencil beam of X-rays swept across the head, and a detector shifted so as to remain co-linearly with it monitored the intensity emerging from its far side. The tube plus detector assembly was then rotated 1° around the patient, and the procedure repeated; here are shown the first and sixtieth scans. **(d)** A transverse CT slice, with one of a number of types of CT artifacts, a "star" caused by a metal aneurism clip; there, the rate of X-ray attenuation changes abruptly from that of soft tissue, causing problems for the numerical calculations of the reconstruction algorithm. Reproduced from Flohr T, Schmidt B, Advances in CT. In: Wolbarst AB, Capasso P, Godfrey DJ, *et al.* (eds), *Advances in Medical Physics*, vol. 4. Madison WI: Medical Physics Publishing, 2012, fig. 4-5 (part a).

the brain, and just about everything else. CT can pick up physically dense objects of the order of 0.1 mm in dimensions, and its general resolution can be better than 0.3 mm. While this is not as good as the resolution in screen-film, CR, and DR, the greatly enhanced contrast may far more than make up for that.

A series of adjacent, thin transverse (axial) slice images can be stacked and melded together, to provide a truly three-dimensional picture (Figure 1.13a). On every slice, a *segmentation* program might automatically locate each interface between bone and soft tissue, say, where the rate of X-ray attenuation changes rapidly, and draw a contour

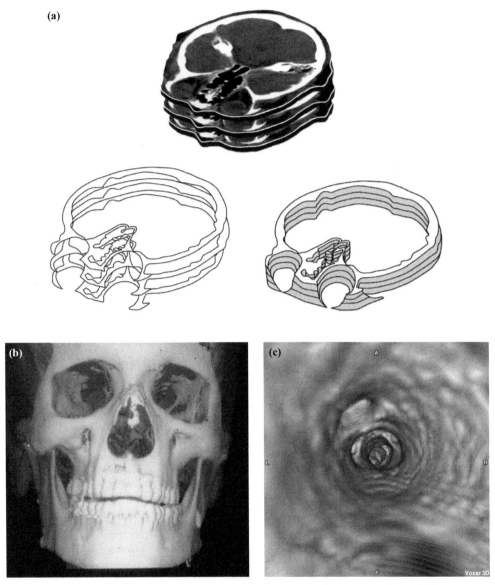

Figure 1.13 Three-dimensional display. **(a)** With CT and MR data acquisitions, slice-images can be stacked upon one another, enabling a reconstruction in three dimensions that can be manipulated (e.g., rotated) so as to offer the best view of a lesion. **(b)** Three-dimensional rendering of the skull (enclosed in 2200-year-old wrappings) of a former resident of Luxor, Egypt, who apparently died of natural causes. He is now part of the permanent mummy collection of the Smithsonian Institution, Washington, DC. Courtesy of Wayne Olan, George Washington University Medical Center. **(c)** Virtual abdominal aorta.

line there. It then assembles the curves in three dimensions, and tiles them optically so as to create a smooth cover representing bone surface. Finally, it can assign degrees of transparency and colors that depend on tissue type, and cast a beam of simulated light through the resulting volumes to give the impression of overlap and depth (Figure 1.13b). It's rather like creating a *papier-mâché* object by plastering paper over a chicken-wire framework, but here it's all done by the computer. Much of the technology that makes all this happen was developed by the animation industry, the military, and others.

The viewer can rotate, dissect, and otherwise manipulate lifelike, three-dimensional images, or display high-resolution coronal or sagittal thin slices. Virtual reality display technologies allow one to observe while traveling down the length of the esophagus, bronchus, intestinal canal, or aorta from within, without actually having to go anywhere near them (Figure 1.13c). It is even possible to watch the heart beating in slow motion, obtaining the images synchronized with the cardiac cycle (cardiac gating) and then replaying the images in a cine loop at the desired speed.

The full power of the approach can be appreciated in an attempt to read the fine details of a cranial fracture. In many cases, there is simply too much visual confusion from overlapping tissue structures to allow the detection and interpretation of slight irregularities with radiography (Figures 1.14). CT can often eliminate the chaos by, in effect, removing all of the body except for a single thin pancake slice of tissues.

MRI can do nearly all of this, too, sometimes providing far better soft-tissue contrast. Still, when either modality can perform a job just as well, then sometimes the considerably lower costs of CT, or the speed of helical, multiple-slice CT, or even just the more rapid access to a CT machine may make it the modality of choice. The major downside of CT is the relatively high radiation doses it involves, which have become a major health concern, especially for infants, children, and women during pregnancy.

Helical, multi-slice CT

In the mid-1970s, the arrival of CT made possible an entirely new way of seeing, and the resulting impact on patient care has been incalculable. Over the past two decades, CT has had to face stiff competition from MRI, which provides clinical information on soft tissues that is usually comparable, and sometimes far superior. This partly explains the development of *helical* CT machines capable of acquiring data much more rapidly by continuously translating the patient table through the gantry opening without having to stop and shoot each slice separately. Soon thereafter, *multi-slice* devices were designed with multiple independent rings, or belts, of tiny X-ray detectors, typically 64 but up to hundreds in some models, which make it possible to create numerous slices simultaneously. Modern helical, multi-slice machines can produce multiple adjacent thin (0.5 mm) slices of a region tens of centimeters long in a matter of seconds, and are now a mainstay of a modern imaging department.

Nuclear medicine, including SPECT and PET: contrast from the differential uptake of a radiopharmaceutical by tissues

Gamma-rays are inherently the same electromagnetic stuff as X-rays and, in medical applications, their ranges of energy overlap. The two, however, differ radically in their origins: gamma-rays are emitted from the unstable nuclei of certain radioactive atoms, while X-rays are created electronically inside an X-ray tube. It is the source of the radiation, not the radiation itself, that distinguishes the two.

Radiopharmaceutical = radionucleus + organ-specific agent

Nuclear medicine provides information that is primarily physiologic or functional in nature, rather than anatomic.

A standard nuclear medicine study makes use of a *radiopharmaceutical*, a chemical substance that consists of two components and displays both of two essential characteristics: one part of the substance is an *agent* that tends to seek out and concentrate preferentially within a particular biological compartment in the body, an organ or tissue of interest. The agent macroaggregated albumin (MAA) protein, for example, consists of microscopic particles (10–90 μm across) that lodge briefly within the patent microvasculature of the pulmonary arterial blood supply, making them suitable for imaging the vasculature (as opposed to the air volumes) of the tissues of the lung.

The other piece of a radiopharmaceutical is the radioactive atom, attached firmly to the agent, that undergoes spontaneous *radioactive decay*, with the creation of, normally, a single, high-energy gamma-ray photon (Figure 1.15a). The characteristics of the particular radionuclide *metastable technetium-99* (Tc-99m) make it just about ideal for imaging, and it has long served as the standard workhorse isotope in nuclear medicine. Tc-99m has an energy sufficiently high to escape the body, but low enough

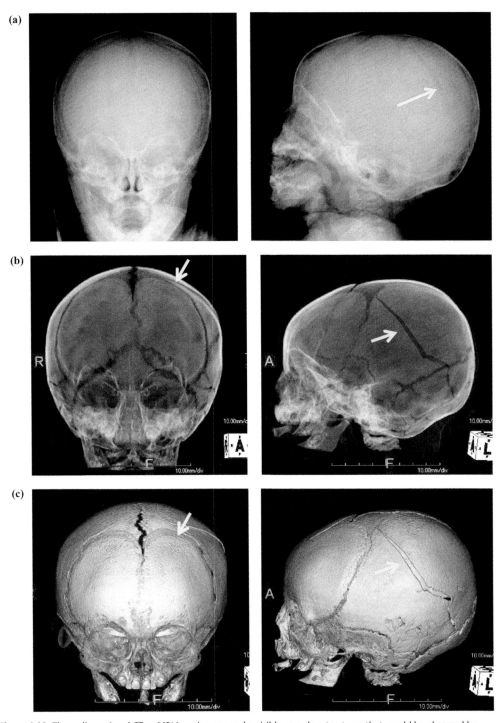

Figure 1.14 Three-dimensional CT or MRI imaging can make visible complex structures that would be obscured by overlying tissues on plain radiography. This case series involves an infant who suffered blunt trauma to the head. (**a**) Initial analysis in the emergency department was performed with AP and lateral radiographs of the skull. Questionable cortical defects on the left side appear on the AP image; these represent a linear fracture of the parietal bone, and are seen more clearly as a radiolucency on the lateral image (arrow). Next, the skull is captured with CT and displayed in both (**b**) a translucent and (**c**) a surface rendering. The CT images show more clearly the same non-displaced fracture extending from the anterior fontanelle across the lamboidal suture (arrows).

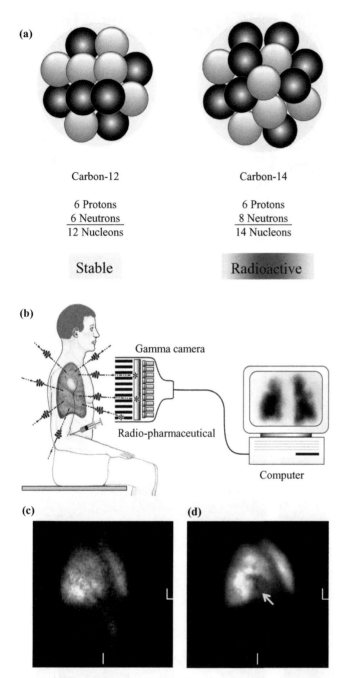

(a)

Carbon-12

6 Protons
6 Neutrons
12 Nucleons

Stable

Carbon-14

6 Protons
8 Neutrons
14 Nucleons

Radioactive

(b)

Gamma camera

Radio-pharmaceutical

Computer

(c)

(d)

L

I

L

I

Figure 1.15 In a nuclear medicine examination, a specific radiopharmaceutical tracer is administered and taken up preferentially by a particular organ or other biological compartment, and from there it radiates gamma-rays. (**a**) The *element* type of an atom is determined solely by its *atomic number*, *Z*, which is the number of protons, hence the positive charge, in its nucleus. The various *isotopes* of a given element are atomic species that all have the same atomic number, but that differ in the number of uncharged, massive *neutrons* in the nucleus. The several isotopes of an element are virtually identical in their chemical, electrical, thermal, magnetic, and other normal properties, but they will differ radically in the behavior of their nuclei. The *radioisotopes* of an element, in particular, comprise a subgroup of its isotopes that are *radioactive*; that is, they undergo spontaneous nuclear transformations with the release of gamma-rays or positrons, or of other emissions that are *not* of interest in imaging. (**b**) Just as an ordinary camera creates photographs out of visible-light photons, a *gamma camera* produces images out of gamma-rays emitted by radionuclides concentrated in biological compartments within the body. (**c**) Normal ventilation and (**d**) irregular perfusion components of a (V/Q) study of the lungs in a patient presenting with acute, stabbing chest pain and shortness of breath, suspected of being associated with a pulmonary embolic event. This diagnosis is nearly confirmed when a perfusion mismatch is demonstrated by the wedge-shaped perfusion defect (arrow) in an area that is fully ventilated.

to interact with the image receptor (a large, fluorescent single crystal of sodium iodide, NaI); a half-life (6 hours) that allows preparation of the radiopharmaceutical and its uptake by an organ, but does not irradiate the patient or others too long after; and the ability to fasten resolutely to a wide range of inexpensive and convenient tissue-seeking chemophysical agents, which are readily available in kits.

Just as a red-hot poker glows in a dark room, a biological compartment containing radiopharmaceutical will "glow" gamma-rays. A *gamma camera* can detect and process them, just as an optical camera captures visible-light pictures (Figure 1.15b), providing a powerful way to evaluate metabolic function of tissues. A gamma camera functions somewhat like an eye. Gamma-rays, unlike light, cannot easily be focused, however, so the role of the lens is played by a *collimator*, a 1 cm thick, highly attenuating lead plate honeycombed with closely-spaced parallel (or nearly parallel) open channels. Behind the collimator is a life-size, thin single, transparent fluorescent sodium iodide crystal. Any gamma-ray that passes straight along a channel of the collimator, and then interacts with the crystal, triggers the production of a *scintillation* (pinpoint burst of light). The crystal is viewed from the back by an *array* of up to a hundred small electronic photomultiplier tubes (PMT), light-sensitive detectors that are attached to a scintillation-location circuitry; together, these play the role of the retinal photoreceptors and neural network of the eye. The photodetector assembly senses each such event and determines its location within the crystal, which corresponds directly to the origin of the gamma-ray within the body, and displays it on the monitor.

Creating contrast through differential uptake of photon-generating radiopharmaceuticals

To summarize: nuclear medicine is based upon *differential uptake* of radiopharmaceutical by various tissues followed by a corresponding spatial *differential emission* of detectable gamma-ray probes.

With a typical *ventilation* (V) study of the lungs, inhaled radioactive xenon gas or aerosolized Tc-99m is evenly distributed throughout the airways to which it has access (Figure 1.15c). The portion of lung air-space containing the radioisotope will glow, with any dark regions revealing volumes where air flow is somehow impaired. No defect is noted in this right anterior oblique (RAO) projection, demonstrating homogeneous ventilation and uptake of the radiopharmaceutical.

In the accompanying *perfusion* (Q, meaning "flow") study, Tc-99m-labeled MAA is injected through a peripheral vein, after which it is briefly trapped within about 1% of the pulmonary capillaries. The radionuclide radiates gamma-rays, and any abnormally dark area may indicate a problem, such as a tumor, and associated regional blockage of blood flow. An area where a blockage exists is evident here, giving rise to a pyramidal defect of hypoperfusion (arrow) (Figure 1.15d). The two parts of this combined V/Q study display a "mismatched" defect, which, while perhaps not visible on a conventional chest X-ray, has a high diagnostic specificity for acute pulmonary embolism.

Nuclear medicine images are of relatively low spatial resolution, typically about 3–4 cm, and reveal only the location, size, and rough shape of the organ or tissue under consideration. But if a part of the organ fails to take up the radioactive material, or is missing, or is eclipsed by abnormal overlying tissues, then the corresponding region of the image will appear dark. Conversely, any part of the organ that takes up an excess of radiopharmaceutical will look unusually bright. So a nuclear medicine image provides information mainly on the physiological status of an organ, parts of which may be affected by a pathology, rather than on the fine details of its anatomy.

SPECT and PET

Just as CT solves the problem of overlapping images in radiography, so also does SPECT in nuclear medicine. In SPECT, several standard gamma-camera heads rotate slowly (∼20 minutes) about the patient (Figure 1.16a), and the accumulated data allow reconstruction of a set of CT-like slices that can either be viewed individually or combined to produce three-dimensional structures.

About half of all SPECT studies are ECG-gated cardiac stress tests for coronary artery disease, and a good fraction of the rest are for bone studies. Applications in oncology are expanding, with increasing numbers of agents becoming available for detection of specific tumor-types (Figures 1.16b). It is increasingly common practice to acquire the corresponding detailed anatomic data with CT or MRI (Figure 1.16c), and superimpose the images.

Photons attempting to exit the body may be absorbed or scattered by outer-lying tissues, of course, compromising the ability to obtain a precise map of differential emission; it is therefore practically essential, to be able to compensate for that effect by computing *attenuation corrections* for both SPECT and PET.

PET makes use of a few unusual and difficult-to-produce atomic nuclei that emit a *positron* (the

(a)　　　　　　　　　　　　　　　**(b)**

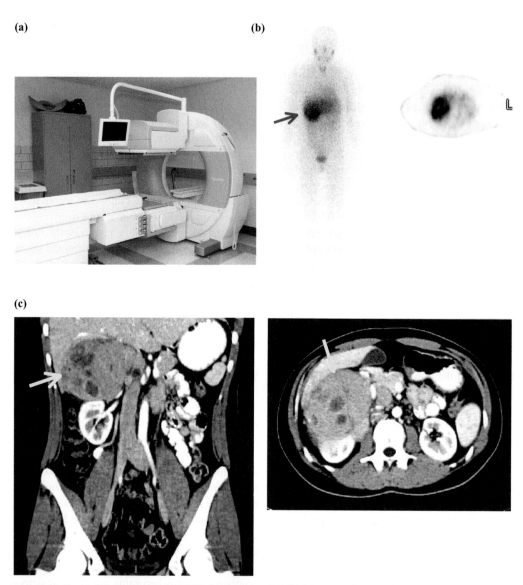

(c)

Figure 1.16 Single photon emission CT (SPECT). (**a**) A two-headed SPECT imager. Alternatively, either gamma camera head, or both together, can serve for a (faster) standard planar study. (**b**) Whole-body 3D scintigraphy with the agent metaiodobenzylguanidine (MIBG) labeled with iodine-123. MIBG resembles noradrenaline and is actively taken up by cells of neuroectodermic tumors. The "hot spot" of activity at the level of the right upper abdominal quadrant (arrow) in this patient with malignant hypertension is caused by a pheochromocytoma. The axial (transverse) SPECT reconstruction confirms the presence of this mass just caudal to the liver. (**c**) Contrast enhanced CT images in intersecting coronal and axial planes show the mass located at the level of the right adrenal gland, representing a pheochromocytoma (arrows).

positively charged antiparticle to the electron) in radioactive decay, rather than a gamma-ray. A positron travels a millimeter or so in tissue before colliding with an ordinary atomic electron, whereupon the two *annihilate* one another, transforming their masses into "pure energy" in the form of a pair of 511 keV *annihilation photons*. (By $E = mc^2$, the energy equivalent of the mass of an electron is 511 keV.) The two photons travel off in opposite directions at the speed of light (Figure 1.17a), and *coincident* (almost exactly simultaneous) detection of many such pairs allows localization of their

(a)

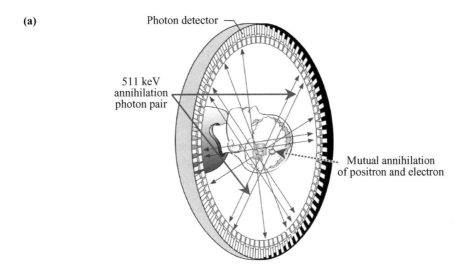

Photon detector

511 keV
annihilation
photon pair

Mutual annihilation
of positron and electron

(b)

PET-FDG   CT   PET/CT

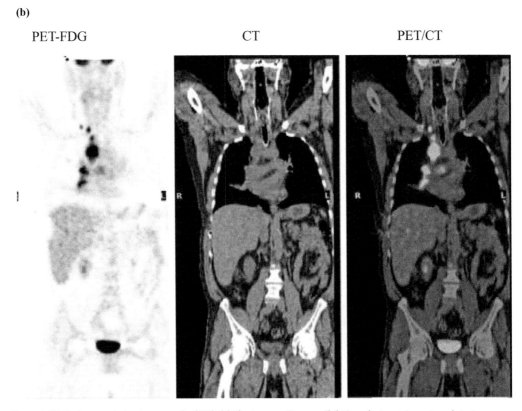

Figure 1.17 Positron emission tomography (PET). (a) The two *positron annihilation photons* trigger two detectors on opposite sides of the patient *in coincidence*; they originated at a point somewhere along the line between them, to within 1–2 mm. (b) To help with anatomic interpretation, PET information is commonly superimposed on a CT (or, still to a much lesser extent, an MRI) study of the same region. In this example, the PET image, to the left, displays foci of metabolic hyperactivity in right hilar and suprahilar masses, indicative of neoplasms. A conventional CT coronal view (re-created from a set of transverse slices) demonstrates the anatomic structures of the chest and abdomen. Superimposing these two and adding a color spectrum scaled to the relative number of positron events, hence to the metabolic activity, demonstrates and localizes the lesions. It also shows the normal metabolic activity within the liver and the absence of any other "hot spots." Courtesy of Robert Hellman, Medical College of Wisconsin, Milwaukee.

region of origin within the body; from that comes the image of the spatial distribution of the radio-pharmaceutical in the body. (Any photons detected one at a time, rather than in pairs, are totally ignored.)

Some of the elements with positron-emitting isotopes (carbon-11, nitrogen-13, and oxygen-15) can be incorporated into physiologically important biomolecules. Most widely employed of these, by far, is the glucose analog fluorine-18 deoxyglucose (^{18}FDG), which tends to concentrate in tumors and other areas of high metabolic activity (Figure 1.17b). Virtually all PET imaging is now *multimodal*, in that the physiological contrast provided by the nuclear medicine study is superimposed on a background of anatomic landmarks obtained at about the same time with a CT machine that is either physically co-joined with the PET device, preferably, or separate from it. New PET devices come automatically with a CT attached.

PET studies are particularly intriguing to neuroscientists and psychiatrists, since ^{18}FDG may indicate the parts of the brain where neural activity becomes notably high when certain mental processes are ongoing. Dynamic PET studies provide information that is similar, but not identical, to those of *f*MRI, and the combination of these complementary modalities (and perhaps with others, such as electroencephalography and magnetoencephalography) shows great clinical potential in the fields of mental health.

Diagnostic ultrasound: contrast from differences in tissue elasticity or density

Unlike the other imaging technologies we have discussed, ultrasonography does not involve ionizing radiation. In fact, the probes involved are not EM radiation of any sort but, rather, high-frequency *mechanical* disturbances that travel through soft tissues in fairly straight lines and at almost constant velocity.

Normal audible sounds consist of waves of compression and rarefaction, of frequencies between 20 Hz and 20 kHz, that flow through air at about 343 m/s at sea level and room temperature. When a drum is struck, for example, its vibrating head alternately increases and reduces the pressure in the air just outside it, which pushes and pulls on the adjacent thin "layer" of air a brief moment later, and so on. The disturbance thus radiates outward as waves of mechanical energy, and a small part of it reaches the ear, driving displacements of the tympanic membrane, and leading to oscillations of the fluid in the cochlea. The actual sound receptors are hair cells within the organ of Corti, sensory neurons attached to microscopic stereocilia of various lengths and weights that resonate naturally over a range of frequencies, and they can be set in motion by vibrations in the cochlear fluid, triggering the cochlear nerve. The transmission of action potentials along the neurons of the eighth cranial nerve to the brain results in the sensation and perception of sound.

Ultrasound waves are similar, except that they are of frequencies far above the audible range, typically between 2 and 10 megahertz (MHz), and they propagate through soft tissues much faster (about 1540 m/s) than does sound in air.

B-mode anatomic imaging

A clinical ultrasound system used for medical diagnosis is similar to active sonar (*so*und *na*vigation *r*anging), developed largely during the Second World War for the detection of submarines. The heart of a US system is the *transducer*, an energy-conversion device that transforms pulses of electrical voltage into mechanical vibrations, and vice versa. The transducer is pressed against the body and, acting somewhat as an audio speaker, produces a narrow, focused beam of pulses of US. In a homogeneous material, such as water or the fluid contents of a cyst, the beam simply dissipates its energy as it penetrates to greater depths, somewhat analogous to the attenuation of a monochromatic beam of X-rays passing through a homogeneous medium. But if a beam passes from one tissue into another, energy is also reflected back at the interface between them (Figure 1.18a).

By analogy, imagine a pair of joined springs of different mass per length or elasticity (Figure 1.18b). When a pulse moving along from one end encounters the junction, some of its energy will continue in the forward direction but the rest will be reflected back as an echo; in an extreme case, with the spring attached to a wall, virtually the entire pulse will be reflected, but returned upside-down. This

(a)

(b)

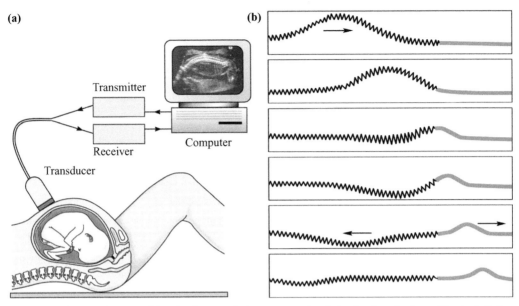

Transmitter

Receiver

Computer

Transducer

Figure 1.18 Ultrasound imaging. (a) Under the control of a computer, electrical pulses from the transmitter, typically 1 per millisecond, are transformed into a narrow, brief beam of high-frequency (2–10 MHz) sound by the transducer. Then, acting in reverse after each pulse, the transducer detects echo signals produced at tissue boundaries and converts them back into electrical signals. Meanwhile, the beam is swept or stepped relatively slowly (30 times per second) across the body, cutting out a thin plane. The computer then untangles all the echoes and creates an image. (b) Echoes arise when US encounters a boundary between tissues of significantly different density or elasticity, much as when a pulse traveling along a spring is partly reflected at a juncture with a different type of spring.

figure is a little misleading, however, in that the displacements of the spring are shown as transverse to the direction of wave propagation; with sound and ultrasound, they are longitudinal, vibrating back and forth along the direction the waves are moving.

After reflection at inter-tissue boundaries, the US echoes are detected by the transducer, now serving as a microphone, and transformed back into electrical signals. The *time of return* of an echo is proportional to the *depth* within the patient of the interface that produced it. The echo's *intensity* depends on the degree of difference in *density* and/or *elasticity* of the materials on the two sides of the interface, as well as on its depth.

Ultrasound is most useful in the study of soft tissues and organs that are radiologically too similar to provide adequate X-ray image contrast, as in Figure 1.19. It is widely used for obstetric/gynecologic, cardiac, and general abdominal imaging. B-mode can assist in diagnosing a wide range of diseases, like pathological changes in the thyroid, gall bladder, pancreas, kidneys, and heart, and in distinguishing a fluid-filled cyst from a solid neoplasm in the

breast or abdomen. Dependent upon the condition being evaluated and the skill of the observer, it can achieve a high degree of clinical precision. US evaluation of an ovarian cystic mass is more diagnostic than direct observation via laparoscopic or open surgical evaluations in some situations, such as if it is inappropriate to take a biopsy specimen. It may also disclose more soft tissue detail than CT, as well as being much faster and less expensive. Ultrasound serves as a guide in carrying out invasive procedures such as the draining of an abscess or other fluid collections, or in approaching a vessel to obtain vascular access. US energy does not pass readily across tissue/air or tissue/bone interfaces, however, and is therefore of limited use for the study of the lung or of the adult cranial cavity.

Doppler imaging of blood flow

A quite different form of US allows the monitoring of blood flow. Wave signals coming from a moving source or detected by a moving observer may be shifted in pitch by an amount proportional to their relative speed and direction, as is evident in the wail

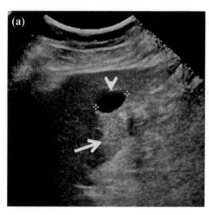
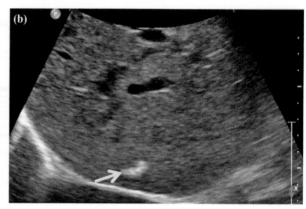

Figure 1.19 In certain situations, the overall US appearance of a lesion can be pathognomonic, characteristic of a specific problem, in which case no further imaging is required. (**a**) Liver with a simple cyst. In the absence of any intrinsic tissue interfaces, the fluid within the cyst transmits the sound waves anechoically, giving the lesion a black appearance (arrowhead). Because little energy was attenuated and removed from the beam within the cyst, the tissues beyond it are brighter than normal, and that part of the image is said to be "enhanced" (arrow). (**b**) US image of a liver containing a hyperechoic rounded lesion, typical of a benign hemangioma (arrow).

of the siren of a fire truck rushing by. That is also the basis for the red-shift determination of stellar velocities, police Doppler radar, and the Doppler ultrasound measurement of blood flow within larger vessels: the faster the blood cells are traveling, the greater the shift in the frequency of the US waves that bounce off them and return to the transducer (Figure 1.20).

It is commonly held that there is virtually no risk to a patient from ultrasound, since no ionizing radiation is involved. At diagnostic intensities, there are no known harmful biologic effects, even to a fetus; this is one reason the modality is used extensively to provide obstetric information and as a visual aid in guiding amniocentesis and fetal surgery. But absence of evidence of health effects from US is not certain evidence for their absence, and one should treat this modality (and all others) with due respect. Indeed, high-intensity US is destructive of tissues, and such beams are used therapeutically to ablate abnormal tissues, or to disrupt crystalline structures such as with nephrolithotripsy. So it is important always to ensure that diagnostic equipment is functioning properly, being operated correctly, and being applied for a medically valid reason, especially when used on the fetus.

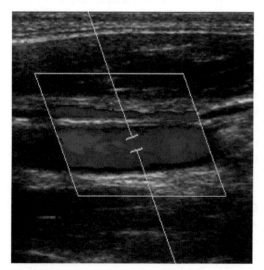

Figure 1.20 In this Doppler image, the red and blue regions indicate blood moving toward and away from the transducer, respectively.

Magnetic resonance imaging: mapping the spatial distribution of spin-relaxation times of hydrogen nuclei in tissue water and lipids

We have already discussed creating contrast through the attenuation of X-rays, the emission of gamma-rays, and the reflections of ultrasound waves. MRI produces contrast in a number of distinct and far more subtle ways, and at times it can provide information on soft tissues that is much more diagnostically useful than the others.

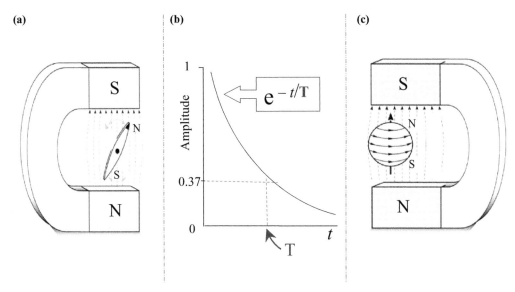

Figure 1.21 The NMR process, central to MRI, can be viewed in several ways. (**a**) With one, spin-relaxation is *analogous* (only!) to the settling down of the swings of a briefly jostled compass needle in a magnetic field, (**b**) with a characteristic *relaxation time*, here called T. (**c**) Like any moving charge, a "spinning" lone proton, the nucleus of a standard hydrogen atom, creates a tiny magnetic field, like that of a compass needle; during NMR, it, too, undergoes a subtle sort of relaxation, but we shall have to provide a good deal more background information to explain it.

MRI not only reveals the structural, anatomic details of the various organs, like CT, but it can also provide information on their physiological status and pathologies, like nuclear medicine. And as with US, there is no risk from ionizing radiation to the patient or staff, since no X-ray or gamma-ray energy is involved. Instead, MRI harnesses magnetic fields and radio waves to probe the protons – in particular, the nuclei of the ordinary hydrogen atoms occurring naturally in water and lipid molecules, within and around cells.

Spin-relaxation times of protons in water and lipids in a strong magnetic field

Imagine a bunch of identical pocket compasses on a table. Each compass needle is itself a tiny bar magnet, and as such it displays two related but different characteristics: it produces its own small magnetic field, and also it tends to align along the Earth's magnetic field.

In your mind's eye, twist all the compasses through 180°, so that they point south, and then release them at the same time (Figure 1.21a). Each will flop back over again, oscillating about north, with an amplitude that diminishes exponentially over time – eventually they all come to rest pointing

north again (Figure 1.21b). The length of time this settling down process takes, as averaged over all the compass needles, is parameterized by their average *relaxation time*, T. For a compass, T is determined largely by the mass and shape of the needles, the nature of the frictional forces such as those occurring at the mechanical pivot points where the needle is supported, and the viscosity of any damping fluid that might surround it.

For protons in water and lipid molecules in tissue, relaxation is a somewhat *analogous* affair, but far more nuanced, interesting, and clinically useful. But first . . .

Fact of life: any electric current gives rise to a magnetic field. If you hold one of our compasses close to a wire that connects a battery to a flashlight bulb, the needle will deflect. It's one of the fundamental wonders that underlie the physical sciences, like the electrical force between charges or gravitational attraction. Physicists can fancy it up, what with descriptions involving quantum mechanics and relativity, but it really doesn't get any more basic.

A proton, the nucleus of a hydrogen atom, behaves somewhat like a rapidly spinning, hence moving, positively charged ball. So it, too, produces its own small magnetic field along its spin axis and, as such, it acts like a tiny compass needle

(Figure 1.21c). In particular, when a patient lies in the extremely strong magnetic field of an MRI device (typically of strength 1.5 *tesla*, some four orders of magnitude (10^4) times greater than the Earth's field), many of the protons in tissue water and lipid molecules will tend to align along it.

It is possible, by beaming in a brief pulse of radio waves of the correct frequency, to make protons in a voxel flip over and point in the opposite (i.e., the "wrong") direction, instead. Immediately thereafter, though, some of these will begin a kind of spontaneous relaxation in which they return to their more comfortable, equilibrium alignment *along* the field. This transition takes place in a manner analogous to (but, on the molecular scale, quite different from) that of a compass needle. The rapidity of the relaxation process for the protons in the voxel is parameterized by its characteristic *nuclear spin relaxation time* known, in MRI, as T1.

The rates of relaxation of excited water or lipid protons within and between cells are exquisitely sensitive to the detailed nature of the local biochemical environments of the protons involved – that is, to the atomic-level friction-like and other physical interactions between them and the nearby biomolecules. The concentrations and biophysical characteristics of these biomolecules, in turn, depend on the type and physiologic status of the tissues, and that will influence the effectiveness of the T1 relaxation mechanism for them. A spatial map of T1 throughout a slice of tissue can therefore produce clinically invaluable anatomic and/or physiologic information.

There is a second sort of proton relaxation process, known as T2, that involves and reflects on quite dissimilar aspects of molecular biophysics, and T2-maps also play a central, and complementary, role in MRI. Indeed, MRI can produce contrast by way of half a dozen totally different physical processes, with countless variations on each theme, and they can all provide useful clinical information.

Mapping the spatial distribution of proton T1 and T2

What MR imaging usually does, then, is to produce a map of variations in the relaxation times of the hydrogen nuclei in the water molecules, primarily, of the tissues (Figure 1.22). T1 or T2 contrast among soft tissues is often much better than that from imaging with X-rays, and it can show subtleties in the physiology of an organ that CT would completely miss. In addition, some forms of MR imaging have no counterparts in other forms of imaging. As seen in the introductory case of Dr. Doe, *f*MRI monitors stimulus-induced local changes in cerebral blood flow and, like PET, can indicate the occurrence of mental processes (Figure 0.5). DTI makes it possible to follow the natural diffusion of water molecules along the axons of neurons, thereby revealing nerve-trunks (Figure 0.6). One can carry out *in vivo* biopsy studies on small volumes of tissue with MR spectroscopy (MRS) (Figures 0.4). It even supports several approaches to MR angiography (MRA) that are non-invasive and do not necessarily involve contrast agent (Figure 1.23).

MRI came onto the scene in the early 1980s, and at first data acquisition was slow, requiring an hour or so per patient. Imaging time has been driven down dramatically and is becoming much less of a major limiting factor; indeed, imaging of the heart throughout the entire cardiac cycle is now routine. Similarly, resolution has improved steadily, and is now better than 1 mm.

MRI is widely and appropriately touted for the absence of ionizing radiation, and it appears that the various strong constant and time-varying magnetic fields involved pose no deleterious physiological effects. Still, one must be ever vigilant for magnetic shrapnel and implants (such as aneurism clips and pacemakers) and for flying screw drivers, oxygen bottles, i.v. poles, hand-cuffs, and the like).

Hopefully these brief sketches have whetted your appetite for a deeper understanding of imaging technologies.

Traditional X-ray filming is still the form of imaging most commonly employed worldwide, and the least expensive. It's also the easiest to describe so, after briefly exploring what a "good enough" medical image means in the next chapter, we shall start off our more in-depth examinations with a reconsideration of radiography.

Appendix: selection of imaging modalities to assist in medical diagnosis

The following is a *sampling* of examples of the selection of common imaging studies of major biological

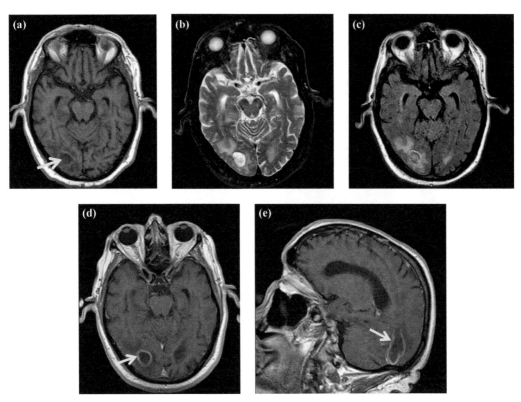

Figure 1.22 A patient known to suffer from AIDS presents with mental status changes, and (a) an initial axial T1-weighted acquisition demonstrates a hypointense, well-circumscribed lesion of the white matter of the right occipital lobe (arrow). The lesion has an isointense rim and is surrounded by hypointense edema. *Note*: One views a transverse/axial tomographic slice-image from the feet upward; the arrow, to the reader's left, is on the patient's right side. (**b**) Axial T2-weighted image at the same level further categorizing the lesion and demonstrating the surrounding edema. (**c**) Axial fluid attenuating inversion recovery (FLAIR) study at the same level, for which the cerebrospinal fluid is dark while the perilesional edema is hyperintense. (**d**) With the intravenous addition of contrast agent (a gadolinium complex), a repeated axial T1-weighted image demonstrates circumferential ring enhancement of the wall of the lesion still surrounded by hypointense edema (arrow). (**e**) This is also demonstrated clearly in an image of a thin sagittal plane through the center of the lesion, where it is seen to be located above the tentorium cerebella (arrow). The overall appearance and contrast enhancement pattern is typical of an abscess and, because of the patient's immunosuppression, the infection was likely to due to *Toxopolasma gondii* (as was proven by biopsy).

systems of the body, based on typical symptoms. It is meant only to provide a few illustrations of possible studies and the order in which they might be chosen, as determined by factors such as diagnostic sensitivity and selectivity. For all the following, diagnostic benefit must be weighed thoughtfully against considerations of safety (especially of the fetus and children), cost, and normal availability of the equipment. Estimated relative cost is indicated by $, $$, and $$$, and dose of ionizing radiation by *D*, *DD*, and *DDD*.

The objective of this appendix is only to illustrate some conventional clinical applications of the modalities discussed in the book. This is obviously very far from complete, and it reflects the opinions of two physicians. It is not intended to serve as medical advice, nor should it be construed as such.

Cardiac versus non-cardiac chest pain

Chest pain presents in two broad categories based on symptomatology and ancillary testing (EKG, cardiac biomarkers, etc.): *cardiogenic* and *non-cardiogenic*.

Cardiogenic chest pain: acute coronary syndrome (ACS) typically presents as:

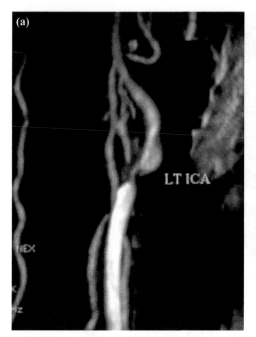
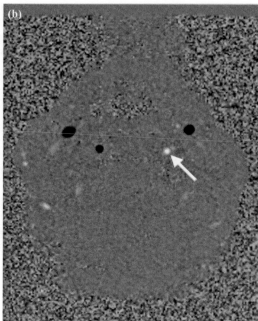

Figure 1.23 Magnetic resonance angiography. (a) Contrast agent (gadolinium) enhanced MRA 3D image demonstrating a stenosis of the left interior carotid artery. After a disruption, protons in most of a thin horizontal slice of soft tissue recover according to relaxation times T1 and T2; with Time of Flight (TOF) MRA, blood within the voxels of a vessel within the slice, however, is refreshed with the inflow of new blood, and spin-change within them is governed primarily by the rate of flow. (b) Phase contrast (PC) MRA differs in that it indicates the direction of flow, as well as the rate. Flow in the left vertebral artery is normally in the caudal-to-cranial direction, and shows up dark; at the arrow, it is bright, indicating retrograde flow, resulting from *subclavian steal*.

Chest pressure (not necessarily sharp pain) with radiation to left shoulder, left arm, left side of neck or jaw;

Associated symptoms of dyspnea and/or nausea and vomiting;

EKG findings of ST-segment elevation corresponding to area of infarct, or ST-segment depression indicating evolving myocardial ischemia;

Elevated biomarkers (troponin-i, creatine kinase-MB (CK-MB), myoglobin) in serum.

Presentation with the classic findings of cardiogenic pain is typically treated with nitroglycerin and thrombolytics, or the patient goes directly to the cardiac catheterization lab for evaluation of coronary anatomy with possible intervention, such as percutaneous thrombolytic coronary angiography (PTCA). Patients with somewhat equivocal findings of cardiogenic type chest pain, however, may benefit from other (less invasive) imaging modalities to determine the etiology of their pain.

Non-cardiogenic chest pain lacks features clinically to be of a likely cardiac source, and therefore follows a different path of investigation. This class of imaging is outlined below for patients who present with chest symptoms (sharp chest pain, isolated dyspnea, chest trauma or mass).

Non-cardiogenic chest pain

Atypical chest pain, dyspnea or chest mass, clinically thought to be not of cardiac origin: imaging the chest in patients with "non-cardiogenic" chest disease typically coalesces around the symptoms or findings of atypical chest pain (sharp, pleuritic, worse with deep breathing), mass, chest trauma, dyspnea or hemoptysis. Diagnoses range from minor to life-threatening (bronchitis to pulmonary embolus).

Chest radiographs (CXR), PA and lateral ($; D): Visualization of pleural membrane and space, lung disease (pneumonia, pneumonitis, interstitial lung disease, atelectasis) mediastinal mass/adenopathy, aortic dissection, cardiomyopathy, lung mass, pulmonary edema, pleural effusion, pneumothorax, pneumoperitoneum, hemothorax, rib fractures, ET tube placement, diaphragmatic integrity, stomach gas, or foreign body. Poor discrimination of hilar versus mediastinal adenopathy or mass; poor sensitivity for evaluation of PE.

Chest CT ($$; DD): Greatly improved sensitivity, specificity, and discrimination of/for: hilar and mediastinal mass; pulmonary disease, pleural disease, and chest wall; staging lung cancer and imaging of lung/pleural mass; cardiac anatomy visualization; chest trauma (tracheal rupture, aortic dissection, pneumomediastinum), pleural/lung disease versus mass, lung abscess versus nodule, interstitial versus infiltrative pulmonary processes. In patients with infectious pulmonary disease, lung abscess versus empyema, rapid evaluation of chest trauma, percutaneous drainage.

Chest CT for PE ($$$; DDD): Suspicion for pulmonary embolus or deep vein thrombosis (DVT) with dyspnea. Requires timely specific IV contrast, minimum 20 gauge, for vascular visualization. 95% sensitive for clinically significant PE.

Chest MRI ($$$; No D): No ionizing radiation: better lung mass characterization and cancer staging, visualization of aorta and mediastinum; discrimination for mediastinal versus hilar mass/adenopathy, vascular invasion in hilum or mediastinum, interstitial versus infiltrative pulmonary disease; congenital heart disease or cardiac tumor. Contraindicated in patients with most pacemakers, intraocular metal, metal clips, cochlear implants, kidney disease (see Box 11.5).

V/Q scan ($$; DD): Evaluation of functional ventilation for dead space, perfusion for shunt. Most scans are intermediate probability for PE, which leads to diagnostic dilemma (20–70% accuracy) giving low specificity for thromboembolic disease. High- and low-probability scans are of excellent sensitivity and specificity.

Chest PET/CT ($$$; DD): Tumor staging for pulmonary or mediastinal, primary or metastatic malignancy. Discriminates benign and malignant mediastinal adenopathy. Metabolic and anatomic information

Cardiogenic chest pain
Chest pain of typical cardiac origin: Substernal pressure with radiation to the left shoulder, jaw, or arm. Although any chest pain or dyspnea (angina equivalent) can be of a cardiac origin, suspicion for ACS is raised when pain posterior to sternum is of a typical cardiac nature.

Chest pain of an atypical nature: With equivocal cardiac testing, such as EKG findings suspicious but not confirmatory of ACS. Imaging in these equivocal cases of borderline historical chest pain associated with other clinical signs and findings potentially consistent with coronary occlusion, coronary artery disease (CAD) involve both cardiogenic and non-cardiogenic imaging strategies. The chest radiograph is the starting point for addressing both types of chest pain or dyspnea. Beyond that, clinical judgment directs testing and imaging.

Myocardial perfusion stress, technetium, thallium ($$$; DD): Typical cardiac pain, atypical chest pain with known ACS, extent of myocardial ischemia. Detection of presence, location, and extent of active ACS/ischemia. Stuttering course of chest pain with uncertain diagnosis; chest pain with equivocal EKG changes and negative cardiac biomarkers; atypical or recurrent chest pain of uncertain etiology.

CT coronary angiography ($$$; DD): Chest pain suggestive of ACS, equivocal EKG changes, negative cardiac biomarkers. Consider direct correlation of observed angiographic stenosis (CAD) with symptoms of coronary lesions. Similar limitation observed with coronary angiography.

Cardiac CT for calcium scoring ($$; D to DD): screening exam for patient with family history, multiple risk factors for ACS, or vague symptoms of possible coronary disease. High score suggestive of coronary stenosis.

Radionuclide ventriculography ($$$; DD): Multigated acquisition (MUGA). Patients with ischemic heart disease and congestive heart failure or cardiomyopathy. Calculation of ejection fraction. To evaluate cardiac output, ejection fraction is determined non-invasively. Difficult to perform if patient has abnormal rhythm.

Abdominal/pelvis imaging
The diagnostic and radiographic therapeutic workup involving abdominal imaging is vast. Abdominal imaging and intervention typically clusters around the symptoms of abdominal pain (sometimes in quadrants) or diffuse abdominal or pelvic pain, abdominal mass/tumor, or vasculopathy (GI bleeding, ischemia, or vasculitis).

Abdominal radiograph ($; D): Screening for abdominal pain, need flat and upright views. Bowel gas pattern for mechanical small bowel obstruction versus ileus; pneumoperitoneum from ruptured viscus or radio-opaque stone (urolithiasis, appendicolith, gallstones). Provides limited contrast.

Abdominal ultrasound ($$; No D): Cystic versus solid lesions of solid organs: hepatic or renal mass/cyst; biliary duct ectasia, cholelithiasis or gallbladder wall thickening; peri-pancreatic fluid of pseudocyst formation; hydronephrosis, hydroureter, abdominal aortic aneurysm, appendiceal inflammation, ascities, or metastatic or primary carcinoma (carcinomatosis). Visualization of pelvic masses, cysts and discrimination from GI source; pelvic masses are best visualized by US (complexity, architecture, thickness of wall). Can guide percutaneous drainage. Best results after 6 hours of NPO. Non-invasive and portable. Bowel gas can obscure; strongly operator-skill dependent.

Abdominal CT ($$; DD for non-contrast study; $$$; DDD for contrast-enchanced multi-phase study: All abdominal and pelvic organs. Small, large bowel obstructions; traumatic injury of any soft tissue organ, abdominal wall mass of injury (hernia); mass, tumor, cyst, or abscess evaluation; obstructive biliary disease, intra-hepatic process; pancreatitis or soft tissue inflammation. Visualization of mesenteric or retro-peritoneal adenopathy or mass. Appendicitis, mesenteric ischemia, urolithiasis or renal obstructive process. Abdominal aortic aneurysm. Uterine or ovarian mass and cancer staging of malignant disease.

IV contrast: Mesenteric ischemia or infarct, aorta, vascular enhancement of solid tumor.

Oral contrast: Rapid increased sensitivity of bowel wall. Excellent spatial resolution not limited by overlying bowel patterns. CT guided drainage or percutaneous biopsy may be possible. Contrast-induced nephropathy.

Abdominal MRI ($$$; No D): Adjunct to CT where superb resolution, tissue contrast, multiplanar views needed; benign versus malignant tumors, mass/tumor such as hepatic, bowel wall, or retroperitoneal. Pre-op staging of abdominal cancers. Subject to motion artifacts, may require IM-glucagon to calm peristalsis; opacification of GI tract not readily available.

Abdominal PET/CT ($$$; DD): Both metabolic and anatomic detail. Primary and metastatic neo-plasms; benign versus malignant lymph nodes; tumor staging, evaluating recurrence.

Mesenteric angiography ($$$; DDD): Small bowel bleeding or mesenteric ischemia can be difficult to isolate by endoscopy or CT alone. For gastrointestinal hemorrhage not amenable to endoscopic evaluation/management; mesenteric aneurysm; vasculitis of splanchnic vasculature; embolization of acute GI-bleeding. Requires femoral artery cannulation and iodinated contrast, maybe sedation.

Radionuclide tagged labeled red-cell ($$$; DD): For slower rates (0.10 mL/min) of upper or lower GI bleeding, intermittent bleeding.

Upper GI fluoroscopy ($$; DD): Gastric and duodenal mucosal inflammation, ulcerations, polyps, mass, hernia, gastric outlet obstruction. Double or single contrast barium technique or gastrografin, water soluble contrast to check for anastomotic leak or perforation. Less expensive/invasive than endoscopy. But lesion identification may not correlate with site of bleeding or pain; barium may hinder subsequent endoscopic procedure, pulmonary edema from aspiration of gastrografin.

Radionuclide gastric emptying ($$$; DD): Functional information about gastric outlet not available by other means. "Dumping syndrome," gastroporesis, inflammatory or neoplastic processes. Establish normal values prior; patient must eat 300 gram meal of liquids and solids.

Radionuclide GI esophageal reflux ($$$; DD): Radionuclide scan evaluates gastro-esophageal reflux disease (GERD) or aspiration pneumonitis. Non-invasive and highly sensitive for GERD, quantification of reflux. But incomplete emptying may mimic GERD.

Radionuclide cholescintigraphy or HIDA scan ($$$; DD): RUQ, excretion of radionuclide into biliary system (biliary ducts, gallbladder, cystic duct, common duct, intestine) with hepatobiliary iminodiacetic acid labeled with technetium-99m (HIDA-Tc-99m). Hepatobiliary system function for suspected cholecystitis, common bile duct obstruction or bile leaks. 95% sensitive and 99% specific for cholecystitis (higher than ultrasound). But does not discriminate obstruction between tumor and stone.

Hepatic angiography { $$$; DDD): Gold standard for hepatic arterial anatomy, hepatic neoplasm. Liver trauma, arteriovenous malformation (AVM), portal vein occlusion. Prior to TIPS procedure for portal hypertension, hepatic transplant. More specific than US for portal vein patency. But requires common femoral artery cannulation for contrast and cardiac monitoring.

Abdominal calcifications: non-palpable but seen on radiograph

Right upper quadrant: Cholelithiasis, renal mass with calcific degeneration, adrenal mass.

Left upper quadrant: Splenic artery calcification or calcified aneurysm, splenic mass or cyst, renal mass or pancreatic tail calcification.

Right/left flank: Urolithiasis and ureteral calculi or calcified mesenteric lymphadenopathy.

Mid-abdomen: Aortic aneurysm or calcified aorta, pancreatic mass, or metastatic lymph node.

Right lower quadrant: Appendolith or distal ureter stone.

Left lower quadrant: Ovarian dermoid, phleboliths, distal ureter calculus.

Pelvis: Uterine fibroids, bladder calculus, ureterovesicular junction stone, ovarian tumor, iliac vessels.

Head and neck imaging

Imaging of the skull, brain, sinuses for CNS infections, headache/trauma, mass, seizure, symptoms of dementia, acute delirium. Other changes in mental status are complex, commonly calling for: plain radiography, CT, MRI, angiography, and PET.

Radiograph: skull, sinus ($; D to DD): Cranial, facial bone fractures; nasal bone, orbital (blowout), Le Fort, mandible fractures, air-fluid levels in sinus. Skull fracture, linear or depressed. Osteomyelitis, several weeks after the process, with areas of lucency. Some tumors (chordoma) may reveal bony destruction or cortical expansion. Mucosal thickening or air-fluid levels in infected sinus.

Head CT – no contrast ($$; D to DD): Initial evaluation of trauma may reveal skull or facial fracture also showing soft tissue injury. Intra-cranial complications: epidural hematoma (convex peripheral high density lesion), subdural hematoma (crescent dense lesion), intracerebral hematoma, subarachnoid hemorrhage, or cranial contusion. A stroke/cerebrovascular accident (CVA) may produce a hypodensity involving a vascular territory in thrombotic CVA, or may be negative in early phases. Intraparenchymal hemorrhage appears as homogeneous dense, defined lesion within cerebral substance. Work-up for headache or possible brain mass may reveal a single heterogeneous mass which may be either isodense or hypodense (as in glioma). Infectious etiology such as meningitis (thrombosis, hydrocephalus, subdural effusion or brain abscess), encephalitis (low-attenuation) or epidural empyema can be visualized. Although non-contrasted head CT may be the first line to evaluate head trauma (acute bleeding and fracture), or CVA (to rule out hemorrhage), IV contrast may help for enhancement of mass, abscess.

Head CT – contrast enhanced ($$$; DD): Contrast enhancement may reveal necrotic tumor core with high-attenuation capsule, differentiates abscess versus tumor, tumor detail (homogeneous lesion with enhanced ring); vascular lesions, such as AVM.

Head MRI ($$$; No D): High T1-/T2-weighted tissue contrast. For neoplasms, image density (darkness) depends on tumor type: T2-*w* images show high density (dark) regions, but T1-*w* isodense (as in glioma). Acute hemorrhage of subarachnoid bleed will show on FLAIR as hyper dense signal. Alzheimer's dementia on MRI similar to CT, with cerebral atrophy and enlarged ventricles. Cerebellar atrophy, multiple sclerosis, seizure disorders, and/or encephalitis all may be best imaged with MRI; likewise with brain abscess versus necrotic tumor. In meningitis, inflammation of the two innermost layers of meninges, versus subarachnoid distention, as well as the etiology of hydrocephalus, are also best seen with MRI. When evaluating thrombotic CVA (after bleed is ruled out by CT), MRI T2-*w* image produces high signal intensity of vascular territory involved.

Duplex color-flow Doppler ($ to $$; No D): Hemodynamic information such as flow velocity for patients with transient ischemic attack (TIA) or CVA.

PET ($$$; DD): Functional pathology of neurodegenerative diseases: Alzheimer's, Parkinson's and Huntington's.

Musculoskeletal imaging

Radiography – extremity or spinal ($; D): Traumatic injury, musculoskeletal pain – typically adequate for uncomplicated fractures, dislocations of bones, joints in appendicular and spinal skeleton. For soft tissue (joint space, muscle) or when sensitivity and specificity not adequate for musculoskeletal pathology.

Radionuclide bone scan ($$$; DD): Whole body evaluation of trauma (occult fracture), primary or metastatic neoplasm, osteomyelitis, arthritis, avascular necrosis, or joint prosthesis. Highly sensitive for osteomyelitis (early), stress fractures.

Bone/joint MRI ($$$; No D): Soft tissue in joint space and bone, except at prostheses; spinal nerve roots, cord, and vertebrae. Primary or metastatic mass involving bone or soft tissue. Soft tissue infections (abscess), marrow disease, or traumatic injury not visualized on plain radiograph or CT. CT may be superior in limited circumstances, such as osteophyte spurring.

Vascular imaging

Vascular imaging for venous thrombosis or patency; arterial stenosis, aneurysm or vasculitis leading to ischemia of a limb or organ system.

Ultrasound ($ to $$; No D): DVT, patency of major venous systems (portal, vena cava). Carotid Doppler for TIA patient with possible thromboembolic event originating in carotid. Vascular bruit, potential arterial stenosis.

Angiography ($$$; DDD): Aorta, major branches for central and peripheral vascular disease. Abdominal aortic aneurysm, thoracic aortic dissection, major arterial stenosis (renal artery, femoral artery). Vasculitis or mesenteric ischemia. Pre-operative evaluation of aortofemoral bypass.

CTA of aorta and major branches ($$$; DDD): Quick evaluation of trauma when aortic dissection or injury is suspected. Assessment of aneurysm.

Vascular MRI or MRA/MRV ($$$; No D): Aortic aneurysm, relation to other major vessels; take-off of renal arteries; pre-op before aneurysm grafting.

References

1 Patton DD. Insights on the radiologic centennial – a historical perspective. Roentgen and the "new light". I. Roentgen and Lenard. *Invest Radiol* 1992;**27**:408–14.

2 Patton DD. Roentgen and the "new light" – Roentgen's moment of discovery. Part 2: The first glimmer of the "new light". 1993;**28**:51–8.

3 Patton DD. Roentgen and the "new light" – Roentgen's moment of discovery. Part 3: The genealogy of Roentgen's barium platinocyanide screen. 1993;**28**:954–61.

4 Seliger HH. Wilhelm Conrad Röntgen and the glimmer of light. *Phys Today* 1995;Nov:25–31.

CHAPTER 2

Image Quality and Dose
What Constitutes a "Good" Medical Image?

This chapter explores the main factors that go into producing clinically good enough medical images. The most important of these is usually the *contrast* among body tissues, and the major categories of modalities differ primarily in the ways they exploit various physical processes and mechanisms in creating it. A second aspect that is often important is *resolution*, the capability to capture fine detail. Both contrast and apparent resolution may be diminished if excessive *random noise* is present, or if non-random patterns of mis-information, *artifacts*, obscure what is there. A comprehensive, routine *quality assurance* (QA) program can confirm that the equipment is operating well, optimizing contrast and resolution while minimizing noise and artifacts, and at the same time ensuring that non-productive dose to the patient and inadvertent exposure of the staff and the public are *as low as reasonably achievable* (*ALARA*).

The creation of medical images with any modality involves the interaction of energetic probes, first with tissues and then with the image receptor. And to paint any sort of meaningful picture of imaging, it is necessary to have at least an elementary understanding of the interactions of various sorts of radiation with matter. Fortunately, you acquired all of what you need in college, and probably most of it even earlier in high school chemistry classes. But for your convenience we begin with a short refresher about some notions about atoms and energy that you have already learned. There is really nothing new here.

The technology of imaging involves electricity and magnetism, and most of it (apart from ultrasound) encompasses the interaction of electromagnetic (EM) radiation with matter as well, so it might be a good idea to begin with...

A brief history of magnetism

The magnetic field is one of the indispensables of modern life. It plays essential roles in generating electricity, powering electric motors, recalling pictures from computer memory and displaying them

Medical Imaging: Essentials for Physicians, First Edition. Anthony B. Wolbarst, Patrizio Capasso and Andrew R. Wyant.
© 2013 John Wiley & Sons, Inc. Published 2013 by John Wiley & Sons, Inc.

on TV and monitor screens, even pumping those hormonic aberrations out of your teenager's stereo speakers.

The ancients were familiar with both electricity and magnetism, but they were unaware of any connection between these two seemingly disparate phenomena. About the only thing known about electricity was the static cling that comes from shuffling across a fur rug, and things stayed pretty much that way until Benjamin Franklin deduced the nature of lightening before taking time off from his scientific endeavors to help convince the British to go home.

Magnetism got off to a faster start. Its discovery was intimately tied to the early working of iron, with the Egyptians and Mesopotamians fashioning ornaments out of small amounts of it from fallen meteorites before 4000 BC. At some point(s), and estimates vary from 2500 BC in China to 800 BC in Greece, people noticed that a certain gray-black, metallic mineral was naturally magnetic. Pieces of the iron ore magnetite (named for the Greek province of Magnesia, where it was mined) cling to un-magnetized iron. Moreover, a magnetized

needle or a piece of magnetite, if suspended by a fine thread or supported by a cork on water, will twist about and always end up aligning north-south. Sailors and scientists learned that wherever and whenever you measure it, any magnetic field has both a specific field strength and a definite field orientation. (An engineer would say it behaves as a *vector* – as opposed to temperature, which has only magnitude and is a *scalar*.) The magnitude and the direction of the field may change from place to place throughout space and over time, but at any particular instant and location, both are well defined and unique. People have long called the end of a compass needle that swings toward the Earth's northern geographic pole, in the Arctic, the needle's "north" pole. So by this convention, the Earth's own internal magnet must actually have a south magnetic pole up there!

A major advance in the understanding of magnetism came in 1820 with the discovery by Hans Christian Oersted, a Dane, that a wire carrying an electric current produced by a simple battery causes a compass needle to deflect (Figure 2.1a).

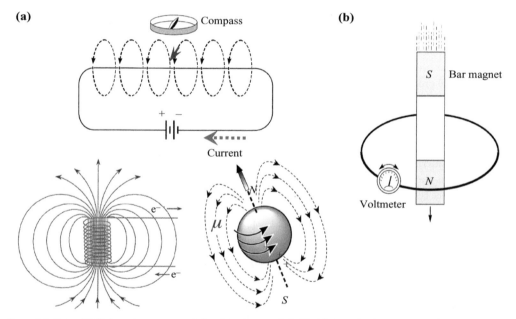

Figure 2.1 Two critically important aspects of electric and magnetic fields. **(a)** A steady electric current along a stretch of wire produces a constant magnetic field that curls around the current and falls off in strength with distance from it. Similarly, a loop of current produces a field, and a coil of *N* loops generates a field *N* times stronger. And an atomic nucleus behaves much like a spinning (hence moving) ball of charge, and the field it creates is parameterized by its magnetic moment, μ. **(b)** A changing magnetic field generates a nearby electric field that can drive an electric current around a wire loop. Both of these phenomena underlie aspects of creating images, especially with MRI.

This demonstrated a second, related but separate, profoundly significant fact of life: not only will a small magnet try to align along a magnetic field already in existence, but also, moving charges such as electrons flowing along a wire will create a magnetic field. A loop of wire can produce a field perpendicular to the plane of the loop, and the field from a coil of N loops will generate a field N times stronger. And an atomic nucleus may be thought of as a spinning ball of positive charge, giving rise to its own magnetic field whose strength is parameterized by its *nuclear magnetic moment*, μ. This is true, in particular, for the nucleus of the hydrogen atom, and is the basis for MRI.

A bit more than a decade later, the great English "natural philosopher" Michael Faraday discovered yet another wonderfully mysterious fundamental reality: a *changing magnetic field* induces a transient *electric field* in the surrounding space. The classic demonstration of Faraday's magnetic induction is to drop a bar magnet through a loop of wire that includes an ammeter or voltmeter (Figure 2.1b). As the magnet passes through the loop, the resulting pulse of voltage and electric field within the wire drives brief currents around it, first one way and then the other (because the magnet's two different poles drive the electrons in opposite directions as they pass by), and the meter pointer swings back and forth accordingly – the world's simplest electric generator!

The stage was finally set for one of the greatest bursts of scientific imagination of all time. Guided by these observations, the Scottish physicist James Clerk Maxwell postulated the existence of the converse phenomenon, in which a *changing electric field* gives rise to a transient *magnetic field*, also verified thereafter by experiment. In 1864, the year of Lincoln's re-election and shortly after publication of *Origin of Species*, Maxwell put all of what was known of electricity and magnetism together into a comprehensive, unified formalism that explained the existence and properties of light and other *electromagnetic waves* – an achievement comparable in significance to those of Isaac Newton, Charles Darwin, and Albert Einstein. Einstein, incidentally, kept three pictures in his office, those of Newton, Faraday, and Maxwell.

In the *Système international d'unités* (SI), the measure of magnetic field strength is called the tesla

(T). The field strength of the Earth itself, viewed as a huge bar magnet, is about 50 microtesla (0.00005 T). Its exact value and direction depend on where you are. The field strength at the surface of the small magnet that holds your favorite finger painting to the refrigerator door is about 0.1 T, a thousand or so times stronger; the fridge magnet may be small, but it is far from weak. MRI is carried out with the principal field typically at 1.5 tesla or, increasingly, at 3.0 T. This is a strong field, by any measure, and it must be stable over time and also uniform, to within a few parts per million, over a volume large enough to accommodate a significant part of the body. The technology needed to produce such a field does not come from the local hardware store, nor is it cheap.

The tesla, incidentally, is named after Nikola Tesla, who was born in Croatia of Serbian parents in 1856 and emigrated to America 28 years later. A dreamer and a man of remarkable and far-ranging genius, Tesla invented (along with much else) major elements of the technology that is used, even now, in generating and harnessing electricity. He and George Westinghouse, who bought a good number of his 700 patents, carried on an extended battle with Thomas Edison regarding the merits of a.c. versus d.c. power. It was Tesla who got it right. Tesla took the occult seriously and, as he grew older, his idiosyncrasies became more pronounced:

> "He couldn't tolerate the sight of pearl earrings, the smell of camphor, the act of shaking hands, or close exposure to the hair of other people. He strongly favored numbers that were divisible by three. He seldom ate or drank anything without first calculating its volume. He counted his steps. He washed his hands compulsively. He never married, but he told a friend he had once loved a particular pigeon 'as a man loves a woman.'"
>
> *New Yorker*, March 4, 1991, p. 28

So much for animal magnetism.

About those probes and their interactions with matter...

Mammography, PET, MRI, and ultrasound use physical probes in examining the body, as was suggested by Figure 1.1 and Table 1.1. The different probes interact with the tissues they traverse in ways that can be highly sensitive not only to the specific physical characteristics of the tissues, but also to the nature of the probes themselves.

Each imaging technology, with its own particular kind of probe, is suitable for the study of only certain kinds of medical problems. A fine crack in a small bone will not show up at all with ultrasound (where the probes are high-frequency sound waves), or with MRI (magnetic fields and radio waves) unless there are associated edematous changes. But it is likely to be fully visible in an ordinary radiograph (X-rays), and in some kinds of nuclear medicine studies as well (gamma-rays). Subtle differences among the soft tissues of the abdomen that cannot be seen with X-rays, on the other hand, may be easy to spot with ultrasound or MRI.

To summarize again: different kinds of probes, different mechanisms of interaction with the tissues, and different methods of detection give rise to different forms of contrast conveying different types of clinical image information, with different degrees of specificity and sensitivity for different disease states.

Energy

All the probes employed in standard imaging are forms of *radiation,* which is commonly defined as energy flowing through space or a medium. A great number of physical phenomena involve the interaction of radiation waves and particles with individual atoms and molecules or with bulk matter, and the resulting exchange of energy among them. The story of obtaining medical images, in particular, is told largely in terms of the transmission, absorption, scattering, reflection, or emission of radiant energy by matter. In any case, it entails physical transformations that can generate contrast of clinical significance.

Perhaps the easiest way to approach energy is through the high-school definition of work energy, as force multiplied by distance. Imagine that you are holding an old and rather squishy apple just above the foot of its tree. Gravity pulls it down, but you hold it up with exactly the same force, so it goes nowhere. Now add in just a tiny bit more of upward force, and cause it to rise slowly. Your arm moves it and, in so doing, performs work on it. As this occurs, the apple's *potential energy* (*PE*), due to its position in the external force field, increases by the same amount.

Energy can be neither created nor destroyed, but in many circumstances it can radically change form. Release the apple, and down it accelerates, acquiring *kinetic energy* (*KE*) of motion. By the fundamental and remarkable law of *conservation of energy* (which is the only reason that the notion of "energy" has any significance), the total energy, *E*, of an *isolated* system (not one being lifted by your hand!) should not change over time. So the apple's final KE as it falls should be exactly the same as its previous maximum PE just before it began dropping. Finally, as it hits the ground, its KE is transformed into the mechanical energy required to splatter it apart all over, the KE of the individual pieces, a small release of heat, and some radiant sound energy – all of which can be quantified. We have learned how to account for it in its various guises and, if we do all the book-keeping correctly, the total amount of it remains exactly the same throughout.

The standard unit of energy is the *joule* (J) but, to an atom, a joule is a galactic amount. That suggests a second, more suitable atomic-scale unit of energy, the *electron volt,* where $1 \, \text{eV} = 1.60 \times 10^{-19}$ J which, along with the kilo-eV ($1 \, \text{keV} = 1000 \, \text{eV}$), appears in any discussion of atomic or molecular events.

Electromagnetic waves

Maxwell's marvelous mathematical theory of electromagnetism revealed, for the first time, how electric and magnetic fields interact and combine to produce waves of EM energy, such as radio waves, microwaves, infrared (heat) radiation, visible light of all colors, ultraviolet, and gamma-rays and X-rays, that can propagate forever through empty space. Figure 2.2a captures in snapshot form the sinusoidal spatial dependence of the electric (*E*) and magnetic (*B*) fields of an EM wave of *frequency, f,* and *wavelength,* λ, propagating at *speed, c,* in the *x*-direction. This, in a nutshell, is how it works: once the wave is under way, a changing electric field creates a changing magnetic field a short distance ahead, which in turn generates a changing magnetic field still further along, which produces a changing electric field beyond that, and so on and on and on. It just keeps on rolling along like tumbleweed.

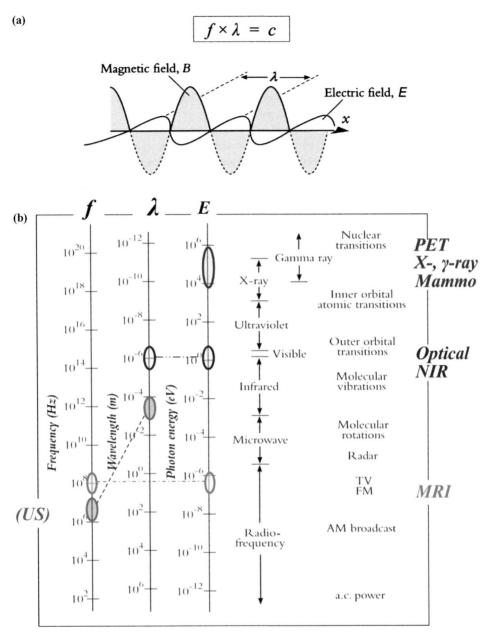

Figure 2.2 Electromagnetic radiation. (a) Snapshot of an EM wave of wavelength λ meters and frequency *f* Hz (cycles per second) traveling in free space in the *x*-direction at the speed of light, *c*. Because *c* is always exactly the same in free space, regardless of how the light is emitted or detected, the frequency, *f*, and wavelength, λ, are inversely related to one another (Equation 2.1a). The electric and magnetic fields, *E* and *B*, point in directions perpendicular to one another, and also to the direction of propagation. (b) The EM spectrum, ranging from high frequency, short-wavelength gamma- and X-rays down through the optical region and to low-frequency, long-wavelength radio waves. Also shown are the energies, *E*, in electron volts of the photons involved in various kinds of imaging, as will soon be explained (Equation 2.1b). Photons of energies from about 19 to 511 keV are employed in X-ray and gamma-ray (nuclear medicine) imaging. Radiofrequency energy is used in MRI. Ultrasound, by contrast, is not a form of EM radiation, but rather a mechanical disturbance propagating through tissue.

As with the notes from a cello, the electromagnetic *spectrum* ranges in frequency and wavelength (Figure 2.2b), but in other respects the radiation is inherently very much alike. How it is produced, the amount of energy it transports, and the mechanisms by which it interacts with matter all do depend on the frequency and wavelength. But the essential physical nature of the radiation itself is common to all forms of it. It all propagates through empty space in straight lines at the speed of light and, in many ways, is described beautifully by Maxwell's formalism.

Like children, waves are constantly moving, but how fast? A child taking $1\frac{1}{2}$ steps per second on average, each with a stride length of $\frac{1}{2}$ m, will shuffle along with a velocity of $(1\frac{1}{2}$ steps/second) $\times$ $(\frac{1}{2}$ meter/step$) = 0.75$ m/s; with shorter steps, the kid can maintain the same speed only by taking more of them each second. The frequency (f), wavelength (λ), and speed of propagation (c) of *any* sort of traveling wave are related in the same simple manner:

$$f \times \lambda = c. \qquad (2.1a)$$

The units of frequency are *cycles per second* (cps) or *hertz* (Hz), and those of wavelength and speed are *meters* and *meters per second*, respectively.

In a vacuum, light travels with a speed of $c = 3.00 \times 10^8$ m/s $= 186000$ miles per second, totally independent of its frequency and wavelength. (Light slows down a little in matter, and its velocity *does* then depend on its frequency, which is how a prism works.) That means that if we double the frequency of the radio waves used in MRI, say, then their wavelength will shorten by a factor of a half. This can lead to an artifact observed when transitioning from a 1.5-tesla machine to 3 T, incidentally, as we shall see. The velocity of ultrasound waves also depends on the material they are going through, but is generally about 1540 m/s in soft tissue, largely independent of frequency.

The crowning achievement in the *classical* (prequantum mechanical) description of EM waves was Einstein's Special Theory of Relativity. This demonstrated, in one of his three great papers of 1905, that electric and magnetic fields are simply two faces of the same entity, the electromagnetic field, but as seen from different perspectives.

Photons

Anything with which we have direct everyday experience behaves either as a particle or as a wave, but nothing acts like both at the same time.

Bee-bees, basketballs, and buses are solid and hard, like particles, and they can really whack into you.

Gentle ocean waves, by contrast, flow unhindered around the piling of a pier and re-radiate circular waves from it. Likewise, waves can pass through one another with no consequences — each emerges from the far side of the event unscathed. In some situations, moreover, waves can combine to demonstrate characteristic *wave interference* patterns. In Figure 2.3a, waves of the same amplitude but slightly different wavelength travel to the right at the same speed. Where two crests overlap, the waves superimpose to form a peak in the combined wave form; conversely, the amplitude of the pattern is low where a pair of peaks of opposite polarity come together. This is even more vivid with the two-dimensional high-school "ripple tank" (Figure 2.3b). Not many similarities, there, with any sort of particle. Once again, particles are particles, waves are waves, and ne'er the twain shall meet. Or so, at least, we thought.

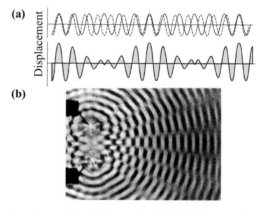

Figure 2.3 Wave interference. **(a)** The superimposing of two one-dimensional waves of slightly different wavelengths, indicating where positive and negative *interference* occur, where their peaks either add or counteract one another. **(b)** Shadows of waves created and interfering when two sticks strike a water surface periodically and in synchrony. What would you see if one lagged a little behind the other? If the frequency of one were a little higher than that of the other?

Several serious difficulties with this view began surfacing at the turn of the twentieth century. It was known experimentally, for example, that light can eject electrons from the surfaces of some metals, a phenomenon called the *photoelectric effect* (which, later, we shall run into often when considering X-ray interactions with matter.) But the classical calculations of those days implied that EM waves should *not* be able to make this happen, any more than an extremely large ocean wave could fling a swimmer out of the water and back onto the pier.

In another of his earth-shaking papers of 1905, Einstein proposed that radio waves, visible light, X-rays, indeed all EM radiation, is comprised of *quanta* (little bundles; from the Latin *quantus*, "how much?") of EM energy, or *photons* (Figure 2.4a). Photons, it became apparent, have the most remarkable property of being able to act in either of two mutually inconsistent, incompatible ways. In some experiments, a photon seems to be a wave of interwoven electric and magnetic fields propagating through space, familiar to us as radio waves and light: diffuse, flowing around things just like ocean waves around a pier, and also undergoing interference, as in Figure 2.3.

In others, a photon acts like a minute, highly concentrated, hard bundle of energy, compactly localized in space. Such particle-like photons, unlike Maxwell's spread-out waves, carry momentum, so that if an atom releases one heading east, the atom will recoil in the westerly direction. The photon, in turn, should be able to collide with an electron on another atom, dislodging and ejecting it from the atom. That would explain the photoelectric effect (Figure 2.4b).

Now wait a second! This really doesn't make any sense at all. Does the energy of ultraviolet radiation, say, or of an X-ray beam exist as particles, in tightly-packed quanta, or is it transported in waves, essentially like those on a lake surface? After all, nothing one can think of in life (try it!) is both particle-like and wave-like simultaneously. Surely EM radiation is one or the other, and there is no middle ground, right?

Well, no. In actuality, electromagnetic energy remarkably seems to exist in both forms, even both

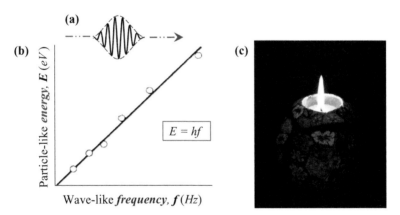

Figure 2.4 The wave-particle duality. (**a**) A rather fanciful rendering/interpretation of a photon of electromagnetic energy. Physicists still do not agree fully on what photons really are, or what it is, exactly, that's doing the waving (it's not just the electric and magnetic fields), but their existence has been re-verified unequivocally in countless experiments. (**b**) Following the lead of the photoelectric effect, Einstein proposed that the energy, *E*, of a *photon* (a *particle*-like concept) is directly proportional to the frequency, *f*, of its *wave*-like doppelganger; and amazingly, the constant of proportionality happened to be exactly the same as the one Planck had found in explaining a quite different, but also atomic-scale, problem – the shape of the energy spectrum of black body radiation. Like the speed of light, Planck's constant, *h*, is one of the fundamental, measured constants of nature; it cannot be derived from anything more basic. (**c**) The unit of energy used in analysis of phenomena at the atomic level is the electron volt (eV). Most biochemical and other chemical reactions require the exchange of a few eV, and the energies of visible light photons are from $1\frac{1}{2}$ to $3\frac{1}{2}$ eV, hence the glow of burning wax. Photons in the 60 to 140 keV range (1 keV = 1000 eV) are absorbed and scattered in normal X-ray and CT imaging, and the *proton* spin-orientation transitions of MRI involve micro-eV photons.

at the same time, depending on what you look for. If you try to measure the wavelength of a photon wave, or find interference patterns, you can. But if you then want to obtain evidence for the same radiation of individual, minute quanta interacting with an atomic electron in a radiation detector, you can do that, too. This totally schizophrenic behavior, known as the *wave-particle duality*, has been mystifying scientists for a hundred years, as has the very nature of the photon.

If all this inconsistency and confusion does not seem totally clear, don't feel alone. After all, nothing in our everyday life behaves as both wave and particle at the same time – what could be the wavelength of a bus? (It has one, but it's much shorter than the diameter of a nucleus!) And what is hard and compact about a ripple on a lake? The only reason for putting any faith in this notion whatsoever or, indeed, for building the glorious cathedral of quantum mechanics upon it, is the absolute and overwhelming support for it from thousands upon thousands of experiments performed over the past century: Nothing has *ever* been found that refutes it. The *wave-particle duality* of photons (and of electrons too) is one of the fundamental tenets, yet most profound unknowns, underlying modern science. Nobody has really understood it, admitted even by Einstein himself.

Nonetheless, guided by the photoelectric studies, Einstein proposed an important linkage between the particle-like and wave-like pictures and properties of photons (Figure 2.4a): the particle-like energy of a photon, E, its clout, if you wish, is always directly proportional to its wave-like frequency, f, that is,

$$E = h \times f. \qquad (2.1b)$$

And the constant of proportionality extracted from the photoelectric data, $h = 4.14 \times 10^{-15}$ eV-s, happens to be the same as the one found earlier by Max Planck in another, very different context having to do with the radiation from very hot objects. It was for proposing the existence of photons, and thereby explaining the photoelectric effect (and not for special relativity) that Einstein was awarded the Nobel Prize in 1921.

Equations 2.1a and 2.1b together provide all the information about electromagnetic waves and/or photons we will need. In particular, they allow us to jump freely among discussions of photon frequency, wavelength, and energy (Figure 2.2b). But while Equation 2.1a is valid for *any* form of wave motion (including ultrasound), Equation 2.1b applies *only* to photons, electrons, *et al.*

A candle flame marks the center of the range of energies that underlie all modern technology and, in particular, the imaging modalities (Figure 2.4c). The visible light it emits consists of photons of about 1.6 eV (red) to 3.4 eV (violet). That suggests, moreover, that the chemical reactions that are producing the light involve the exchange of comparable amounts of energy. The photons of X-ray imaging lie typically between 60 and 140 keV, by contrast, and those of radiation therapy go as high as 25 million eV (1 MeV = 10^6 eV). At the other extreme, the quantum transitions underlying MRI require only 10^{-6} eV. So altogether, the highest energies encountered in medicine are 10^{12} times greater than the least. But in between, the sights and chemistry of everyday life involve energies of only a few eV.

Atoms

By the time Einstein was developing his seismic ideas about photons, many of the rules of chemistry were well established, but there was no explanation of them. Likewise, it was found that when gases are heated white hot, they produced spectra consisting of patterns of discrete lines (Figure 2.5a), rather than a continuum as predicted by the Maxwell theory. This was all quite confusing and distressing, and some felt that only a major conceptual upheaval could bring order to the chaos.

In 1913 the young Danish physicist Niels Bohr was blessed with an essential flash of insight, and took the first serious leap toward a valid theory of the atom. Until recently it had been widely viewed as a positively-charged pudding, embedded with raison-like electrons. Bohr, instead, chose to develop the novel idea that it behaves somewhat like a miniature solar system. Just as relatively light planets orbit an enormous sun and are bound to it by the gravitational force, so also light, negatively charged electrons in an atom orbit a massive, positively charged nucleus, and are held to it by the electric force. As we now understand, an atomic nucleus contains the number Z of positively charged *protons*, called its *atomic number*, which determines

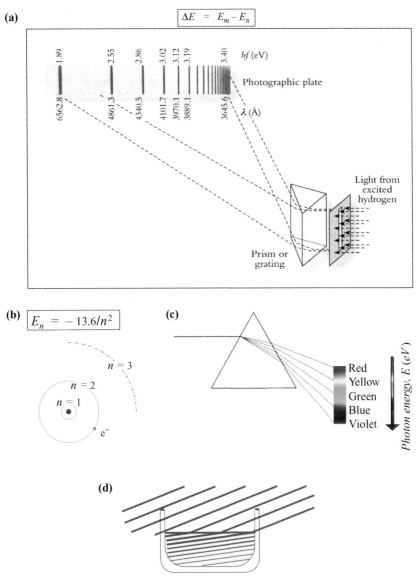

Figure 2.5 Atoms and atomic emission spectra. (**a**) The spectrum of hydrogen gas heated to high temperature is obtained by spreading out the colors of the light it emits with a prism or a grating. The one shown here is a real hydrogen spectrum, recorded on film, displaying a sequence of discrete emission. It was obvious that this pattern of lines was trying to tell us its story, but no one could make sense of it. (**b**) In 1913, physics took a giant quantum leap forward when Niels Bohr, perhaps the greatest Dane since Hamlet, proposed the first theory of the single-electron atom that gave results that agreed quantitatively with much of the previously inexplicable experimental data. While a hydrogen atom is most comfortable with its electron circling in the lowest-lying, $n = 1$ *ground* state, with energy E_1, here the electron has somehow been excited up into the $n = 2$ state, now with E_2; it will very soon drop back down into an $n = 1$ orbital, with emission of a photon of energy $(E_2 - E_1)$. (**c**) How a prism works: refraction. The velocity of an electromagnetic or ultrasound wave changes as it passes from one medium into another, and that alters the direction of propagation of the wave. A prism splits white light into its constituent colors because the decrease of velocity upon entering glass depends on the energy and wavelength of the light photons. (**d**) The path of a ray of monochromatic light deflects when passing from one medium into another with a different wave speed for purely geometric reasons. Waves of different wavelengths and photon energies, hence of different velocities in glass, refract by different amounts.

the atom's element type. An orbiting electron has the same charge as a proton but of opposite sign, and a *neutral* atom has exactly the same number of electrons as there are protons, so the entire atom has no net charge. If an atom or molecule somehow loses or gains one or several orbital electrons, it now carries a net charge, and is called an *ion*.

All nuclei of all elements (except for the lightest form of ordinary hydrogen) also contain *neutrons*, which are about as heavy as protons but uncharged. Virtually all chemical, electronic, and biological properties of an atom are determined totally by its *atomic* number alone, its element type, and the arrangement of its orbiting electrons. But the possible instabilities of a particular nucleus (i.e., radioactivity, the basis for nuclear medicine) and its magnetic properties (i.e., hence its suitability for MRI) depend on the number of *neutrons* in the nucleus, as well. More about that later.

Bohr considered the simplest of all atomic systems, the neutral hydrogen atom, and imagined that its single electron moved about its nucleus, a sole proton, in a circular orbit. Bohr started out by following the mathematical derivation that Newton developed in the seventeenth century to explain planetary motion, but he then made one enormous additional assumption regarding the electron's angular momentum. (Linear momentum is the measure of the tendency of an object to remain in a state of straight-line, constant-speed motion; angular momentum is concerned, rather, with circular or rotational motion, like that of a top or the wheel of a tumbled child's tricycle.) Bohr noted that the units of Planck's constant happen to be the same as those of angular momentum, and he made a wonderfully inspired guess: he imposed a very non-traditional constraint on the calculation, requiring that the angular momentum of the orbiting electron assume values only that are integer multiples of Planck's constant divided by 2π. That is, he insisted that the angular momentum must be of the form $nh/2\pi$, where n, the *principal quantum number*, may assume only the integer values $n = 1$, 2, 3, ...

This radical assumption of quantized angular momentum yielded a remarkable result: totally unlike the case of Earth satellites, both the radii and the *energy levels* available to the orbital elec-

tron of an atom are highly restricted, and precisely *quantized* (Figure 2.5b). That is, the electron can circle only in certain specified orbits, within *shells* at precisely specified distances from the nucleus. Also, it can have only certain discrete energies, parameterized by the principal quantum number as $E_n = -13.6/n^2$ eV. The minus sign is there because the energy of the system, by *convention*, is defined to be zero when its electron is just barely unbound from the nucleus, and moving freely but slowly near it; so the system's energy must be less than that for an orbital electron still *bound* to its nucleus.

When NASA decides to lengthen the lifetime of the Hubble space telescope, it uses a rocket to provide enough energy, ΔE, to push it into a slightly more distant, marginally higher-energy orbit. ("Δ" is commonly defined to mean "a small difference" or "a small change" in whatever follows it – in this case, energy.) And in doing so, it could add *any* increment in energy it chose. An atom is much more selective, however, and the input of energy needed to raise the electron out of the nth bound level and into a higher-energy n'th orbital must be exactly

$$\Delta E = (E_{n'} - E_n), \qquad (2.2)$$

where $E_{n'}$ and E_n can have only the discrete values allowed by the Bohr model. This is also the energy given off, usually in the form of a photon, when an atom drops from a higher-lying to a lower energy state. For transitions among outer-orbital states, as occur commonly during chemical transitions (Figure 2.4c), the emission is typically in the visible range, of a few eV. For higher-atomic-number atoms, in which inner electrons can be very tightly bound, a jump down to a deeper orbital may involve tens of keV, and the resulting high-energy photon is termed a *characteristic X-ray*.

For decades researchers had been tabulating the discrete frequencies of emissions from various excited atoms and, finally, Bohr's model (Figure 2.5b), together with Einstein's expression $E = hf$ (Equation 2.1b), agreed beautifully with the measured data for hydrogen (Figure 2.5a). Each emission line corresponded to the dropping from some n'th state down into the nth level, with the release of a photon of exact energy $(E_{n'} - E_n)$. A transition from an $n' = 2$ orbital down to $n = 1$, for example, would produce a photon of energy $-13.6[1/2^2 - 1/1^2] = 10.2$ eV.

Photons can interact in other ways, incidentally, that do not involve exciting electrons into higher-lying orbits or, in more extreme cases, ionizing the atom. The processes are a little more subtle, and we don't need to go into them, but consider the separation of white light into its constituent colors (Figure 2.5c). A prism, or glass of water, will deflect a monochromatic (single color) geometric ray from its path, regardless of the color. The electric field of a passing electromagnetic wave briefly overlaps that of an atomic electron, which slows down the wave's photons a little. The resulting *refraction* of the ray of (red, in this case) light then occurs for a purely geometric reason (Figure 2.5d): in passing from air into the water, the frequency of the radiation has no reason to change. But as its velocity goes down, the wavelength must decrease as well, by $\lambda = c/f$. As the diagram indicates, however, the wave fronts can remain connected above and below the surface only with an abrupt deflection in the direction of propagation. The same sort of bending phenomenon arises when ultrasound passes at an angle from one tissue into another, with a different velocity of sound, except that the waves are mechanical in nature rather than electromagnetic.

This nicely explains the bending of the light beam, but what about the separation of white light into many colors? Easy! The strength of the photon-electron interaction depends on the photon energy. And in the optical range, the magnitude of that effect happens to increase with photon energy, resulting in a greater reduction in speed. Higher-frequency, and therefore higher-energy ($E = hf$), blue light is slowed down more than red, and therefore ends up deflecting through a greater angle.

Molecules and fluorescent materials

Apart from noble gases, atoms rarely exist alone. They almost always combine, bound largely by electrical forces, to form molecules that can range in size from diatomic hydrogen gas to DNA. Beyond that, vast numbers of atoms or ions come together to create solids, such as the semiconductors and fluorescent materials used to detect and image ionizing radiation.

Atmospheric nitrogen, for example, exists almost entirely in the form of tight, covalently bonded pairs of nitrogen atoms (Figure 2.6a). The two nitrogens stick together because each positively charged nucleus exerts an electric pull on every one of the sixteen electrons of the pair, especially the outer ones that they fully share in common. It's rather like when you and your neighbor's playful pit-bull are pulling from opposite ends of the same arm: you stay together.

For reasons explainable with quantum mechanics, when a few atoms come close together and form molecules, each of the outer *atomic* electron orbitals separates into several *molecular* orbitals (Figure 2.6b). This process goes to extremes when large numbers of atoms conjoin: the molecular orbitals become so numerous and closely spaced that they form, in effect, *electronic energy bands* (Figure 2.6c). The closeness of the *conduction band* to the *valence band* just below it determines the electronic properties of the material: metal (conductor), insulator or, in between, semiconductor.

The band structure is also of great importance in the operation of many kinds of radiation detector and image receptor materials: just as a photon can excite an atomic electron up into a higher-lying level, so also an X- or gamma-ray can excite thousands of electrons from the valence band up into the conduction. If the material happens to be one for which the two bands are separated by a few eV, then readily detectable visible light photons are emitted afterwards, as the electrons relax back down to their more comfortable existence in the lower-lying valence band. This process of X-ray-induced *fluorescence* is what caught Roentgen's attention back in 1895, and it has been central to medical imaging ever since.

The image quality quartet: contrast, resolution, stochastic (random) noise, artifacts – and always dose

Selecting the right technology that employs the most appropriate probe is only the first step in medical imaging. Assuming that a physician chooses the best available diagnostic test, which is likely, the resulting pictures will be of little clinical use unless they are of good enough image quality. While there are other important factors as well, there are four gold standards, mentioned previously, by which images (and the imaging systems that produce them) are most commonly judged: the *contrast*; the *resolution* (also called *sharpness*, or *lack of*

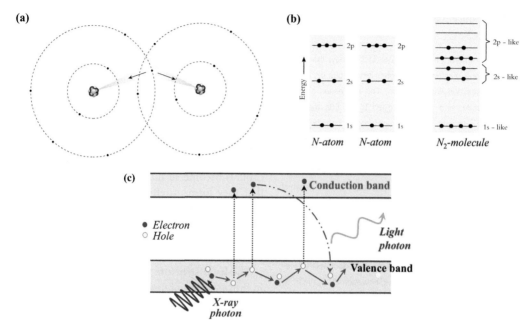

Figure 2.6 Molecular orbitals. **(a)** The two atoms of a N_2 molecule are held together because each nucleus pulls on all 14 electrons, especially the ten in the $n = 2$ shell of each. **(b)** Splitting of atomic energy levels and orbitals when atoms are brought together as molecules. *s, p, d, f, . . .* label atomic and molecular *sub*-shells. **(c)** When large numbers of atoms, molecules or ions are brought close together and coalesce as a solid, their states have to adjust a little. The ultimate result is that the several discrete energy levels spread out into an essentially continuous *band* of energy levels. It is the relationships among the bands that determines whether a solid behaves as a metal, an insulator, or a semiconductor. In this extremely simple case of an idealized insulator, an incident X-ray photon can impart enough energy to the material to elevate thousands of electrons from the filled *valence band* (in which all the near-continuum of super-close states contain electrons), up a few eV into the empty *conduction band*, leaving behind electron vacancies, or *holes*. Electrons residing briefly in the conduction band rapidly drop back down to the valence band, filling the available holes, and giving off visible light in the process.

blur); the absence of visual *random noise*; and *artifacts*, which are deterministic, non-stochastic noise analogous to 60-cycle hum. We would generally like to optimize these, while always keeping radiation dose sufficiently low (Figure 2.7).

Subject contrast

Contrast refers to the degree to which physical differences among materials within a body are revealed in the image.

That is, contrast is an indication of the extent to which an organ, particular tissue, or other object stands out from the background of other, nearby, and perhaps overlapping structures. When contrast is good, clinically significant differences among the tissues show up as visually notable variations in shades of gray or color in the display. But different kinds of contrast are produced by the various modalities, and the most useful, revealing kind can depend strongly on the particular clinical situation. It's rather like apples (Figure 2.8). A bad one may stand out from the rest in the barrel because of its appearance. Or its feel, its taste, its smell, or even its sound when you bite into it. These characteristics are very dissimilar from one another, yet each of them can provide a kind of *contrast* to distinguish the rotten one.

Likewise, there are a number of radically dissimilar tissue attributes and physical processes that can give rise to inherently different kinds of visual contrast, hence distinct forms of diagnostic

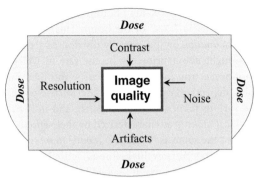

Figure 2.7 The quartet of characteristics of a medical image (or of the device that produces it) that largely determine how effective it will be in supporting diagnosis. The *contrast* refers to the degree to which a tissue or other entity of concern within the *body* is distinguishabe, in the *image*, from background or from other tissues; *resolution* or *sharpness* is the measure of fine detail that the image or system can display; and *stochastic* (random) *noise* and *artifacts* (non-random noise) can diminish both the contrast and the resolution. All the time, the level of radiation *dose* can affect one or more of these, and it is a major objective of imaging with ionizing radiation (gamma- and X-rays) to keep the exposure of the patient, staff, and the public *below regulatory limits* and also ALARA, *as low as reasonably achievable* (a separate but also critical issue), while still ensuring clinically adequate results.

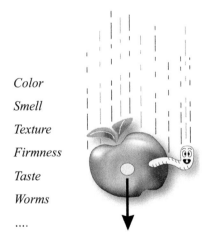

Color

Smell

Texture

Firmness

Taste

Worms

....

Figure 2.8 There are a number of differences between a good apple and a bad one, and the associated forms of contrast (color, smell, etc.) can help you tell them apart.

information. The various modalities produce contrast in different ways, and an important aspect of research, and of clinical training, is in determining which are most effective in investigating specific diseases, and then to discover ways to enhance the contrast itself and to reduce the noise.

The objective of an imaging study is commonly to detect lesions or other irregularities, finding them within the overlapping jumble of patterns originating from the diverse normal tissues. Obtaining adequate contrast is normally the issue of primary concern, and the major developments in medical imaging over the past century have largely come from research efforts to improve contrast of X-ray-based and other technologies. The various imaging modalities create contrast in remarkably diverse ways (Box 2.1).

Box 2.1   Sources of medical contrast for the major modalities

X-ray: radiography, CR, DR, fluoroscopy, DSA, CT

Differential attenuation of high-energy photons by tissues of different thickness, density, chemical makeup, as affected by hf (mechanisms: photoelectric absorption, Compton scatter)

Nuclear medicine, SPECT, PET

Differential uptake of radioactive pharmaceuticals that target specific tissues/biological compartments, followed by differential emission of detectable high-energy photons

Ultrasound, Doppler

Differential reflection of high-frequency mechanical vibrations at different sorts of boundaries between tissues (of different elasticity and/or density)

MRI, MRA, MRS, DTI, *f*MRI

Differences among tissues in environmentally-restricted rotations and other motions of water molecules, hence in proton spin-relaxation times

In X-ray imaging, different materials attenuate high-energy photons by different amounts, casting shadowgrams in a beam transiting the body. But even when there may be little contrast apparent among the soft tissues with X-rays, as is commonly the case, the same organs might show up with dazzling clarity with a nuclear medicine, ultrasound, or MRI scan, and vice versa.

Nuclear medicine monitors the tendencies of a specific organ or other biological compartment to take up a tissue-specific radiopharmaceutical. The emissions of gamma-rays (or, for PET, so-called annihilation photons) by this radioactive tracer can be detected from outside the patient, indicating where it is concentrating (or failing to).

With ultrasound, high-frequency vibrational waves reflect off boundaries between tissues with dissimilar elasticities or densities. Contrast comes from differences among those boundaries for different types of organ interfaces – a far cry from photon attenuation.

And magnetic resonance imaging is highly sensitive, in various ways, to the behavior of the hydrogen nuclei of water molecules, as determined by the local biophysical and biochemical environment. It displays spatial variations in, for example, the rates of rotations and other motions of water molecules loosely bound to macromolecules and cell organelles, and in the flow of water through vessels, and even its diffusion along axon channels.

These diverse phenomena give rise to forms of visual contrast that shed light on totally different aspects of anatomy and physiology.

Two largely independent factors, *subject contrast* and *image receptor contrast*, are responsible for the overall *image contrast* obtained with any modality: subject contrast is brought about by differences in the amounts of interactions of the probes with the various dissimilar tissues of the body. The instrument that then captures the image may degrade or enhance that subject contrast, depending on its image receptor contrast capabilities. Together, the body and the IR generate the final image contrast that the physician sees. This chapter and the next will address subject contrast with X-rays, and Chapter 4 will deal with the rest.

With X-ray imaging, the subject contrast among the tissues comes from differences in the amount that they attenuate X-ray photons along the various geometric "rays" of the beam. This *differential attenuation* by the spatially distributed tissues is brought about primarily by the rate at which photon-electron interactions occur – and that, in turn, depends on *differences* in the *thicknesses* of the various tissues, in their *densities*, and in their *chemical makeup* as characterized by their *effective* (almost the same as "average") *atomic numbers*, Z (Figure 2.9a). You saw this before as Figure 1.6a, but it's so fundamental that it seemed like a good idea to repeat it here. The contrast between bone and the soft tissues of the internal organs is almost always very strong in a radiograph, because bone is so much denser and, even more important, comprised of atoms with higher effective Z. These two factors are characteristic of the *tissues*. There is another important influence on contrast that is a function of the *beam*, rather than of the tissues, namely its effective photon energy, hf; it, too, influences the rate at which contrast-producing photon-electron interactions tend to occur.

X-ray subject contrast can be influenced by modifying the three *technique factors* of the exposure. These parameters – the potential applied between cathode and anode of the X-ray tube (the peak kilo-Voltage, or kVp), the tube current of electrons flowing from cathode to anode (mA), and the duration (*seconds*) – are adjusted by the machine operators in attempts to achieve good enough image quality coupled with low dose. The number of X-ray photons created is directly proportional to the mA-s, the *product* of *tube current* and *exposure duration*, and that significantly influences how noisy an image appears, especially noticeable in CT. The kVp setting determines the effective energy, hf, of the X-ray beam, which has a profound effect on the obtainable contrast: lower kVp yields better contrast in general (Figures 2.9b and 1.6) – but the price to be paid for that is greater patient dose.

Subject contrast of a tissue can sometimes be enhanced artificially by altering its physical properties with a contrast agent. Because iodine and barium atoms are heavier (higher Z) and can be incorporated into compounds in dense fluids, they happen to absorb X-rays particularly strongly. Blood vessels containing intravenously injected iodine compounds tend to stand out clearly from the surrounding soft tissues (Figure 2.9b–d).

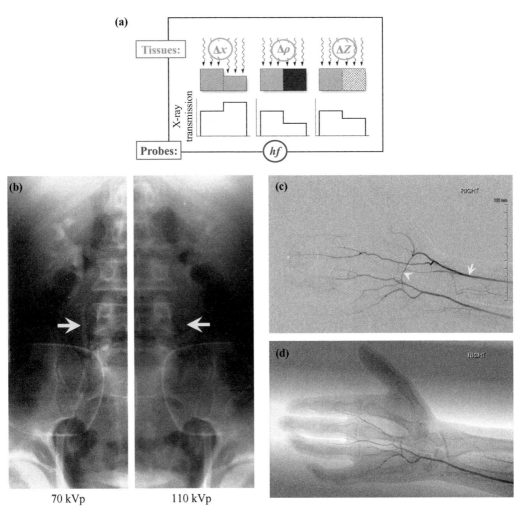

70 kVp   110 kVp

Figure 2.9 Contrast is a measure of the extent to which tissues that are anatomically or physiologically different in the body appear distinguishable in an image. (**a**) In the several forms of imaging with X-rays (radiography, fluoroscopy, digital radiography, digital tomography, CT, etc.), the three primary determinants of contrast among tissues are differences (Δ) in their *thicknesses*, Δ*x*, in their *densities*, Δ*ρ*, such as between lung, muscle, and bone, and in their *chemical makeup*, as parameterized by their effective atomic numbers, Δ**Z**. Another important, and adjustable, influence on image quality in radiography is the effective energy of the photon beam, *hf*; this is determined primarily by the selection of the *peak kiloVolt* (*kVp*), the high electrical potential applied across the X-ray tube. (**b**) Two excretory urograms, or intravenous pyelogram (IVP), were obtained with iodinated contrast medium at 70 kVp, to the left, and 110 kVp. (Most X-ray images, apart from mammograms, are produced in the 60–120 kVp range.) The lower-kVp image shows more clearly the ureters (arrows), which contain urine and iodine-based contrast agent that was administered intravenously and is excreted by the kidneys, and also the renal parenchyma and contrast medium within the renal pelvis and calyces, and the bony structures. Lowering the kiloVoltage commonly leads to better contrast – but the beam is less penetrating, and the amount of radiation dose delivered to the patient is greater. This is one of the many tradeoffs to be considered in imaging. Modified from American College of Radiology (ACR) Teaching File images. (**c**) With the administration of only 7 mL of iodinated contrast medium into the distal brachial artery, the angiographer is able to opacify blood vessels with diameters under 1 mm. A modern digital subtraction angiography (DSA) system easily displays the contours of these opacified arteries (arrowheads) down to the tips of the fingers. Contrast is enhanced greatly with DSA by digitally removing static background structures such as the overlying bone and, at the same time, less contrast agent can be used. (**d**) It is often visually helpful to re-introduce some background anatomy.

(a)

Resolution

(b)

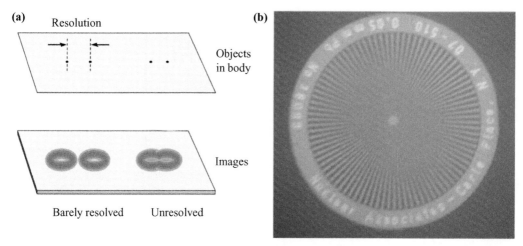

Objects in body

Images

Barely resolved   Unresolved

Figure 2.10 Resolution and sharpness. **(a)** Two small high-contrast objects within the patient's body are lying in a plane parallel to that of the image receptor. When the two are so close together that their images can barely be differentiated, their separation defines the *resolution* of the system in millimeters. **(b)** The smallest distance apart of lines that can be distinguished in this star pattern quality assurance test device describes an X-ray system's resolving power in a related kind of unit: line pairs per millimeter (lp/mm).

Likewise, barium has application for the esophagus, stomach, and intestine (Figure 1.7).

Resolution

As a general rule, medical imaging is concerned primarily with providing adequate contrast, one way or another, to distinguish the object of interest from surrounding tissues. Some kinds of investigations, however, like the search for microcalcifications in the breast, or for slight cracks in small bones, or in the examination of fine, iodine-containing blood vessels, also require high *resolution* (*sharpness*) – the ability to reveal very close objects as being separate and abrupt edges as being sharp, and to display detail on the order of a tenth of a millimeter or so (Figure 2.10a).

X-ray films tend to provide extremely good resolution. With traditional X-ray and fluoroscopic systems, it is quantified in terms of the maximum number of alternating thin strips of X-ray attenuating (such as lead foil) and transmitting (plastic) materials per unit distance that can be made out visually without blending together (Figure 2.10b), and commonly expressed as dark-light line-pairs per millimeter (lp/mm). For digital systems, resolving capability is usually presented in terms of pixel

size (in micrometers, μm), which is closely related: the smaller the size of the pixels in the image receptor, and in a digital display monitor, the greater the lp/mm one should be able to distinguish.

As we shall see, there are several sources of blur that impose limits on the resolution achievable with any modality. Patient (or equipment!) *movement blur* is an important one, for example, and the reason for the inevitable "Take a deep breath and hold it!" (Figure 2.11).

Each modality also has its own operational imperfections that contribute at least a little to blur – in the case of radiography, for example, *penumbra blur* arises from the finite size of the focal spot, the part of the X-ray tube from which the X-rays originate. By analogy, a shadow cast by a tiny bulb, nearly a point-source of light, will be much sharper than one from a flood lamp (Figure 2.12a). Many tubes come with the option of a smaller (but lower intensity) focal spot, which can lead to a significant improvement if fine detail is needed (Figure 2.12b).

A third kind of unsharpness is *image receptor blur*. With screen-film and some kinds of digital radiography, for example, the fluorescent light photons created when an X-ray strikes a fluorescent screen spread out before reaching film (Figure 2.13); that

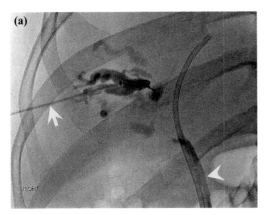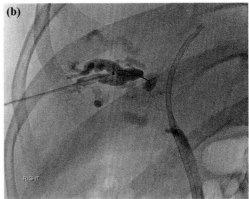

Figure 2.11 Motion artifacts can easily blur the contours of the structures that need to be evaluated. Ways to try to avoid this are through positioning (recumbent giving more stability than standing), breath-holding or restraining (with a support structure), and use of a short exposure time. (a) In the AP image of a percutaneous transhepatic cholangiogram (PTC), iodinated contrast medium has been injected directly into the biliary tract through a small needle inserted intercostally (arrow). Although the contrast agent is seen to extend from the biliary ducts of the right lobe into the common bile duct (arrowhead), the edges are fuzzy due to respiratory motion. (b) Decreased motion with simple breath-hold maneuvers greatly improves the resolution of the bile ducts.

happens less in thinner screens, but the price for better resolution is lower screen efficiency, hence the need for more radiation output from the tube and higher patient dose.

With some kinds of imaging, such as nuclear medicine, the power of resolution is inherently not great; but while PET may get low marks in visualizing anatomic detail, it can often provide other (sometimes much more important) sorts of information, such as on the physiological condition of a compromised organ.

Stochastic (random, statistical) noise and the signal-to-noise ratio

As anyone knows who has ever had a teenager, or been one, noise and messiness come in a remarkable range of forms. In all of its guises, however, noise always has the same practical effect: it obscures messages of importance by interjecting extraneous non-signals that carry no information, or information that is distracting but irrelevant, or (worst of all) information that seems valid but is wrong. Visual noise, in particular, refers to anything that interferes, to some extent, with access to the information content of an image.

Information obtained from an imaging device consists of both useful signal and various kinds of noise energy, all blended together. In an ideal world, signals would be pure and contain only meaningful data, with no junk in there mucking things up. In reality, the issue is to extract as much useful signal as possible out of a background of noise – the amplitude of which may, at times, be considerably greater than that of the signal itself.

Noise is caused in a number of ways and comes in diverse forms, but commonly it is of two general types: *stochastic noise* (also called *random, statistical*, and in some cases *Poisson noise*), which differs from image to image, and *artifacts*, or *deterministic noise*, in which a nearly identical noise pattern may recur among separate images for the modality. Too much of either may render an image diagnostically useless.

A common and sometimes troublesome form of stochastic noise in radiography comes as *Compton scatter radiation*, discussed in the next chapter. When an X-ray photon enters the patient's body and undergoes a Compton interaction with an atomic electron, only part of the photon's energy is transferred to the electron; most of it leaves the scene of the collision as a new, lower-energy *scatter photon*, one that perhaps eventually strikes the image receptor. Such scatter creates a haze (Figure 2.14a), similar to that from silt stirred up near the bottom

(a)

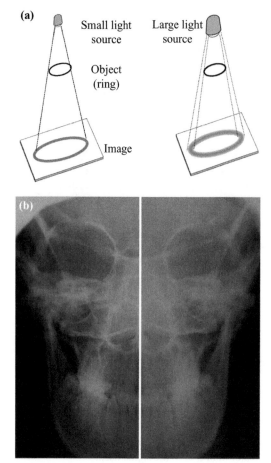

Small light source

Large light source

Object (ring)

Image

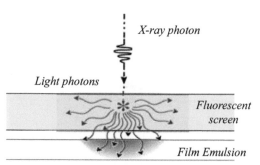

X-ray photon

Light photons

Fluorescent screen

Film Emulsion

Figure 2.13 Another source of blur in radiography is the image receptor itself, such as from the finite thickness of the screen. Scintillation light induced by an X-ray photon bounces around, often at the surfaces of the phosphor grains, and diffuses away from the point of the original X-ray interaction. A thicker screen is more effective at generating light, so less patient dose is involved in creating an image. But there is more room for light to diffuse, and the resolution is lower.

Figure 2.12 Penumbra blur from the finite size of an X-ray tube's focal spot. **(a)** A small light bulb will cast a sharper shadow of a small object than will a large one. **(b)** In exactly the same way, the size of an X-ray tube's focal spot can have a profound effect on the resolution achievable. The image to the left was created with a smaller focal spot size than the other, and consequently displays less penumbra blur. With *any* imaging modality, patient motion and blur inherent to the image receptor also contribute to unsharpness. Modified from American College of Radiology (ACR) Teaching File images.

There is another form of evident random noise that can arise for the converse reason – because insufficient numbers of the "right" kind of information-bearing "quanta" are involved in the creation of an image (Figure 2.14b). That is, if you are going to build an image out of minute dots (or, with digital display, out of tiny pixels of different degrees of brightness or color), as with virtually all forms of medical images, you have to have enough of them for the image to look smooth and not too spotty, or mottled.

Image *contrast, resolution,* and *stochastic noise* have been introduced and discussed separately here, in a scientifically proper, reductionist fashion. Things are not so simple in the clinic, however, as evident in images of the *contrast-detail phantom* of Figure 2.15. For radiography, this is a plate of plastic or metal with holes of various depths and diameters milled into it; the objective is to determine the combinations of contrast (as controlled primarily by hole depth) and resolution (diameter) for which the holes are just barely visible in the image. Here, the test is repeated with two levels of noise, but with the exposure conditions adjusted so that they have the same overall level of darkening. The take-home message from this is that the contrast and resolving capabilities of a system influence one another, and noise can greatly diminish both. It

of a lake that obscures the sharp rocks and snapping turtles you'd prefer to keep a watch-out for. Fortunately, much of it can be removed by way of an *anti-scatter grid*, described below.

With scatter noise, the problem is that there are too many of the "wrong" kind of photons, those that end up darkening the film where they shouldn't.

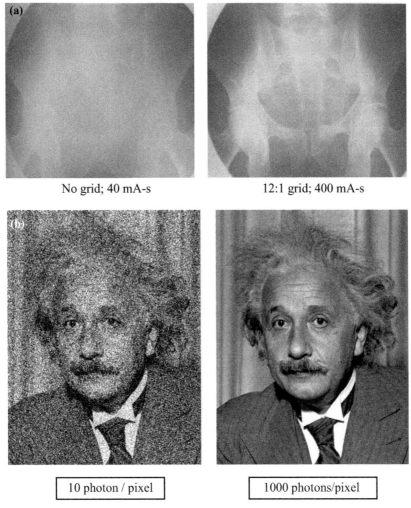

No grid; 40 mA-s   12:1 grid; 400 mA-s

10 photon / pixel   1000 photons/pixel

Figure 2.14 Noise arises from too many bad quanta, or not enough good ones. **(a)** Compton scatter photons produced within the body can land randomly on the image receptor, creating a sort of haze or mist that can substantially reduce image contrast. An anti-scatter grid can eliminate much of the problem, but at the price of much higher patient dose. Modified from American College of Radiology (ACR) Teaching File images. **(b)** Photos created out of 10 and 1000 visible light photons per pixel, respectively, but adjusted so as to display the same average brightness. One finds the same kind of improvement with more information-bearing quanta in fluoroscopy, CT, and nuclear medicine, but more photons and less noise usually translates also into more patient dose. Courtesy of Gordon Cook.

reinforces the important, and not completely obvious, notion that the ability to detect an entity in the body (or a hole in this test phantom) does not necessarily depend on contrast alone, or any of the other factors of image quality, but rather on a complex amalgam of all of them together.

It is of great importance to the creation and improvement of imaging devices that we can quantify noise. Suppose that S is some gauge of the amount of clean, untainted information in a visual Signal; and N signifies the amount of Noise intermixed with it, obfuscating it. Then the signal-to-noise ratio, SNR or S/N, is a simple but valuable indicator of the "quality" and usefulness of the information content of the mixture (Figure 2.16). Many types of studies involve so-called *Poisson*

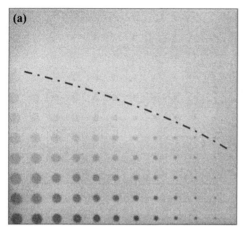
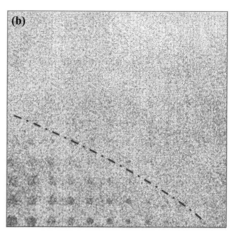

Figure 2.15 The interdependence of contrast, resolution, and random noise is apparent from these film images of a uniformly exposed *contrast-detail phantom*. Such a test device consists of a plate of plastic or metal with holes of different depth and diameter milled (with a flat-ended drill) in it. **(a)** Thousands of X-rays cause the exposure of each small area, or pixel, of the image receptor. In film, say, any particular photon contributes only slightly to the overall darkening, and its individual effect is indiscernible. For the worse appearance of **(b)**, there are two possible explanations: an external source may be creating blotchy noise that is obscuring the real signal. Alternatively, many fewer X-rays are used to expose the film but, to maintain the same overall average level of film brightness, each one of them is made to create a much more visible dab of darkening, resulting in *quantum mottle*. Which do you think is the case here? Modified from American College of Radiology (ACR) Teaching File images.

random processes, for which the signal-to-noise ratio happens to improve proportionately with the *square root* of the signal strength:

$$\text{SNR} = \sqrt{S}. \qquad (2.3)$$

The better image in Figure 2.14b is made up of a hundred times as many microscopic clusters of black silver grains, for example, and its SNR is $\sqrt{100} = 10$ times greater. $\text{SNR} = \sqrt{S}$ also commonly applies to the multiple, small (pixel-size) X-ray detectors of digital radiography, and to those of a CT machine, and in a number of other con-

texts. We shall return in Chapter 4 to Poisson noise to explore how it comes about in so many contexts, the extent to which it reduces the visual detectability of irregularities of interest in the body, and what can be done about it.

The realization that often $\text{SNR} = \sqrt{S}$ underlies a number of approaches to reducing noise in images, and we shall run into it again and again, in one form or another, for all the modalities. MRI images, for example, are usually taken twice, in pairs, with exactly the same imaging parameter settings, and then averaged pixel-by-pixel. There are therefore twice as many information-bearing quanta that add

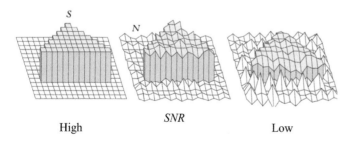

Figure 2.16 Random noise can diminish both contrast and resolution. A useful measure of image quality is the *signal-to-noise ratio* (*S/N* or *SNR*), expressed as the ratio of the average amplitudes of the two. When the SNR is too low, the noise, *N*, may obscure the signal, *S*, of importance.

together coherently, reinforcing the signal; the randomly distributed noise quanta, on the other hand, do not – they somewhat cancel one another out, by chance, as often as they might happen to add. The SNR of the pair of images averaged together is thus a factor of $\sqrt{2}$ higher than for one alone, and the improvement in appearance can be immediately noticeable.

There is another factor to be considered, however, for gamma- or X-ray imaging. $SNR = \sqrt{S}$ indicates that a way to cut the noisy appearance of a CT or fluoroscopic image in half, say, might be to increase the output of the X-ray tube four-fold, producing four times as many X-ray photons. Likewise, to double the SNR of a SPECT image without decreasing patient throughput, you can quadruple the amount of technetium-99m injected. The problem with these approaches is that either also *quadruples* the patient *dose* (not just doubles it!), which is proportional to S, and this may not be a reasonable price if we already have a clinically adequate result. After all, an image only has to be good enough to make a reliable diagnosis; a gorgeous one is nice eye-candy, and the radiographers who person the machines certainly like to present such clear pictures to their physicians – they most likely will not have to take repeats because of poor image quality. But it probably means that the patient is being unnecessarily, perhaps even irresponsibly, over-exposed. It helps to keep in mind Voltaire's timeless observation that "The perfect is the enemy of the good."

Artifacts: non-stochastic noise

Poor design or a malfunction in a stereo system may result in annoying 60-cycle hum or other problems. There are visual analogues of this device-related noise, such as distracting irregularities caused by breathing, even if it is regular, or by the cardiac cycle. You can even find a kind of *non*-random visual *artifact* in the reproductions of radiographs in this book; the pointillistic printing technique involves replacing a smooth gray area with an array of tiny dots, and the larger the dots, the darker a region appears. Look closely, and you can see it. Each modality has its own characteristic set of problematic artifacts when things go wrong – three examples of which appear in Figure 2.17, for CT,

ultrasound, and MRI. We'll see a lot more of them in later chapters.

Quality assurance

X-ray tubes and generators, monitors, computers, CT devices, gamma cameras, and all the other bits and pieces hard at work in an imaging center are usually stable and reliable. But as with any other complex equipment, there is the occasional need for a tune-up or part replacement. It is a well-documented scientific finding, regrettably, that the most frequently used device in any facility is most likely to fail when the patient load is at an all-time high, and when the only staff member who really knows how to fix it is on a two-week lecture and golfing safari in Burkina Faso. And since it may be hard to notice a problem coming on in a device when electrical or mechanical changes are very slow, it is usually good strategy not to wait until bad things happen. An ounce of prevention, etc.

Image quality and radiation safety programs

The simplest, and occasionally the first, way of determining that there may be a difficulty is through signs of dissatisfaction from the viewing physicians or technologists. The level of observer happiness is highly *subjective*, however, and even those with considerable experience may remain unaware of gradual, slight amounts of image degradation.

A second possible approach is *outcome-based*. But by the time the ability of physicians to make correct diagnoses has already been compromised, and the rate of misdiagnosis has climbed by a detectable amount, considerable damage may already have been done.

The third, and best, solution is to routinely carry out *objective* technical assessments as part of a formal, comprehensive, rigorously implemented *quality assurance* (*QA*) program. QA typically consists of two separate but closely related components, the image quality and radiation safety parts (Figure 2.18).

The *image quality* program is designed to maintain and, when possible, to improve the quality of clinical images, ensuring that they are always as

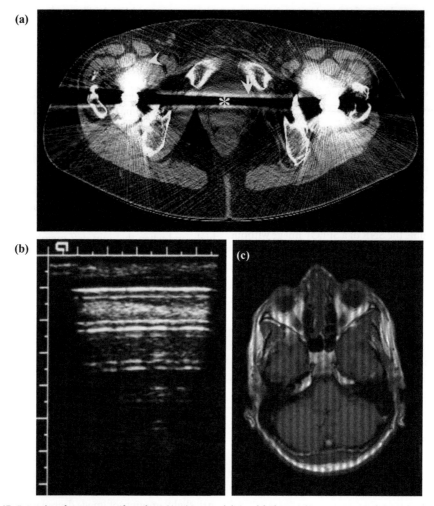

Figure 2.17 Examples of common artifacts found in three modalities. (**a**) This axial/transverse CT of the pelvis in a patient with bilateral metallic total hip prostheses displays three distinct kinds of artifacts: dense metal is much more attenuating of X-rays than are either soft tissue or bone, and here it prevents the transmission of the X-rays through it, completely obscuring portions of tissue (asterisk). In addition, the metal surface introduces a sharp discontinuity in radiological properties that disrupts the computational algorithm that reconstructs the image from raw data, resulting in white streaks emanating from a metallic body in a star-like configuration (arrowhead). Also, metal will preferentially remove lower-energy photons from an X-ray beam, as will be explained in the next chapter; the remaining beam will therefore be of higher average energy, a process known as *beam hardening*, which is responsible for the narrow bands of apparent enhancement linking the two prostheses (arrow). (**b**) Ultrasound reverberates between a flat Norplant device and the transducer, which gives the false impression of multiple parallel, planar structures, with a drop in signal deeper within the tissues. (**c**) This herringbone or criss-cross artifact arose because nearby electronic equipment produced electrical noise that interfered with the MRI device's data processing. Courtesy of Rao Gullapall and J Zhuo.

diagnostically valuable as the apparatus can make them. The technology behind imagers is becoming increasingly complex, and this necessitates more oversight by highly trained and experienced personnel to make certain that equipment problems will be detected and remedied long before they can make a clinical difference, to the extent possible. Also, many clinical studies now fully involve quantitative estimates, above and beyond simple image display, and it is essential the equipment be monitored

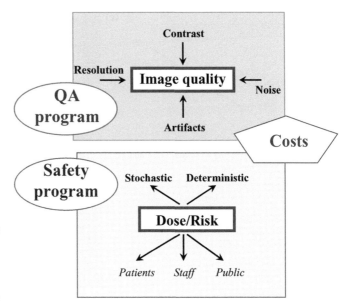

Figure 2.18 A comprehensive *quality assurance* (QA) program routinely demonstrates and documents that *image quality* is diagnostically acceptable, and also compliant with federal and state requirements. Likewise, its *radiation safety* component should keep exposures to patients, medical personnel, and the general public at levels not only below established dose limits but, in addition, ALARA, *as low as reasonably achievable.*

regularly to demonstrate its stability over time for this purpose.

The other part of QA is the *radiation* (and other) *safety* assurance program, set up to keep doses and risks to the patients, staff, and public both ALARA and below federal and state regulatory limits. "ALARA" is a legal construct that applies formally to the exposures of medical staff, nuclear power plant workers, environmental remediation personnel, etc., but the idea can provide protection to patients just as well. Some radiation safety activities are under the control of the *US Nuclear Regulatory Commission* (*US NRC*) and others are monitored by the states, and many are just good, old-fashioned common sense and alertness. It must be explicitly demonstrated, through radiation surveys, that potential doses to the staff and the public, and in a few situations to the patient, are being kept below state and/or federal limits. In addition, there is an ALARA requirement that doses in general be kept as low as reasonably achievable, but it does assume there will be *enough* dose that there will be few re-takes for instrumental reasons. We shall return to radiation safety shortly.

Professional organizations such as the American College of Radiology (ACR), the American Association of Physicists in Medicine (AAPM), and the National Council on Radiation Protection and

Measurements (NCRP) have prepared extensive guidance that describes both parts of QA in suitable detail.

QA programs are usually established and managed by specially trained, PhD- or MS-level physicists or engineers who have chosen to apply their educations and skills in the medical setting. They commonly have obtained certification in a subfield of medical physics by the American Board of Radiology (ABR), and some states are now requiring licensing. Medical physicists also advise management on the selection of new devices; certify that operation of the equipment complies with state and federal technical regulations and other applicable guidelines on an ongoing basis; assist technical aspects of the development of new clinical procedures; and in university settings, participate in the teaching of residents and others, and carry out research.

Some routine elements of the QA program are undertaken daily, weekly, or monthly by the radiographers who normally operate the imaging equipment in patient examinations. The more complex and comprehensive studies, such as the exhaustive acceptance testing and calibration of equipment that is new or that has had a major part replaced, are performed by the medical physicists. So, too, are the annual QA assessments required by state

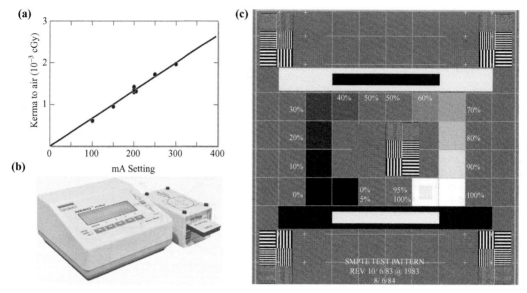

Figure 2.19 Radiographic and fluoroscopic image quality assurance. (**a**) Test of linearity, demonstrating that for a fixed exposure duration and kVp, the measured output of the X-ray tube tracks closely with the tube current (mA) setting. (**b**) An automated, electronic, multi-function beam diagnostics device for non-invasive determination of X-ray beam parameters. It can make a sequence of measurements under computer control, and automatically generate a pre-formatted Excel-based report (www.flukebiomedical.com). (c) The ubiquitous electronic test pattern designed by the Society of Motion Picture and Television Engineers (SMPTE) to assess quantitatively the behavior of electronic display devices, such as liquid crystal displays (LCD), light emitting diode displays, and plasma displays.

and/or federal regulations, and the (less frequent) certification studies called for by the ACR.

A critically important, and sometimes overlooked, aspect of a QA program is the administrative control. The data from QA checks, whether routine or following repair of a malfunction, should be entered into a computer, which then automatically carries out any necessary statistical and other calculations, plots quantitative test data over time, and compares the results with pre-determined requirements. At appropriate times, the chief of the medical physics group should send reports to the physician in charge.

Image QA

A typical image quality program for radiography, say, entails routinely scheduled measurements of a number of machine physical parameters, and the examination of images taken of testing *phantoms* under reproducible conditions (Box 2.2). The tests are intended to demonstrate that every link in the imaging chain is functioning correctly, and that every piece of equipment is properly calibrated.

When the switch setting for the current flowing through the X-ray tube is increased from 50 milliamperes (mA) to 100 mA, for example, does the intensity of the X-ray beam produced actually double (Figure 2.19a)? (If not, a radiographer cannot rely on standardized protocols to produce images with a suitable overall level of darkening and at an acceptable dose level.) Does the X-ray beam penetrate as readily through soft tissue as the kiloVoltage setting on the console implies that it should (Figure 2.19b)? (If the kVp is lower than it should be, the tube is depositing more radiation dose in the patient than is necessary.) Are the focal spot dimensions within specs? (An expanding focal spot reduces achievable resolution, and may indicate a tube that may soon fail.) Does the monitor display the full amount of contrast, resolution, signal-to-noise, brightness, and other attributes that the rest of the imaging chain is capable of extracting (Figure 2.19c)? In the old days, these

Box 2.2   Radiographic system quality assurance

Some of the standard tests one might carry out in an annual QA check, or after replacement of a major part, for a standard screen-film radiographic device, the simplest instrument to be found in an imaging clinic. Those few terms that are not self-evident or discussed here in the text should become meaningful in the next two chapters. The testing of more specialized analog imaging equipment, such as for screen-film mammography, fluoroscopy, or conventional tomography, involves additional studies. The QA of digital devices require jumping into a whole new domain of significantly greater complexity.

Legal postings, warnings
Mechanical, electrical
kVp Accuracy, HVL, wave form
Tube output versus mA-s linearity
X-ray tube output
Exposure reproducibility
Focal spot size, resolution, MTF
Low-contrast detectabiliity
Timer accuracy, linearity
Automatic exposure control
Accuracy of distance indicators
Field size indicators
Light field, radiation field congruence
Radiation field, image receptor centering
Maximum collimator closure
X-ray tube leakage
Film processor, chemicals

measurements would soak up considerable time and person-power, but now with modern, computer-driven instruments, they are faster, more reliable, and (once you know what you're doing) easy to carry out.

Known medical benefits versus potential radiation risks

A high-energy photon that can knock an electron off an atom or molecule, transforming it into a positively charged ion, is known as *ionizing radiation*. X- and gamma-rays (unlike radio waves and visible light) are forms of ionizing radiation, and as such they play particularly important roles in imaging – both in image formation and possibly, as a consequence of causing certain kinds of damage to DNA molecules, in creating a very small, but not ignorable, amount of radiation risk. The next chapter will explore how, exactly, high-energy photons can bring about the ionization of matter, but for now it suffices just to acknowledge that it does happen.

Dose of ionizing radiation

When cooking an omelet or an X-ray tube anode, it is important to keep track of how much *energy*, in joules (J), is imparted to each kilogram of it. Led by this culinary principle, but conscious of the very special properties of *ionizing* radiation, the wise ones have chosen to define the *gray* (*Gy*) as the amount of *ionizing* energy, in joules, imparted to each kilogram of any object, whether it be an egg, an X-ray tube, water, air, a fluorescent screen, a radiation-sensitive transistor, or us (Figure 2.20a):

$$1 \text{ gray} = 1 \text{ J } ionizing/\text{kg}. \qquad (2.4)$$

The milligray (mGy) is, of course, a thousand times smaller. (A unit of dose that is obsolete but still seen in the United States is the *rad*, where 1 rad = 0.01 Gy.) But whatever the units, the essential, operative word here is *ionizing*. Gamma- and X-rays are easily energetic enough to knock electrons off atoms and molecules, and that can lead both to the excitation of the radiation detectors employed in imaging, which is good, but also, occasionally, to very bad things in tissues of patients, or staff.

Pumping 4.5 Gy of ionizing radiation into a 1-liter (1000 cc), 1-kg jug of water will raise its temperature by about 0.001 °C, as would depositing 4.5 J/kg of ordinary heat into it. This is a bit more than the amount of energy given off by a standard 4-watt bathroom night-light in one second. People who receive 4.5 J/kg of ordinary *heat* will not feel the difference – but of those exposed to 4.5 Gy of whole-body *ionizing* irradiation, roughly half will die within weeks (unless they receive specialized medical attention) because of loss of critical leucocyte-forming stem cells. The reason for

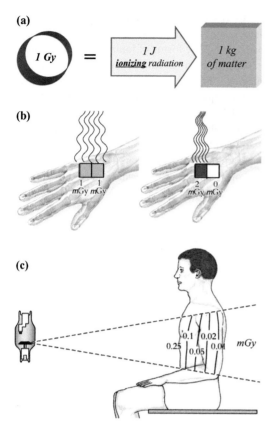

(a)

(b)

(c)

Figure 2.20 The deposition of dose of ionizing radiation is of great importance both in tissue and in the material of an image receptor. **(a)** The *joule* (J) is the standard SI unit of any sort of energy, including its radiant forms. The *gray* (Gy) of radiation *dose* is unique in two important regards: it relates only to *ionizing* radiation, such as high-energy photons and beta particles, which are capable of ejecting electrons from neutral atoms. And it refers not to energy *per se*, but rather to amount of ionizing energy deposited *per unit mass* of matter, the energy density. In particular, 1 Gy is the energy density resulting from the absorption of 1 J of *ionizing* energy by 1 kilogram of any material. **(b)** The spatial distribution of doses throughout the body is rarely uniform. Does 1 mGy + 1 mGy = 2 mGy? It may, or may not. **(c)** Doses in the mid-sagittal plane, at different depths in the body, from a poorly carried out (why?) chest examination. An estimate of the overall radiation *risk* to the patient must account both for the non-uniform dose distribution and also for the fact that the exposed organs are not all equally radio-sensitive.

this great potency of gamma- and X-rays, unlike heat, is that they come as photons that are individually high in energy and sufficiently compact to ionize molecules easily – and that can be biologically harmful or worse. A thrown basketball and an

air-gun pellet may carry the same amount of total kinetic energy ($\frac{1}{2}\,mv^2$), but your hand can readily tell the difference!

At the other extreme, the average American (and even those of us who are a cut or two above average) receives the equivalent of about 3 milligray (0.003 Gy) to all the tissues of the whole body over the course of a year from natural background radiation, and another 3 mGy/y from medical procedures, as averaged over the entire population.

One can be exposed to multiple irradiations, so an obvious question immediately arises: are doses additive? That is, does 1 cGy + 1 cGy = 2 cGy? This is one of the few questions related to the science and art of imaging to which we can provide an unequivocally and absolutely certain answer: it depends. In Figure 2.20b, each of the two adjacent areas of skin on the left separately receives 1 mGy, so the dose is 1 mGy everywhere in the irradiated region. To the right, on the other hand, one area gets 2 mGy and the other gets none, and there is no simpler way to describe the dose distribution. In other words, 1 mGy plus 1 mGy may equal 2 mGy, but then again, maybe it doesn't.

The *mean* glandular dose from a single mammogram is typically 1.5 to 2 mGy, but it is confined to the breast, and it is not deposited uniformly even there: since the body attenuates an X-ray beam, its intensity falls off at deeper depths within, as does the dose deposited. Similarly, the local dose from a standard chest radiograph, the most commonly performed X-ray examination, ranges from about 0.25 mGy in the skin at the point where the beam enters the body to a few percent of that amount where it exits and exposes the radiographic cassette – which must itself receive enough radiation to function properly and avoid an underexposure (Figure 2.20c).

So it is clearly pointless, and misleading, to say that, "the dose to the chest is 0.25 mGy." The *average* dose over the chest, sometimes mistakenly called its "effective dose" (which has an altogether different connotation), is comparable to what it gets from natural background radiation over a matter of days. But the average dose within an organ or tissue is meaningful in an estimate of radiation risk; indeed, dose to each organ separately forms the basis for calculating the widely used *effective dose* (Chapter 5).

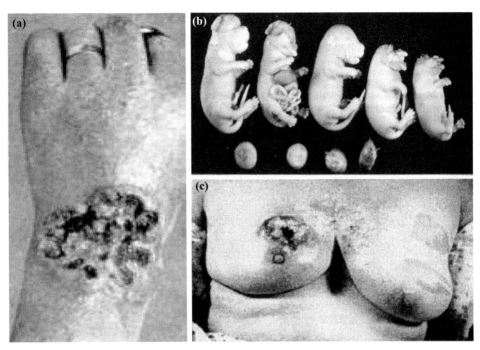

Figure 2.21 There are three generally recognized, broad categories of radiation-induced health effects: radiogenic burns, birth defects, and cancers, and all are believed to arise from disruption of the information content of nuclear DNA.
(a) This severe damage to the skin, or radiation burn, is an example of a *deterministic* health effect; it arose from radiation-induced acceleration of the normal physiological process of apoptosis (programmed cell death) and from the outright killing of so many essential stem cells that the skin tissue could no longer continue to function properly, or repair or replenish itself. It is the possibility of causing unacceptable deterministic complications in adjacent healthy tissues that limits the doses that can be directed at the tumors within radiotherapy patients. Courtesy of Philip H Heintz.
(b) *Teratogenic* effects that may arise from exposure *in utero* share characteristics of both stochastic and deterministic responses. Photograph by Dr. Roberts Rugh, courtesy of Eric J Hall. **(c)** Radiogenic carcinogenesis is a *stochastic*, or probabilistic, effect that may come about because of certain radiation-induced transformations in the genetic material of one or a few cells. This neoplasm was most likely induced by multiple fluoroscopic examinations during the treatment of her tuberculosis; it did not appear until a decade later. Courtesy of Louis K Wagner, University of Texas Medical Center, Houston, TX.

Measurements and tables of patient doses play important roles in determining radiation levels for optimal operation of image receptors. But their primary significance is that they provide the best indication we have of radiation risks to patients, staff, and others.

Possible radiation risks

X-rays and gamma-rays revolutionized the practice of medicine, but early on it was learned that they have their dark side as well. Within a few years of Roentgen's discovery, researchers were reporting cases of horrible "burns" caused by high doses of the radiation, some of which were fatal because of infection (Figure 2.21a). Similarly, irradiation of the fetus by much lesser amounts caused terrible birth defects, including mental retardation, especially with an exposure during the period of most rapid organogenesis (Figure 2.21b). Under the standard conditions used in diagnosis today, however, exposures high enough to cause gross tissue damage are almost completely preventable, and rarely seen, as is radiogenic harm to the fetus. Unfortunately, though, radiation burns and birth defects aren't the only possible problems.

Epidemiological studies of irradiated populations, such as Japanese survivors of the atomic bombs and heavily exposed medical patients, along with experiments on cell cultures and animals, indicate that cancer may be induced (albeit extremely rarely, and by no means necessarily!) even at dose levels far lower than those that cause burns or birth defects (Figure 2.21c). So also can chromosomal damage in gamete cells that may lead to hereditary disruptions. There is, however, a major problem with the cancer-related dose-response studies: the doses at which radiogenic carcinogenesis is unequivocally *known* to occur (0.1 Gy and up) may be a good deal lower than the burn level (tens of Gy), but they are still very high compared to most diagnostic imaging doses (mGy). That is, solid epidemiological data are available only for exposures that are several orders of magnitude greater than what a patient or fetus normally receives in any modern clinical examination. (Exceptions, including negligent and too-aggressive over-exposures from CT and fluoroscopy, have appeared recently on the front pages of the *New York Times* and elsewhere, but presumably these are quite rare.) So direct epidemiological evidence on the real risks from diagnostic amounts of radiation simply does not exist, and it may never: for now we must extrapolate downward from high-dose data and rely on animal and cell studies.

What we do have, though, suggests that the risks from nearly all of today's diagnostic procedures are, fortunately, extremely small — but they cannot simply be discounted.

Radiation (and other) safety QA

The *image quality* component of a proper QA program ensures that the amounts of ionizing radiation produced by or for X-ray, fluoro, CT, PET, etc., machines are sufficiently high to provide clinically useful images. The *radiation safety* part demands, conversely, that the dose to the patients, especially children, not substantially exceed that amount. Imaging centers must also take active measures to make certain that exposures are ALARA for the staff who work around them and the equipment day after day for years, and for members of the general public (e.g., secretaries) who happen to spend time nearby.

The objective of a formal radiation safety program is to determine and control the levels of dose delivered, under the range of operating conditions,

to the patient, to the imaging staff, and to others. More specifically, a radiation safety program for a diagnostic clinic has three interlinked objectives, all embedded in federal and state laws and regulations: It is intended to:

Completely prevent any occurrence of radiogenic *deterministic* effects;

Limit *stochastic* risk to a level considered "acceptable" by public policy setters after careful consideration of the balance of possible risk against known benefits; and

Encourage all staff to strive always to practice and achieve ALARA (Box 2.3, Figure 2.22).

Box 2.3   The objectives of a radiation safety program

Prevent any occurrence of deterministic effects
Limit stochastic risk to an "acceptable" level
Strive always to maintain doses ALARA

We shall pursue radiation safety policies and practices more in Chapter 5, but for now let's introduce four obvious, common-sense *personal actions* which anyone should adopt when working in *any* hazardous environment (Figure 2.22):

Spend as little *time* around the source as possible, while still doing the job properly.

Keep as much *distance* as possible from the source of the hazard; the intensity of radiation, and the risks from many other hazardous situations, fall off with the square of the distance, *r*, from its ori-

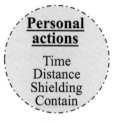

Figure 2.22 Four radiation safety actions anyone can pursue to help keep exposure to any harmful entity ALARA: while still carrying out what needs to be done, minimize exposure *time*; maximize *distance* from source; utilize *shielding*; and *contain* spills.

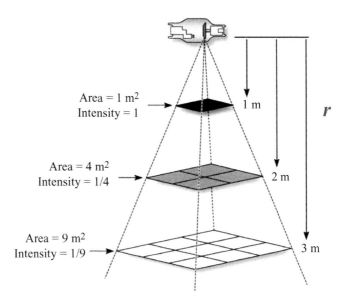

Area = 1 m²
Intensity = 1

Area = 4 m²
Intensity = 1/4

Area = 9 m²
Intensity = 1/9

1 m

2 m

3 m

r

Figure 2.23 The purely geometric basis for the inverse-square rule.

gin, as $1/r^2$ (the *inverse square* rule; Figure 2.23). Farther is better, when you can.

Utilize radiation barriers and *shielding*, such as a lead apron or portable lead-glass shield, when appropriate. The amount of shielding needed depends on the type(s) of radiation, its energy, its intensity at the shield, and the nature of the barrier material.

In case of a spill of radioactive (or toxic) material, such as in a nuclear medicine department, the first line of defense is to *contain* it, stopping it from spreading; also, warn people away to prevent further exposure and to avoid their tramping it around. The second, for any significant accident, is to call the Radiation Safety Officer (RSO) ASAP to check on and perhaps finish off the cleanup effort.

The next time you're around a medical source of ionizing radiation, remember the fundamental mantra that is embedded in the mind of any experienced radiation worker: ***Time***, ***Distance***, ***Shielding***, and, when in a nuclear medicine department, ***Containment***.

In conclusion, there's a fundamental tradeoff between the significantly likely (but not certain) medical benefits from an X-ray or gamma-ray examination, on the one hand, and the highly unlikely (but conceivably possible) radiation hazards, on the other — with analogous issues for the other imaging methodologies as well, even if they do not employ ionizing radiation. Over the years, medical practitioners and public health scientists and officials have learned to strike a reasonable balance between the recognized diagnostic advantages of an imaging study and the possibility (albeit very small) that a radiation-induced cancer might ensue from it.

Ultrasound and MRI are often touted as powerful imaging modalities that utilize no ionizing radiation. No gamma- or X-rays means no cancer induction and no radiation burns. Indeed, it is generally agreed that when these kinds of equipment are maintained properly, by way of a comprehensive QA program, and used with caution, their risks will be exceedingly low. There have been lethal accidents and tissue burns from MRI, however, and it is not completely assured that diagnostic levels of US power are harmless to the unborn. With any imaging modality, as with any other medical procedure, it is important for the practitioner to understand her instrument well, and to operate it only when there are good medical indications to do so, where the anticipated benefits far outweigh the potential risks.

In the coming chapters, we shall have more to say about ways to gauge the risks from high-energy photons and the other imaging probes. At this point, we simply repeat that the estimated likelihood of someone becoming ill from a medically indicated diagnostic procedure is widely believed to be very, very small. The risk should be compared, moreover, with the probably far greater risk from *not* having the procedure performed, in which case a patient's treatment may be considerably less than optimal. So when someone asks "Is this exam *completely* safe?", a good answer is usually: "We don't know for certain, but since it is indicated clinically, it's surely a lot 'safer' than not having the study done."

CHAPTER 3

Creating Subject Contrast in the Primary X-ray Image

Projection Maps of the Body from Differential Attenuation of X-rays by Tissues

Crick and Watson's two-stage transfer of genetic information within a cell has been called the *central dogma of molecular biology*: first the information is transcribed from DNA to messenger RNA, and then it is translated into proteins at the ribosomes.

Had he known about Crick and Watson, Roentgen might well have referred to the process of medical image creation as the *central dogma of radiology*. As an initially uniform X-ray beam passes through the body, information is transcribed into the beam through *differential attenuation* by the various tissues. That information content is then translated into a visual image by a fluorescent screen or photographic plate.

The central dogma of radiology might state that *creation of any medical image is a two-stage process*. In stage I, a set of probes (e.g., X-rays from a tube, an injected radiopharmaceutical seeking a tissue,

Medical Imaging: Essentials for Physicians, First Edition. Anthony B. Wolbarst, Patrizio Capasso and Andrew R. Wyant.
© 2013 John Wiley & Sons, Inc. Published 2013 by John Wiley & Sons, Inc.

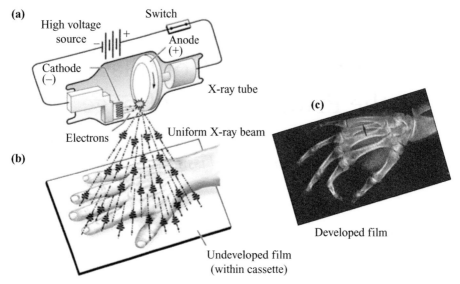

(a) High voltage source, Switch, Anode (+), Cathode (−), X-ray tube, Electrons, Uniform X-ray beam

(b) Undeveloped film (within cassette)

(c) Developed film

Figure 3.1 The standard analog (screen-film) radiographic process.

ultrasound from a transducer, radiofrequency (RF) photons and the magnetic field for MRI) *interacts with the body* and transcribes information about its interior into a pattern, a *primary image*, through their differential interactions with the tissues. In stage II this primary image, after emerging from the body, is captured and translated into a visible image by the *image receptor* (*IR*).

For the particularly simple case of film X-ray imaging, this reduces to:

Pre-I. Generation of a uniform X-ray beam;

I. Interaction of the beam with various tissues of the body, creating a shadowgram; and

II. Capture of the spatially-modulated image on a screen-film IR.

In a little more detail (Figure 3.1 and Box 3.1):

Pre-I. A high-voltage electrical generator and an X-ray tube produce a nearly uniform beam of penetrating X-rays (Figure 3.1a). These emanate from the tiny *focal spot* on the *target* region of the anode of the tube, travel along straight but diverging paths, and expose a portion of the body.

I. This flat beam enters the patient's body, where the atoms of bones and the soft tissues differ greatly in their tendencies to absorb and scatter X-ray photons (Figure 3.1b). The resulting *differential attenuation* imprints a *primary X-ray* shadow *image* onto the previously uniform beam, introducing diagnostic

information into it. A bone attenuates X-rays more effectively than do soft tissues, for example, and casts a deeper X-ray shadow falling onto the IR.

Two kinds of atomic-scale collisions between the incident high-energy photons and atomic electrons, *photoelectric absorption* (*PA*) and *Compton scatter* (*CS*) events, bring about attenuation of the beam. Differential attenuation of photons (by these two mechanisms) in different parts of the beam by the various tissues embeds a non-uniform shadowgram in the remnants of it that emerge from the body. As

---

Box 3.1   The central dogma of radiography

I Various tissues differentially remove photons from uniform beam, creating a shadowgram;

Photoelectric Absorption (PA) and Compton Scatter (CS) produce contrast in it;

Compton scatter photons degrade it;

The *ejected* fast Compton electrons and photoelectrons ionize tissue, deposit dose.

II Photons transmitted through body interact with the IR; primarily through PA;

Photoelectrons excite and activate the IR, which leads to the creation of a visual record.

we shall see, the PA effect is the main contributor to contrast between soft tissues and bones or bullets; CS may be important in the search for lung tumors, which differ significantly from their surroundings in density, but mainly it just introduces visual noise into a radiograph.

An undesirable (in tissue) but inevitable consequence of either kind of photon-electron interaction is the ejection from the atom of the struck electron, which thereupon courses at high velocity through the material. This newly freed electron dissipates its considerable energy in ionizing hundreds or thousands of other atoms and molecules that happen to lie along its path. This deposition of *radiation dose* in tissues causes cellular biochemical changes that almost always are of absolutely *no* consequence. They can occasionally lead to DNA damage, however, including mutations, that might (albeit extremely rarely) cause various sorts of profound biological harm. So all the time, it is important to minimize the radiation exposure of the staff and others, and *un*productive dose to the patient, while still generating clinically adequate images.

II. Stage II takes place in the IR. While an ejected fast electron does no good in tissues, in a radiation detector it is what triggers the instrument. In film radiography, the IR is a radiographic cassette containing a sheet of special photographic film (Figure 3.1b). It captures the spatially modulated pattern of remnant, unabsorbed X-rays emerging from the body, which becomes a visual image through development of the film (Figure 3.1c). The more radiation reaching any part of the cassette, the greater the number of transparent silver halide crystals in the film's emulsion that are transformed into opaque flecks of silver during its development, and the darker that portion of film. Where the body has attenuated the beam more, such as behind a bone, the developed film is pale. So in a sense, an X-ray image is a "negative": it reveals the *primary X-ray image*, the pattern of X-rays that have *not* interacted with the body's tissues, and have *not* been absorbed or scattered there.

So the creation of an X-ray image is a story, with a proper beginning (the generation of a uniform X-ray beam), a thickening of the plot (the interaction of the beam with the bones and soft tissues of the patient, and then with the IR), and a possibly life-or-death denouement (the formation of a visual image that may or may not be capable of resolving a crucial clinical issue).

This chapter describes, a little more richly, phases Pre-I and I of that story. The next chapter will take it up from there.

Creating a (nearly) uniform beam of penetrating X-rays

A wide variety of forms of imaging are built around X-rays: analog (screen-film) radiography and (image-intensifier based) fluoroscopy; digital radiography (DR), digital mammography (DM), digital tomosynthesis, and computed radiography (CR); digital fluoroscopy (DF) and digital subtraction angiography (DSA); and computed tomography (CT). The requisite X-ray beam is generated in much the same way for all of them, and the X-ray photons are removed from the beam by tissues through the same two principal interaction mechanisms, photoelectric absorption and Compton scatter. These modalities differ primarily in the nature of the IR, which captures the pattern of X-rays coming out of the body.

Anatomy of an X-ray tube

Creating an X-ray beam requires an evacuated X-ray tube and a generator that produces direct-current high-voltage and also low-voltage d.c.

There are two electrodes within the tube, the *cathode filament* (a tungsten wire coil) and the *anode* (Figures 3.2a and 1.4a). During an exposure, these are attached briefly to the negative and positive high-voltage poles of the generator, respectively.

The coiled *filament* of resistive wire in the cathode is brought to high temperature when a constant d.c. *filament current* is being driven through it by the generator, so that electrons "boil" off it (Figure 3.2b). As long as the generator's *exposure switch* remains "off," the electric circuit is open and incomplete. Nothing very interesting happens, except that the cathode becomes slightly negatively charged because of the electrons that have escaped it, and it can therefore hold those electrons near to it as a cloud of *space charge* – like a swarm of barnyard flies congregating over their favorite appetizers.

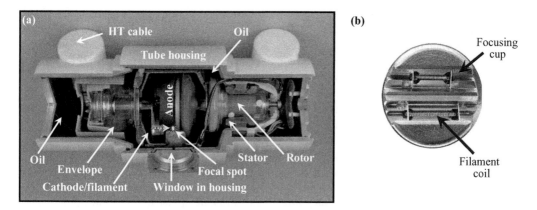

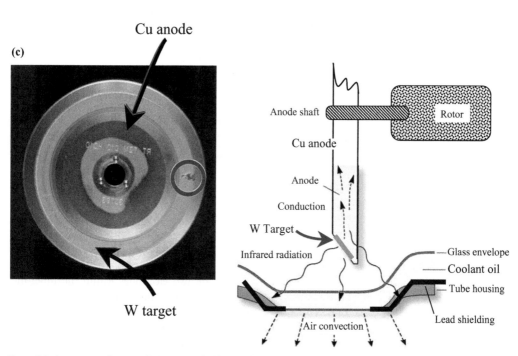

Figure 3.2 An evacuated X-ray tube is surrounded by circulating refrigerated oil for *cooling* and high-voltage insulation, and encased within a *housing* and, outside of that, a few millimeters of lead *X-ray shielding*. (**a**) Within the tube, the *cathode filament* is heated white-hot by low-voltage d.c. from the generator, and electrons "boil" off it. If the *exposure switch* is open, they simply form a "cloud" hovering just above the filament. When the exposure switch is closed, they accelerate toward the *anode*. As these electrons collide with the tungsten-alloy *target* embedded in the surface of the copper anode, one percent or so of their collective energy of motion is transformed into *bremsstrahlung* and *characteristic X-ray radiation* energy. The other 99% is wasted as heat. (**b**) The cathode assembly of a dual-focus tube consists of two coiled filament wires, only one of which is activated at a time, and a separate focusing "cup" influencing its electron cloud. The smaller filament is used for higher-resolution imaging. (**c**) Facing and side views of the annular *tungsten* (unusually efficient X-ray production, extremely high melting temperature) *target* and the copper (very good for conduction of heat away from the target) anode, in which it is embedded. The anode is made to rotate thousands of times per minute by an induction motor consisting of a rotor (supported on ball bearings) within the tube and a stator external to it, which further spreads out the heating caused by the electron bombardment. Infrared radiation from the target and the rest of the anode transports its heat to the cooling oil outside, and air convection then moves it away. While it is commonly the bearings (lubricated with silver powder or, recently, liquid gallium) that give out, pitting of the tungsten target can also occur in a tube, as happened here.

To make an X-ray image, the exposure switch is closed for a few hundredths of a second, thereby applying a short pulse of constant high voltage (and creating a strong electrical force field) between the two electrodes of the tube. The cloud of electrons, having already been thermally driven off the cathode, are now momentarily drawn electrically toward the anode (and replaced by fresh electrons from the cathode). They pick up considerable speed in their fleeting journey, then smash into the tiny *focal spot*, typically on the order of 0.6–1.2 mm across, on the *target* of the anode. The target is a thin annular ribbon of *tungsten* (chemical symbol W, from the ore wolframite) alloy embedded into the surface of the heavy, copper anode disk (Figure 3.2c).

Two things now happen briefly that are both critically significant in the operation of the system: the tube produces X-ray radiation, and the anode becomes scorchingly hot.

Less than 1% of the energy deposited in the target/anode becomes bremsstrahlung and characteristic X-ray radiation

A very small fraction of the kinetic energy of the electron beam is transformed at the target into *bremsstrahlung* and *characteristic X-rays*. These are essentially the same stuff once they are out of the tube – just high-energy photons – but they are created by different physical mechanisms at the target, and they happen to find separate applications: most X-ray studies utilize bremsstrahlung X-rays from a tungsten target, but film mammography exploits the characteristic X-rays of a molybdenum target.

Bremsstrahlung may be translated from the German as "braking radiation," as in hitting the brakes of an automobile, and it refers to a particular energy conversion process: as was predicted by Maxwell's theory, whenever a charged particle suffers an abrupt acceleration or deceleration or change in trajectory, some (and occasionally all) of its kinetic energy is transformed into electromagnetic radiation. Your favorite rockabilly station sends out those joyous melodies by applying a strong a.c. voltage to its antenna, sloshing electrons abruptly back and forth in it, which thereupon emit radio waves – same kind of thing! A bremsstrahlung X-ray comes into existence when a high-speed electron happens to penetrate deep enough into the electron cloud of a tungsten atom and experiences the intense electric attraction of the strongly positive, massive, and relatively immobile nucleus. The electron is violently jerked around (Figure 3.3a), and bremsstrahlung radiation comes into being.

The bremsstrahlung photons produced with a 100 kVp setting, say, range in energy from 0 to 100 keV. That is, the energy, in keV, of the (very few) most energetic photons is numerically equal to the kVp setting. A hypothetical bremsstrahlung *spectrum*, displaying the relative intensity of photon energy produced at each energy, is shown as the dashed straight line, *A*, in Figure 3.3b, for 100 kVp. If a particular 100 keV electron (accelerated through a 100 kVp potential) happens to be jerked completely to rest in a single abrupt collision in the anode, then all its energy will reappear as a single 100 keV photon. But that is a rare event, and nearly all the electrons undergo multiple, less wrenching collisions, resulting in a number of lower-energy photons with an average energy of between one half and two thirds of that peak amount.

For reasons that will soon become apparent, metals and some other materials preferentially absorb lower-energy photons. As a consequence, nearly all low-energy photons that happen to be created below the surface of the target will be soaked up as they attempt to escape it, or while passing through the window of the tube's glass envelope. This causes the downward curvature at the low-energy side of curve *B* in Figure 3.3b. It is standard procedure, moreover to add more filtration to the beam intentionally, *C*, commonly with a thin sheet of aluminum to remove more of the low-energy photons: these cannot pass completely through the patient, so they are diagnostically useless, but they do deposit radiation dose unnecessarily. Since the *inherent* and *added filtration* remove the low-energy photons, this also *hardens* the beam, or shifts its average and peak energies upward toward higher energies, making it more penetrating in tissues.

Characteristic radiation is quite different. It comes from transitions involving inner electrons of heavy atoms, as described in Chapter 2. Unlike the *continuous* spectrum of bremsstrahlung radiation, that of characteristic X-rays consists of sharp, *discrete* narrow peaks occurring at specific energies

(a)

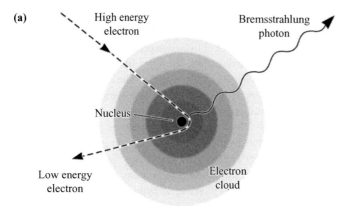

(b)

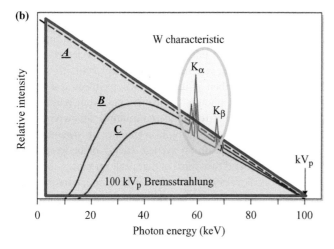

Figure 3.3 Bremsstrahlung X-rays. (a) If a high-velocity electron has sufficient kinetic energy to penetrate deeply into a heavy atom, it may be violently deflected from its path by means of an electric interaction with the nucleus. In the process, the electron may lose some (or, rarely, all) of its energy through the creation of a *bremsstrahlung* X-ray photon. (b) These three spectra reveal the relative intensity of three X-ray beams over a range of X-ray photon energies, all with the generator set to the same kVp. *A*: An idealized 100-kVp spectrum (dashed) of X-rays emerging from a tungsten target, assuming no absorption of photons by it. Discrete peaks corresponding to tungsten (W) characteristic X-rays also appear. *B*: Impact of inherent *filtration* by the anode itself and by the window of the glass envelope of the tube on the spectrum. *C*: With intentional additional filtration, as well.

characteristic of the electronic structure of the element (hence the name). Four peaks of tungsten are apparent in all three curves of the figure.

The efficiency of bremsstrahlung production happens to be proportional to the nuclear charge (i.e., the atomic number) of the target material, and that of tungsten is relatively high ($Z = 74$). The process of producing diagnostic X-rays is *extremely* inefficient; only about $1/2$–1% of the collective energy of the electrons driven from cathode to anode is transformed into X-ray energy at the target. (In metabolizing glucose, by comparison, mitochondria can turn about 40% of the sugar's chemical energy into the high-energy phosphate bonds of ATP, while losing 60%, ultimately, as nonproductive heat.) Efficiency is also linear in the energy of the electron at diagnostic energies, so it is proportional to $Z \times$ kVp. In a 25 MeV radiotherapy linear accelerator (linac), the X-ray production efficiency is considerably higher.

Heat

The second important thing that happens at the anode is that, since the efficiency of bremsstrahlung production is so abysmally low, the remaining 99+% of the combined kinetic energy of the electrons is wasted in the release of vast amounts of non-productive *heat*.

A resistive wire heats up when a battery forces a current of electrons through it, and they give up their energy in banging into atoms. The same thing happens when high-velocity electrons accelerated from the cathode smash into and drive through the target (2500 °C at the focal spot). The tungsten target has a high melting point (3422 °C) and low vapor pressure but, alas, is a poor thermal conductor of heat, nor can it soak up and hold much of it. A thin annular target is therefore normally embedded in a heavy disc of copper, which *is* a very good conductor of heat away from the focal spot region. In addition, the anode is made to rotate rapidly to reduce the likelihood of any spot overheating, giving rise to a faint whirring sound. The heat radiates away from the target and anode as infrared (heat, thermal) radiation, through the vacuum and glass envelope of the tube, and much is then conveyed away by cooling oil circulating around its exterior. Sometimes, however, that's not enough, as indicated by the pitting in the anode of Figure 3.2c. As you can imagine, getting a white hot (1000 °C, on average) anode within a sealed, evacuated vessel to rotate thousands of times per minute, supported on ball bearings with no normal lubricants available, all the while applying 100 000 V or so between the cathode and anode, involves some rather fancy engineering footwork.

It is easy to quantify the rate of heat production, and therefore dissipation. As electrons of charge e⁻ are drawn from cathode to anode, each acquires (eV/e^-) of kinetic energy (in electron volts, eV), by the definition of voltage. Likewise, the current through the tube, the rate at which electrons are flowing through it, is (e^-/s). So the power, P, delivered to the anode, almost entirely as heat, is of magnitude $P = (eV/s) = (eV/e^-) \times (e^-/s)$. This is seen more commonly as $V \times I$, where V is the applied voltage and I is the current. Not all of this energy is degraded into heat; about $^1/_2$–1% of it is radiated away as X-rays – an extremely inefficient process but, for now, it's all we have.

Control of the X-ray exposure: the three technique factors

Here's a similar but different analogy for those readers who do not appreciate cats (Figure 1.5c). (Some, including one of the authors, are inexplicably insensitive to feline charms, commonly pointing out their aloofness – an unfair charge: happy cats are very loof.) A generator and X-ray tube together are rather like a small, closed-loop backyard waterfall (Figure 3.4). An electric pump expends energy from the power company in pushing water to the top of the falls; as it reaches the edge, its drops accelerate downward, with their initial potential energy (due to its position in the gravitational field) being transformed into kinetic energy. And, as they strike the pond below, this becomes sound radiation and heat. The higher the falls (kVp), the more kinetic energy the water droplets will acquire, and the louder the noise from each. Likewise, the greater the flow (mA), the greater overall amount of sound *power* produced. And the longer the pump is working (s), the greater the total sound radiation *energy* delivered.

The three primary controls of the generator for an X-ray exposure, called the *technique factors*, allow selection of the tube potential (kVp, from the earlier, now obsolete, term "peak kiloVoltage"), the

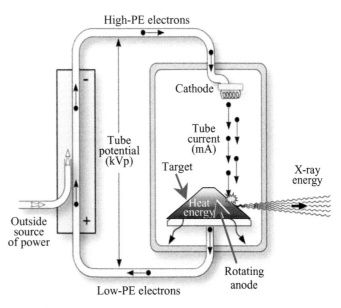

Figure 3.4 A closed-circuit backyard waterfall, masquerading as an X-ray generator and tube.

tube current (mA, in milliAmperes), and the exposure duration (s, in seconds.) The power of penetration of bremsstrahlung and characteristic X-ray energy, and also the amount generated during an exposure (and the resulting darkening of film) increase with the kVp setting. The mA is controlled by adjusting the rate at which electrons boil off the filament; that is, by its temperature. The total beam energy produced is directly proportional to both the mA and the exposure time, hence to mA × s, or mA-s. The total energy delivered by the generator to the anode in an exposure is kV × mA × s, of which only a very small fraction is radiated away as X-rays.

For any particular patient and procedure, the radiologic technologist can select the tube potential, the tube current, and the exposure time (by means of the kVp, mA, and timer controls, respectively) – though some or all of this may be done in part by the device itself with an *automatic exposure control* circuit. These three technique factors affect a number of aspects of the image creation process: the capacity of the beam to penetrate the patient's body; its ability to create subject contrast among the different tissues; to some extent, the tendency of the IR to either enhance or diminish that subject contrast; the overall average level of brightness of the end-product image; and the radiation dose to the patient. Tables of technique factors have been developed for any tube to help optimize the trade-off between diagnostic utility of the image and the patient radiation dose, and modern machines take care of that issue semi-automatically.

Finally, the radiant energy from the focal spot exits through a thin window in the tube's glass or metal envelope, and through another one in the *housing* that surrounds it (Figures 3.5 and 3.2a). The housing provides mechanical support for the tube and for thin aluminum or other metal plates for added filtration. Its adjustable beam *collimator* shutters determine the beam field dimensions; the dimensions of the field are generally made as small as possible, for any particular patient and procedure, to minimize both patient exposure and the amount of image degradation from scatter radiation. A small light bulb and an optical mirror nearly transparent to X-rays are positioned so that a *light field* lies coincident with the tube's radiation field, needed for patient positioning. The housing also serves as a container for circulating refrigerated oil for heat dissipation and electrical insulation; at one end of the tube housing there may be a bellows, moreover, that switches off the tube when the oil becomes too hot and expands past a certain limit. Surrounding *lead shielding* greatly reduces (but cannot completely eliminate) radiation leaking from the tube in any direction except through the window.

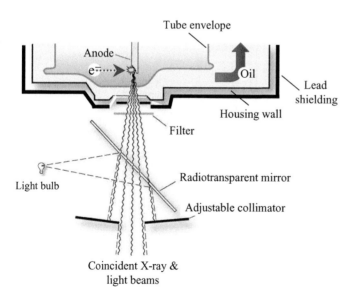

Figure 3.5 Constraining the beam. The tube housing and attached collimator assembly allows the control of the beam size, to minimize both patient dose and degradation of image contrast from scatter radiation produced in the body. Note the lead shielding everywhere except at the beam-exit port. During patient set-up, a small light can illuminates the area to be exposed.

Interaction of X-ray and gamma-ray photons with tissues or an image receptor

The attenuation of an X-ray beam in passing through matter can be viewed from both of two different but equally important viewpoints. From a simple experiment, one can determine that globally, the intensity, $I(x)$, of the beam falls off (ideally) *exponentially* with the thickness of the material, x, it travels through; the rate of attenuation is parameterized by the *linear attenuation coefficient, μ*. Alternatively, it is possible to consider the nature of the collisions of individual photons with the atomic electrons of the medium on the microscopic level, and get to exponential attenuation and μ that way. The two approaches are essentially equivalent.

The global picture

Exponential attenuation of an ideal X-ray beam by an ideal medium

Electromagnetic radiation can interact with matter by various mechanisms. The relative probability that a particular type of interaction will take place depends on the energy of the photons and on the nature of the material, and physicists have expended much of their efforts over the past century learning about those processes, suggested in the far-right column of Figure 2.2b.

The *attenuation* by matter along an extremely narrow beam, or geometric "ray," of X- or gammarays is a process easily studied by experiment (Figure 3.6a). The intensity of the beam, $I(x)$, is monitored as different *thicknesses*, x, of the attenuating material

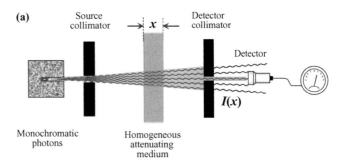

Figure 3.6 Exponential attenuation of X-rays by matter. (a) Experimental setup for the study of the interaction of a narrow gamma- or X-ray beam with matter. In the ideal case, there are four constraints on the experiment: The beam is monochromatic, so no beam hardening in the material occurs; the pair of beam collimators keep (lower-energy) scatter photons away from the detector; the attenuating material being studied is homogeneous; and the distance from source to detector remains fixed, so there is no inverse-square effect. (b) This particular beam in this specific medium is undergoing exactly exponential attenuation, with a half-value layer (HVL) thickness (over which beam intensity falls by a factor of $^1/_2$) of 1.8 cm. (c) A plot of an exponential function on ordinary linear graph paper. (d) *Semi-log* paper is designed specifically to plot out an exponential function as a straight line.

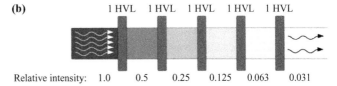

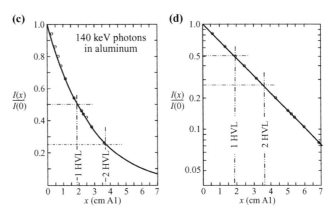

are inserted into the beam path. $I(0)$ is the intensity when there is no attenuating material in its path, $x = 0$. The more material the beam has traversed, the more probable it is that any particular photon will have interacted with some atom and thus be culled from it, and the lower the detector reading. Thus the greater the *thickness* of the body part being imaged, or the more obese the patient, the less the amount of the incident X-ray energy that makes it all the way through.

In Figure 3.6b, the intensity of a non-diverging 140 keV *monochromatic* (of single energy, as from a radioactive material, as opposed to the continuous band of energies from the target of an X-ray tube) photon beam from a distant technetium-99m point source is monitored as increasing amounts of homogeneous material are inserted between source and detector. In this particular study, the beam is measured to fall by a factor of a half when 1.8 centimeters of aluminum is used; 140 keV radiation is therefore said to have a *half-value layer* (HVL) thickness of 1.8 cm in aluminum. The intensity of the beam falls by another half in passing through a second 1.8 cm thick plate of Al, then by yet another half at the next plate, and so on. After passing through two or three HVLs, the beam will be only $\frac{1}{4}$ and $\frac{1}{8}$ as intense as when it started out, respectively. Thus the same *fraction* of what remains is absorbed or scattered in each identical thickness of material, and the beam is said to be undergoing *exponential attenuation*. A beam transiting a thickness x of material will pass through x/HVL half-value layers, so the intensity can be shown as an explicit function of x, namely $I(x)/I(0) = 2^{-x/HVL}$.

It would be fine to work with powers of 2 as above, but by convention, exponential attenuation is normally written to the base e $\equiv 2.71828\ldots$, instead. Just as π is ubiquitous in trigonometry, so also "e" is a fundamental numerical constant that is of central importance in calculus and, in terms of it, the attenuation expression assumes the form (Figure 3.6c)

$$I(x)/I(0) = e^{-\mu x}. \qquad (3.1a)$$

μ is a *parameter* known as the *linear attenuation coefficient*, and it is essentially equivalent to the HVL – it may entertain you briefly to show that $\mu \times HVL = 0.693$. Just as the units of HVL are centimeters, those of the attenuation coefficient must

be cm^{-1} for the entire exponent to remain dimensionless; after all, what could e$^{-3\,cm}$ possibly mean?

Suppose, as an example of Equation 3.1a and Figure 3.6b, that the attenuation coefficient μ of a beam of a certain energy in a given medium is tabulated to be 0.231 cm^{-1}. The fraction of its intensity remaining after passage through 5.0 cm, say, is then $I(5\,cm)/I(0\,cm) = e^{-[0.231\,cm^{-1} \times 5.0\,cm]} = 0.32$.

All the interesting information about the nature of the attenuating material and of the photon beam is completely wrapped up in the specific numerical value of μ or, equivalently, of the HVL. μ is, ultimately, the measure of the spatial *rate* at which photoelectric and Compton interactions are taking place in a medium, whether it be the tissues of the patient, the materials of the IR, or the concrete or lead of radiation shielding. The exponential shape, on the other hand, is a result of elementary bookkeeping, and it pops up in a surprising number of quite diverse situations. It applies to any process in which the amount of something remaining present changes by exactly the same *fraction* (such as $\frac{1}{2}$) every additional centimeter, every second, every unit of dose, whatever. Here it keeps track of what happens when you add more and more attenuating material; that is, when you increase x, regardless of what μ or HVL happens to be.

Because exponentials are encountered so commonly, some clever soul designed *semi-logarithmic* graph paper, which plots out any exponential function as a straight line, the slope of which is μ. Before the advent of computers, semi-log provided a quick and dirty way to determine if a data set did, in fact, really follow an exponential form (Figure 3.6d). A curve on linear graph paper may be suggestive of many functional forms, but straight is straight! Even now it offers a compelling and convenient way to display data that are exactly or nearly exponential, or that cover a wide range of numerical values.

So far, we have been addressing a rather ideal situation. The bremsstrahlung beam from an X-ray tube is not monochromatic, however, nor one of good geometry in which scatter is rejected. And unless you're examining a compressed jellyfish, a real body is neither homogeneous nor of uniform thickness. It is the variations in tissue materials (in particular, their densities and chemical makeup) and thicknesses at different points in the body that give rise to the patterns seen in X-ray images. Still, attenuation is often *approximately* exponential with *x* in reality, and the model is conceptually valuable.

Let's attempt to shed a little more light on the true meaning of μ. If you remember a little calculus, it's easy to find (just take the derivative of $e^{-\mu x}$) that

$$\mu = -[\Delta I/I]/\Delta x. \qquad (3.1b)$$

μ appears here to represent the small *fraction* of the cohort of photons lost, $\Delta I/I$, when a beam passes through, say, a *small* amount of material, Δx, like a millimeter of it, say. Alternatively, but equivalently, $\Delta I/I$ may be viewed as the *probability of any one photon* undergoing a photon-electron interaction over that small distance. μ is commonly expressed in units either of fractional decrease in intensity, or of probability of interaction, per millimeter. Each interpretation has its benefits.

The microscopic view

The interaction of electromagnetic radiation with matter depends on the energy of the photons and on the makeup of the material

Photons across the spectrum of frequencies and energies come into being in different ways, and they also interact dissimilarly with matter (Figure 2.2b).

Visible-light photons are absorbed in raising outermost-shell electrons of atoms to vacant, slightly higher-lying energy states. And photons of these energies are likely to be emitted when the just excited atoms and molecules relax to their ground states. Absorption and re-emission of photons striking a smooth metal surface occur so rapidly that they are said to be reflected. Non-radiative relaxation mechanisms exist at these energies as well. Light energy hitting black cloth is absorbed and degraded into heat. In photosynthesis, de-excitation of an optically excited chlorophyll molecule involves many electrochemical steps, through which some of the original photon's energy ends up stored in the high-energy phosphate bonds of ATP.

Infrared, or heat, photons are of lower energies (0.1–1.8 eV) than those in the visible range, and are absorbed and emitted principally through changes in the quantized vibrational states of molecules or solids. As an example, the environmental green-house effect occurs because visible sunlight easily passes through the atmosphere and is absorbed by the Earth's surface. Most of this energy is transformed into heat in the process, but some is re-emitted back away from Earth as lower-frequency infrared radiation, and is subsequently absorbed by carbon dioxide, water, methane, and certain other atmospheric gases, since it causes transitions among their vibrational states. Too much of this will lead to a continuing warming of the air, melting of glaciers, rise in sea level, large-scale climate changes, and, if unchecked, environmental catastrophe. It's no more complicated than putting a heavier blanket (more anthropogenic CO_2) onto something that gives off energy (re-emitted sunlight): everything gets hotter, just as predicted by the voluminous work of virtually all independent climate scientists.

Microwave photons, in the gigahertz (GHz, 10^9 Hz) range, induce and are generated in transitions among the vibrational and rotational states of molecules. The radiation in a microwave oven excites such modes in water molecules, for example, resulting in the "frictional" heating and cooking of food.

With *radio waves*, in the lower-frequency regions of the spectrum, it is the wave-like attributes that are most apparent, which is why the physical dimensions of a radio antenna are usually comparable to the wavelength of the radiation coming from the transmitter. Below 100 MHz or so, in particular, there exists a window into the body through which EM radiation can pass readily. This radiofrequency (RF) radiation can, in highly special circumstances involving the application of a strong external magnetic field, be made to interact with atomic nuclei (especially the nuclei of ordinary hydrogen atoms, i.e., lone protons) by means of the nuclear magnetic resonance (NMR) phenomenon – which is the basis for MRI.

On the other, high-energy side of the visible and ultraviolet, it is collisions of predominantly particle-like *X-ray* and *gamma-ray photons* with *orbital electrons* of atoms in tissues and in IRs that underlie the formation of images.

The most and the least energetic of these radiations differ in energy by about twelve orders of magnitude – by a factor of 10^{12} – but they are inherently all the same kind of wave-particles. They are produced in radically dissimilar ways, however, over the possible range of their energies. Also, they interact with matter by way of very different physical mechanisms, again depending on their energies and on the properties of the materials they come across.

This chapter will concentrate on *ionizing* EM radiation – X-rays and gamma-rays. The issue of underlying importance in X-ray imaging (apart from patient dose) is the relationship between the rate of attenuation of a beam along a geometric ray – which is to say, the spatial rate at which X-ray photons are interacting with the atoms of tissues or IR materials with the thickness or depth, *x*, that they traverse. The six curves of Figure 3.7, obtained in the manner of Figures 3.6, are all near-exponentials (Equations 3.1), straight lines on semi-log paper that plots intensity, $I(x)$, against *x*. The slope ($\Delta y/\Delta x$) of each is the linear attenuation coefficient, $\mu = -[\Delta I/I]/\Delta x$.

There are two distinct monochromatic photon energies considered in the figure, 40 keV and 80 keV, and for all three materials being examined, lung,

muscle, and bone, the 40 keV curve is steeper: for all three of them, $\mu(40 \text{ keV}) > \mu(80 \text{ keV})$. Indeed, as a general rule with an important exception, the lower the beam effective energy, the greater the rate of interactions and the faster the attenuation.

What about the materials? Normal lung tissue is biochemically almost the same as other soft tissues, such as muscle, but it is typically one third as dense, which explains the factor of three difference in μ at each of the two energies. The difference between muscle and bone is due partly to their densities, but even more so to their chemical makeup, notably the greater *Z* of the calcium within the bony cortex. But to make sense of this, we shall need to examine the two key mechanisms by which X-rays interact with atomic orbital electrons.

Two principal mechanisms for the interaction of gamma- and X-ray photons with atomic electrons: photoelectric absorption and Compton scatter

Diagnostic-energy X-ray photons (20–150 keV) can interact with atoms and thereby be removed from a beam in several ways, but normally only two of them are significant in image formation: photoelectric absorption and Compton scatter. For each of these, it will be valuable to find explicit expressions relating how the linear attenuation coefficient (hence the spatial rate of attenuation of a beam) depends on the density, ρ, and effective atomic number, *Z*, of the material, and on the effective beam energy, E: $\mu = \mu(\rho, Z, E)$.

In a PA interaction (encountered also in the previous chapter, but for light and albeit at much lower energies), an incident photon of high energy, hf_{in}, from an X-ray tube (or a gamma-ray from a radioactive nucleus) collides with an unwary atomic electron, in tissue, or in the radiosensitive material of an IR, etc., and the electric field of the photon interacts strongly with that of the charged electron (Figure 3.8a). Apart from some of the photon's energy expended in breaking the electron's bond to its nucleus, E_b, nearly all of its energy is conveyed to the ejected *photoelectron* as kinetic energy, KE_{PA}: high-energy photon in, high-energy photoelectron out, and that's it:

$$hf_{\text{in}} = E_b + KE_{\text{PA}}. \qquad (3.2a)$$

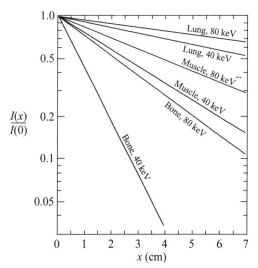

Figure 3.7 When a beam of high-energy photons passes through a block of material, the relative amount of X-ray energy that is transmitted through, or removed from, it is determined by three characteristics of the *matter*: its *thickness*; its *density*; and its *chemical makeup*, in particular the effective atomic number, *Z*. Transmission also depends on the *energy* of the *photons*, *E*. These six curves, straight on semi-log paper, demonstrate idealized exponential attenuation by two soft tissues of different densities (muscle and lung) and by bone, all obtained at two monochromatic photon energies.

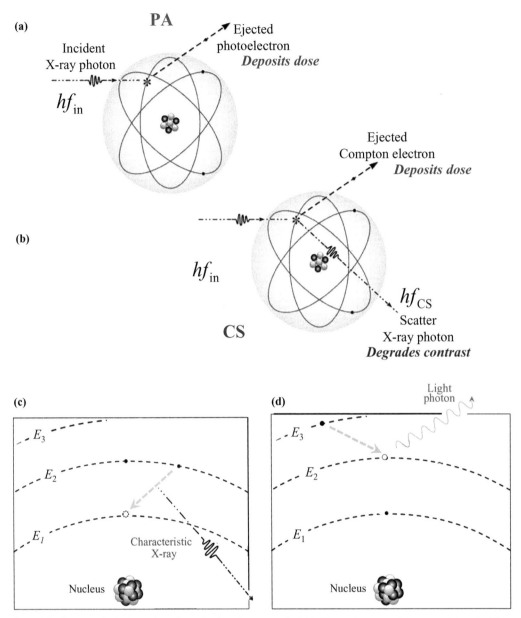

Figure 3.8 The two principal atomic-scale mechanisms by means of which diagnostic-energy photons can interact with the atomic electrons in matter. (**a**) In a *photoelectric absorption* (PA) event, an incident gamma- or X-ray photon of energy hf_{in} collides with and transfers practically all its energy to an orbital electron, ionizing the atom. In so doing, the photon is removed from the beam, contributing to the creation of the primary X-ray image. Also critically important but for another reason, the photon ejects the electron (hereafter called a *photoelectron*), which leaves the scene of the encounter at very high velocity and kinetic energy. Any photon that manages to pass through a patient is highly likely to interact with the image receptor (IR), by way of a photoelectric event, and excite it. (**b**) A *Compton scatter interaction* (CS) is similar, except that only some of the incident photon's energy ends up as kinetic energy of the ejected *Compton electron*; most, in fact, goes to a newly created *Compton scatter photon*, hf_{CS}. Some such scatter photons from tissues may escape the body and strike the IR at random locations, creating scatter noise and degrading image contrast. (**c**) After a photoelectric or Compton event, the just-ionized atom will be in an unstable "excited" state, with an electron vacancy in some shell; it immediately de-excites with the emission of a *characteristic X-ray* or (**d**) if only outer orbitals are involved, of visible light.

As we shall see, it is the PA interactions that are primarily responsible for the creation of contrast in an image produced with X-rays. And nearly all the energy of the photoelectron ends up as radiation dose, deposited either in tissue or in the IR.

With the *Compton scatter* interaction of Figure 3.8b, the incident photon transfers a part of its energy to the ejected *Compton electron*, and most of it goes to a somewhat lower-energy, newly created *Compton scatter photon*: X-ray photon in, Compton electron *and* high-energy Compton scatter photon out,

$$hf_{in} = KE_{CS} + hf_{CS}. \qquad (3.2b)$$

Because Compton interactions commonly involve outer-lying, loosely attached outer atomic orbitals, the binding energy is negligible. CS interactions do not contribute much to the creation of contrast, except in lung where the tissue density differentials can be substantial; indeed, they are notable mainly for the hazy noise imparted to a radiograph by the randomly scattered photons that happen to reach the IR. And Compton electrons, like photoelectrons, deposit dose.

Soon after any PA or CS event, the just-ionized atom is left in an unstable "excited" state, commonly with an electron vacancy in an inner shell, in this case the $n = 1$, K shell (Figure 3.8c). The atom de-excites when an electron from a higher (e.g., $n = 2$) orbital drops into the vacancy, with the emission of a *characteristic X-ray*. If there remain vacancies in further-out orbitals, a downward cascade of atomic electrons will continue within the atom, concluding typically with the emission of a visible light photon (Figure 3.8d).

There is a third photon-electron mechanism, known variously as *Rayleigh, elastic, coherent,* and *classical scattering*; a photon approaches and enters an atom but flies away in a new direction, like a comet swinging around the sun. It is a weak event, and negligible except for the very low photon energies of mammography; it adds slightly to scatter, but deposits no dose.

The rate of beam attenuation increases with density

Again, the four factors that determine μ and how effectively an organ will imprint a clinically meaningful pattern in the X-ray beam emerging from the patient are: the local thicknesses, densities, and chemical compositions of the tissues, and the effec-

tive energy of the photons: $\mu = \mu(\rho, Z, E)$, as was suggested in Figures 1.6a and 2.9a. The implications of this are apparent from Figure 3.7.

For both photoelectric and Compton interactions, the rate of beam attenuation, as parameterized by μ, is directly proportional to *tissue density*: $\mu \sim \rho$.

Suppose a block of healthy lung, or of foam rubber, is x cm thick, and you compress it to one third its original thickness, so that it ends up with three times the starting density (Figure 3.9a). The product (ρx) becomes $(3\rho \times x/3)$, which is unaffected by the compression. In addition, because the total number of atoms in the beam path is the same, the attenuation by the block, $I(x)/I(0)$ of Equation 3.1a, is also unchanged, as is $e^{-\mu x}$ and therefore (μx), as well. But if both (μx) and (ρx) remain fixed during compression, the same must be true of their quotient, $(\mu x)/(\rho x) = [\mu/\rho]$. Finally, $[\mu/\rho]$ is constant during compression if and only if $\mu \sim \rho$. The ratio $[\mu/\rho]$ in which the density is divided out, is a sometimes useful entity known as the *mass attenuation coefficient*.

It is the dependence of μ on ρ alone that is often responsible for the detection of higher-density tissue irregularities in lung (Figure 3.9b,c).

Figure 3.10a displays the linear attenuation coefficient as a function of monochromatic photon energy, $\mu(E)$, for four materials of interest: lung, muscle, bone, and lead used for radiation shielding. At an energy of about 20 keV, say, the attenuation coefficient of muscle, in particular, is μ_{muscle} $(20\ keV) = 0.9\ cm^{-1}$. This is three times that of lung: $\mu_{lung}(20\ keV) = 0.3\ cm^{-1}$, which is the same as the ratio of their densities. No surprise here! You will find this same ratio for muscle and lung at all other photon energies as well. Values of μ for bone and lead are greater, and this is due, in part, to their greater densities – but not entirely. Something else very important is going on as well, involving their chemical makeup!

The photoelectric linear attenuation coefficient, μ_{PA}, depends on the chemical composition of the tissue or image receptor and on the effective energy of the beam; the Compton coefficient, μ_{CS}, is virtually independent of both

Some images reveal tissues, by way of both the PA and CS effects, that differ primarily in terms of their densities, as with lung tumors or regions

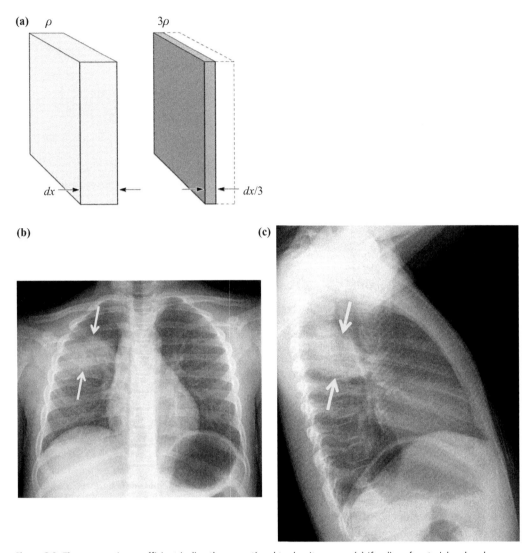

Figure 3.9 The attenuation coefficient is directly proportional to density, $\mu \sim \rho$. (a) If a slice of material such as lung or foam rubber is compressed, (ρx), $I(x)$, and therefore (μx) remain the same, so the ratio $[\mu/\rho]$ must do so, as well, which means that μ is linearly proportional to ρ. (b) This patient presented with a productive cough, fever and chest pain. His physician, suspecting a pneumonia, ordered an upright chest X-ray in the PA and (c) left lateral projections. The whitish density within the right lung field represents a focus of infection or pneumonia of the posterior segment of the upper lobe (arrows). The infection fills the otherwise air-filled alveoli with fluid (either exudative or purulent), giving it a density similar to that of the heart, since the density of the fluid is significantly higher than that of the normal adjacent alveoli. The pair of orthogonal views enables one to localize the infiltrate precisely.

of pneumonia (Figure 3.9b,c). (Muscle and water are radiologically similar.) Differences in density and thickness always contribute at least somewhat to contrast, but in the many situations the PA effect happens to play the dominant role, and contrast may be affected even much more by the chemical composition of materials and the photon energy.

With muscle, for example, μ_{total} is partitioned into μ_{PA} (red and yellow) and μ_{CS} (blue and yellow) in Figure 3.10b. It appears that $\mu_{\text{total}}(20 \text{ keV}) = 0.9$ cm^{-1}, and $\mu_{\text{CS}}(20 \text{ keV}) = 0.2$ cm^{-1}. So, although it is difficult to read from the graph, it must be from their difference that $\mu_{\text{PA}}(20 \text{ keV}) = 0.7$ cm^{-1}.

Let's first address the Compton component for muscle, μ_{CS}, since it is simpler. In fact, apart from

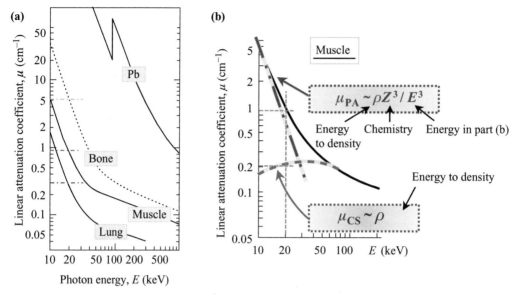

Figure 3.10 The nature of the interaction of high-energy photons with matter is determined by the density and chemical composition of the medium and by the energy of the photons. (a) $\mu(\rho, Z, E)$ is plotted against monochromatic $E = hf$ for lung and muscle soft tissues, bone, and lead, with values indicated for $hf = 20$ keV. Compare the ratio of $\mu(20$ keV) values for lung and muscle with that of their densities. (b) The separation of $\mu(E)$ for muscle into its photoelectric and Compton components. $\mu_{CS}(\rho, Z, hf)$ is nearly independent of Z and E, but is linear in tissue density: $\mu_{CS}(\rho, Z, hf) \sim \rho$. The photoelectric coefficient is of the form $\mu_{PA}(\rho, Z, E) \sim \rho\, Z^3/E^3$.

the factor of ρ, μ_{CS} is virtually the same for all substances. It depends only very weakly on Z, and we can pretty much forget about it: the whole blue dotted curve will be scaled and shifted up or down by the density, but it is otherwise nearly oblivious to the material. In addition, for the energy region of interest, $\mu_{CS}(E)$ is a flat and horizontal function of photon energy, E, as well. To summarize: at diagnostic energies,

$$\mu_{CS}(\rho, Z, E) \sim \mu_{CS}(\rho) = \rho\times\text{constant}_{CS}. \quad (3.3a)$$

The photoelectric effect has a more interesting narrative. Recall that a prism splits apart the constituent colors of white light because the degree of interaction of the incident photons with the atomic electrons in the glass depends on their energy (Figure 2.5c). Likewise for the PA interactions of gamma- and X-rays with the inner (primarily) orbital electrons in tissues and other materials. The general rule is that *more* energetic photons are *less* likely to be absorbed. $\mu_{PA}(E)$ falls off rapidly with energy for muscle as the red and yellow dashed line in Figure 3.10b. This plot has been made on *log*-

log graph paper, the virtue of which is that it shows *power-law* functions as straight lines; note the scales on the two axes. In this case, $\mu_{PA}(E) \sim 1/E^3$, where the power (the exponent, 3) has been learned easily because it is the slope of the straight red and yellow dashed line.

X-ray photons are more inclined to interact by way of the PA effect, moreover, with atoms of higher effective atomic number. Indeed, the photoelectric coefficient happens to vary approximately with the third power of Z:

$$\mu_{PA}(\rho, Z, E) \sim \rho Z^3/E^3. \quad (3.3b)$$

Finally, the curve for lead (Pb) in Figure 3.10a displays a perhaps unanticipated discontinuity. Lead's *absorption K-edge* occurs exactly at the ionization/binding energy of the element's innermost, most tightly held, K-shell electrons. X-rays with energies less than the K-edge cannot eject these electrons from their orbitals, but those with energy even slightly greater than it *can* do so – a new interaction mechanism is now available, in effect, namely K-electron photoelectric events, and so

μ as a function of E jumps abruptly upward there.

This K-edge phenomenon can be put to good use in designing X-ray contrast media. Iodine happens to have a large absorption edge at 33.2 keV, and for photons above this, the element suddenly becomes significantly more attenuating. A photon with energy above the edge that is incident on a blood vessel containing a high concentration of iodine therefore has a particularly high probability of undergoing PA. And since the edge occurs in the middle of the bremsstrahlung energy range for typical kVp settings, much of the beam will be removed by the vessel (but not by the surrounding soft tissues). So the K-edge, with its jump in the rate of attenuation at 33.2 keV, is a major reason, along with its high atomic number (Z = 53) and density, that iodine is so widely adopted as a vascular contrast agent. Likewise, barium (Z = 56) has a K-edge at 37.4, and serves often as a contrast agent for the gastrointestinal tract.

Now to put it all together – literally. Fact of life: the probabilities of mutually exclusive events are additive. Imagine that 2 of the 100 used cars on a lot are gorgeous, American-made Corvettes, and 4% are ugly dirtbag Porches; then the total odds of your selecting one or the other of these two types at random (i.e., with your eyes closed) would be 6%. Now, recall that μ was defined earlier not only as a spatial rate of attenuation, but also the *probability of interaction per unit distance*. A photoelectric absorption event and a Compton scatter are mutually exclusive – a given incoming photon cannot do both at the same time. (A Compton scatter photon, of course, can undergo a subsequent CS or PA interaction, but that's a different matter.) So the attenuation coefficients for the two processes are simply additive:

$$\mu = \mu_{PA} + \mu_{CS}. \qquad (3.3c)$$

And that, in turn, is why we can consider the two processes completely separately, combining their impacts here, at the end.

Why the rate of photoelectric absorption declines so rapidly with photon energy

One last thing, before we leave the topic of attenuation mechanisms. It may have surprised you that the photoelectric coefficient depends so strongly on Z and E, while the Compton does not.

Here's a quick, hand-waving explanation. As is usually the case with billiards or pool, a Compton collision is a three-body event, involving the incident photon, the ejected Compton electron, and the newly-created CS photon. And as with billiards, both momentum and energy are conserved during the event, and for scattering through any angle.

Now consider a photoelectric event involving a free, unattached electron far off in outer space. This would be a two-body affair: the incident photon would transfer all of its energy to the liberated photoelectron. While such a thing can be OK with pool, it simply cannot occur for a photon and an electron: the electron has mass and the photon does not, and therefore it happens that momentum and energy cannot be conserved simultaneously in this two-body event, so it just never occurs. (Check it out – the momentum of a photon is E/c.)

Since simple one-photon, one-electron events are forbidden, any interaction between a photon and an electron must involve a third body as well. And in practice, a normal PA event actually *is* a three-body collision: the struck electron is bound to the nucleus, with which it can share energy and momentum. The catch is that the greater the photon energy, hf_{in}, the less relevant is the attachment of the electron to the nucleus, and the more the situation resembles that of a free electron, which is forbidden – and the probability of interaction decreases. Conversely, the greater the Z, the more the inner-orbital electrons are *un*like free ones, and the greater $\mu_{PA}(Z)$ becomes.

In short, Compton interactions hardly care what an electron is attached to; they just go for it, and the greater the density of atomic electrons (electrons/cc), the better. Photoelectric events, however, favor lower energy photons, and inner-orbital electrons on higher-Z atoms. CS interactions become prevalent in lower-Z tissues and at high energies – not because μ_{CS} increases, but rather because PA occurrences become so scarce.

What a body does to the beam: subject contrast in the pattern of X-rays emerging from the patient

Contrast is usually the issue of paramount concern for any sort of medical imaging. For the X-ray modalities, it comes from *differential* attenuation by the various tissues. And while strong attenuation by any one tissue, or by all of them, does not necessarily imply high contrast, the two are related – and we can manipulate aspects of the photoelectric and Compton effect probabilities to increase the contrast and the clinical utility in a diagnostic procedure.

Figures 3.10a and b indicate that Compton scatter is the principal photon-electron mechanism at higher energies and in soft (low Z) tissues, and that contrast among them comes from density differences, as with lung neoplasms and pneumonia.

The PA effect is dominant at lower E and in higher-Z materials, and it is largely responsible for subject contrast between soft tissues and bone, pieces of metal, microcalcifications in breast, and other objects composed of "heavier" elements.

Differential photoelectric absorption produces most of the subject contrast in the primary X-ray image

The X-ray beam entering the patient's body is nearly uniform and relatively strong. What emerges from the far side is weak and spatially modulated, containing an X-ray (as opposed to visible light) pattern that indicates what lies within. In a typical chest radiograph, roughly 99 out of every 100 X-ray photons that enter the body are absorbed or scattered by its atoms and removed from the beam. Thus, only about 1% of the beam's original photons

pass through the patient unscathed. (Several times that amount of CS radiation may have been created in and leave the body, but that normally contains no useful information.) Embedded in this remnant beam, however, is an X-ray shadow, the *primary X-ray image*, which indicates the spatial distribution of the variously attenuating tissues or other objects within the body.

Image contrast describes the ability of an image or imaging system to somehow distinguish different adjacent tissues from one another through visible differences. It is determined by two largely independent factors: *subject contrast* in the pattern of X-rays emerging from the patient, and *image receptor contrast*, a term that covers any attribute of the equipment that gives rise to an amplification or loss of subject contrast. This chapter will consider only the subject contrast itself, as caused by the body; the next will consider IR and image contrast.

Unlike the situation of the "attenuation coefficient," there is no single correct way to define "contrast" between two regions of tissue – the best you can do is find something that works for your purposes. In Figure 3.11a, we can adopt about as straightforward an expression as possible for *image contrast*: the strength of the optical brightness or luminance, L, on the monitor coming from the

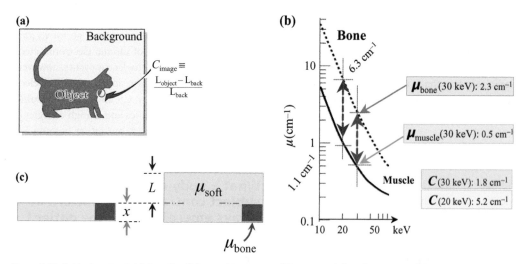

Figure 3.11 Subject contrast. (a) Equation 3.4a provides one possible way to define the contrast. (b) At energies where the photoelectric effect is significant, subject contrast generally improves with lower kVp. (c) You may wish to convince yourself that adding a layer of soft tissue of thickness *L* causes a rise in attenuation throughout, but by itself does not affect contrast; the additional material provides opportunity for more Compton scatter, however, which *does* decrease contrast.

object of interest is L_{object}, and that from background is $L_{background}$, so we might set:

$$C_{image} \equiv (L_{object} - L_{back})/L_{back}. \qquad (3.4a)$$

Working backward from this image contrast suggests that *before* the X-rays reach the IR, it might be appropriate to define *subject contrast* as, say,

$$C_{subject} \equiv (I_2 - I_1)/(I_2 + I_1), \qquad (3.4b)$$

in terms of the X-ray intensity, I, exiting the body at two nearby points. Even more simply,

$$C_{subject} \equiv (\mu_2 - \mu_1), \qquad (3.4c)$$

might do, assuming that the two materials of interest are equally thin. Again, none of these is *the* definition of contrast, but rather examples of several that may happen to work for our purposes.

Consider, for example, the contrast between a bone and the adjacent soft tissue (Figure 3.11b). With 30 keV photons, the linear attenuation coefficients for bone and muscle are 2.3 and 0.5 cm^{-1}, respectively, so the subject contrast, by Equation 3.4c is $C_{subject}(30 \text{ keV}) = \mu_{bone}(30) - \mu_{muscle}(30) = 1.8 \text{ cm}^{-1}$. Repeating this for 20 keV gives the considerably greater $C_{subject}$ (20 keV) $= 6.3 \text{ cm}^{-1} - 1.1 \text{ cm}^{-1} = 5.2 \text{ cm}^{-1}$. Either way, adding a uniform-thickness overlay of muscle (or anything else) will increase the attenuation everywhere by the same amount, so *that* alone will not affect the contrast – but the additional material will generate more Compton scatter, and that can diminish the effective subject contrast (Figure 3.11c).

The moral of this little tale is one of great practical importance in X-ray imaging: in situations where the photoelectric effect is assuming the dominant role, lowering the photon energy generally yields higher subject contrast! Need a clearer image? Then turn down the kVp. This is the reason that mammography is often carried out with the 19 keV characteristic X-rays from a molybdenum target. An important exception to this rule is when imaging with iodine or barium contrast agents, where it is often better to raise the kVp to take advantage of the greater attenuation above their K-edges.

The price to pay for lowering the photon energy, of course, is less beam penetration, and therefore more dose deposition, as will soon be seen. In such cases, it must be felt that more is gained in quality of diagnostic information than lost in radiation risk.

Compton scatter mainly reduces subject contrast in the primary X-ray beam...

Blue skies and hazy days result from the scattering of light by air molecules and fine droplets of water vapor. Otherwise, the sun would shine brightly white against a star-flecked black backdrop, as could the morning moon. Similarly, the bottom of a lazy river is lost from view if too much light becomes scattered by its suspended silt.

Just as the stars actually do vanish at sunrise, and the features of the river bottom disappear in murkiness, so also radiologic images are obscured by CS photons. The X-ray photons that emerge from a body and reach the film cassette can be thought of as falling into two general categories. *Primary* photons have undergone no interactions whatsoever within the patient, and it is the faint X-ray shadow they transport that can be captured and transformed into visual information. Compton-*scattered* photons, on the other hand, leave their scatter points heading every which way, and a number of them may strike the IR randomly and in oblique trajectories, adding a mist of visual noise and degrading contrast significantly. The effect of scatter on subject contrast was apparent in Figure 2.14a, a radiograph of the pelvic region before and after a large fraction of the scatter radiation is removed by means of a grid.

A simple parameter useful in discussing scatter is the scatter-to-primary (*S/P*) ratio, which is the level of scatter radiation energy relative to that of the image-forming primary radiation in an X-ray shadowgram pattern. The reduction of subject contrast with too much *S/P* can be expressed as $C_{subject} = C_P / (1 + S/P)$, where C_P refers to contrast in the primary X-ray image, without scatter. An important objective of radiography clearly must be to keep scatter to as low a level as possible, but without loss of too much image-bearing, primary radiation.

As much as 90% of the photons exiting a body may be scatter. The factors most important in determining the amount generated in a patient are the cross-sectional area of the beam, the thickness of the body part being imaged, and the kVp. The dependences on beam size and on thickness of (or depth within) the patient, for example, appear in Figure 3.12a for a 100 kVp beam. With a very small field and thin patient, little scatter is produced, and the *S/P* ratio is close to zero. *S/P* at the center of the field (Figure 3.12b), point **A**, grows rapidly with increasing field size, however, and subject contrast drops

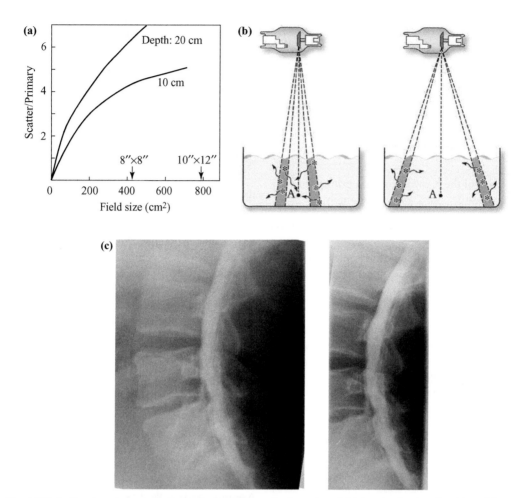

Figure 3.12 Scatter degrades contrast. The scatter-to-primary ratio depends on field size, the depth and position of the point of interest within the body, and the energy of the beam. **(a)** The field-size dependence of the *S/P* ratio, between scatter radiation intensity and image-bearing primary radiation along the central axis at two depths for a 100 kVp beam. **(b)** The intensity of *primary* photons at point A is independent of field size, but that is not the case for scatter. When the field has already become large, however, additional scatter volume brought into play by enlarging it further does not affect the dose to point A much, because most Compton photons do not scatter that far. **(c)** Improvement in contrast with reduced field size for a lateral myelogram of the lumbar spine. Overall patient exposure has not scaled down linearly with width, however, because with less scatter reaching the cassette, it was necessary to increase the tube current by 50% for sufficient irradiation of it, to yield an adequate overall level of darkening. Modified from American College of Radiology (ACR) Teaching File images.

off; more tissue is exposed, as also in Figure 3.12c, and there is more irradiated tissue producing scatter. The ratio levels off for wider fields of dimensions that exceed the mean free pathlength of the scatter photons – when a field is already quite large, additional scatter photons will be created at the field edges with a further increment in size, of course, but few of them will reach point **A**.

There are several ways to cut back on the amount of scatter radiation produced in the first place. The most obvious is to minimize the field size of the beam, while still covering the full region of clinical interest, so that less tissue is irradiated; this not only reduces scatter production, but also the volume of tissue at potential stochastic risk from irradiation. The immediate benefit of reduced field size on image quality is evident in Figure 3.12c for a pair of lateral myelograms of the lumbar spine. The contrast and visibility of detail improve considerably with tighter beam collimation.

In addition, the scatter radiation dose to health-care staff may be considerably less, especially during fluoroscopy, and the overall dose deposition to the patient may be lowered – even if the tube current has to be increased somewhat to maintain an adequate average level of apparent image brightness.

A second approach is to set the kVp to lower values, decreasing beam penetration, hence scatter creation near the beam-exit side of the patient, but at the expense of higher dose. Another, as is done routinely in mammography, is to compress the tissue, reducing its thickness; other benefits of compression are that it diminishes dose, keeps down motion blurring, and spreads out the tissues being viewed so as to reduce the overlapping of the various signals produced at different depths in it.

Fortunately, much of the scatter that does exit the body can be removed by an *anti-scatter grid* before striking the film cassette.

... But a grid can remove much of the scatter radiation, at the price of more patient dose

It is possible to reduce the amount of scatter, once it exists, that eventually reaches the IR. An *anti-scatter grid* acts somewhat like a Venetian blind and can remove 85% or more of the Compton photons (Figures 3.13 and 2.14a). Consisting of thin lead louvers separated by nearly radio-translucent spacer material like fiber or aluminum, an ideal grid lets through only those X-rays that have not undergone scattering within the patient, and are

still traveling along the straight and narrow in their original direction; those that come in at an angle, after scattering, are absorbed in the lead strips. The shadows of the lead sheets in a static grid may appear as thin parallel lines in the image, but a *Bucky grid* is moved rapidly a few centimeters during an exposure to blur them out. There are other techniques of scatter reduction, as well, such as introducing an *air gap* between patient and IR that provides space for some scatter photons to escape to the sides of the beam. Similarly, with a *scanning slot* method, a thin fan beam and a narrow collimator and the IR are moved in synchrony, but relatively slowly, along the patient, and provide some scatter rejection.

The downside of a grid or air gap is that the mA-s must be raised to compensate for the reduction in the number of X-ray photons striking the IR, with a corresponding increase in patient dose.

What the beam does to a body: dose and risk

We have already discussed *photon-electron* (PA and CS) interactions at some length. There is a different, but equally important, kind of atomic-scale interaction, and it is *not* between an incident X-ray *photon* and an orbital electron. It involves an *electron-electron* collision, rather, between a high-energy photo- or Compton electron (ejected during another, slightly earlier PA or CS event nearby) and an atomic orbital electron. Such electron-electron collisions are the basis of dose deposition in tissues,

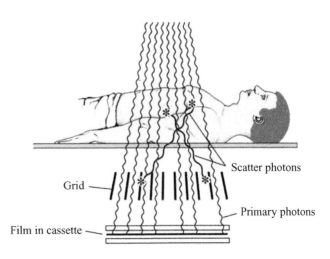

Figure 3.13 A grid reduces the loss of contrast caused by scatter. Most of the primary, image-bearing X-ray photons run nearly parallel to and between the lead leaves of the grid, and reach the film; with a "focused" grid, the lead sheets are aligned to account for the natural divergence of the X-ray beam. Most CS photons from the body enter the grid at an angle and are absorbed by the leaves. The effectiveness of a grid is determined largely by the length, thickness, and separation of the lead sheets, as is the amount by which the mA-s must be raised when the grid is adopted.

Scatter photons

Grid

Primary photons

Film in cassette

which is always undesirable, but also in IRs, which is absolutely essential to their functioning.

In tissues, all the dose is deposited by ejected high-energy photoelectrons and Compton electrons (but in a high-Z image receptor, only by photoelectrons)

Ejected at high velocity from its atom by a single photon, a newly-liberated photo- or Compton electron flashes through matter and interacts with many *thousands* of atomic electrons that it passes, via the electric (Coulombic) force between charged bodies (Figure 3.14a). Again as with pool balls, a very fast electron enters an atom at high velocity, and it and another electron leave immediately, at odd angles and at somewhat lesser speeds. In this manner, the incident electron and those it sets in motion all rapidly disperse their energy in ionizing hundreds or thousands of other atoms along their tortuous tracks (Figure 3.14b). They deposit their energy as radiation dose, and this has vitally important consequences, for both worse and better, in two very different settings – in the patient's tissues, and in the IR.

First, the "for worse." As will be considered more deeply in Chapter 5, even small amounts of *ionizing* radiation can cause *stochastic* transformations in cellular DNA in ways that may lead, albeit extremely rarely, to radiogenic carcinogenesis. In addition, an improperly maintained or utilized piece of diagnos-

tic equipment may put out much more dose than it should, even occasionally giving rise to skin burns and other *deterministic* health effects. So while it is critical to employ enough radiation to form clinically adequate images, at the same time patient (and staff) dose should be maintained ALARA.

Now for the "for better": as discussed in the next chapter, a photon emerging from the patient will usually interact with an IR by way of the PA mechanisms, because it is commonly composed of high-Z materials. The ejected fast photoelectron will ionize and excite the IR's active material, such as a fluorescent screen that emits a tiny burst of detectable visible light (Figure 2.6c). Too little dose will lead to too few points of light and thus a noisy, mottled image. Too much exposure, on the other hand, may give terrific pictures, but at the price of far too much patient dose. Radiographers prefer to avoid an underexposure, which requires a re-take, so they tend to give their physicians nice pictures by intentionally turning up the mA-s a little (or, sometimes, a lot) more than needed. This approach is not possible with film – the whole sheet turns black – but it is with digital. Despite the excess patient dose, this is becoming a fairly common practice with digital systems, and has given rise to the slightly callous expression "*Burn, don't return*." It is necessary to counteract this phenomenon, known as *dose creep*, and attitude through proper training and oversight, and a solid quality assurance and radiation safety program.

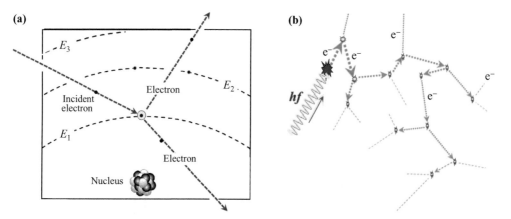

Figure 3.14 Critically important role of the ejected photoelectric and Compton electrons. **(a)** While PA and CS events are the first step in image formation, **(b)** the liberated photo- and Compton electrons then act out their own critically important parts – not in image creation but in dose deposition (in tissues and/or in the IR).

Selection of the kVp: the great contrast versus dose tradeoff

There is an important tradeoff between subject contrast and patient dose that comes up frequently in selecting the kVp. An IR such as a screen-film combination tends to be a good deal less sensitive to the kVp setting than is $C_{subject}$, so selecting the best technique factors for a radiograph might seem straightforward: choose a kVp for which the relative differences among the attenuation coefficients of the tissues of importance are greatest, then find a suitable screen-film combination, and finally dial up an mA-s to result in a visually pleasing overall average level of brightness. That would mean using as low a kVp as you can get away with. Reality, of course, is never so simple, and the main complicating factors here are the patient thickness and the patient dose.

When the kVp is too low, the beam is not adequately penetrating, and its intensity will fall off too fast. The intensity entering the body therefore has to be made high for enough X-rays to transit and exit and produce an acceptable average radiation level at the IR – and that means a great deal of radiation dose being deposited along the way, suggested by the area under the red line in Figure 3.15a. But increasing the beam energy to reduce the dose, under the blue line, also means lowering the subject contrast. A major tradeoff! The kVp needs to be low enough for adequate (but not necessarily best possible) subject contrast, but sufficiently high for good penetration, hence acceptable dose.

With a bone chip in a 23 cm thick part of a patient, for example, the middle curve and the right-hand scale of Figure 3.15b record the steady

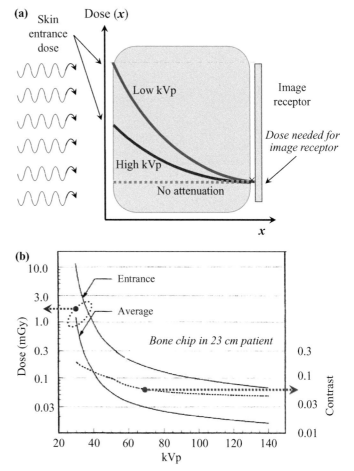

Figure 3.15 The tradeoff between contrast and dose. (a) The higher the kVp, the more penetrating the beam, and the less the intensity at the entrance skin surface needed to provide the exposure level required to activate the IR. And the amount of ionizing radiation deposited in the tissue as dose will therefore also be lower. (b) The dependence on the kVp of the entrance and average doses to soft tissue (scale to the left) in a 23-cm thick subject, and on the contrast of a 1-mm thick bone chip. The contrast improves as the kVp is lowered, but the entrance dose (averaged over the top 1 cm of tissue) and the average dose (over the full 23 cm) increase much more rapidly. These curves suggest that it might be reasonable to set the balance in the 60–80 kVp range. Modified from Bushberg JT, Seibert JA, Leidholdt, Jr. EM, Boone JM, *The Essential Physics of Medical Imaging*, 2nd edn, Philadelphia, PA: Lippincott, Williams, and Wilkins, 2002, fig. 6-21.

decline in contrast as the applied voltage increases. The two other curves reveal that, as expected, both the entrance skin dose and the average body dose for the region fall off with kVp. Imaging centers normally prepare *technique factor charts* to standardize the technique factors to be used by the radiographers for routine examinations, based on studies like those of the figure, but much of that business has become automated for digital devices. A general rule for dealing with the kVp is that when the subject contrast is intrinsically strong, as in the imaging of a bone or barium-coated bowel or a thick iodine-filled vessel, dial in as high a tube potential as possible while preserving adequate clinical contrast.

In mammography, conversely, the contrast is naturally poor, and there is a need to squeeze as much of it out of the system as is possible, so one has to work at lower potentials (about 20 keV). Except for very large breasts, the thickness will not be excessive under compression, and the dose and assumed risk will generally be acceptable relative to the benefit of a good examination.

In conclusion, physicians who read images have a range of needs for what constitutes "good enough" contrast, with which they can feel comfortable and confident making a diagnostic call. The operative phrase is "*clinically good enough.*" In digital imaging, in particular, it is always possible to improve the contrast-to-noise balance and generate a "perfect" image that physicians will love, but at the price of much higher level of irradiation. An image has to be good enough to be clinically trustworthy, but going much beyond that, to the aesthetically pleasing phase, is generally not a good thing for the patient.

CHAPTER 4

Twentieth-century (Analog) Radiography and Fluoroscopy

Capturing the X-ray Shadow with a Film Cassette or an Image Intensifier Tube plus Electronic Optical Camera Combination

We have just considered the production of a nearly uniform X-ray beam, and the subsequent interaction of its high-energy photons with materials within a body. The primary objective, in most cases, is to generate a clinically adequate degree of subject contrast in the emerging X-ray shadowgram. That part of the story is nearly the same for all forms of X-ray imaging: screen-film radiography, intensifier tube-based fluoroscopy, computed radiogra-phy, digital radiography, digital fluoroscopy, digital subtraction angiography, conventional or digital planar tomography, computed tomography, and others. What differs among them is not the creation of the X-ray shadowgram but, rather, the way in which that shadowgram is captured and made suitable for display.

The image receptor (IR) still employed most widely throughout the world is radiographic film

Medical Imaging: Essentials for Physicians, First Edition. Anthony B. Wolbarst, Patrizio Capasso and Andrew R. Wyant.
© 2013 John Wiley & Sons, Inc. Published 2013 by John Wiley & Sons, Inc.

within a cassette. Perhaps the second is fluoroscopy making use of an image intensifier (II) tube plus an electronic optical camera combination. Here we shall deal with these two analog forms of imaging, and turn to the digital ones in subsequent chapters.

Recording the X-ray pattern emerging from the patient with a screen-film image receptor

Because X-rays cannot readily be focused as light can, an X-ray image receptor must be comparable in size to the object being studied. Such can be the case with radiographic film, of course, and commercial II tubes are up to 40 cm (16 inches) across. Just as with the body's tissues, it is the thickness, density, and chemical composition of the radiation-sensitive materials in the IR, along with the beam energy, that determine how successful it will be capturing a pattern of X-ray energy emerging from the patient, and the information it carries.

Film alone is relatively insensitive to high-energy photons, however, and it takes a lot of them to produce an image. This imparts a fair amount of dose to the patient, which is both undesirable and nearly always avoidable. It is energetically much more efficient, and imparts much less dose, to employ fluorescent screens in addition to the film; indeed, the most important purpose of employing a cassette, by far, is to reduce the patient dose significantly (Figure 4.1).

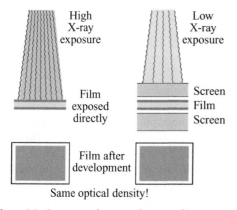

Figure 4.1 The primary function of a screen-film cassette is to reduce patient dose. Also, exposure times can be shorter, largely eliminating motion blur, and lower heat production in the anode lessens thermal stress of the tube, lengthening its life. Screen blur does increase, however, with screen thickness.

Image capture takes place in a two-step *indirect-detection* process:

The primary X-ray image, or pattern of X-rays remaining after passing through the patient, is first transformed into a nearly identical pattern of visible light by the two fluorescent screens within a radiographic *film cassette*;

It is this light that then actually exposes the film (Figures 4.2a and 1.6b).

This approach can reduce patient dose, and thus the estimated risk of stochastic health effects, by a factor of from 10 to 100. Because so much less radiation is needed to get adequate response from the screen cassette, moreover, the exposure can be much shorter, diminishing blur from patient motion. Also, lower exposures are less demanding on both the X-ray tube and its generator. The only downside (which in most situations does not matter) is that the resolution of the system goes down.

A fluoroscopic screen reduces patient dose but diminishes resolution

Film darkens if silver halide microcrystals in its emulsion are sensitized by radiation and subsequently transformed into flecks of opaque silver metal when the film is developed (Figure 1.9).

X-ray photons might be allowed to expose a sheet of radiographic film directly, as is done with some bite-wing dental imaging and occasionally when especially fine detail is required. In this case each photon that strikes a silver halide microcrystal fully sensitizes it, readying it for the chemical transformation into a speck of pure silver during development. The limitation is that one X-ray photon can strike only one silver halide crystal and trigger its transformation. So to achieve adequate darkening, many, many X-rays must strike the film. And that means lots of patient dose!

It is much more dose-efficient to expose the film when it is in a cassette (Figure 4.2a). A standard cassette consists of two *intensifying screens*, each consisting of a flat layer of compacted microcrystals of fluorescent material, or *phosphor*, held in place by an inert, translucent bonding material (Figure 4.2b). Between them is sandwiched the sheet of radiographic film. Early on, the phosphor in nearly all intensifying screens was calcium tungstate ($CaWO_4$). Since the 1970s, however, more sensitive *rare earth* screens have come into widespread use.

(a)

(b)

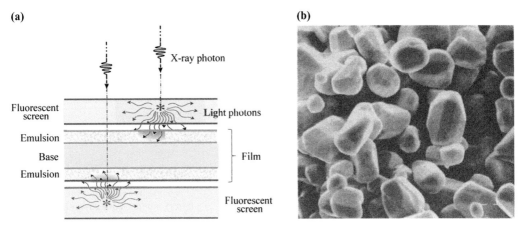

Figure 4.2 **(a)** A screen-film cassette is normally comprised of a pair of fluorescent screens in a light-tight, mechanically rigid housing; the cassette can be opened in a darkroom to insert or remove film from between the screens. An X-ray photon interacts with and excites a microscopic fluorescent crystal in a screen; the microcrystal immediately relaxes with the emission of thousands of visible light photons, and the resulting pinpoint of light exposes the film. **(b)** This fluorescent screen is composed of microcrystals of the rare earth phosphor $YTaO_4$:Nb, and the average crystal is about 6 microns across. Rare earth screens, such as this and those of gadolinium oxysulfide (Gd_2O_2S) or lanthanum oxybromide (LaOBr), are faster than the traditional standard, calcium tungstate, in part because, with their lower K-absorption peaks, they more readily intercept X-ray photons in the range of energies important in image formation. They also convert X-ray energy to light more efficiently. Reprinted from Brixner L, Holland RS, Kellogg RE, *et al.*, Low print-through technology with rare earth tantalite phosphors. In *SPIE* vol. 555, Medical Imaging and Instrumentation '85, p. 84, 1985, with permission from the International Society for Optical Engineering.

An X-ray photon striking a grain of fluorescent material in a screen excites it, and the excited crystal immediately de-excites back down to its comfortable ground state with the emission of a pinpoint burst of many thousands of visible-light photons (Figure 2.6c). Unlike the situation with X-ray photons, however, a half dozen or so visible light photons must strike a silver halide microcrystal to sensitize it – but there are so many of them released from a screen microcrystal from a single X-ray photon that it's not a problem; indeed, one X-ray can indirectly sensitize hundreds or thousands of grains in this fashion, producing a cluster of that number of silver grains, rather than just one.

Fluorescent materials and their close relatives find use in many modalities, including screen-film, II-based fluoroscopy, CR, some DR and DF, CT, planar nuclear medicine, SPECT, and PET, as well as in some display monitors and radiation dosimetry instruments. Since we'll be seeing much of them, it may be worthwhile, for the more curious reader, to say a little more about them.

A single X-ray in a screen leads to a cluster of hundreds of silver grains on developed film. Their numbers fall off from the center as a nearly Gaussian (normal) bell-shaped curve. If one 50-keV X-ray is absorbed by a crystal, for example, it ideally might release some 20 000 2.5-eV optical photons, give or take a few, which can sensitize a cluster of a few thousand silver bromide crystals a small fraction of a millimeter across, and result in the creation of that number of silver flecks with development.

The *image receptor efficiency* (*intensification factor*) of a screen-film combination is the overall measure of its dose-reduction capability. Factors that influence it include the *quantum detective efficiency* (QDE) of the screen; its *intrinsic phosphor* (*light emission*) *efficiency*; the *screen escape efficiency* for light; and the *optical efficiency* of the light sensitive part of the image receptor (Figure 4.3a).

The QDE of the screen refers to the fraction of those X-ray photons that reach it that are then actually detected; that, in turn, depends strongly on both the attenuation coefficient of the screen material and its thickness, in accord with Equations 3.1. The QDE of calcium tungstate ($CaWO_4$), for a long time the standard screen material, is less than that of rare-earth compounds such as gadolinium oxysulfide (Gd_2O_2S, or GOS), lanthanum oxybromide (LaOBr), and yttrium tantalate ($YTaO_4$).

(a)

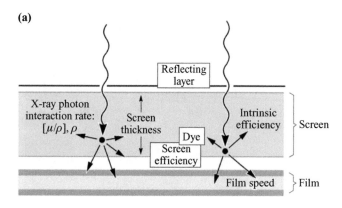

(b)

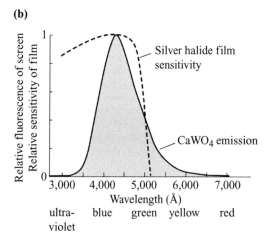

Figure 4.3 Parameters that determine the image receptor efficiency (intensification factor) and speed of a screen-film or other fluorescence-based X-ray image receptor (IR). **(a)** These include the X-ray capture efficiency (also known as quantum detection efficiency, QDE), the intrinsic phosphor (light-emission) efficiency, the screen escape efficiency, and the efficiency of the optical component of the IR (in this case, film) in capturing the light from the screen. The numerical scale of screen speeds is established by setting a "par-speed" calcium tungstate screen to 100. **(b)** The spectra for calcium tungstate light emission ($CaWO_4$) and for light sensitization of plain silver halide. This combination was the standard for much of the twentieth century before the advent of rare-earth screens and their specialized films. $1 \text{ Å} = 10^{-10}$ m.

Rare earth screens, with their K-edge absorption peaks at lower X-ray energies, are superior in part because they more readily intercept X-ray photons in the range of energies important in image formation.

The *intrinsic phosphor efficiency* relates the optical energy (and number of light photons) released per unit of X-ray energy absorbed. Phosphor efficiency is up to 20% for newer rare earth phosphors, largely due to the presence of trace amounts of impurities added intentionally, such as terbium (Tb), thulium (Tm), europium (Eu), and niobium (Nb).

The *screen escape efficiency* determines the fraction of the optical photons emitted that escape the screen heading toward the film. It is influenced by light scatter, diffusion, and absorption by the phosphor grains, which depends on their sizes and optical surface properties, and typically it is a good deal smaller than $1/2$. Dye added to the screen materials will cut back on the spreading out of light over long distances, thereby improving resolution but diminishing the intensification factor. A reflecting layer at the back of a screen has the opposite effects.

The *optical efficiency* is best when the emission spectrum of the screen and the absorption/sensitization spectrum of the film material overlap, as is the case of a calcium tungstate screen and standard silver halide (Figure 4.3b and Box 4.1).

The exposure and development of radiographic film

Radiographic film is similar to standard black-and-white photographic film. It is built on a flat polyester *base* 150–200 microns thick ($1 \text{ } \mu\text{m} = 10^{-6}$ m) that provides mechanical structure. The base must be nearly transparent, although it may be lightly tinted to reduce eye strain associated with the light produced within viewboxes by fluorescent tubes. It also has to be strong so as not to tear, and rigid enough to remain flat on the viewbox, yet sufficiently flexible to wend its way around the rollers of an automatic film developer.

Box 4.1   Parameters that influence the effectiveness of an X-ray image receptor

Quantum detective (X-ray capture) efficiency (QDE)
    attenuation coefficient, μ
        K-edge peaks
    thickness
Intrinsic phosphor (light-emission) efficiency
    dopants
Screen escape efficiency
    reflective layer
    dye
Optical efficiency
    silver flecks deposited per incident optical photon
            screen-emission/film-absorption spectral overlap
            silver halide microcrystal dopants, manufacture
        photodiode voltage output per optical photon, etc., for digital system

The film is coated normally on both sides (but only on one for mammography, and with a single screen, for better resolution) with a 10–20 μm layer of emulsion. Emulsion is a gelatinous medium within which are suspended vast numbers of microscopic, translucent grains of the active ingredient, silver halide. The halide concentrations are typically 90–99% bromide and 10–1% iodide, plus trace amounts of other odds and ends. During produc-

tion, the crystals are heated in an atmosphere of a sulfur compound that create tiny AgS *sensitivity specks* on their surfaces that enhance their responsiveness to irradiation by *light* from a screen. The microcrystals are of the order of 1 μm across, and there may be billions of them per square milliliter of emulsion. When struck by at least a half dozen or so visible light photons from the screen during the exposure, a crystal becomes *sensitized*, and transforms into a fleck of black silver under film development. More X-ray photons reaching a small pixel or area in the screen cause more scintillations of light there, and more clusters of pure silver will eventually darken the corresponding spot in the film. The development process is much like that of ordinary film photography.

In a little more detail: ±10% iodine ions are added during the manufacture of silver halide crystals; with an ionic radius larger than that of bromine, these cause structural strains that force some silver cations into interstitial positions in the lattice, where they are held exceptionally loosely. Also, AgIBr crystals start out surrounded by a negatively charged *bromine barrier* that drives anions and electrons away. Every X-ray-induced pinpoint of light from the screen exposes a cluster of transparent silver halide grains. In any one of them, a visible light photon can knock an electron off some Br⁻ ion (Figure 4.4a), after which the now neutral Br° atom is only slightly bound to the lattice; it can escape the crystal and then diffuse out of the emulsion. The freed electron migrates to the crystal's sensitivity speck, which, in turn, becomes negatively charged (Figure 4.4b). The now negatively charged sensitivity speck attracts a nearly free interstitial Ag⁺ ion to it (Figure 4.4c). A grain that is struck by at least a half-dozen or so visible light photons attracts multiple

Figure 4.4 Development of photographic/radiographic film. (a) A visible light photon from the screen, or its resulting photoelectron(s), strikes a bromine ion in a transparent silver halide crystal; the now-neutral bromine atom diffuses away from the crystal, and its electron is free to be drawn toward the sensitivity spot created in the crystal during film manufacture. (b) The sensitivity spot now carries a negative charge and (c) attracts one of the silver cations that happens to be relatively free to move about. (d) Enough silver deposited in this fashion will form a breach in the negative "bromine barrier" around the crystal, through which the developer, an electron donor, delivers more electrons, greatly accelerating the process.

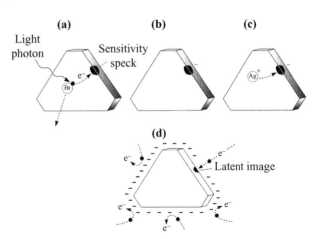

silver ions to it and, in this fashion, is *sensitized*, and a "gap" is created in the crystal's electric surface bromine barrier (Figure 4.4d). Developer molecules (which are electron donors) can now bring more electrons to the sensitivity speck from outside the crystal and hasten along the process of attracting silver ions. Eventually, a sensitized grain is transformed completely into a fleck of black, metallic silver (Figure 1.9). Where more X-ray photons have passed through the patient, more clusters of silver will darken the developed film.

A thin *supercoat* affords physical protection of the emulsion, but it must be permeable to the chemicals involved in developing the sensitized grains and in *fixing*, or dissolving, those that were *not* sensitized, and then *washing* them away; otherwise they would slowly transform into silver on their own, and blacken the film over time.

Optical density of developed radiographic film and the characteristic curve

A viewbox produces the intensity L_0 of white light and, of that, the lesser amount L_t is transmitted through some area of the developed film (Figure 4.5a). The *transmittance* there is defined as L_t/L_0, the fraction of the light incident on the film that is transmitted through it. This ranges from a value of 1, for a perfectly clear developed film, to 0, for one that is completely opaque. The transmittance decreases with greater exposure of the patient and the IR, and either too little or too much radiation will produce a useless film (Figure 4.5b).

It is convenient, and the generally adopted convention for film, to express the darkening of a portion of it in a completely equivalent form, in terms of *optical density* (*OD*) there. The OD is really just another way of expressing the transmittance, and is defined through $L_t/L_0 \equiv 10^{-OD}$. If the OD is 2, the film attenuates the light by a factor of $L_t/L_0 = 10^{-2} = 0.01$. As its name suggests, the OD is a number greater than zero that increases with the amount of silver laid down during development. The more opaque the film becomes and the "denser" it appears optically (i.e., the more it blocks light), the greater the OD.

In practice, useable ODs range from about 0.25 to 2.5, with light transmittance in film of between 0.5 (which shows up very bright on the viewbox) and 0.003 (nearly black). On a standard lightbox,

the eye can readily distinguish patterns and details for ODs between about 1.0 and 1.5; outside the range of acceptable ODs, the film is either under- or over-exposed – but a *bright* or *hot light* may work to find patterns in dark regions. For two superimposed OD = 2 films, each decreases transmittance by a factor of 0.01, so the total decrease is 0.0001, or OD = 4; thus while you multiply factors of L_t/L_0, you add ODs. The OD is often defined in a totally equivalent form as OD $\equiv \log_{10}(L_0/L_t)$.

The *response*, or *characteristic*, or *H&D curve* (after F. Hurter and V.C. Driffield, who first published one) of a screen-film system indicates how much OD any particular amount of radiation will generate. A complete characteristic curve can be generated rapidly and easily in the clinic by tracking the ODs obtained by stepping the *air dose*; that is, the dose in air immediately at the front face of the cassette, required to produce each (Figure 4.5c). By convention, a logarithmic scale is used for the radiation level, so that each additional step by 0.3 along the *x*-axis corresponds to another doubling of the air dose. The shape of the characteristic curve depends on the output spectrum of optical photons from the screen, the precise recipe for manufacture of the silver halide crystals in the emulsion, details of the film development process, etc.

The characteristic curve of a screen-film system consists of three parts. At very low doses, the *toe* of the curve emerges from the *fog* that occurs normally in developed film even with no exposure to radiation. Above the toe lies the nearly straight *linear part* of the curve, where imaging is carried out, in which changes in OD are proportional to changes in the logarithm of the dose to the cassette. The linear portion terminates in a *shoulder*, or *saturation* region, above which the curve flattens out in a maximum-OD, black plateau.

There can be significant contrast only where the slope of the curve is fairly steep; that is, in the linear region. The way to bring about this desirable condition is to provide a reasonable tube current and exposure duration for the given kVp. The intensity of the X-ray beam scales directly with the tube current and with the square of the applied potential, so it is really the product $(mA\text{-}s)(kVp)^2$ that must be selected correctly.

Over- and underexposures of screen-film (or digital X-ray) images are rarely problems now because of *automatic exposure control*. An AEC system is built around one or several radiation detectors that are nearly radio-translucent and positioned somewhere up- or downstream of the patient, as in Figure 4.5d; when the X-ray detector reaches a pre-determined level of exposure, it switches off the tube.

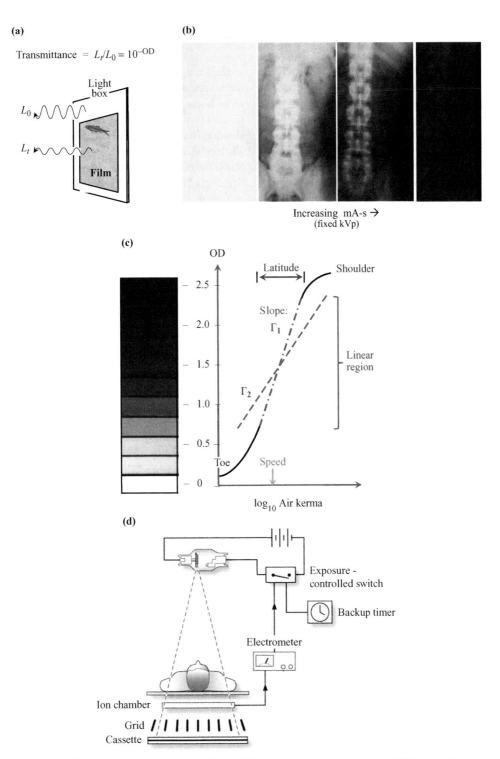

(a)

Transmittance $= L_t/L_0 = 10^{-OD}$

Light box

L_0

L_t

Film

(b)

Increasing mA-s →
(fixed kVp)

(c)

OD

Latitude   Shoulder

Slope:
Γ_1

Linear region

Γ_2

Toe   Speed

$\log_{10}$ Air kerma

(d)

Exposure - controlled switch

Backup timer

Electrometer

Ion chamber

Grid

Cassette

Figure 4.5 Quantifying the darkening of a region of film. (**a**) *Transmittance* and *optical density* (OD) are nearly equivalent (but numerically different) measures of the transparency of the film. The OD increases with film opacity, where more silver has been laid down and less light is transmitted through, L_t. (**b**) Increase of average OD with mA-s, when all other factors (in particular, the kVp) are held constant. An increment of 10 kVp darkens the film roughly as much as doubling mA-s. (**c**) For the *characteristic curve* of a screen-film combination, the optical density is plotted against the logarithm of the dose (or equivalently, kerma) to air. (**d**) An *automatic exposure control* (AEC) or *phototimer* system takes much of the guesswork out of exposures. It tracks the radiation being deposited in a dosimeter in front of or behind the cassette, and it switches off the X-ray tube after delivery of a pre-determined amount that is known to work well for the IR.

Every X-ray IR has a characteristic curve relating the strength of its response to the air dose at its input. It commonly provides more information than is needed, and usually it is sufficient to know only the *contrast* or *gamma*, the *latitude*, and the *speed* of the IR.

Contrast of a screen-film IR refers to the difference in OD at two points in an image that comes about from a difference in the exposure. For optimal contrast and reproducibility, it helps to work in the *linear* portion of the characteristic curve, where it is steepest.

The *latitude* is the range of exposures over which the film is clinically useful, where the characteristic curve is nearly straight and where the OD is typically between about 0.25 and 2.5.

Speed refers to the amount of radiation needed to reach a point near the middle of the useful OD range. It is commonly defined, somewhat arbitrarily, as the inverse of that value of exposure or air dose required to achieve an OD of 1 above fog level; the smaller the exposure needed to reach the reference OD level, the *faster* the system. Increasingly sensitive screens and/or films (with decreasing resolution capability) are labeled *detail*, *par*, and *fast*.

The concept of optical density of a portion of film is itself becoming obsolete, being displaced by measures of brightness on electronic display monitors. But some of the ideas that grew out of it (e.g., latitude, contrast) are still in widespread use.

Unlike a film-screen combination, the IRs for digital planar imaging have responses that happen to be linear in exposure; that is, their characteristic curves are completely straight, with no toe or shoulder. It is therefore commonplace to intentionally modify a (linear) characteristic curve electronically, introducing film-like curvature into it, for the display of digital radiographs. This lets physicians trained and experienced with the traditional, film-like appearance read them more easily.

Prime determinants/measures of image quality: contrast, resolution, random noise, artifacts, . . . and, always, patient dose

The previous chapter described the way in which a nearly uniform X-ray beam enters a patient and, in passing through, is transformed into an information-bearing primary X-ray image. The present one began by saying more about the way in which a screen-film image receptor captures that primary X-ray image and converts it into a permanent visual record.

Picking up where Chapters 2 and 3 left off, we return to the issue of what is needed for an X-ray image to be clinically useful: good image contrast and resolution, low noise, and no artifacts (Figure 4.6). Let's start with the effect of the

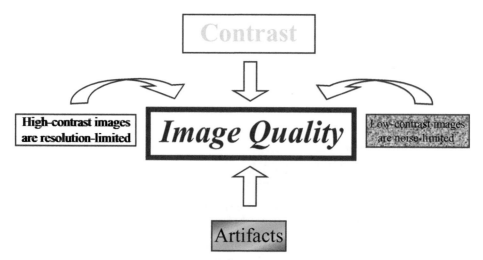

Figure 4.6 The four simple, standard measures of image quality: contrast, resolution, noise, and artifacts, all of which can often be improved, but usually at the cost of more patient dose.

image-receptor itself on contrast, and how it combines with subject contrast to yield overall image contrast.

Subject contrast, image-receptor contrast, and image contrast

Psychophysics studies have revealed that the eye can distinguish something like 50 levels of gray, running from black to white. Fewer levels of gray could lead to a checkered look but, because of physiological limitations on retinal discrimination, more than 50 would do little to improve the appearance, and it might cost more. Visual contrast between two regions in an image would be greatest if they were represented as black and white, of course, but this would not help much with the nuances of a real medical image. How to make best use of 50 shades of gray to portray physical differences within the body?

The ability of a screen-film combination to capture and depict contrast between two points in a patient is determined by two things. The first is simply the difference in air dose reaching the screen at the corresponding two points, as determined by the *subject contrast*, $C_{subject}$. The second is the system's *image receptor contrast*, C_{IR}, the sensitivity of the IR to variations in exposure. The rate at which the optical density changes with the log air dose for film, the slope of the linear portion of the characteristic curve, is a kind of IR contrast, and is commonly labeled Γ. This is known variously as the *gamma*, the *maximum gradient*, and, more generally, *image-receptor contrast*. Screen-film systems typically have Γ-values between 2 and 3.5.

More simply and generally, C_{IR} may be expressed as the rate of change of IR electrical output, or perhaps of monitor luminescence, L, with IR-input dose:

$$C_{IR} = \Gamma = \Delta L / \Delta D. \qquad (4.1b)$$

Combining this with our expression for $C_{subject}$ yields a flexible and powerful expression for the overall image contrast, one that applies to all imaging modalities (Figure 4.7a):

$$C_{image} = C_{subject} \times C_{IR}. \qquad (4.1c)$$

(a)

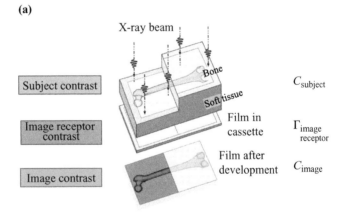

(b)

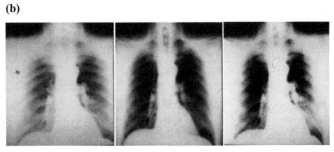

Increasing Γ →

Figure 4.7 Contrast is quantified in terms of the relative difference in the level of optical density, or radiation intensity, or some other relevant parameter, between two regions, or between a region and background. (a) Overall, *image contrast* is determined by both the *subject contrast* and the *image receptor contrast*. (b) Image contrast, with same subject contrast and overall soft-tissue OD, but different values of IR contrast, Γ.

Subject contrast is thus "amplified" by the image receptor contrast, C_{IR}. It may be necessary to modify the definitions of all three terms in Equation 4.1c somewhat for other modalities, but the basic idea remains meaningful.

It is evident in Figure 4.5c, by the way, that the greater the gamma for a film, the smaller the latitude. If a high gamma is required to accentuate contrast in one part of a film, the range may be so limited as to leave other important regions too dark or too transparent. Three great advantages of a digital radiographic system are that the response of the IR (unlike that of film) is linear over a very wide range of exposures, so that there are no toe or shoulder problems; the gamma can be adjusted separately for any region of interest of the image; and the gamma and latitude are unlinked.

Subject contrast can depend strongly on kVp (Figure 2.9b), but the response of a screen, and in particular its value of gamma, are determined primarily by the materials and details of its construction. IR contrast is almost always greater than 1, and it augments the subject contrast in the X-ray pattern falling on it by the factor of C_{IR} (Figure 4.7b). For $C_{subject}$ = 2.5 at the chosen kVp, and with a screen with C_{IR} = 2, say, the subject contrast would be amplified by a factor of 2, ending up with an total image contrast of C_{image} = 5, by Equation 4.1c.

Resolution: causes of unsharpness

The resolution of an image or of an imaging system is a measure of its proficiency at revealing that small, close-together objects in the body, or thin lines in a test device, are actually separate, and its ability to reveal fine structure and sharp edges. It can be expressed rather loosely either in terms of a separation distance of objects that just barely appear distinct (e.g., 0.5 mm) or as a spatial frequency, the inverse of a distance, such as 2 line pairs per millimeter (2 lp/mm) (Figure 2.10). These are not exactly the same thing – indeed, they refer to somewhat different gauges of the power to capture detail – but they are closely related. (When

considering resolution quantitatively, incidentally, it is necessary to clarify what is actually meant by "separate," since the image will have some blurriness at the edges; are we assuming 10% overlap of the edges of images as assessed by eye? 30%?)

A good "detail" screen plus film combination may achieve 10 lp/mm, while film alone may be capable of 20 lp/mm and more, not that resolution on the order of 0.05 mm is frequently required. With digital systems, resolution is limited ultimately by pixel size of the IR, and the width of one pixel pair is comparable to that of a line pair.

Resolution is closely related to, albeit somewhat different from, sharpness. "Sharpness" commonly refers to the boundary at an abrupt interface, such as the edge of a long bone. It might be expressed as the rate of change of OD in a film, $\Delta OD/\Delta x$, or in the primary X-ray beam itself, as $\Delta D_{air}/\Delta x$. It can be strongly interlinked with apparent contrast: while an unsharp border may be visible if the contrast is high, it may be difficult to make out even a very sharp edge with a low-contrast system. Indeed, the degree of available contrast, the resolution, and the sharpness present are all involved in determining the blur in an image.

There are four important determinants of the unsharpness or *blur*, b, within an X-ray image and, likewise, of the resolving capabilities of any X-ray system. These are the inherent shapes of the objects within the body that are being examined; patient or equipment motion; the finite size of the focal spot on the anode from which X-rays emanate; and the thickness of the cassette screen (Figure 4.8).

Objects within the body with sides that diverge with the beam may give rise to images with the sharpest edges (Figure 4.9a). A round entity may be harder to detect, with the blur inherent in its shape reducing apparent contrast and edge sharpness.

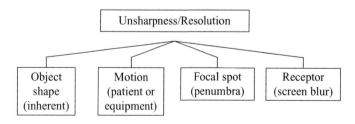

Figure 4.8 Contributors to unsharpness in a screen-film exposure include the inherent shape of the object being viewed, motion of the patient or imaging device, the penumbra or geometric blur from the finite size of the focal spot, and that introduced by the image receptor itself.

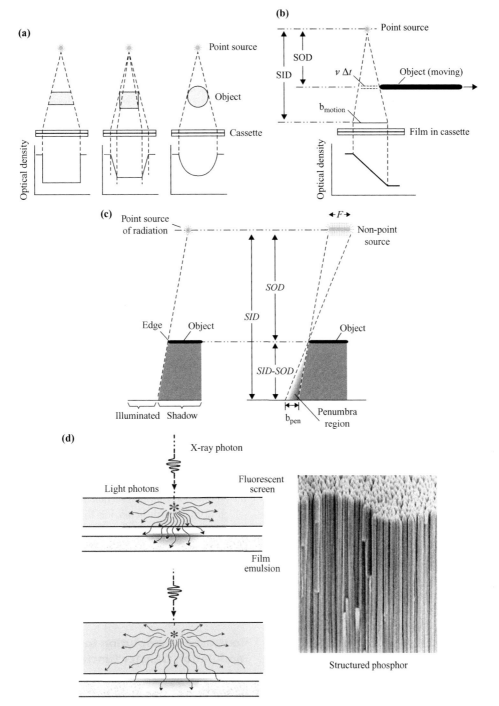

Figure 4.9 Again, four contributors to unsharpness in a screen-film exposure. (a) Inherent shapes of the objects within the body that are being examined. (b) Patient or equipment motion; if the two are moving at velocity v relative to one another during an exposure of duration Δt, this introduces a (magnified) blur of dimension $b_{motion} = (v\,\Delta t)(SID/SOD)$, where SID is the screen-to-IR distance and SOD is the screen-to-object distance. (c) The finite size of the focal spot on the anode's target, from which X-rays emanate. A point source of radiation can cast a sharp shadow of a sharp-edged object but with an extended source there appears a region of blur, or *penumbra*, at the edge of the shadow image. Again, by similar triangles, the width of the penumbra blur region at the IR depends on the dimensions of the source, F, and on the distances of the object from it, SOD, and from the image plane, (SID – SOD), as $b_{focal} = F$ (SID – SOD)/SOD. (d) The thickness of the cassette screen. If the screen is thin, so that all interactions are close to the film, there results a more compact cluster of silver microcrystals, hence the potential for better resolution; but the dose will have to be higher for a thin screen to lead to the same overall average OD as a thick one. The columnar crystals of a *structured phosphor*, such as this one of cesium iodide, reduce image degradation caused by the scatter of light within the screen. Similar considerations arise for some digital IRs. Courtesy of Ehsan Samei, Duke University.

Relative motion of the patient and the imaging equipment can cause loss of resolution in an X-ray film unless the exposure time, Δt, is sufficiently short (Figure 4.9b). Motions of less than 0.1 mm during exposure usually do not contribute to *motion blur*; those greater than 1 mm commonly dominate blur.

A perfect pinpoint focal spot would cause no blurring, on the left in (Figure 4.9c). The finite size, F, of a real source of X-rays, however, causes unsharpness known as *penumbra, geometric*, or *focal spot blur*. Just as the shadows of your hand cast in a dark closet by a floodlight are fuzzier than those from a tiny bulb, likewise the millimeter or so dimensions of a real focal spot will cause a blurring. By similar triangles, the width of the *focal spot blur* region, b_{focal}, depends on F and also on the source-to-object (*SOD*) and source-to-IR (*SID*) distances. For high-resolution imaging, most tubes allow selection of a smaller cathode filament-coil; in addition, one can adjust the SID and SOD to diminish the unsharpness, bearing in mind the effects on magnification, scatter, and patient dose. Because the dimensions of the focal spot source can increase with tube aging, the National Electrical Manufacturers Association (NEMA) has set QA tolerances for various nominal focal spots sizes.

Absorption of an X-ray photon in a phosphor crystal of a screen results in a scintillation that sends thousands of visible light photons off in all directions. In their travels, light photons will be scattered multiple times at the surfaces of other phosphor crystals, diffusing outward (Figure 4.9d). By the time the light pulse finally emerges from the screen surface adjacent to the film, the photons will have spread considerably; the area of film they fall on, creating a cluster of silver grains, will be a great deal larger than the size of a single silver halide crystal. So while we started with an infinitesimal X-ray collision area, the response from the image receptor is enlarged to size b_{IR}, the *image receptor blur*.

There is a reciprocal relationship between the speed and the resolution of a screen, since faster screens of a given fluorescent material are thicker (so as to contain more phosphor crystals per unit area). With a thinner screen, however, the phosphorescence events all occur closer to the film, and the bursts of light will have less room to spread out within the phosphor before exposing it. But a thinner screen is less sensitive, absorbing a smaller fraction of the incident X-ray beam, and a higher X-ray exposure and patient dose are required to achieve an acceptable optical density.

The diffusion of light within the phosphor can be reduced, and higher resolution obtained, with a *structured phosphor* consisting of close-packed, crystal needles aligned perpendicular to the plane of the screen. When an X-ray interaction produces a minute flash of light, the thousands of resultant optical photons will travel up or down it, reflecting off the interior surfaces of the crystal as with an optical fiber. This confinement cuts down radically on the lateral spread of optical photons, improving system resolution, and it allows the deposition of a thicker layer of phosphor, for greater sensitivity.

Each component of an imaging system makes its own contribution to the overall unsharpness and loss of contrast of the image. The three dominant controllable contributions for planar radiography are blurs from patient or equipment motion (b_{motion}), from the finite size of the focal spot (b_{focal}), and from the image receptor (b_{IR}). One might expect that correction of one aspect of blur might overcompensate for the blurring effect of another, but such is not the case. Different kinds of blur do not necessarily line up in the same direction, so one cannot obtain the total unsharpness simply by adding their b values together. The statistical theory of error propagation suggests that they tend to combine, rather, as

$$b_{total} = \sqrt{(b_{motion}^2 + b_{focal}^2 + b_{IR}^2)}. \quad (4.2)$$

If one of the three is noticeably larger than the other two, then it will easily dominate, helped along by the 2 in the exponent, and little benefit comes from trying to reduce either of the others.

There is a simple quantitative approach, called the *modulation transfer function* (MTF) formalism, which does a much better job than this in assessing not only a system's powers of resolution, but its ability to deal with contrast, as well. The MTF is a very powerful and widely used metric for assessing and describing the performance of any imaging modality, and it plays a central role in QA programs for all of them.

Contrast and resolution together: the modulation transfer function

Images are generated, processed, stored, and transmitted by imperfect systems. Some components of an imaging train are more imperfect than others, however, so there is a need for ways to determine and describe the extent to which any one degrades the images created in it or passing through it.

Resolution was introduced as a fairly crude yardstick – a single number (e.g., lp/mm) to define what is actually a rather complex phenomenon

(Figure 2.10). Likewise, contrast is a straightforward construct until, that is, you consider objects of small size, also seen in the figure. The MTF goes far beyond the two separate image quality ideas of contrast and resolution, quantitatively combining them in a fashion that allows useful numerical evaluations and comparisons of a broad range of pieces of equipment.

The MTF is not a particularly complicated subject, but it does take a bit of space to describe it, so we'll only sketch it here, and relegate the more technical details to advanced texts.

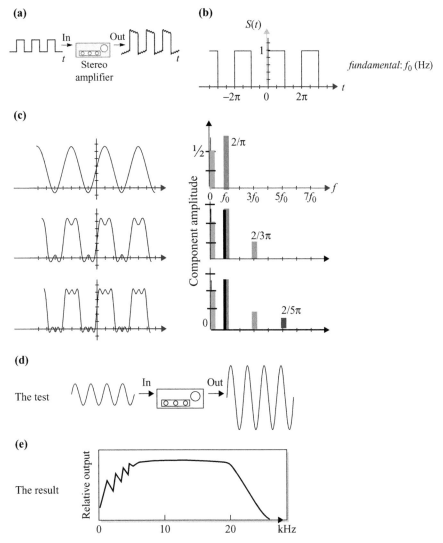

Figure 4.10 Fourier analysis of your antique stereo. (**a**) When you input a square-wave signal, something altogether different comes out. (**b, c**) The Fourier decomposition of a temporal square wave of amplitude 1 and frequency f_0. The combination of the constant $1/2$ plus a single sine wave $(2/\pi)$ sin $(2\pi f_0 t)$ provides a very crude approximation of the square wave. Adding a term of amplitude $(2/3\pi)$ and frequency $3f_0$ flattens off the tops and bottoms a little, and including higher harmonics does better yet. The set of peaks to the right, one for each harmonic, is a fully equivalent representation of the square wave, called the *Fourier spectrum*. (**d**) To study the poor performance of the stereo more systematically, you input a set of many monochromatic (single-frequency) sine-wave signals one at a time, all of the same unit amplitude but for a range of frequencies, and (**e**) plot the output versus frequency, *f*. The MTF is, in essence, the corresponding graph for sinusoidal *spatial* patterns passing through an imaging device.

Background: the Fourier representation

The general problem is one sadly familiar to all of you Bach and Beatles aficionados. The *Goldberg Variations* just haven't been sounding quite so effervescent on your paleolithic stereo lately. Likewise, Lucy isn't glittering as brightly in the sky. So you pump a square-wave test input voltage signal into the amplifier and examine the output on a monitor, and your worst suspicions are confirmed. The stereo is clearly doing something not right, leading to significant tonal distortion (Figure 4.10a). It is not apparent from this study, however, exactly where the difficulties lie.

An image, unless it is pure abstraction, is a representation of some aspect of reality. An ordinary photograph, painting, or sculpture may sometimes even be visually indistinguishable from the original. An angiogram, on the other hand, may well provide the vital information needed, but it doesn't look much like the patient.

An image can itself have a representation, which is thus a representation of a representation. The type of representation that is perhaps easiest to conceptualize is the digital (Figure 1.11), which will be explored in Chapter 6 and encountered often thereafter. You can scrutinize a CT scan because a computer has transformed a set of numerical measurements into a quantitative representation of the slice that, in turn, guides the monitor in the creation of a visual representation. Once the quantitative representation exists, moreover, it can be stored, transmitted, processed, even analyzed electronically; a mathematical representation, even a very elementary one, makes many things possible.

There are other good ones, as well. In 1815, not only did the Duke of Wellington roundly thrash Napoleon at Waterloo but also, perhaps of as great lasting significance, Jean-Baptiste-Joseph Fourier demonstrated that just about any mathematical function or curve in time or space can be represented as (be decomposed into) a combination of sine and cosine waves of the appropriate frequencies and amplitudes.

Creating such a Fourier representation of a curve turns out to be particularly easy if it is *periodic*, like the square wave of Figure 4.10b, and varies repeatedly over time at some *funda-mental frequency*, f_0. The interval between repetitions of the pattern, the time of passage through one cycle, is the *period*, of duration $1/f_0$ second. The *Fourier representation* of the square wave, $S(t)$, is expressed as a simple sum of sine contributions whose frequencies are *harmonics* (integer multiples) of f_0 (Figure 4.10c). The trick is to get the respective *amplitudes* of all the harmonic terms right, and that is the job of the mathematical technique known as *Fourier analysis*.

There is no need to describe here how a Fourier decomposition is performed, to determine the amplitudes of the separate harmonic terms, but in practice it usually involves some straightforward math and a computer-based process known as the fast Fourier algorithm (FFA); suffice it to note that it can all be done easily with the right computer programs.

Let's consider again the square wave with signal strength, $S(t)$ that steps back and forth between 0 to 1 with frequency f_0 (Figures 4.10b and 4.10c). The closest we can get to that with a *single* sinusoidal term is $S(t) = 1/2 + (2/\pi) \sin (2\pi f_0 t)$, where the constant $1/2$ causes the sine wave component to stick up a bit above the flat top of the square wave. The fundamental and the constant plus a third-harmonic component of frequency $f = 3f_0$ and amplitude $2/3\pi$, that is, $1/2 + (2/\pi) \times \{\sin (2\pi f_0 t) + 1/3 \sin (6\pi f_0 t)\}$, is nearer to the original, and throwing in the right higher order harmonics is even better. The terms get smaller, but the more of them you add, the more the Fourier sum becomes like the real thing and, in theory, the infinite sum should provide a perfect replica. The *spectrum* to the right of each wave indicates the magnitudes of the fundamental and harmonic contributions that are added together to generate it, and is a concept we'll return to on a number of occasions.

In practice, of course, it is not possible to manipulate all the terms in an infinite series, or to handle infinitely high-frequency harmonics, and so one must *truncate* it, or cut it off, at some point, converting it into a *finite* Fourier series. The truncation frequency must be high enough to capture all the detail of interest in the signal, and to prevent unacceptable distortions in the process. But the more Fourier components included, the broader is the *frequency bandwidth* required of the equipment to handle them all; but more bandwidth also means that less noise can be filtered out. Also, since the signal is to be digitized, the longer the computation and transmission times are, and the greater the cost. Fortunately, the higher-frequency contributions to the Fourier sum almost always tend to become vanishingly small rather quickly, and one can truncate the series when they become too tiny, or too time-consuming, or too computer-costly to deal with, and retain only those of essential lower frequencies.

The fact that a complex sound can be expressed as a combination of the right sine waves suggests a systematic way to analyze the stereo's behavior (Figure 4.10d). We enter, one at a time, a trial set of unit-amplitude pure sine waves (forget about square waves hereafter), and see how the amplitude of the output varies with the frequency of input (Figure 4.10e). The *gain*, or amount of amplification, should be constant over the range of audible frequencies, and the gain curve flat. The frequency response actually measured may be able to tell a good deal about how well the amplifier is working and, in this case, it seems that something is grievously wrong at the low-frequency end. Since no one seems able to fix these things anymore, it's probably time for the old heave-ho and buy a replacement from Asia.

A *spatial* pattern or image in one, two, or three spatial dimensions can be expressed as a Fourier combination of sine waves of different spatial frequencies, amplitudes, and phases, as well, in which spatial frequency is expressed with the symbol k, in cycles per millimeter, rather than f, in cycles per second. One can perform exactly the same kind of analysis in multiple dimensions for an imaging system or any of its constituent parts. Such Fourier manipulations are essential in the image reconstruction for CT, SPECT, PET, MRI, and other tomographic modalities.

Modulation is contrast

Fourier analysis also underlies the MTF method of assessing image quality. The MTF of an imaging system is, roughly, the spatial counterpart to the stereo amplifier's frequency-response function. It provides a powerful tool for determining and displaying the extent to which a piece of equipment preserves or degrades the quality of images passing through it. In particular, it allows us to assess and interpret, simply and quantitatively, its combined contrast and resolution capabilities.

Suppose we are interested in how much, and how, an imaging device might degrade the input signal in carrying out its appointed information-processing task. Inspired by the success of our analysis of the stereo's behavior, we realize that it might help to systematically examine the response of the imaging system to a range of monochromatic sinusoidal input signals, all of the same amplitude, and obtain the system's frequency-response curve. It simplifies matters to view this in terms of a variation on the notion of the contrast we have already explored.

A good way to proceed is to follow the lead of a.m. (*amplitude modulation*) radio. Audio information, typically in the range of 20 Hz to 20 kHz, is superimposed on a radiofrequency (RF) carrier of, say, between 520 and 1610 kHz (for commercial a.m. broadcasting in the USA). Most of the power is conveyed by the carrier, and its frequency is what you tune to; but the signal of interest, such as a 4 kHz tone, is sculpted out of the carrier energy. In Figure 4.11a, for example, the input is 75% modulated, which is to say that $3/4$ of the available carrier is used to convey information, and only $1/4$ of it is wasted; modulation of the output signal, on the other hand, has been reduced to only 50% by the device.

The contrast C of an object in an image can be defined as the difference in signal strength (or pixel value, or brightness, etc.) between it and a fairly uniform adjacent background area, as in Figure 3.11a. The image of an organ can be expressed as a sum of sine waves in space, and one can think of the carrier itself as a kind of "background"; then we can view the modulation, M, as the contrast, C. In passing through the apparatus, the signal of Figure 4.11a doubled in amplitude, which is nice – but more importantly, the modulation declined from 0.75 to 0.5. That means that less information is conveyed per unit of power expended – less bang for the buck. It is conventional to define the MTF for a device and frequency as C_{out}/C_{in} or, equivalently, as M_{out}/M_{in} which, in this case is $0.5/0.75 = 0.67$.

For clinical purposes, the MTF describes the extent to which an imaging system or component degrades the contrast, or modulation, of a *spatial* sinusoidal pattern at any *spatial* frequency value, k, as a signal passes through it:

$$MTF(k) \equiv M_{out}(k)/M_{in}(k). \qquad (4.3a)$$

(For a spatial frequency of $k = 3$ cycles/mm, say, the signal will progress through three cycles [2π each] over a span of 1 mm; equivalently, the period of the wave pattern is $1/k = 1/3$ mm.) Here "background" is no longer a carrier wave, but rather has its usual meaning. Figure 4.11b shows how one might create such a sinusoidal pattern of X-rays with a specially designed undulating attenuating filter. (Note, incidentally, that we want to generate a sinusoidal primary X-ray beam, so the attenuator itself can*not* be sculpted in a sinusoidal manner: attenuation through it is exponential with thickness, not linear.)

MTF$_{IR}$ for a screen-film image receptor

The greater the $MTF(k)$ is at high spatial frequencies, k, the more adept it is at capturing fine detail.

To record the MTF for a screen-film IR, let the system view spatial X-ray patterns of sine waves of different spatial frequencies, k, in cycles per cm, and check to see what occurs at the

(a)

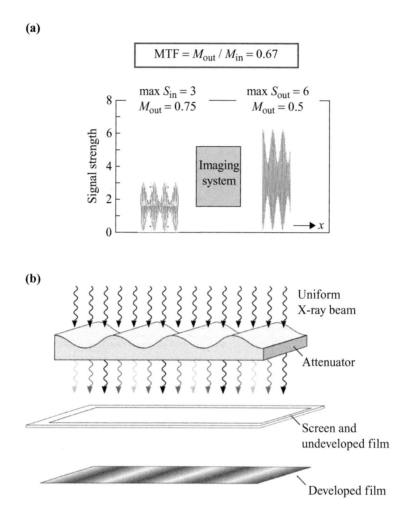

(b)

Uniform X-ray beam

Attenuator

Screen and undeveloped film

Developed film

Figure 4.11 Modulation. **(a)** The input and output audio signals at this frequency are of 0.75 and 0.5 modulation, respectively, and the MTF is 0.5/0.75 = 0.67. **(b)** After passing through this wavy metal filter, the spatial pattern of intensity of the resulting X-ray beam is sinusoidal, $S_{in}(x, k) = 1 \sin (2\pi kx)$, where k refers to the *spatial frequency* of a wave, in units such as cycles/mm.

output (Figure 4.12). For simplicity, we have arranged for all the input signals at all frequencies to be of unit modulation, $M_{in}(k) = 1$. In the top row, for $k = 1$ cm^{-1}, the signal has been amplified by the apparatus, but the modulation is unchanged (Figure 4.12a). In Figure 4.12b and c, at $k = 2$ cm^{-1} and 3 cm^{-1}, respectively, $MTF(k)$ has fallen to 0.5 and 0.33, as recorded in Figure 4.12d.

For a perfect device, the MTF would be a constant for all k, the dashed horizontal line, and there would be no image degradation. But a real imaging system, like a stereo, is nearly always more adept at handling signal components at some frequencies than at others. The response is usually best at low spatial frequencies, and the MTF typically falls off from a maximum

value near $k = 0$. Studies of observer performance suggest that what we call "limiting resolution" typically corresponds to the spatial frequency (in cycles/mm or line-pairs/mm) at which $MTF(k)$ has fallen to about 0.1.

But why is the $MTF(k = 0)$ unity for long wavelengths, but drops at frequencies above some sort of higher-frequency threshold value?

Consider a screen-film image receptor. Imagine that a very narrow (e.g., 10 μm) needle-beam *input* of X-rays, of dimensions described by $S_{in}(r)$ where r is the distance from the center of the needle-beam, strikes the screen (Figure 4.13a, to the left). Such a beam might be produced by shining a standard X-ray beam on a thick metal plate with a pinhole drilled in it.

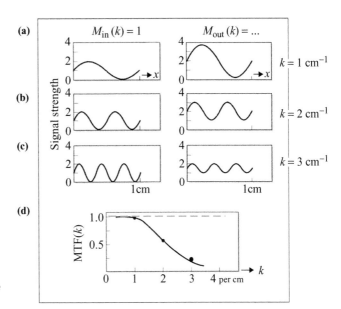

Figure 4.12 Creation of an MTF curve. (a-c) Obtaining the modulation at several spatial frequencies, and (d) generating the MTF(k).

The visible light photon *output* in the screen will radiate outward from the interaction point in all directions, giving a circularly symmetric area of brightness that falls off relatively slowly with r, primarily because of light scattering at screen grain boundaries. The resulting curve of output brightness versus r is bell-shaped, and is referred to as the *point spread function, PSF(r)*. It is described largely by its amplitude (height) and its *full width at half-maximum (FWHM)* amplitude. The PSF of the screen-film system is as important a notion as its characteristic curve, but it has quite different applications.

Now let's remove the plate with a hole in it, and expose the image receptor, instead, to a long-wavelength pattern of X-rays

produced by the specially designed attenuating filter of Figure 4.11b, where the wavelength $1/k$ of the input signal happens to be much greater than the FWHM of the PSF (Figure 4.13b). The dimensions of the $PSF(r)$ will be too small to have much effect on the slowly varying output image, and the MTF_{IR} for the image receptor at that spatial frequency will remain close to 1. But as the wavelength of the input becomes comparable to the FWHM, and then even shorter (Figure 4.13c), the output image will be spread out by the same effects that gave rise to the width of $PSF(r)$; this will be reflected as a roll-off in the $MTF(k)$ at the higher spatial frequencies. A thick screen may be more sensitive to X-ray photons, capturing more of

Figure 4.13 The significance of the full width at half-maximum (FWHM) of the *point spread function* (PSF). (a) For a circular, needle-thin beam of X-rays incident on a screen-film image receptor, the output image has a much broader, bell shape, the OD (darkness) of which falls off with radial distance, r, from its center, as described by $PSF_{out}(r)$. (b) When the wavelength of the input signal, $S_{in}(x,k)$, is long (i.e., for a low spatial frequency, small k, signal), the width of the PSF has no bearing on the output, and the MTF is not affected. For short-wavelength, high-spatial-frequency signals, however, the factors that blur out the PSF have the same effect on the details of $S_{in}(x,k)$, and image quality is diminished by the screen.

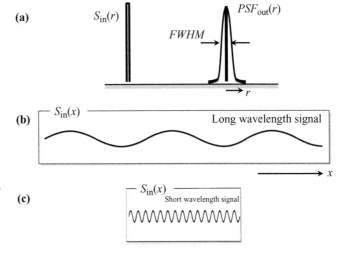

(a)

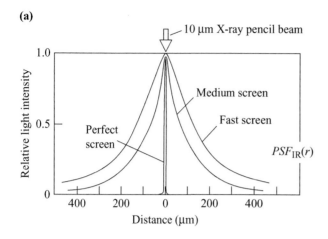

(b)

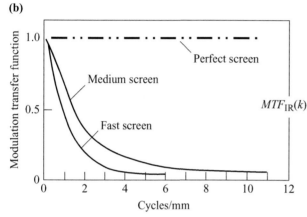

Figure 4.14 PSF and MTF for image receptors of three different spatial resolutions (sharpnesses). (**a**) The outputs, $S_{out}(r) = PSF(r)$ for IRs with high, medium, and low spatial resolutions, all with a 10-micron needle-beam X-ray input. (**b**) Although it may not be obvious why, the $MTF(k)$ for each is obtained simply as the Fourier transform of its PSF.

them than a thinner one, but its spatial resolution is also lower (Figure 4.9d).

There is a direct, simple, and important linkage between the PSF of a system and its MTF. As a general rule, the thicker the phosphor, the broader the PSF, and the more rapid the roll-off of the $MTF_{IR}(k)$. If the IR had no degrading effects on the signal, the output would also be a narrow peak, like the input, as with the PSF marked "perfect" in Figure 4.14a. Its spectrum would show the amplitudes at all frequencies as unity, just as with the input (Figure 4.14b). But a real imaging device diminishes the quality of a signal, and the result is a broadening and re-shaping of the PSF. The Fourier spectrum of the output signal no longer exhibits frequency components all of the same unit amplitude, moreover, but rather their amplitudes fall off at higher frequencies, as reflected in the MTF. We can put this in another, very useful way.

One way to determine the entire $MTF_{IR}(k)$ curve for a device would be to design and employ a set of pattern filters for many spatial frequencies of the type of Figure 4.11b. A much simpler and faster approach, based on the above argument, is to return to the needle beam's $PSF(r)$ function and simply take its Fourier transform,

$$MTF(k) = \mathbf{FT}\{PSF(r)\}. \qquad (4.3b)$$

It's not hard to demonstrate this but a little lengthy, and maybe the 2nd edition will be allowed more pages, but for now, "It can be shown that…" will have to do. Meanwhile, Figure 4.14 demonstrates this invaluable relationship with the same needle-beam X-ray input but screens of different thicknesses.

MTF_{focus} of an X-ray tube focal spot

Similar arguments allow the calculation of the MTF associated with other aspects of an imaging system. In addition to the IR, factors that affect the output signal in a radiographic imaging system include the size and shape of the tube's focal spot (Figure 4.9c), and any relative motions of patient and equipment (Figure 4.9b).

The source of X-rays is the small *focal spot* on the anode, where the high-velocity electrons strike, and where the high-energy bremsstrahlung and characteristic photons originate. In an ideal world, a focal spot would be minuscule and circular, and its X-ray beam could be said to have originated from a *point source*. Such is not the case for a real X-ray tube. Because the electrons that strike the target come from a wire coil that is a thick line source and are guided to some extent by a focusing cup (Figure 3.2b), the focal spot is not circular, but rather like a pair of bananas, elongated and of finite size, giving rise to *focal spot penumbra*, or *geometric blur*.

By means of a *pinhole camera* (Figure 4.15a), one can capture the two-dimensional image of a real focal spot on film (Figure 4.15b), and map out the intensity of radiation coming from the various points on it as a two-dimensional $PSF_{focal}(x,y)$ (Figure 4.15c). This map can be Fourier analyzed to provide a two-dimensional $MTF_{focal}(k)$ (Figure 4.15d), which falls off from the center with increasing spatial frequency, k.

The rectangular shape and finite dimensions of an X-ray focal spot normally have little discernible impact on a normal radiographic image. Problems can become evident, however, when the highest resolution is required, as with hairline fractures in bone, thin contrast-filled blood vessels, and breast calcifications, because the blurring may obscure high-frequency (that is, very small) components of the object being examined. While this difficulty may be largely eliminated by switching to a finer coil, it may worsen if the tube has aged and degraded enough for its blurring effects to become excessive.

Similar arguments allow the calculation of the $MTF_{motion}(k)$ associated with patient motion, and with other aspects of the imaging chain.

The MTF of a whole system is the product of the MTFs of its parts

The MTF is useful not only for examining focal spots, image receptors, and other items in the imaging process, but also for determining how the overall performance of an imaging system is influenced by the behavior of its separate components. If the imaging system consists of separable stages in series, where the output of each serves as the input to the next, then the behavior of the entire system at each spatial frequency, k, may be described as the product of the $MTF(k)$s of the various components. For our example,

$$MTF_{system}(k) = MTF_{focal}(k) \times MTF_{IR}(k)$$
$$\times MTF_{motion}(k). \quad (4.3c)$$

The MTF is a generalized description of the behavior of an imaging system, of what happens to the contrast and resolution together over a range of spatial frequencies (Figure 4.16). And it often can indicate if, why, or at least where, there is a problem.

The $MTF_{system}(k)$ of Equation 4.3c is more than just an extension of Equation 4.2. But like that equation, it suggests that if one of the three sources of unsharpness is noticeably more degrading than the other two at a certain frequency, then it will easily dominate the resulting blur in the image. That is, the largest contributor of blur controls the overall unsharpness of the image, and improvement in the other contributions won't help much. Similarly, if

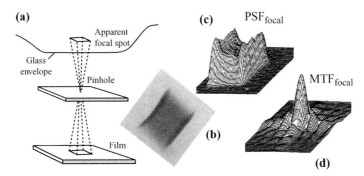

Figure 4.15 Study of the focal spot of an X-ray tube. **(a)** By means of a pinhole camera, the pattern of X-rays emitted from the focal spot exposes a high-resolution detector. **(b)** Scanning and measuring the response of the detector in two dimensions yields **(c)** a detailed two-dimensional PSF_{focal}. **(d)** The Fourier transform (spectrum) of the PSF is the MTF. Modified from Wagner RF, Weaver KE, Denny EW, Bostrom RG, Toward a unified view of radiological imaging systems. *Med Phys* 1974;**1**:11–14 (part d).

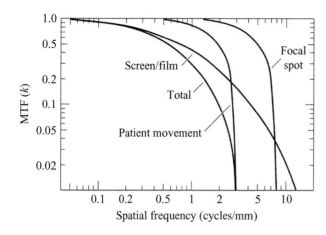

Figure 4.16 The MTF for this screen-film system is comprised of three constituent sub-MTFs that deal, respectively with focal spot penumbra, motion, and IR blur. It is calculated by way of Equation 4.3c.

any one component has a low MTF at some frequency, then the MTF for the entire system will be at least as low there. The imaging chain is only as strong as its weakest link. From the perspective of the design engineer, if the weakest link can process or display information with a spatial (or temporal) resolution comparable to a wavelength of $1/k$, then the other components in the chain need to perform well only up to a frequency of a few times k.

Another measurable construct, the *detective quantum efficiency* (*DQE*), combines the idea of the MTF with ways to quantify noise interference. The MTF and the DQE are the two standard measures of system overall performance. The DQE is somewhat more complicated, however, and we shall not pursue it here.

Stochastic noise and lesion detection

Even after one has made heroic efforts to optimize contrast and achieve acceptable resolution in an X-ray image, all the while keeping the dose to the patient (and everyone else) ALARA, the level of noise may simply be too great for a study to be clinically satisfying, as suggested by the contrast-detail image of Figure 2.15. One immediate response is to enhance the signal level somehow, in particular by increasing the mA-s and/or the kVp – and, as a possible consequence, the dose. The essential question is, of course, how much to do so. And might there be other ways to reduce the noise, as well?

Noise is rarely an issue for screen-film or digital radiography, but it certainly can be for analog or digital fluoroscopy, CT, and all forms of nuclear medicine, ultrasound, and MRI. Here the problem

is usually not the addition of unrelated random non-signals, as in Figure 2.14a, but rather the lack of sufficient "quanta" of information (Figure 2.14b), whether they be individual X- or gamma-ray photons, or echo vibrations, or radiofrequency photons in MRI signals.

This section provides brief examples of two related but different approaches to the issue of detecting low-contrast lesions in the presence of background noise, and both of them are built around the Poisson statistics mentioned in Chapter 2.

Poisson noise

A highly specific but frequently encountered category of random processes is named after the French mathematician Simeon Poisson. In 1837, Poisson derived a statistic that accounted accurately for the yearly variations in the number of Prussian officers kicked to death by cavalry horses. (No doubt it worked equally well for horses kicked to death by Prussian officers.) If it were found, over the course of several decades, that the mean number of officers dispatched in this fashion was $\mu = 3.2$ per year, then Poisson's formulas revealed that the probability of exactly 4, say, being killed in any randomly chosen year is 18%.

A *Poisson process* is one that involves discrete, countable (i.e., an integer number of them), statistically independent events; in addition, they must occur relatively infrequently, but at a fairly constant and/or uniform rate over substantial intervals of time, distance, or other relevant continuous parameter. This may sound extremely restrictive, and rather esoteric, but in fact Poisson processes are ubiquitous in life. We bring this up because surprisingly large numbers of physical and biological processes are of the Poisson type, and Box 4.2 lists some of the ones associated with imaging.

Box 4.2   Each of these is a Poisson process, and the numbers of events per unit of distance, size, time, etc., obey Poisson statistics

Poisson process	Number of . . .
Emulsion manufacture	AgBrI grains/100 μm^2
Digital image receptor	X-ray photons/pixel
Radiopharm. conc.	Radionuclei/mm^3 tissue
Scintillations in NaI(Tl) IR	Light photons/gamma
Ultrasound noise	Scatter points/voxel
Electronic noise	e through transistor/μs
MRI signal intensity	Protons/voxel
Tissue homogeneity	Voxel T1
Mammogram dose	Average μGy/exposure
Cell killing	Cells alive/colony
Car accidents, noon	Arrivals at ER/h

A Poisson distribution (e.g., number of Prussian officers rendered defunct per year versus probability) has an amazing, and not intuitively obvious, characteristic that can simplify and shed considerable light on many situations involving noise. Unlike the Gaussian (normal) curve, the Poisson can be described *fully* in terms of a *single* parameter, the *mean*, μ, alone; not only that, but also, for a Poisson process with an *average* of μ events per unit of area, time, dose, etc., the *standard deviation*, σ, happens *always* to be numerically equal to the square root of the mean:

$$\sigma = \sqrt{\mu} \qquad (4.4a)$$

For a Poisson process, then, the signal-to-noise ratio is $\mu/\sigma = \mu/\sqrt{\mu} = \sqrt{\mu}$, or

$$SNR = \sqrt{\mu} \qquad (4.4b)$$

seen earlier as Equation 2.3.

For nearly any Poisson process of interest, the Poisson distribution can be *approximated* by a traditional Gaussian/normal function, but where the mean and standard distribution *must* have the values μ and $\sqrt{\mu}$, respectively. It is then possible to fully exploit the well-known, tabulated probability information on the Gaussian, in particular that of Box 4.3. Suppose that in a region of a multipixel image receptor, it is found that $\mu = 36$ X-ray interactions per pixel, on average, for a certain exposure. This is a Poisson process, and its distribution is nearly Gaussian in shape, so we can immediately assert that *about* 67% of the pixels underwent between 30 and 42 ($\mu \pm \sqrt{\mu}$) photon-electron events (nearly all of which are photoelectric). Conversely, 5% of the pixels enjoyed either fewer than 24 or more than 48; that is, outside the ($\mu \pm 2\sqrt{\mu}$) range. This kind of argument happens to be a valuable guide in efforts to reduce Poisson-type noise.

Box 4.3   If a statistical data set is distributed at least approximately in a normal (Gaussian) manner with a mean of μ and a standard deviation of σ, then about 68%, 95%, and 99.7% of the data points lie within $\mu \pm \sigma$, $\mu \pm 2\sigma$, and $\mu \pm 3\sigma$, respectively. Alternatively, a single data point (measurement) has these probabilities of lying within the corresponding ranges

Range	Probability
$\mu \pm \sigma$	0.68
$\mu \pm 2\sigma$	0.95
$\mu \pm 3\sigma$	0.997
$\mu \pm 4\sigma$	0.99996

4σ and detecting a small nodule or bone chip

To detect a particular small anatomic feature, it must stand out perceptibly from background noise. For it to be clinically useful, that is, the signal-to-noise ratio must be sufficiently high – but, again, how high is that? How likely, or unlikely, it is that anyone would catch the small nodule in Figure 4.17? It's all a matter of playing the odds!

For concreteness, we'll assume an II tube fluoroscopic system pulses once briefly and is observed by a charge-coupled device (CCD) electrical optical camera that feeds via computer into a monitor. Imagine that a narrow row of tissue is partitioned into

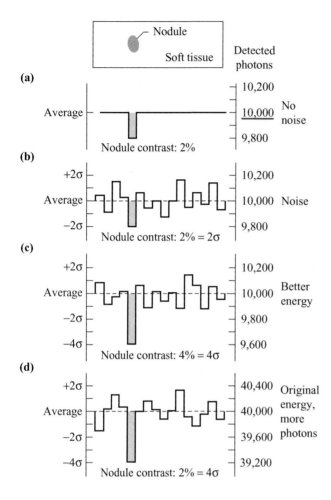

Figure 4.17 Effect of noise on the detectability of a small nodule, 1-voxel (2 mm) across, that attenuates 2% more than the surrounding soft tissues. Suppose that on average, 10 000 X-rays pass through every voxel apart from the one with the nodule during an exposure. (a) In the (unrealistic) case of no random noise, the 2% nodule stands out clearly. (b) The standard deviation of counts, $\sigma = \sqrt{10\,000} = 100$ happens to be numerically the same as 1% of the mean value, so the 2% contrast corresponds to (is of the same magnitude as) a 2σ spontaneous random variation. Gaussian statistics informs us that $2\frac{1}{2}\%$ of the voxels will lie naturally 2σ or more below the baseline, or norm, so the probability is only 1 in 40 that such a voxel contains a real nodule, which is not convincing evidence of its presence. How to increase the likelihood of obtaining a correct diagnosis? Either (c) enhance the contrast of the lesion (e.g., lower the kVp, utilize contrast agent) or (d) improve the statistics with four times as much mA-s.

2-mm-wide voxels, and that something more attenuating resides in one of them. It might be a tiny bone chip, for example, or a very small lung nodule, or even a small, iodine-filled blood vessel seen in cross-section. In any case, suppose that 10 000/mm X-ray photons traverse the typical voxel during the pulse, while only 9800 pass through the irregular one; there is a deficit of 200 photons there. Subject contrast, $C_{subject}$, is of the order of (10 000–9800)/10 000 or 2%. If magically there were no Poisson variations present – that is, in the absence of random noise – the voxel will stand out clearly from background and should be easy to detect (Figure 4.17a).

In reality there *will* be noise, of course, since the numbers of X-rays transmitted through the patient and striking pixels obeys a Poisson statistical distribution. The Poisson standard deviation is $\sigma = \sqrt{10\,000} = 100$, which means that the 2% deficit caused by the nodule, and the resulting contrast, is numerically just about equivalent to 2σ. So if you saw a 2% darker spot in an image, you could not tell whether it came from a nodule

there or just from a random count variation of amplitude 2σ (Figure 4.17b). (The vertical axis to the right records the number of X-ray photons per pixel that eventually show up on the monitor, and on the left this is expressed in multiples of σ.) By Box 4.3, about 95% of all the pixels will experience a number of photons within the range from $(\mu - 2\sigma)$ to $(\mu + 2\sigma)$ photons, from 9800 to 10 200. A full 5% of the soft tissue pixels, or 1 in 20, will transmit 9800 to 10 200 photons, and for 2.5% pixels, or half of these, the count will be *lower* than 9800 Thus the 2% change caused by the nodule can easily become lost in the noise fluctuations, which are of comparable amplitude and occur in 2.5% or 1/40 the pixels. It would be very easy to miss a 2σ-deep irregularity under these conditions, and a test with that many potential false positives is diagnostically of little help. So what's to be done to make the odds better?

We need to increase the SNR or, as they say in the trade, improve the statistics. One possibility is to increase the inherent contrast of the nodule by, say, reducing the kVp and effective

photon energy to a level that might make the voxel more attenuating relative to the tissue by a factor of two, say, thereby
doubling its contrast to 4% (Figure 4.17c). After adjusting the
mA-s to achieve the same background noise level as before,
the number of counts for the nodule is now 4σ below the mean,
at 9600. By Box 4.3, there is about a 0.00003 probability of
that occurring by chance – very good odds of it being a true
positive, indeed.

Another option is to go back to the original photon energy
but quadruple either the mA or the pulse time, so that now
40 000 photons transit each voxel of soft tissue, on average
(Figure 4.17d). We're back with 2% contrast again, but the
deficit is now 800; σ is now 200, and C is therefore equivalent
to $\sim 4\sigma$. And again, there is only about a 0.003% probability
that so great a divergence (4σ) from background would have
occurred by chance. In other words, 4σ of contrast is very likely
to be from a real nodule, and it should be next to impossible
to miss.

As we shall see in Chapter 6, there are various
computer programs for smoothing out noise, and in
other ways processing digital images. While sometimes much more can be gained than lost this way,
such efforts can also reduce signal strength too, so
they must be used with full understanding.

To summarize the point of Figures 4.17: the
greater the number of interaction events per unit
area, on average, the smaller the relative magnitudes
of the variations that will naturally occur randomly
from pixel to pixel. If random noise diminishes the
utility of an image, and perhaps obscures an object
of interest, a solution to the problem may be to get
better statistics with more photons. Alternatively,
it may be possible to enhance the contrast artificially as, for example, with iodine contrast agent
injected into a blood vessel. Either way, one of the

two issues of importance is the magnitude of the
clinically significant signal relative to the level of
background noise. The other is the dose. Back to
the old tradeoff.

Low-contrast, larger lesions and the Rose criterion

Poisson statistics has just provided a way to explore
the detectability of a single, voxel-sized irregularity.
It can also guide us with large, low-contrast lesions.
For variety's sake, let's examine a simple planar
nuclear medicine scan; the argument for radiography would be much the same.

Contrast in nuclear medicine comes from the
differential uptake of a specific radiopharmaceutical by a target tissue, followed by the corresponding
differential emission of high-energy photons. When
the concentration of the radiopharmaceutical in the
lesion ends up being either significantly greater or
less than that in the surrounding tissues, then this
will be notable as a hot-spot or dark area on the
display. Poisson statistics and the capabilities of the
eye place lower bounds on possible combinations
of lesion size, contrast, and numbers of gamma-
rays for which such an irregularity can be detected
(Figure 4.18).

With a correct setting of the display monitor's controls, the
brightness and apparent smoothness of a region are determined ultimately by the average number of gamma-rays
detected and displayed per square centimeter of normal background tissue, $(N/A)_{back}$. With a corresponding term for the
lesion, $(N/A)_{les}$, a definition for the lesion contrast cries out and
thrusts itself upon us:

$$C_{les} \equiv [(N/A)_{les} - (N/A)_{back}]/(N/A)_{back}.$$

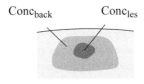

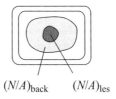

Figure 4.18 Subject contrast within the body in this nuclear medicine study is a measure of differential concentrations
of radiopharmaceutical (in effect, a radioactive contrast agent) in organs or other biological compartments relative
to the background (back) level. Image contrast refers to the corresponding variations in brightness on the display. The
detectability of a lesion (les) depends critically on its subject contrast (which is strongly affected by the random variations in
the number of gamma-rays detected per unit area of the crystal of the gamma camera, i.e., the noise level) and on its size.

Gamma camera image quality tends to increase with number of counts – rapidly, at first, but then with diminishing returns. The increase can come either from use of a greater amount of radiopharmaceutical or from a longer imaging period. The first will increase dose to both patient and staff. With longer imaging times, the likelihood of motion blur goes up, and patient throughput declines,

An average emission rate of the order of 1000 counts/cm^2 at the camera face is commonly held to represent a good balance. In a low-contrast image, $(N/A)_{les}$ does not differ much from $(N/A)_{back}$, and (apart from in the definition of C_{les}) we can call them about the same, here: $(N/A)_{les} \sim (N/A)_{back} = (N/A)$, and delete the subscripts.

Suppose that an average dimension of the lesion is d_{les}, so that its area is d_{les}^2. The average number of counts for an area of background of this size is $N_{les} = d_{les}^2(N/A)$. For the spontaneous, random variations in number of counts that will occur in a lesion-sized area and with this average number of background counts, Poisson statistics informs us that the standard deviation is $\sigma = N_{les}^{1/2} = d_{les}(N/A)^{1/2}$. The relative variation, also known as the *noise contrast,* is

$$C_{noise} \equiv \sigma/N_{les} = 1/N_{les}^{1/2} = 1/d_{les}(N/A)^{1/2}.$$

Multiple psychophysics studies have shown that humans are generally capable of visually detecting objects (that are not too large or small) amid noise when the image satisfies the *Rose criterion*: the lesion contrast must be at least three to five times the noise contrast:

$$C_{les}/C_{noise} = C_{les}d_{les}(N/A)^{1/2}$$
$$= [(N/A)_{les} - (N/A)_{back}]d_{les} / (N/A)^{1/2} > 3 - 5.$$

$$(4.4c)$$

Not too surprisingly, Equation 4.4c is like an expression for a signal-to-noise ratio for minimal detectability. If a lesion is anticipated to be small or of low subject contrast, then the camera must accumulate a larger number of counts to overcome the loss of image signal amid the statistical noise, as common sense would dictate. This can be achieved either by imaging for a longer time (increasing the likelihood of motion blurring) or with higher radio-pharmaceutical activity and subject contrast (and dose to the patient).

Deterministic noise and other artifacts

Unlike the digital modalities, screen-film displays few artifacts, or forms of deterministic noise.

One that occurs rarely, but is obvious when it does, arises from physical damage to undeveloped film, such as from electrostatic electricity (Figure 4.19a).

Another, which is slightly more subtle, is the distortions that come, in all projection modalities, from differential magnification of objects within the body that are not at the same distance from the IR (Figure 4.19b). The dimensions of a projected image, *I*, depend not only on the size and shape of the *Object*, *O*, but also on the *Distances* of the object from the (nearly) point *Source* of radiation (*SOD*), and from the *Source* to the *Image* receptor (*SID*): the magnification, MAG, is

$$MAG = I/O = SID/SOD. \qquad (4.5)$$

Special requirements for mammography

Breast cancer is the most common potentially lethal malignancy affecting women, and one in eight will be diagnosed with the disease during her lifetime. A total of 180 000 new cases of invasive breast cancer will be diagnosed this year in the United States, and these will lead to the deaths of 40 000 people.

Women between 20 and 24 have the lowest incidence rate, 1.4 per 100 000. The risks increase above that age, however, reaching 100, 200, and 300 per 100000, respectively, by ages 40, 50, and 60, with a maximum at about 75. The median age at time of diagnosis is 61, and 95% of cases and 97% of deaths occur in women 40 and older. Above 45, the incidence rate is higher for Caucasian women than for African Americans, but African Americans have a greater probability of dying at all ages. Incidence and mortality figures are lower among women of other racial and ethnic groups. Fewer than 1% of breast cancers are diagnosed in men [1].

Mammograms are notoriously difficult to read. Most breast cancers manifest radiographically as low-contrast changes in the lobules and ducts of glandular tissues that are sometimes adjacent to adipose tissues, and these faint irregularities are easily obscured by the visual complexities of overlapping normal breast tissues, and little subject contrast can be achieved. Fibrous, ductal, and glandular tissues of the breast have nearly the same radiological properties as water, and the density of fatty tissue is only

(a)

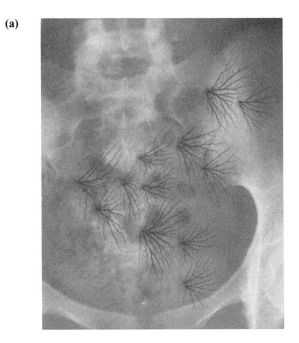

Figure 4.19 Artifacts. (**a**) The effect of static electricity on undeveloped film. (**b**) Identical circular coins lying in a plane (the object plane) will produce, in a parallel image plane, images that are circular and all of the same size. But those in different planes will be magnified by different amounts, and this effect can lead to distortion artifacts in a clinical image. Likewise, balls and circular coins not lying parallel to the image plane will produce images that are neither circular nor the same size, even if their centers are all at the same height above the image plane. It is because of this *parallax* effect that interventionalists always attempt to center the field of view on the region of interest, to minimize distortion due to differential magnification.

(b)

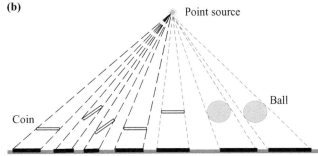

10% or so lower. The widely used Breast Imaging Reporting and Data System (BI-RADS) of the American College of Radiology offers a qualitative assessment of breast density, with four categories: (1) almost entirely fat; (2) scattered fibroglandu- lar densities; (3) heterogeneously dense; and (4) extremely dense (Figure 4.20).

Some breasts also display the other major telltale sign of a potential lesion, characteristic patterns of *microcalcifications*. These are flecks of calcium

Figure 4.20 Representations of the four Breast Imaging Reporting and Data System (BI-RADS) breast density qualitative and quantitative assessments. (**a**) BI-RADS 1, almost entirely fat; (**b**) BI-RADS 2, scattered fibroglandular densities; (**c**) BI-RADS 3: heterogeneously dense; and (**d**) BI-RADS 4: extremely dense. Reprinted with permission from *Journal of the National Comprehensive Cancer Network*.

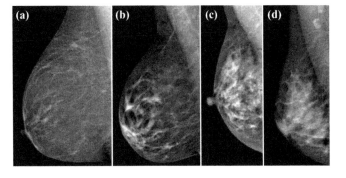

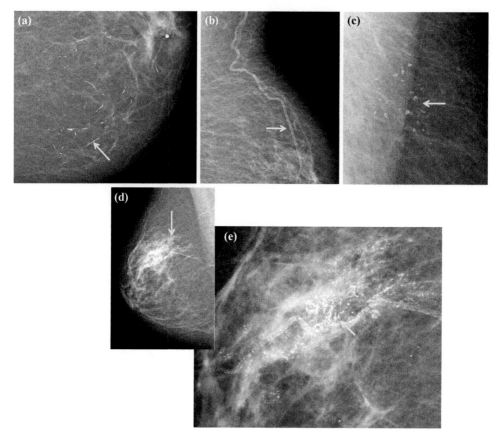

Figure 4.21 The spatial distributions and specific configurations of microcalcifications in the breast may be diagnostic of cancer. Screening examinations must also be as sensitive and specific as possible so as not to miss an early, small neoplasm, and also to avoid additional unnecessary examinations (and dose!) when dealing with benign etiologies. (**a**) Craniocaudal view of the left breast, demonstrating a cluster of microcalcifications of benign configuration extending throughout the quadrant. These smooth, spindle-shaped small crystals of calcium-based material are typical of plasma cell mastitis or secretory disease (arrow). (**b**) Medial-lateral oblique (MLO) view of the same left breast demonstrating linear, parallel-track calcifications following the distribution of an artery, representing angiosclerotic changes (arrow). (**c**) A magnified, focally (locally) compressed MLO view of the upper portion of the left breast in another individual, demonstrating a cluster of rounded and polygonal calcifications with lucent centers. These are typical of benign skin calcifications associated with degenerative metaplastic changes (arrow). All three of these types of microcalcifications are considered benign and do not require further evaluation. (**d**) In a third patient presenting for a screening mammogram, this MLO view reveals a cluster of irregular microcalcifications within the upper outer quadrant of the right breast (arrow). (**e**) With a magnified view, the microcalcifications appear irregular and sometimes branched (arrow), typical of a focus of comedocarcinoma. The calcifications within the branching ducts of the breast follow metaplastic changes of the cancer cells themselves.

salts, commonly hydroxyapatite or calcium oxalate, visible when as small as 0.1 millimeter, that vary in shape and spatial distribution in diagnostically informative ways (Figure 4.21), and there is a BI-RADS classifications scheme for them, as well.

Fortunately, mammography can, in most cases, reveal the disease while it is still at an early stage, sometimes long before a neoplasm has grown large enough to be palpable – and five-year survival for stage I patients is over 95%. Hence the obvious value of routine, high-quality screening. BI-RADS provides a seven-level assessment scheme by means of which a reader can score the likelihood of breast disease for a particular set of patient images: 0, incomplete; 1, negative; 2, benign finding(s); 3, probably benign; 4, suspicious abnormality; 5, highly suggestive of malignancy; 6, known biopsy – proven malignancy.

The dedicated mammography system: particularly high contrast and resolution are essential, along with very low dose

Mammography is a form of radiography specialized and refined specifically for imaging the breast. One is normally searching for lesions that are small and very similar radiologically to the surrounding breast soft tissues, and also for microcalcifications. Both excellent contrast and exquisite resolution are essential, and that requires a radiation exposure high enough to achieve an acceptable signal-to-noise ratio. At the same time, the breast is sensitive to ionizing radiation, so it is also critical to keep dose as low as reasonably achievable for reasons of safety.

Achieving an optimal balance between creating clinically adequate images, while at the same time keeping the risks "acceptably" low, is difficult with all forms of imaging with ionizing radiation, but it is especially so for the breast. None of contrast, resolution, noise, and dose objectives is particularly easy to achieve separately, and producing a single imaging device that can satisfy them all simultaneously has required heroic design ingenuity (Figures 4.22a and b). First to achieve this was screen-film mammography, with low-energy molybdenum (Mo) characteristic X-rays (rather than bremsstrahlung) generated by a special tube with particularly small focal spots on a Moly target and detected with special mammography film, with emulsion on one side only for better resolution, within a single-screen cassette (Figure 4.22c). These efforts have culminated in the *full-field digital mammography* (FFDM) system (Chapter 7).

Because of the subtlety of the signs of disease, there is need in mammography both to optimize the subject contrast (through an optimal choice of kVp and achieving low noise with enough mA-s) and to obtain a high degree of spatial resolution (by way of a small focal spot and an extra-high-detail screen or digital IR). The latitude of the image receptor must be broad enough to accommodate the low-intensity beam emerging from the thick tissue near the chest wall, moreover, and also the much greater number of X-ray photons that pass through the skin at the anterior edge of the breast. And, of course, the dose should be kept low to minimize both radiation risk and patient anxiety. A modern dedicated mammographic unit is designed to achieve the best possible balance among these somewhat conflicting requirements, and is made up of a specially designed mammographic X-ray tube and generator, breast compression device, grid, and a unique screen-film or digital IR.

The utility of a mammogram depends, ultimately, on its ability to allow the clinician to discriminate among the various normal and abnormal breast tissues. The attenuation properties of glandular, adipose, muscle, skin tissues, and neoplasms are alike, and often differences are not visible with standard projection radiography. Contrast among the radiologically similar soft tissues of breast is enhanced by imaging with a very low-energy X-ray beam produced with specialized targets, windows, and filters. Attenuation by all tissues is higher and the beam penetration is poorer at low energies, which is not desirable since it leads to greater dose deposition in breast tissues; but the relative *differences* in attenuation between tumor and normal breast are accentuated, and so also is the contrast, which is crucial.

A screen-film mammographic X-ray tube generally has a rotating *molybdenum* (*Mo*) anode/target; operated commonly between 23 and 34 kVp, it provides a suitable beam composed of molybdenum-characteristic X-rays (at 17.5 and 19.6 keV) and a small amount of bremsstrahlung (Figure 4.23a). The beam emerging from the tube is then filtered, as in standard radiography, to remove its diagnostically nonproductive components. Molybdenum is the material of choice for the beam filter, as well as for the target. Any element is relatively transparent to its own characteristic X-rays, but not to those a bit higher (Figure 4.23b). (Why?) An Mo filter allows Mo characteristic X-rays to pass through readily, but heavily attenuates lower- and higher-energy (hence less eliciting of contrast) bremsstrahlung.

Tubes commonly provide a second, alternative anode target-track made of rhodium or rhenium, with slightly higher characteristic X-ray peaks, or tungsten. Tungsten operated at low kVp yields a somewhat higher-energy beam than molybdenum, for dealing with larger, denser breasts, where there is need for more penetration. The most advanced systems select the target material, filter, and kVp for a patient automatically, after a trial, low-dose exploratory exposure.

(a)

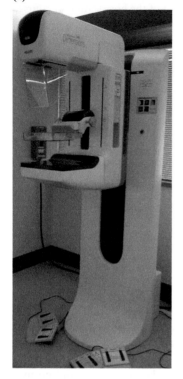

(c)

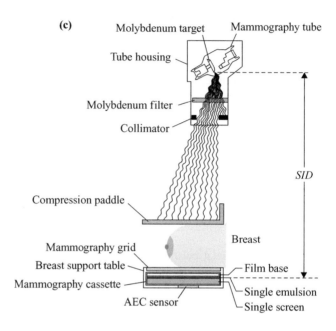

(b)

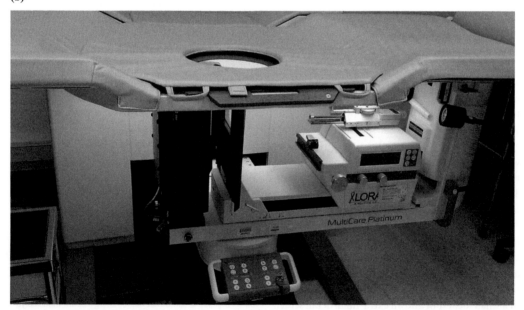

Figure 4.22 Mammographic imaging. (a) A modern mammography unit. (b) Mammographic stereotactic needle biopsy system for patient in the prone position. (c) Schematic of the components.

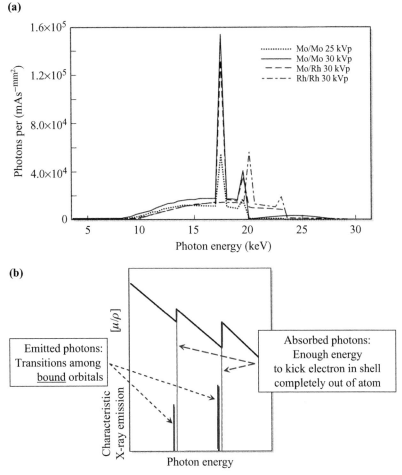

Figure 4.23 The mammographic beam. **(a)** While virtually all other kinds of X-ray imaging employ higher-energy bremsstrahlung radiation from a tungsten target, screen-film mammography does better with the low-energy characteristic X-rays from a molybdenum (or, less frequently) a rhodium- or rhenium-alloy target, with a matching Mo, Rh, or Re filter. The choice of filter is important because **(b)** an absorption edge for a material occurs at an energy slightly higher than the corresponding characteristic X-ray emission lines for the same material. Molybdenum characteristic X-ray photons pass through molybdenum more readily, for example, than do photons of a bit higher energy. A molybdenum filter can therefore be used with a molybdenum-target mammography X-ray tube to pass molybdenum characteristic X-ray photons, while cutting out higher-energy bremsstrahlung photons, which are less effective in extracting image contrast, and therefore would degrade the image. The filter also removes very low-energy bremsstrahlung photons, which are clinically useless but which do contribute to patient dose.

A mammography tube has two small focal spots to select from. The smaller of them, nominally about 0.1 mm across, serves in magnification imaging. (With *magnification*, the image receptor is moved away from the breast, rather than in *contact* with it; this leads to a larger image because of the geometric divergence of the beam [Equation 4.5], and to less scatter radiation striking the IR, because of the air gap, but at the price of a dose that increases to compensate for the inverse-square law loss in intensity.)

One of the more unpleasant aspects of mammography, from the patient's perspective, is compression of the breast between a pair of parallel, flat paddles translucent to X-rays (Figures 4.22 and 4.24). But compression reduces the thickness of the block of tissue being imaged, and therefore less penetration is needed, making a lower kVp feasible. It also lessens the amount of radiation required for the image, so less dose is deposited; likewise, less is scattered toward the IR, which also helps with contrast. It sets the tissues to a constant thickness,

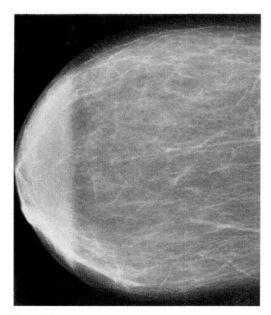

Figure 4.24 Compression of a breast in the cranio-caudal projection, with the edge of the paddle evident. Compression spreads out otherwise overlapping tissues for clearer visibility, produces uniform thickness and therefore fairly even average optical density, holds the breast immobile to reduce motion blur, diminishes scatter and, because the compressed breast is thinner, reduces dose. Courtesy of TG Langer, University of Virginia Health Sciences Center.

which gives the image a mostly uniform average brightness, for better visualization. It also spreads them out over a large area, so that their shadows are un-stacked, reducing the visual confusion from their overlapping, and improving contrast. And firmly holding the breast in place prevents blurring from patient motion, which improves resolution.

The cassette contains only one rare earth screen, and high-contrast film with photographic emulsion coated on one side. The X-ray pattern from the breast passes first through the film base, then the emulsion, and finally into the intensifying screen; this arrangement minimizes the screen blur, since many X-ray interactions occur near (and the most light quanta come from) the proximal surface of the screen, immediately adjacent to the emulsion. The resulting resolution can be of the order of 15–20 lp/mm.

The switch to digital image receptors, in particular the flat panel imagers of DR with electronic readout, has been rapid. While fewer than 10% of mammographic units in the US were digital in 2005, more than 70% of the devices now in operation are.

QA and the Mammography Quality Standards Act

Because of a quirk in the Atomic Energy Act passed more than half a century ago, we are all protected from improper use of X-ray equipment almost exclusively by laws and regulations of the individual states. The sole major exception, for now, is that of mammography, as implemented in the federal *Mammography Quality Standards Act of 1992* (*MQSA*), amended by the *Mammography Quality Standards Reauthorization Act* of 1998 (*MQSRA*), together commonly called simply "the MQSA." The MQSA instructs the FDA to set and enforce detailed minimum federal quality standards for mammography facilities in their regulations, readily accessible at Title 21 of the Code of Federal Regulations, Part 900, Section 12 (21 CFR 900.12) and other parts (www.fda.gov/radiation-emittingproducts/mammographyqualitystandardsactandprogram/default.htm).

All mammography units must pass an initial MQSA equipment evaluation before being put into clinical service. The MQSA regulations include standards for equipment capabilities, the quality control program, image quality, and acceptable levels of radiation dose for a specified phantom. Every facility that performs mammography must be certified by the FDA, and approved by an accrediting body such as the American College of Radiology (ACR), which offers guidelines and requirements for performing high-quality mammography. By the MQSA regulations, the lead interpreting physician is responsible for the QA/QC program, and the mammography physicist directly oversees it, although many parts of it are carried out by the mammography technologists who produce the images. The MQSA also specifies minimum requirements for the training and continuing education of interpreting physicians, medical physicists, and mammography technologists, including extensive instruction, hands-on, supervised initial practice, and frequent experience.

Interpreting mammograms is surely one of the most demanding tasks in medicine, one for which specialized training is imperative. But the diagnosis by a radiologist, no matter how skilled and experienced, is limited by the quality of the images produced by the technologists and the equipment. And it is disturbing that studies from some clinics make

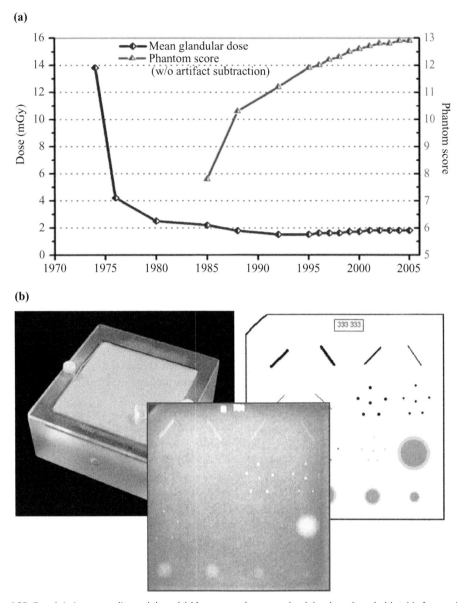

Figure 4.25 Trends in image quality and dose. (a) Mammography mean glandular doses have held stable for nearly three decades, while imaging scores on test phantoms are only now leveling off. Courtesy of David Spelick, FDA. (b) The FDA's MQSA phantom and a high quality mammographic image of it. Embedded in the phantom are test points, rods, etc., of precisely manufactured dimensions and attenuation properties. The smallest microcalcifications (<1 mm) are the ones of greatest concern. Modified from American College of Radiology (ACR) Teaching File images.

only barely minimally passing scores on the image quality tests given during accreditation reviews and federal inspections. Still, studies of image quality with test devices designed by the FDA and by other means, and of the associated doses, both show encouraging trends (Figure 4.25a).

A special MQSA "phantom" designed by the FDA plays a central role in the QA program (Figure 4.25b). The phantom is a 4.2 cm thick block of material with the attenuation properties of an equal-parts homogeneous mixture of glandular and adipose tissues. Within it are embedded tumor-like masses, fibers, and clusters of specks of bone-like material, all of various sizes; it is necessary to detect a minimum number of each.

Image intensifier-tube fluoroscopy: viewing in real time

When Roentgen placed his hand in an X-ray beam and beheld the bones of his fingers on a fluorescent screen, he was creating the first *fluoroscopic* image. Within months, medical practitioners around the world were employing essentially the same approach in their clinics. They did this in a darkened room by projecting a beam through the patient, with the X-ray image appearing directly on the screen. They first had to adapt their eyes to the dark for perhaps half an hour, and even then the images were faint and of low contrast. So with the steady flow of improvements to conventional film radiography, medical fluoroscopy fell largely by the wayside.

Analog fluoroscopy = X-ray tube + image intensifier tube + solid-state CCD or CMOS electronic optical camera

Because of two major advances in vacuum-tube electronics, however, fluoroscopy enjoyed a renaissance, and it is once again a standard means of allowing the viewing of dynamic X-ray images *in real time*. One of these was television.

Ever since Samuel Morse telegraphed "What hath God wrought!" from Washington to Baltimore on May 24, 1844 and, three decades later, Alexander Graham Bell's assistant heard the first intelligible words sent by telephone, "Mr. Watson, come here. I want you," people dreamed of transmitting pictures, too, over wires or through the air. (Nearly as memorable as Bell's summons was the reaction, soon thereafter, of Pedro II, Emperor of Brazil, to a demonstration of the new marvel: "My God! It speaks Portuguese!") It was not until 1927, however, that a fully electronic television system was finalized. A year later, General Electric began transmitting experimentally from a station, under call letters W2XB, from Schenectady, NY, and the BBC began public high-quality broadcasting in 1936. Spurred on by the wartime effort to perfect radar, television had acquired sufficient spatial and contrast resolution, low noise, and reliability by the 1950s for

millions to share in the good and the rot that TV hath wrought. But generally more constructively, it allowed radiologists to display visual medical information in real time.

The other critical technical advance was the development, at about the same time but specifically for radiological application, of the X-ray *image intensifier* (II) – an electronic vacuum tube device that can transform a faint, life-sized pattern of X-rays emerging from a patient into a small, bright visible-light image (Figure 4.26a).

An analog fluoroscopy system is similar to one that produces radiographs, with the replacement of the cassette with the II tube and optical cameras (Figure 4.26b). Still and cine film cameras and television were long the standards for observing the output of the II, but they have been superseded by solid-state CCDs or *complementary metal-oxide semiconductor* (CMOS) imagers (Figure 4.26c). These electronic optical cameras differ in design, but behave much alike, and act as the eyes of nearly all digital cameras and camcorders. The video signal from the CCD or CMOS camera passes into the computer for processing, storage, and instant display.

The principal components of an II tube are the large input screen (15–35 cm across); the focusing electrodes; the anode; and the small (3 cm in diameter) output fluorescent screen (Figure 4.26a). The X-ray pattern emerging from the patient strikes the *input phosphor* of the II tube, typically cesium iodide (CsI) in the structured form (Figure 4.9d), producing pinpoint bursts of visible light photons. The interior surface of the input screen is coated with a thin veneer of photosensitive cesium-antimony metal alloy, the *photocathode*, from which the scintillations of light (not the X-rays!) eject photoelectrons. The spatial configuration of these freed electrons closely resembles that of the initial primary X-ray image. As the electrons accelerate through the vacuum toward the *anode*, they are squeezed closer together by the *focusing electrodes*, without losing the shape of their pattern. On striking the small fluorescent *output screen* (e.g., ZnCdS:Ag, Gd_2O_2S:Tb, etc.) at high velocity, each electron produces a bright point-flash of light. It thereby re-creates the original primary X-ray image, only shrunk to a size suitable for recording by an optical camera, thousands of times brighter than the one originally produced on the input fluorescent screen, and capable of capturing motion. The light image is transferred by lenses and perhaps fiber optics to the CCD, where it is transformed into an electronic signal to be

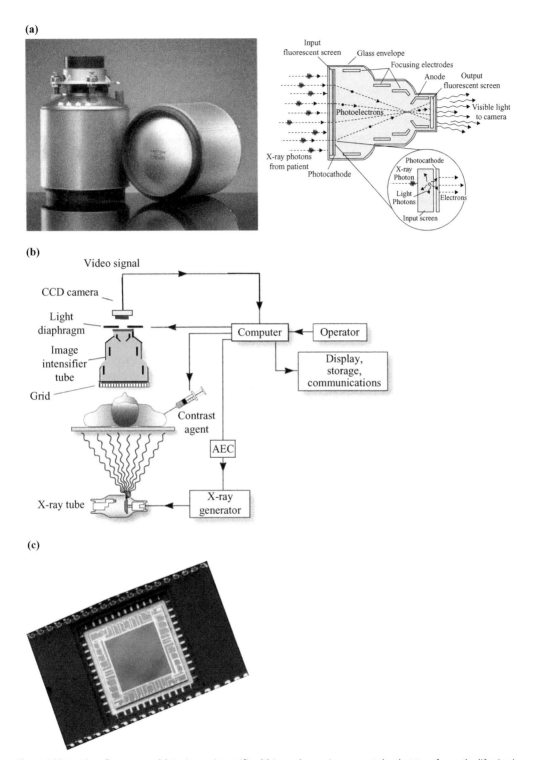

Figure 4.26 Modern fluoroscopy. (**a**) An image intensifier (II) is an electronic vacuum tube that transforms the life-sized X-ray shadow pattern emerging from a patient into a small, very bright optical image ready to be viewed by an electronic optical camera and fed into a computer. (**b**) Block diagram of a modern II-based fluoroscopic system, where everything is under computer control. (**c**) A small solid state electronic optical camera, such as a charge-coupled device (CCD), that observes the output of the II tube and sends its signal to the computer.

digitized and sent to the computer and monitor. As a rule of thumb, a good II tube with a structured-CsI phosphor input screen has an overall resolution about half of what is achievable with screen-film. The capacity of an II tube to reproduce subject contrast, on the other hand, is relatively poor, partly because of the low radiation exposures involved and the resulting high statistical noise and weak SNR.

An important component is the feedback loop of the automatic brightness control (ABC) or automatic exposure control (AEC) sub-system: the intensity of the light emerging from the II tube is monitored either by a beam splitter (a partially silvered mirror) and photocell, or from the average video signal of the CCD camera; should the average light level go down, for example, a signal is fed back to the generator, which can increase the X-ray tube mA or kVp or the X-ray pulse duration. The X-ray tube current is normally something like a few mA, incidentally, which is a hundred-fold lower than that for a single radiograph; but in fluoro mode, the X-ray tube may be pulsing rapidly for minutes at a stretch, and it is necessary to control both patient dose and anode heating.

The X-ray beam is pulsed repeatedly, 30, 15, 7.5, 3.75, or even fewer times per second, making possible continuous, live imaging. Real-time viewing has proved invaluable in reducing fractures, surgically removing shrapnel and other foreign bodies, and guiding the progress of catheters and other devices. The sharply visible patterns of an injected radiographic contrast agent flowing along through blood vessels can be observed and recorded as they occur and then re-played immediately – not after long minutes of waiting for motion picture film to be developed. The movement of swallowed contrast agent past a constriction in the throat can be watched as it takes place, and re-viewed again and again as needed. While slow pulsing can lead to somewhat jerky motions of catheters, boluses of iodinated blood, etc., it can also cut down significantly on patient dose, which is particularly significant for pediatric examinations. There may also be advantage in frame-averaging, moreover, in which some temporal resolution is lost in exchange for images with lower spatial noise, and in other forms of combining information from several frames at once. Alternatively, last-image-hold imaging, or frame-freezing one at a time, can provide the needed information with few frames and at extremely low dose.

Long after the II tube and television established fluoroscopy in the imaging clinic, more sophisticated solid-state technology and computers elbowed their way in, with profound consequences. The II tube plus electronic optical camera combination is being displaced by the solid-state *active matrix flat panel imager* (AMFPI). This computer-driven, pixelated image receptor, which is somewhat like a body-sized CCD that detects X-rays rather than light images, has found wide acceptance in interventional angiography and cardiology, albeit still at notable cost. More about that in Chapter 7.

Fluoroscopy QA

Quality control for fluoroscopy starts out much the same as for radiography, with some obvious extensions to cover the II tube, the optical camera, and the monitor display. There are a number of electronic test signals to be sent directly from the computer to the *monitor*, for example, without the involvement of any imaging device, that can reveal its contrast and resolution (i.e., its MTF), noise, and brightness performance, as was seen in Figure 2.19c.

Radiation safety has to be more comprehensive, because local doses may be much higher (commonly over 250 mGy for a large patient), and there are risks of deterministic health effects as well as of the stochastic. Over 200 radiation injuries have been reported in the literature. Usually attributable to insufficient physician training or experience, these include hair loss, erythema, rashes, and extremely painful burns and ulceration. The burns, unlike those from heat or chemicals, may not appear for a while after the exposure, and bad ones may never fully heal. Many of these complications occur not in the region being examined, but rather in an arm or breast that happens to be in the way and, because of the inverse square effect, receives a much higher dose. Ways to minimize dose and risk include utilizing the last-image-hold feature; monitoring dose at the beam input to skin and/or at the entrance to the IR; turning to high dose rate only when essential; maximizing SID; choosing 7.5 frames/s if dose/frame is independent of dose rate; intermittently re-directing the beam to new areas of skin; and ensuring that any excess-dose warning systems are activated. By FDA regulations, the entrance skin dose should be under about 100 mGy/min, except under special conditions when it can rise to about 200 mGy/min.

Conclusion: bringing radiography and fluoroscopy into the twenty-first century with solid-state digital X-ray image receptors

With screen-film, the same entity – a piece of photographic film – serves to capture and display the image. Because they are so rigidly linked, one cannot separately optimize the capture, processing, and display steps. The film's latitude and contrast are fixed, moreover, so some parts of it may be so over- or underexposed, or so poor in image contrast, as to render it clinically useless; the only way around this problem is to shoot another film with different technique factors.

A film is stored in racks, moreover, or, if you *really* need it, it's hidden deep in a pile in Dr. Green's office, and she happens to be spending the month searching the Loire valley for the perfect Sancerre. If ever found, moreover, it will have to be transported or communicated by hand or snail mail. Similar considerations apply for fluoroscopy. Finally, the only way to analyze the information content of an analog image is for a physician to examine it visually. That generally works well, but after a while, any film reader cannot help but become bleary-eyed, and perhaps slightly distracted by phone calls from her teenage children or from charming malpractice insurance salesmen.

All that is undergoing rapid change, brought about by the take-over of imaging systems by computers, as will be discussed in Chapter 6. Screen-film cassettes and II tube plus CCD combinations are giving way to fully digital solid-state active matrix flat panel imagers, which can directly transform a pattern of X-rays into a voltage signal and send it to a computer instantaneously. In nearly all situations, the innate image quality in digital radiography and fluoroscopy (R/F) systems is at least comparable to that of the analog units.

But beyond that, digital *image processing* can work wonders in enhancing contrast, in eliminating both stochastic (random) and deterministic (systemic) noise, and in sharpening up edges. The acts

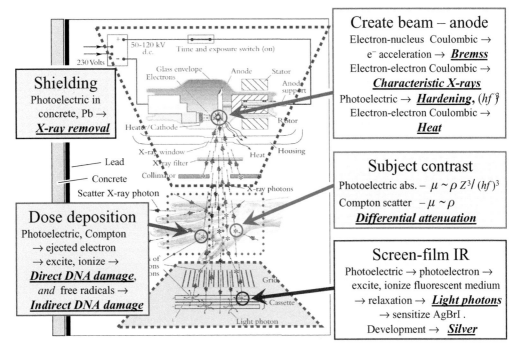

Figure 4.27 The works.

of image acquisition, massage, and rendition are now *un*linked, so one can tune the technique factors to maximize subject contrast, and then separately adjust the image processing parameters for best image receptor contrast on the display. The outcome will surpass what can be achieved by trying to optimize both on film at the same time. And by sending the final image to a *picture archiving and communication system* (*PACS*) (Figure 0.2), it can be recalled in seconds, or sent down the hall or around the world in the same amount of time.

One of the most exciting, but debated, aspects of computers in imaging involves their capabilities in pattern recognition. *Computer-assisted detection* (CAD) is now widely employed with digital mammography as a "second pair of eyes," and it can increase a physician's rate of cancer detection by 20%, and is an approach more cost-effective than obtaining a second reading from a different radiologist. CAD also finds application in the search for lung nodules, and in a few other niches. But the subtlety of many of the clinically significant variations in detail and contrast, together with the great range in normal and abnormal patterns occurring among different individuals, makes the general problem of automated CAD and diagnosis highly challenging.

Where research in pattern recognition and other forms of artificial intelligence will lead, in medicine and elsewhere, is uncertain. But what is clearly evident is that computers will progress far beyond their currently limited role of offering second opinions on a few special medical conditions, and that they will move on toward full computer-aided decision-making, providing increasingly reliable probabilistic differential diagnoses. This process will not displace physicians for the foreseeable future, but it may require them to acquire some radically new skill sets.

* * *

We've covered a lot of territory so far, and a good deal of it will come up again in future chapters. You can re-assure yourself of how much you have already taken in by re-capping the story of the creation of an X-ray image (Figure 4.27). Enjoy!

Reference

1 American Cancer Society. Breast Cancer Facts and Figures, 2009–2010. At www.cancer.org/Research/Can cerFactsFigures/BreastCancerFactsFigures/f861009-final-9 -08-09-pdf. Accessed October 22, 2012.

CHAPTER 5

Radiation Dose and Radiogenic Risk

Ionization-Induced Damage to DNA can cause Stochastic, Deterministic, and Teratogenic Health Effects – And How To Protect Against Them

Imaging with gamma- and X-rays has saved countless lives over the past century, but medical radiation is a double-edged sword.

Our exposure to ionizing radiation has doubled over the past few decades

In the earliest days, those who experimented with X-rays and radium were largely unaware of the harm that ionizing radiation can cause. The radiation-induced effect observed most commonly among those pioneers was a reddening of skin; some even used this *erythema* to gauge X-ray exposure. But many cases of severe and irreversible radiogenic burns and carcinomas of the dermis were soon reported. And over the years, physicians and others have provided extensive and tragic evidence of the dangers of excessive irradiation.

Until recently, most of the ionizing radiation to which we are all exposed was naturally occurring. It comes primarily from three sources: *cosmic rays*, which are highly energetic protons and other particles bombarding Earth from outer space,

Medical Imaging: Essentials for Physicians, First Edition. Anthony B. Wolbarst, Patrizio Capasso and Andrew R. Wyant.
© 2013 John Wiley & Sons, Inc. Published 2013 by John Wiley & Sons, Inc.

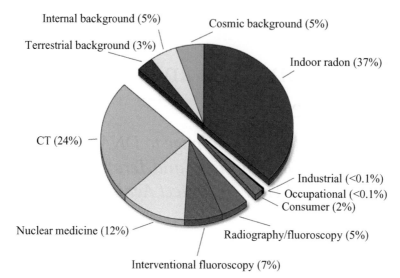

Figure 5.1 Relative contributions from natural background, medical, and other sources to individual effective dose in the US for 2006. Natural background radiation varies greatly from place to place, but in the United States it averages to the equivalent of gamma- or X-ray dose of about 3 mGy. A critical point is that the total average dose – the overall size of the pie – has about doubled from when it was last published, and most of the change is due to medical studies, in particular CT. Because of the numbers of people exposed (especially with CT), medical imaging now presents to the population the same risk of cancer and hereditary effects as does background radiation, even though diagnostic exposures are usually localized to only a small part of the body. Redrawn from NCRP [1], fig. 1.1, with permission from the National Council on Radiation Protection and Measurements. http://NCRPonline.org.

mostly from the Sun; *radioactive materials* in the soil and rocks around us (primarily radium-226 coming from the decay of uranium-238) and in our bodies (potassium-40) that emit gamma-rays; and *radon* (Rn-222), a noble gas originating with the decay of radium in the soil that then seeps into our basements. The average American receives the risk equivalent of about 3 milligray (mGy) of high-energy photons to the whole body over the course of a year. The best *estimate* of lifetime risk from lifetime exposure to *natural background ionizing radiation* is that 1 in 100 of us will die prematurely because of a cancer induced by this background. At the same time, roughly one in four of us will suffer some other fatal "spontaneously occurring" cancer caused by an unrelated mechanism.

Over the past few decades, that state of affairs has changed radically. In 2009, the *National Council on Radiation Protection and Measurements* (NCRP) produced an updated report on the average exposure of the US population to ionizing radiation [1]. Their principal finding is that now, on average, each of us gets the equivalent of an additional body exposure of 3 mGy/yr of high-energy photons

(Figure 5.1). By comparison, the dose from a standard chest radiograph ranges from about 0.25 mGy to skin at the point where the beam enters the body to a few percent of that amount where it exits and exposes the image receptor (Figure 2.20c) – so the dose averaged over the chest (not the whole body!) is similar to what the same volume of tissue gets normally from natural background radiation over a matter of days.

The largest part of diagnostic medical irradiation (not therapeutic, which is not of great concern as a significant contributor to cancer risk) comes from CT, in large part because of supplier-induced demand, self-referral, and the understandable desire to practice clinically and legally "defensive" medicine. At many facilities patient doses are unnecessarily high as a result of lack of awareness of the seriousness of the radiation risks by physicians, inadequate training and credentialing of staff, and the absence of certification of machines and facilities. Increasing pressure from the American College of Radiology (ACR), The Joint Commission (TJC), and the Intersocietal Accreditation Commission (IAC), and from other directions, is helping to turn that situation around. Many in the radiology community, moreover, understand that excessive exposure is potentially a significant health problem, and are actively taking steps to reduce the doses from CT and other sorts of examinations, especially for children.

Also contributing to the difficulty is the ugly reality of *digital dose creep*: with digital imaging equipment such as DR, CT, SPECT, PET, *et al.* (and unlike film), more exposure always leads to less noisy pictures – and those who produce and use this kind of information often select higher exposures to produce higher image quality, even when it is not clinically required. Not surprisingly, many physicians demand *excellent* pictures, rather than being satisfied with ones that involve significant dose and risk reductions but are "only" *clinically adequate.*

Radiation health effects are caused by damage to DNA

The pizza, beer, and friends were great, and you ended up $10 ahead, but come 2:00 in the morning, you're desperate for the antacid. After rummaging through the medicine cabinet in the pale light, you chew a few, meander back to bed, and fall asleep again before your head hits the pillow. It probably does not cross your mind, during all this, that your night-light uses a 4 watt bulb (Figure 5.2).

Four watts is very little power. Leaving the light on for exactly one second releases four joules (4 J) of light and heat energy – a watt is defined to be one joule per second. And a joule, itself, is not much. Four joules is enough to lift 1 kilogram of tissue about a foot upward, or to raise its temperature something like 0.001 °C. A second's worth of energy from the bulb imparted to every kilogram of standard man (70 kg) would elevate his temperature by that amount.

If, instead, a source rapidly deposited 4 or 5 J of X- or gamma-radiation to each kilogram of a human, rather than light or heat, the odds are about 50% that he would die of radiation sickness within 60 days. Recalling the definition of *gray* (Gy) of dose as 1 joule of *ionizing* radiation per kilogram of matter (Equation 2.4 and Figure 2.20a), we can rephrase this as: $LD_{50/60} = 4–5$ Gy for a uniform, acute gamma- or X-irradiation. $LD_{50/60}$ is the *Lethal*

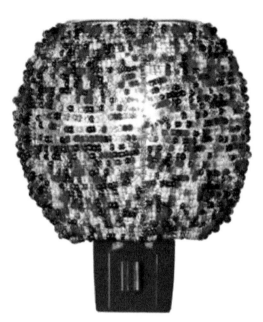

Figure 5.2 A 4 watt night-light. If you exposed every kilogram of your body to a 4 W source of *ionizing* radiation for a few seconds, it would kill you. Courtesy of www.Lampsplus.com.

Dose for 50% of the population, without specialized medical care.

Why the difference? It's like the tossed basketball versus the shot bee-bee pellet mentioned earlier. They may carry the same total energy, but only the one in the concentrated and compact form will sting. Likewise, only a *high-energy* photon, such as an X- or gamma-ray, carries sufficient energy to eject a photoelectron or Compton electron from an atom, ionizing it, and possibly leading ultimately to health problems. As long as *one joule* of **ionizing** photon radiation ends up in *one kilogram* of the medium, that's *one gray*. The *rad*, incidentally, is an older unit still employed somewhat in the US but being phased out; 1 rad = 0.01 Gy = 1 cGy.

Radiogenic damage to DNA

The problem is clear and inescapable: the very photon-electron event that removes a photon from the beam, and thereby contributes to image formation, also give rise to a high-energy photo- or Compton electron. As it blazes through tissue, this ejected electron dissipates its considerable kinetic energy over a millimeter or so by exciting and

(a)

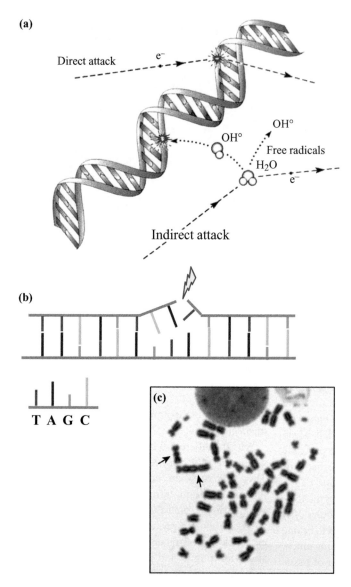

Direct attack

e⁻

OH°

OH°

OH°

Free radicals

H₂O

e⁻

Indirect attack

(b)

T A G C

(c)

Figure 5.3 Radiation damage to DNA molecules. **(a)** *Direct attack* by a fast electron on a DNA molecule, and *indirect attack* by way of hydroxyl (OH°), hydrogen (H°), and other *free radicals*. **(b)** One of the numerous possible forms of DNA damage that can occur to either the sugar-phosphate chains or to the purine or pyrimidine bases; here there is a break in one chain, and it may be fully reparable – or not. **(c)** Metaphase spread of cultured lymphocytes, with radiation-induced dicentric chromosome aberrations indicated by arrows. Courtesy of Dr. Gordon Livingston, Radiation Emergency Assistance Center/Training Site (REAC/TS), Oak Ridge, TN. Reproduced from Wolbarst *et al.* [6], fig. 5a, with permission of the Radiological Society of North America (RSNA) (part c).

ionizing hundreds or thousands of molecules lying along its erratic path (Figure 3.14). In so doing, it may directly or indirectly excite or ionize DNA molecules, inducing chemical changes that give rise to alterations of base sequences or other damage. That can cause gross tissue harm, if too many cells or their precursors are killed or incapacitated in this manner. Or, very occasionally, mutations in the genetic makeup of one or a few cells may lead to carcinogenesis, or to genetic damage expressed in one's offspring. The cellular barriers and transport mechanisms that exclude some chemical and bio-

logic agents cannot prevent the intrusion of high-energy photons and electrons, and all organs and tissues are vulnerable to their effects.

Radiogenic harm to DNA comes primarily in two ways, known as *direct* and *indirect attack* (Figure 5.3a).

With *direct attack* on a DNA molecule, a fast electron passing nearby will directly excite or ionize some part of a strand of DNA and leave it in an unstable, chemically vulnerable excited state, DNA*:

$$\text{DNA} + \text{energy} \rightarrow \text{DNA}^*. \qquad (5.1a)$$

Alternatively, the typical mammalian cell is 80–90% water, and in an *indirect attack*, a high-speed electron transfers some of its kinetic energy to a water molecule, commonly just splitting it into hydrogen and hydroxyl *free radicals*, H$^\bullet$ and OH$^\bullet$,

$$H_2O + energy \rightarrow H^\bullet + OH^\bullet, \qquad (5.1b)$$

or any of a number of similar entities. A free radical is a molecule or ion that contains an orbital electron with a spin that is not *paired* with that of another orbital electron. For non-obvious, quantum mechanical reasons, an atom or molecule strongly prefers to have all of its electrons paired up, with their spins pointing in opposite directions. In attempts to rectify this awkward situation, a radical will undergo chemical reactions far more rapidly and vigorously than do ordinary molecules.

A hydrogen cation – that is, an isolated proton – can combine with a stray electron to produce a neutral hydrogen atom, which also happens to be a hydrogen radical, H$^\bullet$, with an unpaired electron. Likewise, the hydroxyl radical has eight paired electrons and one unpaired. Since both of these radicals have odd numbers of orbital electrons, pairing of electrons within either is not an option. (Similarly, ordinary oxygen gas, O$_2$, in its ground electronic state is one of the most reactive of molecules, in part because it happens to hold two *un*paired electrons.) Either H$^\bullet$ or OH$^\bullet$ will readily combine with any nearby DNA molecule through reactions such as

$$DNA\text{–}CH_3 + OH^\bullet \rightarrow DNA\text{–}CH_2^\bullet + H_2O.$$
$$(5.1c)$$

This leaves the DNA molecule in a chemically unstable state, just as a direct attack does. As such, the DNA molecule is now ready itself to undergo a reaction that may well be self-damaging.

The net effect is that the information content of the DNA may be altered. The resulting disruption may come through that of an oxidative or alkylation attack on one of the complementary partners of a base pair, for example, in which the composition or structural geometry of the purine or pyrimidine base is altered. This can result in a localized point mutation that extends over one or two (such as in the formation of a thymine dimer) base pairs. It is estimated that about 80% of chromosomal damage from fast photo- and Compton electrons (originating from high-energy photons) is brought about through such rearrangements of nucleotides.

Then again, radiation may cause a tear in one of the two sugar-phosphate backbone chains, creating an isolated *single-strand break* (Figure 5.3b). Much less frequent with gamma- and X-rays, but also less readily repaired, is a *double-strand scission*. Damage of these sorts may lead to cross-linkages within one strand of DNA, or between the two strands, or between DNA and a protein. While usually subtle, the damage can sometime lead to observable chromosomal aberrations (Figure 5.3c).

Such events tend to follow a well-defined general sequence, summarized in Figure 5.4. Fast Compton- or photoelectrons or free radicals attack a DNA molecule, causing a structural transformation (Figures 5.3). If too many essential cells in a tissue are killed or rendered non-functional, the irradiation will lead to a *deterministic health effect*

Figure 5.4 Sequence of events in the radiation damage in cells. Cells that undergo radiogenic harm may undergo complete repair. Note the feedback loops involving error repair. Alternatively, they may die or become non-functional, and if this happens to too many of them, the tissue will display a *deterministic* health effect. Many cells are repaired partially and survive, and some of these may have experienced a sort of alteration of the information content genetic material that leads to carcinogenesis, known as a *stochastic* health effect.

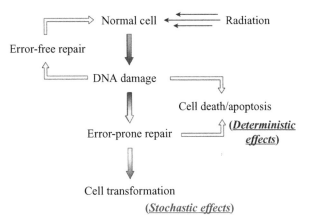

in the tissue as a whole. Conversely, certain kinds of damage to the genetic material of one or a few cells may result in a *stochastic health effect*, such as a cancer or, if the affected cell is a germ cell, a *transmitted genetic effect*. Finally, irradiation during rapid cell growth and organogenesis, as occurs in humans approximately from weeks 3 to 11 weeks of gestation, may also lead to congenital anomalies from changes in the growth parameters of the affected cells.

Many kinds of radiogenic cell damage can automatically be repaired by way of complex biochemical processes that involve numerous enzymes and other biochemical feedback loops. Some are so highly efficient at fixing things that they are called *error-free repair* mechanisms. Others that are more error-prone include non-homologous end joining, homologous recombination repair, and illegitimate recombination repair. The difference is somewhat analogous to error-free versus lossy data compression techniques in computer data storage. Regardless of the mechanism, most repair of cellular aberrations occurs with no obvious sequelae.

Stochastic health effects: cancer may arise from mutations in a single cell

In imaging, we are almost always concerned primarily with stochastic (probabilistic) health effects that may arise at low doses, rather than deterministic "complications" that may come at much higher doses, as in radiation oncology.

Stochastic (probabilistic) radiogenic health effects

It is widely assumed (but not proven) that even a *small* dose of ionizing radiation can occasionally cause genetic mutations that substantially corrupt the information content of the DNA of one or a few cells (Box 5.1). Such a *cell transformation* may turn on an oncogene, or switch off the suppression of one, resulting in uncontrolled mitosis. Malfunctioning DNA can also lead to *stochastic effects* other than carcinogenesis, such as genetic effects manifesting in one's progeny or, in the case of irradiation of the fetus, growth restriction, microcephaly, mental retardation, and other congenital abnormalities.

Box 5.1   General characteristics of stochastic (of primary concern in X- or gamma-ray imaging), deterministic (which can arise almost entirely in radiation therapy or in radiologic accidents), and teratogenic health effects in the unborn

---

Stochastic/random, e.g., cancer, hereditary mutations in oncogenes of DNA of 1 or a few cells

      loss of cellular control

risk of occurence proportional to dose (D)

      data: Hiroshima/Nagasaki, $D > 0.1$ Sv

Deterministic, e.g., burns, RT complications too many cells, stem cells killed

      loss of tissue/organ *functionality*

severity of harm increases with D above $D_{threshold}$

Acute radiation syndrome (ARS)

Teratogenic, e.g., congenital defects, retardation elements of both stochastic and deterministic organogenisis: weeks 3–11 of gestation

---

The word *stochastic* refers to events that occur randomly and independently, for which it is only their *probabilities of occurrence* that can be estimated. Radiogenic cancers and genetic errors are said to be stochastic, in the sense that they are brought about by random collisions of high-energy photons and electrons with atoms. Such health effects are not certain to occur even at high exposures, but their probability of occurrence does increase with dose, at least at higher doses (>0.1 Gy). It appears that, unlike the case of cell killing or apoptosis, no critical number of cells have to be transformed for this to occur, and it may (or may not) be that there is no dose threshold below which there is no risk.

The severity of a problem, should one arise, does not increase with the dose, as it does with a deterministic effect; cancer is cancer, regardless of how much dose was imparted in causing it. Again, it is only the *likelihood* that a cell will switch into a cancerous form that depends on dose, not the *severity* of the outcome of the change.

At the low doses employed with radiography, however, epidemiological data are absent, and the shapes of any dose-response relationships (in particular, whether or not there do exist dose thresholds) are not known with certainty – and unfortunately, that is the dose region of real diagnostic clinical interest. One must bear in mind, of course, that the absence of evidence of very low-dose health effects is not evidence for their absence.

But in any case, and most fortunately, the probability of cancer induction during a normal radiographic examination is extremely small. A patient's calculated radiation risk from an appropriately prescribed diagnostic procedure would almost inevitably be much lower than the far more certain risks from forgoing the study and suffering the medical consequences. Virtually all experts would agree that if a radiological study is clinically indicated, and carried out properly, its expected benefits will greatly outweigh the small possible risks, and that the odds strongly favor the patient who undergoes the study. The nature of the balance in screening millions of patients with very low doses, on the other hand, is not as clear.

The sievert (Sv) of equivalent dose: accounting also for stochastic biological risk

"Dose" refers to ionizing radiation delivered to anything at all, animal, vegetable, or mineral, and it is quantified in terms of grays. It has been helpful to contrive several other entities that relate to the induction of stochastic (*not* deterministic) health effects in human tissue. The two most important of these are *equivalent dose* and *effective dose*, and these both come in units known as sieverts (Sv) (Table 5.1).

A number of parameters affect the response of cells or tissues to irradiation. Some of these are their normal rate of cell turnover (i.e., frequency of mitosis), the degree of cell differentiation, the stage of the cell cycle at the time of irradiation, and the presence of naturally occurring or synthetic chemical radiation sensitizers (in particular, oxygen) and protectors. The most important radiation-related factors are the dose, the dose rate, and the pattern of the ionizations it produces. In particular, when charged particles pass through matter, whether they be Compton electrons or carbon-12 ions from a specialized radiotherapy treatment machine, they leave trails of ionizations behind them. The spatial rate at which they deposit their energy along their paths, $\Delta E/\Delta x$, is called the *linear energy transfer* (LET).

Electrons are very light, and when set in motion in tissue by incident X-rays or gamma-rays, they are knocked about vigorously in collisions with atomic electrons. They move fast and don't linger near any individual atoms, and they parcel out their energy to widely separated clusters of a few ions each. Compton and photoelectrons (and by extension, the gamma- and X-rays that liberate them) are therefore said to be *low-LET* (Figure 5.5a). When a low-LET particle passes close to a DNA molecule, ionizations of the medium will tend to occur at points so far apart that immediate damage will almost always be confined to only one base or one sugar-phosphate strand. Cells have an armamentarium of defensive enzymes and other factors to repair many such faults, generally over minutes or hours.

Protons and alpha particles, by contrast, are thousands of times heavier than an electron and, with the same kinetic energy, move perhaps a hundred times more slowly. They snowplow their way through matter, and produce dense contrails of closely spaced ionizations and free radicals (Figure 5.5b). They transfer energy to the medium in this particularly effective fashion, and they are

Table 5.1 Quantities used in the measurement of ionizing radiation, and both SI and traditional units.

Quantity	SI unit	Traditional	Relationship
Dose	gray (Gy) = J-kg^{-1}	rad	1 Gy = 100 rad
Exposure	C-kg^{-1} in air	roentgen (R)	1 R ~1 cGy in air
Equivalent dose	sievert (Sv)	rem	1 Sv = 100 rem
Effective dose	sievert (Sv)	rem	
Committed dose	sievert (Sv)	rem	
Activity	Becquerel (Bq)	curie (Ci)	1 Ci = 3.7 × 10^{10} Bq

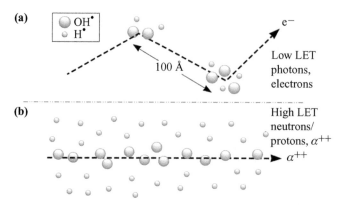

Figure 5.5 A major determinant of the amount of biological harm from a particular form of radiation is the closeness, or spatial density, of the ionizations it produces; this is parameterized by the *linear energy transfer* (LET), the spatial rate at which it lays down energy along its path through the tissue, d*E*/d*x*. **(a)** High-energy photon, photoelectron, Compton electron, and beta particle events occur in small clusters spaced far apart; these forms of radiation are all considered low-LET. **(b)** Alpha particles, protons (and the fast neutrons that may liberate them), and heavy ions produce much denser ionization trails, and are high-LET. They are far more likely to cause double-strand breaks in DNA and other forms of possibly non-reparable damage, and are more adept at causing biological harm.

termed *high-LET* particles. High-LET radiation is much more probable than low-LET to cause double-strand breaks and certain other forms of complex damage in DNA that are resistant to complete cellular repair. It is therefore more likely to have an adverse biological effect in tissue per unit absorbed dose, because of which high-LET radiation is said to display a high *relative biological effectiveness* (RBE). High-LET, high-RBE particles have greater ability both to kill cells and to cause cancer.

The sievert, the SI unit of *equivalent dose* to tissue or organs, is a modification of the gray that accounts for the differences in the radiosensitivities of tissues to various kinds of radiation. (Just as the gray is displacing the older rad, likewise the sievert is pushing aside the *rem*, where 1 Sv = 100 rem.)

The equivalent dose in sieverts is related to the deposited dose in gray by means of a *quality factor* (QF), which is a cruder version of the RBE: equivalent dose (Sv) = QF × *D* (Gy). By convention, ordinary X-rays are commonly taken to serve as the reference radiation, so for them and gamma-rays QF = 1. It is for this reason that for virtually *all of imaging,*

$$1\,\text{Sv} = 1\,\text{Gy} \quad (\text{gamma-, X-rays}). \qquad (5.2)$$

Units of grays are more familiar to medical practitioners, except for CT doses, which are reported

in mSv, by unfortunate convention. Sieverts play the dominant role in radiation protection, where high-LET radiations may also be present; during a nuclear power plant or weapon disaster, people may be exposed not only to high-energy photons and beta particles but also to neutrons or to alpha-emitters, so the "dose" there is most appropriately expressed in sieverts.

Finally, for reasons that need not be discussed here, the X-ray radiation falling upon skin or the input to an image receptor is sometimes reported as mGy of *air kerma*. For medical purposes, 1 mGy of air kerma is identical to 1 mGy of dose to air at the same location. An older unit, the *roentgen* (R), which is nearly 0.01 Gy to air, is also rapidly becoming extinct.

The critically important linear no-threshold dose-risk assumption, and estimates of [*Risk/Dose*]

As mentioned at the beginning of the chapter, it is estimated that we all have about a 1 in 100 chance of dying from a cancer induced by the 3 mSv/year of natural background radiation. To compute this, we need two pieces of information: one is the amount, or dose, of radiation actually deposited in the irradiated tissues. The other is the risk, or probability of cancer mortality, per unit of radiation delivered.

The product of these two factors provides an overall estimate of the risk:

$$Risk = [Risk/Dose] \times [Dose]. \qquad (5.3a)$$

This essential *linear, no-threshold* (*LN-T*) assumption underlies virtually all of *radiation protection* at the present time. It incorporates two important points: first, the risk rate, [*Risk/Dose*], is a *constant* and independent, in particular, of the dose. Second, the radiation risk is linearly proportional to the dose, [*Dose*], and there is *no* threshold dose below which very low levels of exposure are risk-free (Figure 5.6a). This implies that the risks for one person receiving 0.01 mSv per day for 365 days, and another who gets 3.65 mSv in a single day are the same. This may well be valid at low doses, or only approximately so, or outright wrong, and perhaps for some biological tissues but not others. But, in any case, LN-T is considered by the leading risk-assessment and regulatory bodies to be the best approach for the development of radiation safety guidance and regulations.

The best *estimate* from the available data is that the probability per sievert of low-LET ionizing radiation causing a fatal cancer is about 5% Sv^{-1}, or

$$[Risk/Dose] = 5 \times 10^{-5} \text{ mSv}^{-1}. \qquad (5.3b)$$

It can be computed, then, that the accumulated risk of mortality from natural background radiation over a 70-year lifetime is something like (3 mSv-y^{-1} × 70 y × 5 × 10^{-5} mSv^{-1}) = 1%. Roughly the same numbers of people presumably suffer radiogenic neoplasms associated with ionizing radiation exposure from medical procedures. Either way, the rate for *incidence* of radiogenic cancers is a factor of about 1.5 times higher than that.

The most trusted quantitative data available at present come from epidemiological studies of people who received considerably higher doses, in particular the survivors of the atomic blasts at Hiroshima and Nagasaki in 1945. Studies of two hundred thousand of the surviving inhabitants of those cities, begun shortly after the end of the war and still ongoing more than half a century later, indicate that those who received doses significantly higher than background level experienced higher probabilities of eventually being stricken with cancer. Similar data come from follow-up studies of patients who underwent (also generally long ago)

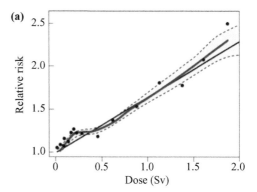

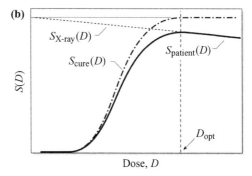

Figure 5.6 Dose and stochastic health effects. (a) A dose-response curve fit to some of the available data. The straight black line describes the linear no-threshold (LN-T) model for radiogenic cancer mortality, commonly *assumed* in the preparation of radiation safety public policy; with this assumption (about which there is considerable ongoing debate), our best *estimate* is that the lifetime risk of cancer induction is about [*Risk/Dose*] = 5 × 10^{-2} Sv^{-1}, or 5% per Sv, a value explicitly recommended for general use in Publication 103 of the International Commission on Radiation Protection (ICRP) [5]. (b) In an imaging study, one attempts to optimize the overall probability of patient survival. The optimal imaging dose is that for which the overall probability of cancer survival, $S_{patient}(D)$, goes through a maximum.

irradiation of the spine for ankylosing spondylitis, of the breast for postpartum mastitis, and of enlarged thymus in children, and repeated fluoroscopy during management of tuberculosis. Further information came from the experiences of uranium miners, radium dial painters, and others. To summarize all this work succinctly: it clearly appears *within the higher-dose data* (0.1 Gy and up) that the probability of cancer induction is proportional to the dose received (Figure 5.6a).

But such exposures are far greater than what a patient receives in nearly any modern radiological examination. At the lower exposures encountered in practice, the radiogenic cancer incidence and mortality data are easily swamped by the *statistical noise* from the normal variations and fluctuations in the vastly greater number of cancers that occur "spontaneously." This is the case primarily because radiogenic cancers are extremely rare, and they cannot in any way be distinguished from those that arise from other causes; there is no known marker, no fingerprint, to distinguish the relatively small number of cases that happen to be brought about by ionizing radiation.

The lack of data where it actually matters, in the diagnostic range, is but one of a number of difficulties. There is considerable variability among specific subpopulations that is related to differences in age, race, gender, smoking, local environmental chemicals, socioeconomic status, diet, occupation, even nationality – the Japanese have a low natural incidence of breast cancer and high incidence of stomach cancer, for example, while the converse is true for Americans. Such confounding factors, which often overlap, can affect the estimation of both the radiogenic and the "spontaneous" cancer rates. This is further complicated by the long latency period between exposure and the appearance of a malignancy. While leukemia (especially among children) may show up within a few years of exposure, many solid tumors take one or two decades, making it hard to establish a link with any potential causal agent. Powerful statistical arguments and tools must be employed to tease out the numbers of excess radiogenic cancers, and they have their own limitations.

The radiation protection community in general deals with this conundrum by extrapolating the argument from the high-dose linear relationship, for which a fair amount of data exists, down into the low-dose region that is of importance in imaging. The first and most severe problem in trying to do this is, quite simply, that we really do not know how hazardous small additional amounts of ionizing radiation are. There are no low-dose epidemiological data from which to discern the shape and slope of the low-dose part of the dose-response curve with any assurance – and quite possibly there never will be any. There is evidence from cell-culture and other studies, moreover, that there may be thresholds below which radiogenic carcinogenesis

normally does not occur. Still, at present, the LN-T is widely accepted by public health physicians and officials as a prudent working hypothesis upon which to build public health policy and regulations for protecting patients, medical staff, and others from radiation dangers.

The validity, or lack thereof, of the standard LN-T assumption is *the* critical question in the field of radiation safety and protection. It is the subject of much scientific debate (along with some that's not quite so scientific), especially among environmental scientists and policy makers; the costs of cleaning up contaminated nuclear power plants and Department of Energy weapons-production facilities run into the hundreds of billions of dollars; this is to weighed against the *possible* protection (if radiogenic carcinogenesis really *does* occur at very low doses) of the thousands living on-site or nearby after remediation. While the finances may not be so staggering in medicine, it is obviously still an issue of great importance there, as well.

Adoption of LN-T has been endorsed by the Biological Effects of Ionizing Radiation (BEIR) committee of the National Academy of Sciences (NAS), the United Nations Scientific Committee on the Effects of Atomic Radiation (UNSCEAR), the International Commission on Radiological Protection (ICRP), the National Council on Radiation Protection and Measurements (NCRP), and other major scientific advisory bodies. These organizations have examined not only radiogenic cancer incidence and mortality, effects of *in utero* exposure, and genetic effects in the offspring of those irradiated, but also other illnesses such as cardiovascular, digestive, and other diseases [2, 3].

Oh, by the way, one last thing. The NCRP and the ICRP suggested that the [*Risk/Dose*] factor obtained with high-dose epidemiology be reduced at low lowest doses by a *Dose and Dose-Rate Effectiveness Factor* (DDREF) of 2, to account for those two influences; the [*Risk/Dose*] = 5×10^{-5} mSv^{-1} of Equation 5.3b already includes that correction [4]. So whether or not there is no threshold, the curve is definitely *not* linear – the slope presumably drops by half at lowest doses. And the dose rates for a film or DR are certainly quite different from those of a CT or a PET scan, and it is not clear what should be done about that. So much for LN-T – which, nonetheless, is still the only game in town.

Optimal dose for patient survival of both the disease and the diagnosis

Any diagnostic procedure that involves ionizing radiation must deposit at least a little dose to provide a benefit, and sometimes more than a little. But that possibly leads to an associated risk. So how does one find the dose that is most likely to provide a positive overall outcome?

Let us illustrate the dose optimization problem with a very simple hypothetical case study. Suppose that a patient presents with symptoms of a disease that is lethal if untreated, and for which there is a reliable gamma- or X-ray imaging tool that can reveal how to treat it properly. The probability of successfully detecting and analyzing the lesion, thereby making it possible for the patient to Śurvive the disease, $S_{cure}(D)$, is likely to be a sigmoidal function of patient dose, D (Figure 5.6b). At too low an exposure, noise will be too high, yet the use of very high doses won't improve things. (Indeed, with a screen-film system, say, too much dose to the IR will turn the film entirely black.) The symbol S is adopted to emphasize the point that it represents the probability of subsequent patient Śurvival of the illness.

At the same time, the probability that the patient will suffer a lethal radiation-induced cancer from the diagnostic procedure itself is assumed to follow the linear no-threshold dose-response relationship; equivalently, the probability that the patient will Śurvive the possibly deleterious effects of the diagnostic procedure decreases from unity, falling off linearly and extremely slowly as $S_{rad}(D) = [1 - \alpha D]$ for some small α.

The overall probability of patient well-being, $S_{patient}(D)$, the likelihood that the patient will survive both forms of harm (i.e., be cured of the disease and yet not incur a radiogenic cancer during the diagnosis) is therefore given by the product of the two independent probabilities, $S_{patient}(D) = S_{cure}(D) \times S_{rad}(D)$. This product passes through a maximum at some "optimal" exposure, D_{opt}, and, if the objective is to cure the patient and do no irrevocable harm in the process, then D_{opt} is the best amount of dose to employ. At lower exposures, the increased risk from the disease would more than compensate for the reduced hazard of the radiation itself, and the converse is true above D_{opt}.

Our little exercise is interesting philosophically, but perhaps its most important conclusion is that such an analysis need not be carried out in practice for diagnostic imaging of symptomatic patients. The radiation risk is nearly always extremely small, and $S_{rad}(D)$ edges downward so very slowly with D. This suggests that the approach normally taken by cautious physicians is correct: one should employ sufficient radiation to obtain the necessary diagnostic information, but not go much beyond that. And, of course, one should take all reasonable radiation safety actions to reduce avoidable doses to patients and staff.

Although the individual radiation risk from a radiographic procedure may be quite small, the collective risk within a large population being screened may be substantial. An approach that works in the emergency room may or may not be suitable in, say, mass screening for breast cancer. In that case, $S_{patient}(D)$ must be reconsidered in greater detail – and in particular, the applicability there of the linear no-threshold assumption.

The effective dose (in Sv) is currently the least bad predictor of cancer risk S

Having just discussed the $[Risk/Dose]$ term in estimating $Risk$, we shall now return to the $[Dose]$ component.

The *effective dose* (ED) is widely viewed as the least bad available method to estimate the stochastic risk for a person who is exposed non-uniformly. Formerly known as the effective dose equivalent, the ED is a risk-weighted average over the local doses to the various organs and *Tissues*, as parameterized by the index T.

Effective dose accounts both for the organ/tissue dose, $D_{T,}$ and the relative radiosensitivity of each, with a tissue risk-weight of w_T (Table 5.2):

$$ED = \sum w_T D_T. \qquad (5.4a)$$

Table 5.2 Organ dose weighting factors, w_T, for use in calculating effective dose (Equation 5.4). Such values have been generated by the International Commission on Radiological Protection (ICRP) [5], the NCRP, and the federal government, and may evolve over time (see the Code of Federal Regulations at 10CFR20.1003, and Subparts C and D).

0.12	0.08	0.04	0.01
Breast	Gonads	Bladder	Bone surfaces
Colon		Esophagus	Brain
Lung		Liver	Salivary glands
Red marrow		Thyroid	Skin
Stomach			
Remainder[a]			

Remainder: adrenals, extrathoracic tissue, gall bladder, heart wall, kidneys, lymph nodes, muscle, oral mucosa, pancreas, prostate, small intestine, spleen, thymus, uterus/cervix.

The sigma indicates summation over T. Every cancer has to have occurred in *some* organ, so the sum of the weighting factors themselves is forced to unity,

$$\sum w_T = 1. \tag{5.4b}$$

Like Equation 5.3b, these w_T values come from the Japanese bomb data: of those who received a uniform whole-body dose and acquired a cancer, about 4% occurred in the liver, so w_T is set to 0.04 for that organ.

The corresponding total risk, from Equation 5.3a, is then

$$Risk = ED \times 5 \times 10^{-5} mSv^{-1}. \tag{5.5c}$$

The idea is that if a person is exposed *non-uniformly* and the ED is calculated to be 4 mSv, say, then the total stochastic risk will be the same as if the patient received a whole-body, *uniform* dose of 4 mSv. Even though it uses only (low-LET) gamma- and X-rays, radiology has borrowed the ED construct from the radiation protection community and reports dose in sieverts, not grays, for CT in particular.

Representative doses for diagnostic studies

Although there are numerous sources of guidance on estimated organ and effective doses from various medical procedures, two of the most useful at present are the NCRP report no. 160 [1], and a series of reports prepared by the NEXT program (Nationwide Evaluation of X-ray Trends) managed by the Center for Devices and Radiological Health (CDRH) of the FDA and the Conference of [state] Radiation Control Program Directors (CRCPD).

Table 5.3 reproduces representative EDs for some standard imaging procedures in the United States, as compiled from a number of sources. The X-ray technique factors or quantity of radiopharmaceutical employed for a particular study in any given imaging center will depend on the patient's body size and shape, on the rigor of QA practiced there, on radiation measurements made perhaps a while ago, and other factors, so the dose to an individual may differ substantially from these numbers. Beware that some publications confuse ED (in mSv) with organ dose (in mGy).

Stochastic health effects in children

The use of CT has been increasing exponentially over the past decade, for children as well as adults,

Table 5.3 Representative effective doses (mSv) from non-CT (the last two of which are nuclear medicine studies) and CT procedures, compiled by the authors from a number of sources. Those from CT will be discussed further in Chapter 8, and committed effective doses from nuclear medicine diagnostic examinations in Chapter 9. Some imaging studies are reported in the literature in terms of milligray of *dose* to local organ; these are not to be confused with *effective dose* in mSv, which averages risk-weighted exposures throughout the entire body – for much of which D_T may be zero. Some authors confuse the two.

Typical Effective Doses (mSv)	
non-CT	
Dental bitewing	0.02
Chest radiograph	0.02
Mammogram (both breasts, 2 views)	0.5
Abdomen	1
Lumbar spine radiograph	1
Barium enema exam	5
Coronary angiogram (diagnostic)	5
Sestamibi myocardial perfusion	5
Thallium myocardial perfusion	10
CT	
Head	2
Chest	5
Abdomen	5
Pelvis	5
Abdomen and pelvis	10
Coronary angiography	10

and the escalating dose from pediatric CTs is now seen as a major public health issue. Children are of greatest concern regarding dose, for three important reasons:

Infants and children are biologically different from adults, and they require special care during *all* forms of imaging. For one thing, their tissues are inherently more radiosensitive: they have relatively more cells that are rapidly dividing, so there is greater opportunity for uncorrected errors to arise and be propagated. Red bone marrow, for example, is found throughout the neonate's body, and it is a highly radiosensitive tissue. Also, the cells of the young appear to be less effective at repairing the mutations that may be caused by ionizing radiation.

In addition, the lifespan of a child, during which a cancer may be expressed, is several decades longer, increasing their risk of occurrence.

Finally, kids are frequently over-exposed because the technologists choose, or have been instructed, to continue carrying out pediatric procedures with technique factors originally designed for larger people. Because a child is usually much thinner than an adult, far less intensity of the *input* beam is needed for a sufficient dose to arrive at the image receptor (Figure 5.7a). So one can turn down the mA-s, or turn on the automatic dose control that all CT vendors provide, and obtain images that may not be perfectly smooth and noise-free, but that are just as adequate clinically – and that impart half as much overall dose or less.

The point is that kids may currently be getting far more dose than they should, or is needed. Parts, and sometimes all, of their bodies are commonly irradiated unnecessarily. But there are ways to reduce the dose significantly, especially for CT.

The region being examined should be kept as small as possible; in CT, the scan should be no longer than what actually has to be viewed. In addition, when an X-ray study is called for clinically, children should wear thyroid shields and lead aprons, where possible.

Many conscientious physicians refrain from calling for a CT scan when an ultrasound or MRI would be clinically adequate, and involve no ionizing radiation. Also, it is usually possible with children to avoid CT exams that require multiple scans from different phases of contrast enhancement (*multi-phase examinations*). Along the same vein, one can diminish the number of scans by burning a DVD of a study carried out at a community hospital following a trauma, say, and transferring it to an appropriate recipient when the child reaches the specialized trauma center. A little coordination can reduce unnecessary patient dose, delays, and cost.

The FDA, the ACR, and just about everyone else have come together to form the Alliance for Radiation Safety in Pediatric Imaging and to support the development and implementation of the *Image Gently* campaign (Figure 5.7b). The strategies mentioned here and many others are described in their web site (www.pedrad.org/associations/5364/ig). Similarly, the *Image Wisely* program continues to raise awareness among medical professionals of the need for improved radiation protection for adults, as well.

Deterministic health effects at high doses: radiation killing of a large number of tissue cells

Cell death is of no importance if only a few cells are so affected, except in the early embryo. But, as a result of exposure to a *high* dose of radiation above a tissue-specific *threshold dose*, adequate repair may not take place; too large a fraction of the cells in the tissue may undergo radiogenic acceleration of the normal physiological process of apoptosis or be killed outright (Box 5.1). The tissue or organ as a whole may then become partially or totally non-functional, giving rise to a *deterministic* health effect, such as the "radiation burn" seen in Figure 2.21. Above the dose threshold, the severity of the damage increases with the number of cells disabled or killed, hence with the amount of radiation absorbed.

Deterministic radiogenic health effects

In 1904, Bergonie and Tribondeau noted that the radiosensitivity of a cell increases with its reproductive activity, and the length of the period of its mitosis, but decreases with its degree of differentiation (Box 5.2). As has been verified numerous times in the years since, tissues with cells that normally undergo rapid proliferation or self-renewal are commonly more sensitive at elevated doses (far above the diagnostic range) to radiation-induced cell killing and the resultant deterministic effects. Rapidly dividing cells such as the epithelium of the GI tract, skin and hair cells, erythroblasts, spermatogonia, and lymphocytes are typically highly sensitive due to the large fraction of time spent in the M-phase of the cell cycle. And ionizing radiation depletes the supply of stem cells – it either kills them outright or inhibits their mitosis – so that they can no longer replenish the tissue at a rate sufficient to maintain its proper functioning. Cells with high metabolic activity, for example, exocrine glandular cells such as those of the salivary, are also very radiosensitive. Muscle and nerve cells, by contrast, are relatively resistant to radiation damage.

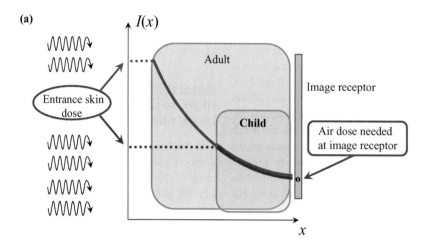

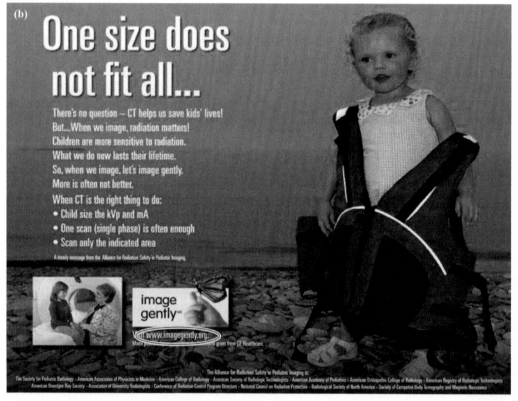

Figure 5.7 Protecting children from *unnecessary* radiation. (a) A large fraction of the X-ray energy incident on an adult is attenuated by the time the beam reaches the far side of the body, but much less so for a child. So to achieve a specified dose to the front of the IR, the intensity and dose at the skin on the beam-input side of a child should be correspondingly lower. (b)The *Image Gently* campaign is helping physicians become more aware of the need to make extra efforts to keep doses to children *as low as reasonably achievable* (*ALARA*) while still obtaining the necessary clinical information. With permission from the Alliance for Radiation Safety in Pediatric Imaging and the Image Gently campaign (http://www.pedrad.org/associations/5364/ig/) (part b).

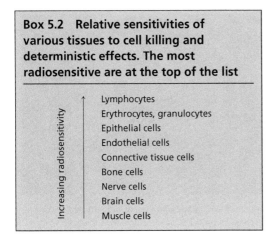

Box 5.2   Relative sensitivities of various tissues to cell killing and deterministic effects. The most radiosensitive are at the top of the list

Increasing radiosensitivity ↑

Lymphocytes
Erythrocytes, granulocytes
Epithelial cells
Endothelial cells
Connective tissue cells
Bone cells
Nerve cells
Brain cells
Muscle cells

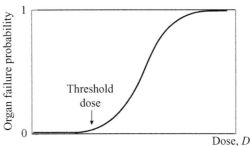

Figure 5.8 A dose-response relation for a *deterministic* effect in an organ or other tissue (as opposed to that for stochastic transformations in single cells) is typically sigmoidal in shape. At low doses, little if any damage occurs. Above an effective *threshold level* that is specific to the type of radiation, the tissue and biological end-point, and the individual, the damage increases with dose until the tissue is fully non-functional.

As with the human response to many other hazards, the very old and the very young are more susceptible to certain radiogenic deterministic injuries and illnesses.

Deterministic effects that manifest after months or even years, such as cataract formation, are said to be *late* effects. Those that become apparent within hours, days, or weeks of an intense irradiation are known as *acute* or *early* effects, such as radiation erythema. And a sufficiently high exposure over a short period of time will rapidly give rise to one or more forms of *acute radiation syndrome* (ARS), which can be life threatening. Radiation burns and other such deterministic effects still arise occasionally in diagnostic patients, but they are almost always preventable.

A non-stochastic health effect will manifest, with a reasonable degree of certainty, if an organ- and individual-specific threshold dose level (typically of the order of 1 Sv when delivered over a short period of time) is exceeded (Figure 5.8). The severity of the response, unlike the situation with stochastic effects, almost always does increase with the dose, once the threshold is exceeded. Factors that determine the extent and severity of a radiogenic non-stochastic health effect include the total amount of dose imparted, the rate at which that occurs, and the radiosensitivity and amount of the tissue covered. Doses of 10 Gy can be applied to a small area of skin with little danger, for example, while greater doses to the same region can cause irreparable severe damage that may even lead to death through infection.

Deterministic effects should almost never arise from diagnostic studies. And when a physician, technologist, or physicist sees severe erythema or a skin burn, it inevitably means that someone is either intentionally over-exposing the patient or failing to monitor the radiation output of a machine.

Radiotherapy is different. A typical course of 20 or 30 radiotherapy treatments may require the total delivery of 50–60 Gy in multiple *fractions* spread out over the course of a month or so, but usually only to a small part of the body and not all at once. It is the potential for causing concomitant unacceptable deterministic complications in healthy neighboring tissues that limits the therapeutic doses that can be delivered to the region of the lesion. Depending on the type and location of the tumor, there can be radiation sequelae ranging from the barely noticeable to the catastrophic: erythema, desquamation, or ulceration of the skin; sterility; opacification of the lens of the eye; fibrosis of the lung;ulceration of bowel and esophagus; renal failure; paralysis from destruction of a segment of the spinal cord, and others. So while the patient and radiation oncologist may desire to treat aggressively, they must balance this against the likelihood of producing unacceptable and irreparable deterministic complications.

Teratogenic effects in the unborn

Much of this section is based on the classic by Eric Hall and Amato Giaccia, *Radiobiology for the Radiologist*, 7th edn, Philadelphia, PA: Lippincott, Williams, & Wilkins, 2011.

Epidemiological studies indicate that the incidence of childhood malignancies caused by irradiation *in utero* increases with dose, but that the risk is small. The primary concern is with non-stochastic harm.

In those few, higher-dose cases where teratogenic effects have arisen, damage includes both congenital physical defects manifested as growth-restriction and microcephaly, and a lowering of intelligence to the point of severe mental retardation. Two primary determinants of the extent of radiogenic damage in the womb, as learned largely from studies on mice and rats and to some extent from the atomic bomb survivors, are the dose received and the timing of the exposure. With regard to radiation harm, gestation may be partitioned into three distinct periods: pre-implantation, organogenesis, and fetal. Pre-natal death can be induced at any time by a sufficient dose, but the threshold for this increases with embryonic/fetal age.

For doses greater than 0.1 Gy, the most significant risk to viability is from an exposure during the *pre-implantation period*, which lasts from conception until the implantation of the embryo into the wall of the uterus, about 10 days after conception. If radiogenic injury is significant during this interval, the result may be fetal loss and spontaneous abortion, typically an all-or-none phenomena, and embryos that survive rarely display ill effects.

After implantation, the major organs form and develop during *organogenesis*, in which the cells are rapidly dividing and differentiating and are therefore particularly radiosensitive. During this period, generally taken to extend through the first trimester of pregnancy, an embryo is highly vulnerable to gross structural congenital malformations. Even relatively small amounts of ionizing radiation may interfere with the normal proliferation of neurons near the cerebral ventricles, and with their subsequent migration to the neocortex (Figure 5.9). So even typical diagnostic levels of irradiation (tens of milligrays or less) may be harmful to the embryonic and neonatal central nervous system. For irradiation during the period of greatest susceptible to the onset of severe mental retardation, during weeks 8 through 15, its incidence (often accompanied by microcephaly) appears to be linear in dose: a 1-Gy exposure at that time increases the likelihood of occurrence of severe retardation by 40%. For the 16–25-week period, the risk is lower, and it appears that there may be a threshold at 20–30 mGy. With

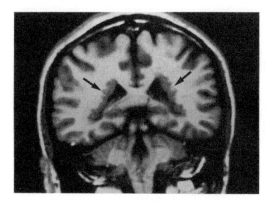

Figure 5.9 MR image of a 41-year-old retarded man who received about 0.7 Sv at Hiroshima, 8 to 9 weeks post-conception. The irradiation appears to have interrupted periventricular neuronal migration, and anomalies include gray matter clumping around the ventricles (arrows) and a thinning of gray matter peripherally around the brain, as can be observed with other disease processes such as tuberous sclerosis. The narrowing of the cortex is directly associated with the partial interruption of neuronal migration from the highly vascularized germinal matrix located in the periventricular portion of the cerebral hemispheres. It has been hypothesized that deterministic harm to blood vessels occurring during the fetal stage decreases oxygen and nutrient availability, and thus damages the migrating neurons and their migration pathways. This decreases their overall number and leads to migration disturbances. Courtesy of Wm. J. Schull, University of Texas Health Science Center, Houston, TX.

greater dose, a subtle downward shift of intelligence has been noted: IQ test scores seem to decrease by about 30 points per Gy of fetal exposure.

Organogenesis is followed by the *fetal* stage. Many studies have indicated that adverse fetal effects are generally negligible at less than 100 mGy.

For a woman known to be pregnant, or thought possibly to be so, many physicians would consider it prudent to put off an examination that might significantly irradiate an embryo or fetus. Alternatively, they might select a different modality that does not involve ionizing radiation. The recent development of tests that can detect a pregnancy shortly after conception, however, now allows the physician and patient a far greater degree of flexibility regarding irradiation if she is of child-bearing age. In the case of a severely injured maternal patient, appropriate management should almost always trump concerns of possible radiogenic injury to her unborn. A most

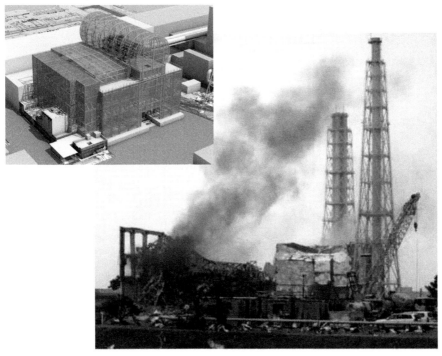

Figure 5.10 Fukushima Dai-ichi Reactor No. 3. The insert displays the cover installation erected subsequently, to reduce the hazards in removing the remaining fuel and other radioactive materials from Unit 3. Used with permission from Tokyo Electric Power Company (TEPCO).

important predictor of fetal well being is maternal well being; hence if a study is necessary because of a mother's condition, then it should be carried out.

Acute radiation syndrome

This section has absolutely no application to the normal usage of radiation in diagnosis or therapy, and hopefully you will never have cause to turn to it, except out of general interest. Also, since the material in it has been published recently in much expanded form and that provides extensive references, it will be kept very short [6].

It is possible that people may receive excessive whole-body irradiations from, for example, an industrial accident, a "dirty bomb" that widely disperses large amounts of highly radioactive materials, an extreme reactor failure, or even detonation of a nuclear weapon. A small number of high-dose events have occurred in the past, perhaps the most widely known of which were at Hiroshima and Nagasaki. This page is being written on the 25th anniversary of the explosion of the Chernobyl nuclear reactor near Kiev – and the Fukushima Dai-

ichi power plant on the north-east coast of Japan is still smoldering, following the earthquake and ensuing tsunami that devastated the region (Figure 5.10). Monitoring and environmental pathway modeling indicate that the wind is carrying radioactive dust from Fukushima far from the site, contaminating the ground, crops and fodder, and surface water. Irrigation water and rain, both heavily contaminated, are leaching fission products recently deposited in the topsoil deep into the groundwater, which is needed for drinking by humans and animals and for irrigating crops and fodder. Locally obtained meat, milk, fish, and vegetables cannot be consumed at present. This is not only a tragedy on an epic scale for those poor souls who live nearby, but also possibly a major regional environmental threat.

Some of the unfortunates affected were far enough from the epicenters of these events to survive the blast and thermal injuries, but nevertheless suffered varying levels of *acute radiation syndrome*. ARS consists of a complex of distinct deterministic effects caused by radiation damage to specific

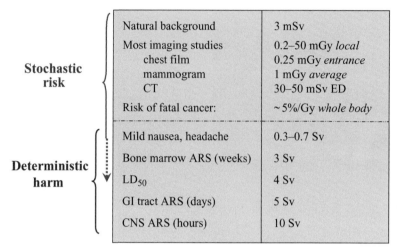

Stochastic risk	Natural background	3 mSv
	Most imaging studies	0.2–50 mGy *local*
	chest film	0.25 mGy *entrance*
	mammogram	1 mGy *average*
	CT	30–50 mSv ED
	Risk of fatal cancer:	~5%/Gy *whole body*
Deterministic harm	Mild nausea, headache	0.3–0.7 Sv
	Bone marrow ARS (weeks)	3 Sv
	LD$_{50}$	4 Sv
	GI tract ARS (days)	5 Sv
	CNS ARS (hours)	10 Sv

Figure 5.11 Symptoms and health effects that arise at various levels of acute exposure. The levels of dose that give rise to deterministic effects depend on the type of radiation (i.e., high- versus low-LET), the tissue type, the biological endpoint of concern, and the general state of health of the individual. Listed are typical doses for various radiobiological effects that arise from a rapid whole-body exposure. In case of an exposure of the order of a gray or more, *deterministic* effects may begin appearing, initially with symptoms like nausea and headache. Without specialized medical care, LD$_{50}$ (Lethal Dose for 50% of those exposed) is 4–5 Sv. These numbers are estimates by the authors, based on a number of sources.

organ systems, namely the bone marrow (the most radiosensitive), the lining of the small bowel, the skin and, at very high doses, the microvasculature that supports the nervous system. A common set of symptoms including nausea, vomiting, diarrhea, and headache, may manifest within minutes or not for days, and these can be brief or long lasting. There follows a "latent" period during which the patient may feel and appear healthy. But the same symptoms return after that, along with new ones like loss of appetite, fatigue, fever, and, for the most intensely exposed, seizures and coma. The severity and speed of onset of the symptoms increase with the amount of damage caused, which, in turn, increases with the dose imparted (Figure 5.11).

An acute, whole-body exposure of 3–5 Sv or more may lead to the *hematopoietic* or *bone marrow syndrome* as a result of significant damage or sterilization of the stem cells of the marrow. Blood-forming tissues normally renew their cell populations at a rate faster than 1% per day, making them highly radiosensitive. The cells that are lost first and foremost from an irradiation are the peripheral circulating lymphocytes; the rapidity with which the lymphocyte count drops, and the level to which it falls in the first 12–48 hours following an incident, can be a clinically useful indication of dose imparted. As the dose increases, with progressive marrow hypoplasia and then aplasia occurring at

5–6 Sv, adverse health outcomes may include pancytopenia, with ensuing infections and hemorrhaging associated with the significant decrease of white blood cells, red blood cells, and platelets (Figure 5.12).

Death may occur within weeks or months, when the circulating white cells die out and are not replenished. It is commonly stated, because of the dose range of the hematopoietic syndrome, that without specialized medical attention, the lethal dose to 50% of a population is of the order of 3.5–4 Sv of whole-body exposure, although published estimates vary between 3 and 5 Sv. At the higher end, but with the best of care including antibiotics, transfusions, intensivist monitoring, and expert nursing, life may be preserved with exposures of up to 7 Sv – and occasionally even higher, with a bone marrow transplant. There are no reliable reports of anyone surviving a whole-body exposure of 10 Sv.

Higher doses give rise, in addition, to the *gastrointestinal syndrome*. It results from damage to the epithelial lining of the small intestine, the killing of epithelial stem cells in crypts of the microvilli, and the loss of the microvasculature that supports the mucosal lining of the GI tract. Radiation-induced damage to the GI mucosa can cause electrolyte disturbance, profound fluid losses, diarrhea that may be bloody and lead to frank hemorrhaging, and to malabsorption that causes malnutrition and cacexia. Severe diarrhea alone can be fatal, due to loss of fluids, protein, and electrolytes. Also, bacteria and other infectious agents traversing the denuded bowel epithelium may cause

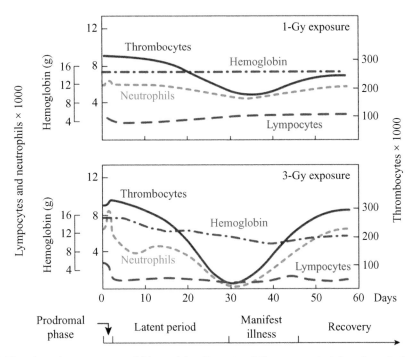

Figure 5.12 Time-dependent response model for peripheral hematopoietic components. A time-dependent response model of the various peripheral hematopoietic components to an acute 1 Sv (upper graph) or 3 Sv (lower) whole-body dose. At higher doses, the concentration of neutrophils, in particular, passes through a potentially lethal nadir about a month after exposure. The timing of the processes indicated here depends strongly on the dose and on the prior state of health of the individual. Reproduced from Wolbarst et al. [6], fig 4b, with permission of the Radiological Society of North America (RSNA).

lethal septicemia, a phenomenon exacerbated by the concomitant depletion of lymphocytes and neutrophils. Finally, volume depletion in itself may result in hypotension and cardiovascular collapse, with secondary renal failure or hepato-renal syndrome. Severe GI syndrome can lead to death within days or weeks.

Damage to the hematopoietic and GI systems may be accompanied by *cutaneous radiation injury*. Such an injury may become apparent within hours or may not be seen for weeks, depending on the dose. At low doses, there may be itching, tingling, and edema. Acute skin surface doses as low as 2–3 Gy may cause erythematous changes locally. The threshold dose for temporary depilation is on the order of 3–5 Sv, and that for erythema is 5–6 Sv. Above 10 Sv localized to part of the skin, the injury progressively worsens with increasing dose, advancing from dry desquamation, wet desquamation, and bullae (blister) formation, to ulceration and necrosis. Such a *radiation burn*, resulting from depopulation of the basal layer of skin, may be debilitatingly painful, and also life threatening because of concomitant infections and fluid loss. Radiation skin damage differs from the kind caused by extreme heat or

by chemicals in that it appears as a delayed effect, and there may be recurrent skin breakdown even after a scar forms.

The *central nervous system, cerebrovascular*, or *neurovascular syndrome* occurs at much higher doses than the others, above 50 Sv (although there may be symptoms at 20 Sv). While the fundamental cause of the hematopoietic and GI syndromes is clear – the depletion of critical populations of stem cells essential for the replenishment of the circulating blood cells or of the epithelial lining of the gut, respectively – the exact cause of death from the CNS syndrome is not yet understood well. It is probably related to damage associated with increased intracranial pressure caused by edema, vasculitis, and meningitis. Initial symptoms include severe vomiting, confusion, disorientation, ataxia, even seizures, and coma sets in quickly, perhaps within hours of the exposure. Death will follow within days or less, possibly before other findings of radiation sickness appear.

Whether tissues can recover from radiation exposure depends strongly on the dose-rate; that is, the dose imparted per unit time. A whole-body exposure of 6 Gy of X-radiation received in one day or less, for example, would mean almost inescapable death. On the other hand, a total of 6 Gy delivered in daily increments over a period of 30 years would amount to an annual dose of 0.2 Gy. This is just four times the federal occupational exposure limit of 50 mSv/year, and it may lead to a small increased risk of cancer, but it will not produce any deterministic effects.

The *Four Quartets* of radiation safety

As indicated at the end of Chapter 2, the objectives of a radiation safety program are to: prevent the occurrence of any radiogenic *deterministic* effects; limit *stochastic* risk to a level deemed "acceptable" by public policy setters; and encourage all staff to strive always to practice and achieve ALARA.

Doses can be quite high to medical personnel who fail to make conscious efforts to keep them down. Fluoroscopic exposures to some interventional physicians, for example, tend to be higher than necessary. To avoid this happening, operators can try to cut down the beam-on time (without compromising clinical effectiveness, of course), such as by utilizing a slow frame rate, pulsed technique with frame-hold. Also, they can get into the habit of wearing lead aprons with thyroid shields, and to put lead glass shielding in place when possible.

Personal actions

There are four personal actions one can undertake to minimize risk when working around *any* hazardous entity: while still doing the job properly,

Time: minimize the *time* spent around it;

Distance: maximize the *distance* from it, bearing in mind the *inverse square* rule;

Shielding: utilize available radiation *shielding* and barriers; and

Containment: with a spill of radioactive (or toxic) material, *contain* it, keep people away, and call the Radiation Safety Officer for guidance.

These are the first of what may be thought of as, with apologies to T.S. Eliot, the *Four Quartets of Radiation Safety* (Figure 5.13).

Department activities

A second quartet concerns the activities that an imaging clinic or department can do (and may,

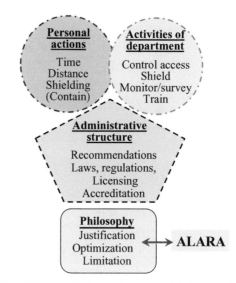

Figure 5.13 A radiation safety program is built on a solid *philosophical foundation*, and consists of *personal actions* and *imaging center activities* that are guided, or required, by the components of the *administrative structure*.

in fact, be legally required to do) to further this effort. These activities involve the design of new or reconfigured imaging suites; controlling access to radiation areas; routinely monitoring workers and surveying work areas; and training:

Design. In building or renovating an imaging suite, it is imperative to design protective walls and barriers at the outset to be consistent, now and for future possible uses, with applicable regulations. Radiation exposures must be below state and federal regulations in the control area for the imaging suite, in nearby patients' waiting rooms, at the secretary's cubicle, residents' lounge, etc. (Figure 5.14a). There must be enough barrier material in place for the potential exposure on the protected side to be below federal and state exposure-rate limits. Apart from the 511-keV annihilation photons from a PET patient, a few feet of high-density concrete or a millimeter or so of lead will usually suffice – but excessive, unnecessary amounts of shielding can increase the cost of construction, and waste valuable space. The design of shielding for an imaging suite or the rooms around it requires the services of an experienced medical or health physicist or engineer; it is also a good idea to consult with your building's structural engineer *and* your regulatory agency

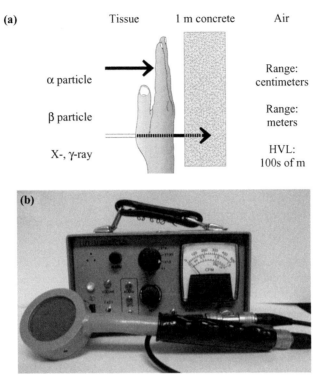

(a)   Tissue   1 m concrete   Air

α particle

β particle

X-, γ-ray

Range:
centimeters

Range:
meters

HVL:
100s of m

(b)

Figure 5.14 The design and surveying of radiation shielding barriers. **(a)** Shielding of rooms that contain imaging equipment protects people from gamma- and X-rays. Charged particles give up their kinetic energy more or less continuously, ionizing the tissue or barrier molecules they pass by; they run out of steam at about the same depth, and have a finite range, and rarely cause serious shielding problems in medicine. High-energy photon radiation, conversely, does not have a specific penetration distance, but rather the intensity falls off roughly exponentially with tissue or barrier thickness, decreasing to half its value over the half-value layer (HVL) thickness. The objective is to reduce the exposures on the far side of a barrier to below legal limits. Procedures are available from the NCRP and others for determining the thicknesses of concrete and/or lead sheeting required for various photon energies. **(b)** After a shielding wall of an imaging suite has been built, it is necessary to perform radiation surveys to confirm its effectiveness. A portable, highly sensitive ion-chamber detector can monitor the adequacy of the walls, doors, vents, ceilings, and floors of imaging suites. Likewise, a portable Geiger counter can scan areas for trace amounts of contamination with radioactive materials. Devices such as this one are also employed routinely to check hands and feet of people leaving areas where they might have inadvertently become contaminated with unsealed radioactive materials. With thanks to Walter Miller.

before you begin anything. And then survey the area at proper intervals of time afterwards (Figure 5.14b) [7].

Area control. Allow access to certain areas only to authorized personnel; post warnings, put in interlocks, etc., where radiation may be present. In *uncontrolled areas* with unlimited access, such as patient and visitor waiting rooms and areas for employees who do not work routinely with radiation (e.g., pediatric nurses' offices adjacent to the X-ray suite), no one should receive exposures in excess of 1 mSv/yr, on average, or 0.02 mSv/hr for brief periods.

Monitor staff and survey areas. Routinely survey radiation personnel and the areas where they or others might possibly be exposed. A radiation worker wears a film badge, thermoluminescent dosimeter (TLD), optically stimulated dosimeter (OSD), or other device, (Figure 5.15a), and perhaps an additional radiation sensor when there is a chance of a higher rate of exposure (Figure 5.15b). Radiologists, cardiologists, radiological and dental technologists, and others both within and outside medicine are allowed by law to accumulate no more than an annual whole-body *occupational* (from their work) exposure of

(a)   **(b)**

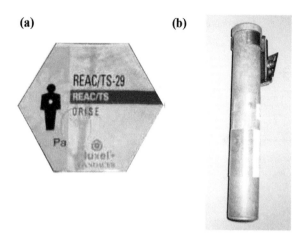

Figure 5.15 Personal dose monitoring. (**a**) Virtually everyone directly involved in producing X-ray or gamma-ray images wears a film or other badge that keeps track of the (normally) very small amounts of radiation received over the course of a month or so. Courtesy of Doren Christensen, Radiation Emergency Assistance Center/Training Site (REAC/TS), Oak Ridge, TN. (**b**) A worker who might be getting significant amounts of radiation during a task should also carry a pocket dosimeter, which records doses deposited over minutes or hours. With thanks to Walter Miller.

50 mSv (Table 5.4). (Nearly all European countries have reduced the limit to 20 mSv, averaged over 5 years.) Most medical personnel in the USA actually receive a fiftieth of the limit or less, and the resulting 0.1% incremental lifetime risk is comparable to that of dying in a natural catastrophe, such as a tornado, flood, or earthquake; the odds of being killed in an auto accident are an order of magnitude greater. In addition, areas where exposures may occur to anyone must be monitored periodically to ensure that annual doses to occupants are below legal limits. And the monitoring devices themselves must be checked and re-calibrated periodically.

Train. Instruct and regularly refresh all personnel on the basics of normal and emergency radiation safety – and make certain that they continue to comprehend, and know how to use, what is needed for safe operation. The price of safety is eternal and active vigilance and, for that to occur, people have to fully understand what is required of them.

Table 5.4 The ICRP, NCRP, and other bodies provide *recommendations* on annual dose limits that apply to normal occupational exposure of workers and to members of the general public. In the United States, these strongly influence the *legal regulations* that the federal government imposes at 10 CFR 20 (see 10CFR20 Subparts C and D). These effective and equivalent doses do not include natural background radiation, or that delivered to a patient because of an intentional medical exposure. Special measures must be taken to protect the fetus of a worker who has declared herself pregnant, and also to deal with emergency situations. These recommendations and regulations may evolve slowly over time.

Limit on exposure	10 CFR 20 (mSv-y^{-1})	ICRP (2007) (mSv-y^{-1})
Occupational		
Stochastic (effective dose)	50	50[a]
Deterministic (equivalent dose)		
to lens of eye	150	150
to skin, extremities	500	500
Embryo-fetus	5 during pregnancy	~ same as for member of the public
General public		
Stochastic (ED)	1	1[b]
hourly rate	0.02 mSv h^{-1}	
"infrequent exposure"	5	

[a] No more than 20 mSv y^{-1} (2 rem y^{-1}) averaged over 5 years
[b] Exceptionally, higher than 1 mSv y^{-1} (0.1 rem y^{-1}); but no more than 1 mSv y^{-1} averaged over 5 years.

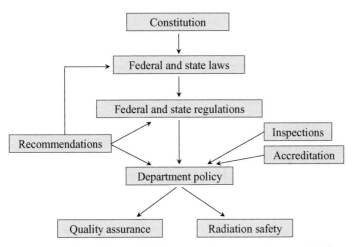

Figure 5.16 The legal framework of recommendations, regulations, and enforcement tools that combine to push an imaging department or clinic toward establishing strong and effective image QA and Radiation Safety programs.

Administrative structure: recommendations, laws, regulations, licensing, accreditation

High quality and safe operation is motivated by good intentions and ensured by an administrative structure that involves a number of parties who provide *recommendations*, *laws* and *regulations*, *licensing and enforcement*, and *accreditation*.

Recommendations. Several non-government organizations provide extensive and highly regarded guidance and suggestions for safe operation around ionizing and other forms of radiation. Many of the laws, regulations, policies, and practices described here originated from such recommendations, and continue to evolve because of changes in them. Among the most influential of them are in reports of the ICRP and the NCRP, e.g. [5,8,9].

Laws and regulations. The Constitution explicitly describes the process by which Congress and the President pass federal *laws*, also known as *statutes*, and the states follow similar procedures for their own laws (Figure 5.16). A federal or state law may authorize and/or require some federal or state *agency* (FDA, EPA, a state's Department of Health, etc.) to prepare a *regulation*, or *rule* that provides specific, comprehensive instructions for its implementation. The development of a federal regulation involves the agency working openly with public stakeholders, and responding fully to feedback from them, and progress is reported

from time to time in the *Federal Register*. Upon its completion, the new or revised rule is incorporated into the *Code of Federal Regulations* (Figure 5.17).

Of particular importance in the management of radiation is the part of the Code at *10 CFR 20*, a section that concerns fundamental regulations of the Nuclear Regulatory Commission (US NRC) [10]. This is a detailed NRC directive, which draws largely from ICRP/NCRP recommendations, for the day-to-day control of radiation exposures from those radioactive materials that the Commission controls under the authority of the Atomic Energy Act of 1946 and 1954 (AEA), such as the radiopharmaceuticals of nuclear medicine. The rule also serves as the principal model for regulation by all the states of *all* (including X-ray) radiation exposures of workers and members of the public.

The NRC ultimately controls the use of *radioactive materials* for diagnostic or therapeutic purposes. It is willing to delegate this responsibility and authority, however, to the *NRC Agreement States* that assent to enforce the rules as rigorously, primarily through the issuance of state licenses and state inspections; as of 2012, there were 37 of them and counting. As noted above, moreover, for historical reasons, the AEA does not authorize any federal agency to oversee the use of X-ray machines, or of linear or other accelerators. The states have filled in this gap by establishing their own safety laws and regulations designed almost entirely around 10 CFR

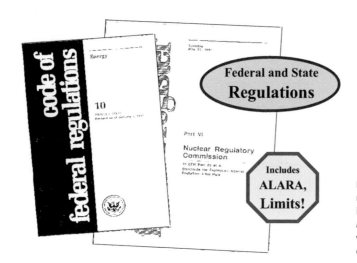

Figure 5.17 Changes in the NRC or other regulations that govern the use of ionizing radiation appear first in the *Federal Register* (published daily), after which they are compiled in the *US Code of Federal Regulations* (*CFR*).

20, although the degree of vigor with which they do so depends strongly on the level of their financial well being.

An exception is the Mammography Quality Standards Reauthorization Act (MQSRA) of 1998 (Chapter 4), through which the FDA established and watches over a federal program specifically for X-ray breast imaging (21 CFR 900.12). Another important job of the FDA, incidentally, is to certify that all medical imaging devices meet its safety and effectiveness requirements before they leave the factory door; once in the clinic, however, the FDA is usually out of the picture.

Licensing. A federal or state regulatory body needs to make sure that every facility under its purview is following its regulations properly. To do that, it may issue a specific *license* that spells out in gruesome detail exactly what that particular facility must, can, and cannot do. Licensing can be a drawn-out procedure, but it serves to avoid misunderstandings. The agency in authority may carry out routine unannounced inspections to ensure that the site remains in compliance, but often this just serves to check that necessary records are all up to date. For some states that are undergoing especially hard times financially, inspections may come rather infrequently, unless there is an obvious need for them.

Accreditation. The American College of Radiology (ACR), The Joint Commission (TJC), the Intersocietal Accreditation Commission (IAC), and others may offer to accredit departments or individual imaging machines with a valu-

able seal of approval. This is becoming more than just a nicety, however, since leading insurance companies have agreed to reimburse studies performed on CT, MRI, ultrasound, and other machines at stand-alone facilities only if they have gone through the ACR accrediting process, which ensures that at least minimal performance requirements are met. It is to be expected that this requirement will soon apply to larger facilities, as well. The ACR accreditation of a single CT unit, for example, consists of four parts: extensive paperwork on the education and certification and/or licensing of the physicians, technologists, and medical physicists who use or work on the machine; submission of a number of sample images obtained with typical site protocols, to be inspected by outside volunteer radiologists; testing and recording of various aspects of image quality, obtained by a medical physicist with a specially designed CT test phantom; and several specific dose measurements made on a so-called CTDI (CT dose index) phantom.

The philosophy of radiation protection

Finally, radiation safety programs around the world rest firmly upon three philosophical pillars, the ideas of justification, optimization, and limitation. (OK, so this one's not a quartet.) And, in practice, the backbone of a state or federal radiation safety program is its intension and effort to implement these three principles:

Justification means that there should be no exposure of anyone unless there is a good reason for it, with the expectation of a net benefit; who benefits versus who assumes the risk can sometimes be a subject of debate.

Optimization is, in most situations, just another name for ALARA, and it may be thought of as the medical Golden Rule of protection from *any* hazardous source: always strive to keep all doses to all people to a minimum, consistent with good image quality and proper medical care. Indeed, much of staying ALARA is simply a matter of being alert and continually exercising common sense. But the practice of ALARA is more than just a very good idea: it is made mandatory in the US by the NRC and its Agreement states, as engraved in their compilations of regulations like the US CFR. Locally, a medical facility's Radiation Safety Officer (RSO) is required to establish and enforce an active ALARA program.

Limitation. The real teeth of a state or federal radiation safety program are in the requirement to *limit* radiation dose to staff and the public and, in a few instances, to the patient. As just discussed, in the United States, most of the limits involving medical practice may be found published in 10 CFR 20, and these are summarized in Table 5.4.

Image QA and radiation safety are considered by some to be not particularly glamorous. And since maintaining image quality and safety takes time and money – sometimes considerable amounts of both – clinic chairs and administrators occasionally make the "mistake" of skimping on them. But to do so is a practically, ethically, and sometimes criminally bad decision. Failure to implement and manage a rigorous and effective QA and safety program is known from unhappy experience to sometimes spell absolute disaster, both personal and financial, for patients, facilities, and physicians.

References

1 NCRP. *Ionizing Radiation Exposure of the Population* of the United States, report no. 160. Bethesda, MD: NCRP, 2009.

2 National Research Council. *Health Risks from Exposure to Low Levels of Ionizing Radiation*: BEIR VII. Washington, DC: National Academies Press, 2006.

3 United Nations Scientific Committee on the Effects of Atomic Radiation (UNSCEAR). *Effects of Ionizing Radiation*. New York: United Nations, 2006.

4 Brooks AL, Eberlein PE, Couch LA, Boecker BB. The role of dose-rate on risk from internally-deposited radionuclides and the potential need to separate dose-rate effectiveness factor (DREF) from the dose and dose-rate effectiveness factor (DDREF). *Health Phys* 2009;**97**:458–69.

5 ICRP. 2007 Recommendation of the International Commission on Radiological Protection, ICRP Publication 103. *Ann ICRP* 2007;**37**(2–4).

6 Wolbarst AB, Wiley A, Nemhauser J, *et al.* Medical response to a major radiological emergency. *Radiology* 2010;254:660–77.

7 NCRP. *Structural Shielding Design for Medical X-Ray Imaging Facilities*, report no. 147. Bethesda, MD: NCRP, 2004.

8 Proceedings of the First ICRP Symposium on the International System of Radiological Protection. **Ann ICRP** 2012;**41**(3–4). Available at www.sciencedirect.com /science/journal/01466453. Accessed October 23, 2012.

9 NCRP. *Radiation Dose Management for Fluoroscopically-Guided Interventional Medical Procedures*, report no. 168. Bethesda, MD: NCRP, 2010.

10 US Nuclear Regulatory Commission. Standards for Protection against Radiation. US Code of Federal Regulations, 10 CFR 20, 2007.

CHAPTER 6

Twenty-first Century (Digital) Imaging

Computer-Based Representation, Acquisition, Processing, Storage, Transmission, and Analysis of Images

Medicine is becoming ever more computerized, and this is especially true of clinical imaging.

For some of the older analog modalities such as fluoroscopy, planar nuclear medicine, and ultrasound, computers are enabling their successors to produce and display enhanced diagnostic information whose quality and flexibility their inventors could not have imagined. Computers now support programs for drawing out contrast that previously was invisible (Figure 6.1); radically diminishing the level of visual noise that earlier would have overwhelmed anything of interest; sharpening up edges and producing better resolution; combining the information content from multi-ple, adjacent two-dimensional slice-images to generate a composite three-dimensional display; even overlaying image information from two distinct sources, such as CT and PET, greatly enhancing the usefulness of either alone through their synergy. Computers make possible not only extraordinary forms of image processing and quality improvement, but also the capacity for instantaneous archiving and retrieval, and transmission to the ICU or across the continent at light speed. And, at their cutting edge, *computer-assisted diagnosis* (CAD) systems even undertake the automated analysis and diagnosis of certain pathologies.

Medical Imaging: Essentials for Physicians, First Edition. Anthony B. Wolbarst, Patrizio Capasso and Andrew R. Wyant.
© 2013 John Wiley & Sons, Inc. Published 2013 by John Wiley & Sons, Inc.

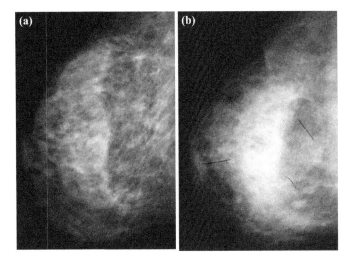

Figure 6.1 Digital mammography versus film. (**a**) The digital image provides more contrast and less noise, allowing the visualization of clinically relevant masses and calcifications in dense-tissue regions than does (**b**) a screen-film study.

While computers greatly improve some modalities, for others, like CT, PET and SPECT, and MRI, they are absolutely essential, *sine qua non* for their very existence. One cannot simply acquire CT, PET, or MRI data and display it, as with film, fluoroscopy, planar nuclear medicine, or ultrasound; it is necessary first to transform the data completely, turning it inside out mathematically, to *reconstruct* an image out of seemingly random data (Figure 6.2).

Digital computers

A computer is a machine that processes information according to the precise dictates of a stored set of instructions, or program. The computer accepts input data from a source, such as an imaging device; acts on them in a way determined by the program to, for example, diminish the level of visual noise in its images; and generates an output that might be displayed on a monitor, or serve as the input for

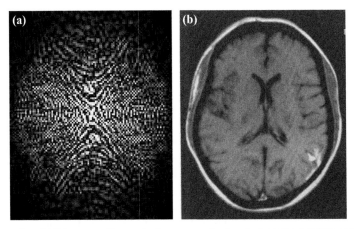

Figure 6.2 Reconstruction. (**a**) This apparently meaningless menagerie of squiggles is the raw data, expressed as a so-called *k*-space representation, from an MRI study of a head. (**b**) Following the application of an extensive and complex set of mathematical transformations known as *reconstruction*, something appears that seems quite substantive – but appearances can be deceiving! We are not seeing a photographically realistic portrayal of the physical tissues here, but rather a map of proton T1 relaxation times within them.

another program or computer. The sets of stored programs and the blocks of data operated on are contained in program (instruction) files and data files, respectively.

Most of the things we experience around us are in a sense *continuous*. Distances, the passage of time, mountain roads, rapid pressure variations on your eardrums, ocean surfaces and AM radio waves – all of these are smoothly varying and connected. Signals with this property are said to be *analog*, and a few highly specialized *analog computers* have been built to operate on them.

Digital computers, on the other hand, make use of messages that are not continuous in nature, but rather are made up of separate parts. "Digital" comes from the Latin *digitus*, or finger (not necessarily on the other hand), and from the notion of counting, at least up to ten. Hard to imagine, but at some point in the distant past, one of our direct ancestors was the very first creature on earth to signify exactly seven or nine bison by holding up his hands. (For larger herds, he'd have to take off his sox.) Digital information is made up of discrete pieces that can be counted. When we invented writing, whether with pictograms or alphabets, that was also a kind of digital signaling, too.

While most things are normally continuous, often we can communicate about them only digitally. We measure the height of the wheat in terms of feet: this year's crop is already about 1.5 meters tall, which is a good sign. And the farmer's weight has grown to 280 pounds, which is not. Here, the tape measure and the scale, together with someone to read them, to within some degree of accuracy, serve as *analog-to-digital converters*. In obtaining information from the outside world, computers use A/D converters all the time, because they can cogitate only digitally.

A bit about bytes

A computer thinks and communicates in bits. A *bit* (*bi*nary dig*it*) is the smallest quantity of information needed to respond to a simple yes-no question. "Is it raining?" can have only two answers ("sort of" doesn't count), and the correct one can be supplied with a single bit of data.

The answer to the question can be shown on paper by a checked or empty box, a blue or red stripe, a picture of a chicken or of a fruitcake, the numbers 256 and 1024, the letters *b* and *β*, or even by the words "oui" and "bu shi." Any one of these will do, or any other pair of entities, as long as everyone agrees on what the two mean.

The answer can also be stored electronically by way of a single *binary switch* with *two possible physical states of being*: open or shut, on/off, low/high-voltage, and so on. Again, the two states can represent, or be represented by, anything you wish. The states of a binary switch can be indicated by the two English words "yes" and "no," or by the pair of numbers "0" and "1." A single zero or a one then conveys a bit of information, as long as people know the coding convention.

A computer's microprocessor and memory consist of billions of interconnected, microscopic electrical on-off switches built into a silicon chip. The number of bits in a message, of course, is totally unrelated to its importance. It might take a million bits to store a trashy novel, while a single zero or one in the wrong place conceivably could start an unintended war – well, at the least, it could crash your PC at the wrong time.

"Is it raining, and is it cold?" is a two-part question that requires a two-bit reply, such as 01 or 11, where the order matters. The first digit in a pair may be defined to refer to the "raining" query, and a "0" to a "no." More complex queries may demand more bits for a complete response.

Combinations of bits can not only answer multiple yes-no questions, but also signify numbers, letters of the alphabet, and even abstract symbols and concepts in messages. This also requires agreement upon codes, or conventions, to translate ideas and symbols into strings of bits and back again – and the basis for the codes used in computers is the *binary number system*, built out of only 0s and 1s. Nearly all computers are designed to operate with programs and input data conveyed in binary numbers.

The year that Sergeant Pepper changed the world can be expressed in the ordinary *decimal* system as a specific four-digit combination of integer multiples of 1000s, 100s, 10s, and 1s; that is, of powers of 10: $(1 \times 10^3 + 9 \times 10^2 + 6 \times 10^1 + 7 \times 10^0) = 1967$, where the right-hand side is a shorthand notation for what is on the left. We could include powers of 10 from $10^0 = 1$ up through 10^7, with that glorious year becoming 00001967, but common practice is to drop leading digits that happen to be zeros.

Likewise, one can equally well decompose a "real" digital number into powers of 2. The decimal integer 92, the atomic number of the heaviest chemical element naturally occurring on Earth, might then be represented in powers of 2 from 2^0 to 2^7, say, as $(0 \times 2^7 + 1 \times 2^6 + 0 \times 2^5 + 1 \times 2^4 + 1 \times 2^3 + 1 \times 2^2 + 0 \times 2^1 + 0 \times 2^0)$, which can be abbreviated as the specific 8-bit sequence 01011100. Each 0 or 1 in this binary sequence is a *bit*, and you have to know the rule, the prescription, for translating a sequence of 1s and 0s into (in this case) a decimal number.

A sequence, or block, of precisely eight bits is a called a *byte*. Unlike the decimal system, leading zeros within a byte are retained. Thus, while the atomic number of uranium may not be presented as 0092 too often, it is perfectly appropriate to represent it as the single binary byte 01011100.

How many distinct, different bytes can there be? In other words, how many different symbols can the complete set of all possible bytes correspond to? Consider, first, what we can do with one bit: there are only two options, namely 0 and 1. With an *ordered* pair of two bits, there are four options. The first can be either 0 or 1, and so also for the second, so altogether there are $2 \times 2 = 2^2 = 4$ possibilities, which comprise the set $\{00, 01, 10, 11\}$. These four combinations can stand for $\{0, 1, 2, 3\}$, respectively, if you like, or $\{1, 2, 3, 4\}$, or $\{\alpha, \beta, \gamma, \delta\}$ or even $\{17, \yen, \text{chicken}, \text{chicken}\}$. Likewise, an ordered triad of bits has 2^3 possible combinations: $\{000, 001, 010, 011, \ldots, 111\}$, corresponding to eight possible symbols. The maximum possible number of different 8-bit *bytes* is $(2 \times 2 \times 2 \times 2 \ldots \times 2) = 2^8 = 256$.

The interpretation of any byte is determined solely by convention or agreement. Perhaps the most elementary and common system for assigning individual meaning to the 256 possible distinct bytes is to count with them beginning, say, with zero (Box 6.1). Another one found commonly is the "ASCII" code for numbers, upper- and lower-case letters, and a number of symbols.

Box 6.1

One simple assignment of meaning to the 256 possible different forms for a single byte. A byte consists of a sequence of 8 bits of information. The first can be either 0 or 1, as can the second, up through the eighth, so there are $2 \times 2 \times 2 \ldots \times 2 = 2^8 = 256$ distinct possibilities. While the complete set of bytes can represent any 256 (or fewer) things you wish, one common and elementary application is just to list the first 256 decimal numbers, in which the bytes 00000000 through 11111111 correspond to, say, decimal 0 through 255.

Binary	Decimal
00000000	0
00000001	1
00000010	2
00000011	3
00000100	4
00000101	5
00000110	6
00000111	7
00001000	8
00001001	9
...	
1111 1110	254
1111 1111	255

It is possible to devise a convention, for example, that detects errors that may occur in a byte or word: an *even-parity* byte code might include information in the low seven places, but sets the *parity bit* (farthest to the left) in such a way that it plus the others add up to an even number: the byte 00110110 is thus legitimate, but 10110110 is not. There are many variations on this theme, including codes (Hamming, Hadamard) that not only find errors, but even correct them.

Here's an interesting but easy bit of entertainment for you. A linear protein molecule consists of a sequence of amino acids, uniquely determined by a corresponding sequence of *codons* in a strand of DNA; a codon is a short string of nucleic acid bases that codes, ultimately, for a single amino acid. There are 20 different commonly occurring amino acids out of which proteins are built, and four different nucleic bases for making codons. What is the smallest possible size of (number of bases in) a codon, assuming that all codons contain the same number of bases? (Hint: 3.) What are the implications of the fact that more codons are available than needed?

A permanently connected grouping of two or more bytes is called a *word*. With the simple decimal-number counting convention of Box 6.1, there are $2^{16} = 65\,536$ distinct 2-byte words, ranging from $(00000000)(00000000) = 0$ to $(11111111)(11111111) = 65\ 535$, which is commonly written 64k in computerese. For nearly all applications, a small modern computer will manipulate 4-byte and even 8-byte $= 64$-bit words (not to be confused with the 64 in 64k). The purpose of this is not to let us define $2^{64} = 18M$ symbols, but rather to make arithmetic calculations much faster.

Hardware and architecture

A computer, designed to think in bytes and words, consists of tremendous numbers of microscopic, solid-state binary switches, each with only two possible states. Different combinations and sub-groups of these switches carry out a range of different activities by means of which the machine functions. It undertakes the acquisition and processing of digital medical image data, the brief or longer-term storage of data and information, logical and arithmetic operations, and displaying the results of all that effort.

The architecture of a digital computer system appears, in most rudimentary form, in Figure 6.3. The computer is built around a *central processing unit* (CPU), commonly called *the processor*, and some associated, ultra-fast *cache* memory, both on a solid-state, silicon-based microchip. Directly attached to the CPU/cache chip are additional chips that provide gigabytes (GByte) of immediately and rapidly accessible *random access memory* (RAM); these temporarily store the programs and data that the CPU is currently working with. Feeding into the CPU/memory unit by electrical *buses* are the *input devices*, such as medical image acquisition instruments, touch-screens, and keyboards. Typical *output devices* are a workstation with monitors, a PACS, or a *local area network* (LAN). A facility will typically also install enough short-term *temporary storage*, such as DVD-like magnetic and optical discs, to allow fairly fast access to the studies performed, say, over the past 30 days, plus what is needed for ambulatory cases. Finally, a large facility

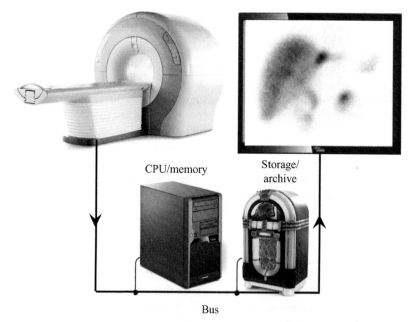

Figure 6.3 Architecture of any medical imaging computer system consists of four parts: a *central processing unit* (CPU) and super-fast *cache memory* all on a chip, and billions of bytes (GBytes, 10^9 bytes) of very fast solid-state *random-access memory* (RAM); a source of data input (e.g., an image acquisition device); output (LCD monitor, PACS, hard-copy, Internet link); and terabytes (TBytes, 10^{12}) of slower, cheaper archive storage, or long-term memory.

may produce hundreds of terabytes (TByte, 10^{12}) of data per year, and all of that must be held long-term in on- or off-site *mass archiving* systems that are orders of magnitude slower, but also vaster and much cheaper. The coming of so-called *cloud computing* and *cloud storage* may greatly expand a facility's capabilities for all of this.

Driven and synchronized ultimately by a system *clock*, the CPU fetches, decodes, and executes the software instructions coming from the operating system and application programs. Computer speed is commonly measured either in clock speed (e.g., GHz) or in *millions* of *instructions* carried out *per second* (MIPS).

Computer RAM comprises billions of individually addressable *registers*. The simplest register comprises a block of memory, consisting of eight transistor switches and capable of storing a single byte of data. A computer might write the byte 01011100 into a block, say, by setting its eight switches to the configuration of Figure 6.4. It later could read back

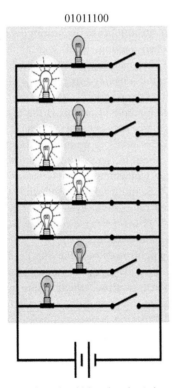

01011100

Figure 6.4 A register, in which a closed switch and its light being on are taken to represent a "1" bit. Starting at the top, this register happens to be storing the binary number 01011100.

the register by trying to send currents through all eight switches and seeing which ones conduct.

Back to the CPU for a moment. It performs not only *arithmetic* computations that involve numbers, but also *logical* operations on abstract symbols. Consider a combination of switches that test the truth of the compound statement "it is cool **AND** sunny," where each of the two component statements, "it is cool" and "it is sunny," may be either TRUE or FALSE. Suppose that the phrase "it is cool" is represented by switch **A**, which is closed when the statement is TRUE, and open when it is FALSE (Figure 6.5a), and so also for switch **B** and "it is sunny." It is possible to build the needed AND circuit out of a battery, a light bulb, and two binary blade switches in series, and the circuit can exist in four different states (Figure 6.5b). Current flows around the complete circuit (causing the bulb to light and indicating that the compound statement "it is cool **AND** sunny" is TRUE) only when both the component statements are separately TRUE, as indicated by the *truth table* of Figure 6.5c. This is an extremely simple application of *Boolean algebra*, the branch of mathematics that underlies logical computation.

What makes such tedious and simple-minded machinations useful is the phenomenal speed with which a computer takes its tiny steps. Individual switches can be made to open and close billions of times a second, in synchrony with the computer's internal master clock. So even a process that requires hundreds of thousands of separate switching events may still be carried out in under a millisecond.

The ultimate wizardry of the computer stems ultimately from the fact that the very *commands* that tell switches to open and close can themselves be represented by combinations of bits just like data, held in registers, moved around, and even altered during operation. A program is a sequence of such commands that together lead to the performance of some set of logical or arithmetic tasks, and the program itself is stored in the computer's memory, along with the data.

Digital acquisition and representation of an image

The actual creation of an image at an acquisition node begins with the generation of an analog

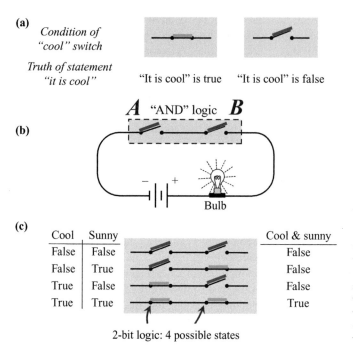

(a)

Condition of "cool" switch

Truth of statement "it is cool"

"It is cool" is true   "It is cool" is false

A "AND" logic B

(b)

Bulb

(c)

Cool	Sunny		Cool & sunny
False	False		False
False	True		False
True	False		False
True	True		True

2-bit logic: 4 possible states

Figure 6.5 Representation of a simple AND logic circuit to determine the truth of a compound statement. (a) A closed switch means that its corresponding statement is TRUE. (b) 2-bit logic circuit, with only four possible configurations. (c) Compound statement "It is cool and sunny" is TRUE, with a bright light, only when the individual statements of which it is comprised are both TRUE. (Incidentally, what's wrong with this figure?)

(almost always) voltage signal by a signal receptor. In digital angiography, the detection system might be an image intensifier tube coupled to a CCD electronic optical camera; or with the more advanced systems discussed in the next chapter, it would be the X-ray sensor for each of the millions of pixels of a flat-panel detector array. In CT, the image receptor comprises thousands of solid-state X-ray detectors lined up in multiple rings, and in MRI, antennas detect radiofrequency waves and transform them into signal voltages. And an ultrasound transducer does the same with acoustic waves. In each case, the radiation-induced signal is a continuous, analog voltage that reflects on some aspect of tissue characteristics at a point, along a line, over an area, or throughout a volume within the patient, and it has to be digitized.

A medical image comprises one million pixels, give or take a factor of ten: digitizing a radiograph

The voltage from a signal detector must be sampled sufficiently frequently, and its magnitude at each sample transformed into bytes by an analog-to-digital converter. (A glass thermometer and you, together, nicely illustrate the idea of digitization; the length of the mercury column varies continuously with the temperature but, in sampling it, you read it off as a discrete number to the nearest degree.) For a continuously varying signal, such as that from a single MRI signal-pickup coil or an ultrasound transducer, the *sampling rate* may be many thousands of times per second.

A simple example of all this is the *digitization of a radiographic film*. Let's say a thoracic surgeon in Los Angeles needs to examine a patient's film taken last month in New York City, and she needs it right away. Unfortunately, the New York clinic is still pre-PACS, and it takes a good while to locate the required radiograph. Eventually, it is entered into a *film scanner/digitizer*, a computer-controlled laser-plus-photodetector system.

Within a light-proof box, the film lies flat on a horizontal glass plate. The computer plus optical imaging system partitions the film into an imaginary *matrix* of millions of tiny square film pixels, typically 0.1 mm on a side, and assigns a digital *pixel address* to each, corresponding to its physical location on the film, as in Figure 6.6 (an expansion of Figure 1.11a).

After that, the system's computer directs a narrow laser beam to sweep rapidly across and slowly down the film in a precise raster pattern, one horizontal line (indicated in red) at a time (Figure 6.7a). At

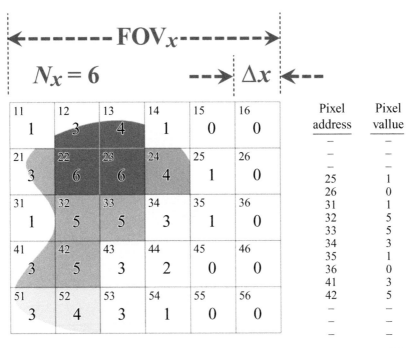

Pixel address	Pixel vallue
–	–
–	–
–	–
25	1
26	0
31	1
32	5
33	5
34	3
35	1
36	0
41	3
42	5
–	–
–	–

Figure 6.6 Digital representation of an image. The image is partitioned by an imaginary grid into tens of thousands to millions of very small square pixels. Every point on the image is assigned a unique pixel address, and its shade of gray is expressed as the pixel value. The image can then be represented as a listing of pixel addresses and corresponding pixel values. The number of pixels in an image, $\mathcal{N}_{image}$, is related to the field of view (FOV) as $\mathcal{N}_{image} = \mathcal{N}_x \times \mathcal{N}_y$, where $FOV_x = \mathcal{N}_x \, \Delta x$ for a voxel of width Δx.

every point on the film, it already knows the pixel address, which was used to aim the laser. A light-sensitive photodetector continuously assesses the intensity of light passing through film, as the beam travels continuously along the straight line on it (Figure 6.7b), and generates a corresponding analog voltage (Figure 6.7c). This continuous voltage is sampled to the nearest millivolt at the center of every film pixel, then transformed by an analog-to-digital converter (ADC) to a numerical *pixel value* (Figure 6.7d).

Thus the system measures the degree of darkness of film in each pixel, and translates it into a numerical pixel value, and tabulates the result (Figure 6.7e). The relationship between the pixel value at any address and the corresponding pixel brightness and/or color is known as the *gray scale*, and the long string of all the digital pixel addresses and values produced in this fashion is called a *bit map*. In summary, keeping track of the brightness or color of an image while scanning it along a raster path is a simple and effective way to transform a two-

dimensional spatial image into a one-dimensional sequence of digital numbers.

The computer now sends these stored numbers to California electronically where, by reversing the whole process, the surgeon can generate a visual reproduction of the film and get to work (Figure 6.7f). After she enters the data file of digitized pixel addresses and values into her computer, it now knows both the position and the expected amount of brightness everywhere on the monitor. The program goes to its first pixel location, creates the appropriate amount of light there, and then proceeds on to the next pixel. With a matrix several thousand pixels on a side, the image she will view on a large monitor will be nearly indistinguishable from the original X-ray film.

Determinants of image quality: resolution, pixel size, matrix dimensions, and field of view

The four basic measures of quality of a film, namely resolution, contrast, noise level, and artifacts, are

(a)

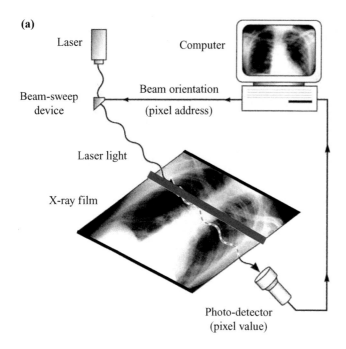

(b)

(c)

(d)

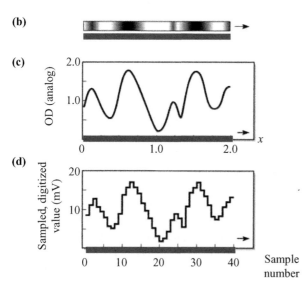

(e)

Address	Value
—	—
—	—
15	14
16	12
17	10
18	8
19	5
20	3
21	2
—	—
—	—

Stored image

(f)

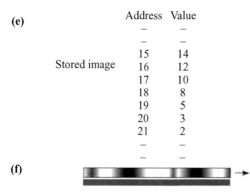

Figure 6.7 Digitizing an X-ray film. (a) The system scans a laser beam along a raster pattern of straight horizontal lines, while sampling the brightness of the light transmitted through the film at every pixel. (b) This pixel-wide strip of film corresponds to sweeping along the red line, and (c) the resulting analog voltage is read from the photodetector. (d) The voltage from the photodetector is digitized, and sent to the computer, (e) which organizes all the data as a long string of digital pixel-addresses and pixel-values. (f) The image can be recovered, on a monitor or laser printer, by feeding this pixel address and pixel brightness information to the display device.

just as relevant for digital images, and we can couch some of these ideas in computer-friendly language. Regardless of how a digital image is produced, its information content depends on the fineness of its spatial detail, on the subtlety of the variations in shadings of gray or color that can be distinguished in the display monitor, and on the level of visual noise. The smaller the pixels, the more gray levels of shading, and the quieter the random fluctuations, the more faithfully a digital representation can capture and reproduce reality. There are, however, inherent limits to the spatial resolution and contrast achievable by any imaging technology and, ultimately, by the viewer. At the same time, the amount of computer time and power required to process, store, and ship an image will increase, not too surprisingly, with the amount of information content, and so, too, will the expense.

With regard to resolution, it is necessary to distinguish between the innate capabilities of the imaging device, of the display, and of the eye. Ideally, the three would be about the same, and sometimes the design engineers are clever enough for that to be so. Let us assume here that this is the case. Then how small does a voxel (a cube or elongated cube of tissue within the body to which a pixel on the display corresponds) have to be, relative to the objects we are examining? At the other extreme, as pixel size grows on display, when does it start looking pixelated, or comprised of little squares, rather than smooth?

The smaller the pixels and the greater their number, up to a point, and the greater the number of gray levels employed in displaying, also up to a point, the more faithfully can a representation capture the original. MRI studies are commonly carried out with a 512×512 pixel matrix, and a gray scale of 2^8 to 2^{12} shades (Figure 6.8a); the histogram records the gray-scale pixel values, with a sagittal view, as a function of position as you move along the short bright line we have focused on within the pons.

Inadequate resolution will result from too few, too large pixels (Figure 6.8b). More pixels and gray levels per image, on the other hand, mean slower image reconstruction and processing, and greater storage and communication costs. Thus an impor-

tant objective in designing or purchasing imaging equipment is to create a system with somewhat more than enough ability to accomplish the requisite clinical tasks, but not too much beyond that, so as to keep cost and time down. The best the eye can resolve, for example, is about 0.1 mm with close viewing; there is little point in paying (a lot) for a more complex image receptor or a more powerful computer or display screen that go far beyond this if the "improvements" they bring are barely perceptible. In addition, we are now finding that coarser images, with less resolution, often can still provide adequate diagnostic information. This would lead to reductions in cost, time of acquisition and processing, radiation dose, and even the amount of contrast agent administered. And that may lower movement artifacts, decrease the deleterious effects of ionizing radiation and iodinated contrast media, and help with the financial impact of the examination.

The ability to resolve fine detail is limited, ultimately, by the cones of the fovea centralis. The fovea is about $1/3$ mm across, and within it are 50 000 densely packed, atypically slender cone cells. These cover only 1% of the retinal surface, and they provide focused, high acuity vision for no more than a few degrees from the center, but they connect to fully half the cells of the visual cortex. As a result of all this, the best visibility with normal viewing of $2/3$ meter from the monitor is no better than 0.2 mm, and, with close viewing from half that distance, 0.1 mm. The eye can discern only 50 to 100 distinct shades of gray, moreover, which is spanned with a gray scale depth of 6 or 7 bits. The use of color, of course, complicates things a little.

MRI and CT usually can provide less spatial resolution than can digitized film, or than can DR, CR, and DSA, and often there is little harm in adopting a coarser pixel matrix, such as 512×512, for both image acquisition and display. (This is partly a result of the tradeoff among technical capability, cost, and, for CT, patient dose; indeed some experimental MRI and CT machines do work at 1024×1024 and, for small-animal studies, at even sharper resolution.) Nuclear medicine generally requires less fineness. Fewer pixels and gray levels per image means faster image reconstruction

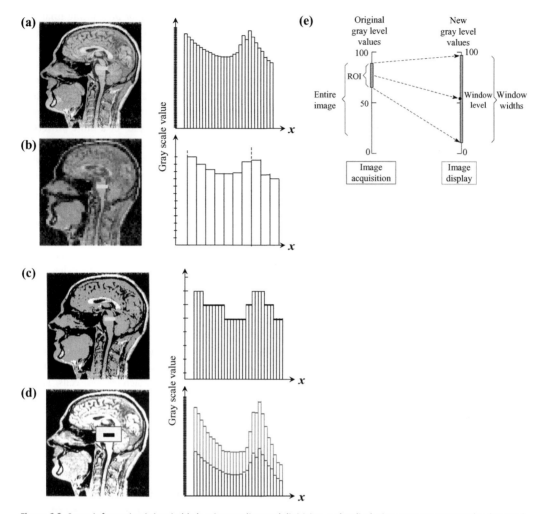

Figure 6.8 Some information is inevitably lost in sampling and digitizing and redisplaying, so a system must be designed to ensure that images are not overly degraded. It is essential, in particular, that pixels be sufficiently small and numerous, and that there be enough shades of gray. (a) A typical, good state-of-the-art clinical MRI sagittal image of the head, with a 512 × 512 pixel matrix and 256 shades of gray. The histogram to the right shows the digitized pixel values as a function of position along the short, bright line within the pons. (b) The same image, but reconstructed on a 64 × 64 grid, in which the pixel dimensions are a factor of 8 larger; this is exaggerated here for emphasis, but the pixelation could be noticeable even at 256 × 256. Features will be missed, moreover, if the pixels are too large relative to the details of the entity being viewed. (c) Likewise, despite good resolution, there must also be enough distinct gray levels available to prevent a blotchy appearance. (d) Even with an adequate pixel matrix and gray scale, the image may appear over- or under-exposed unless the levels of gray are properly scaled by way of the *windowing* process; the light blue histogram resulted from doubling the *window width*, which would bring the image closer into alignment with Figure 6.8a. (e) Altering window central level and/or window width can make an image more suitable to the eye. Photos courtesy of WS Kiger, III, Massachusetts Institute of Technology.

and processing, and less storage and communication capabilities, and it may lead to perfectly adequate image quality.

The number of pixels, $\mathcal{N}$, needed to capture a given *field of view* (FOV) in a two-dimensional image depends on the resolution required (Figure 6.6). The FOV_x in the x-direction, say, increases linearly with the corresponding number of pixels, $\mathcal{N}_x$, and with pixel size, Δx as

$$\text{FOV}_x = \mathcal{N}_x \times \Delta x. \tag{6.1}$$

The entire image will, of course, be composed of $\mathcal{N}_x \times \mathcal{N}_y$ pixels.

Back to our digitized radiograph. Suppose it is partitioned with a matrix that is 3000 pixels across, and that the field of view is 30 cm. $\Delta x = FOV_x/\mathcal{N}_x$ reveals the pixels to be $(300 \text{ mm})/(3000) = 0.1$ mm across, about the resolving capability of the eye, which is why it looks so good.

Aliasing and the Nyquist theorem

How small must voxels and pixels be for an image to be of sufficient resolution and to appear smooth? Resolution in an image has been defined as the distance between very small, point-like high-contrast objects in the body that can just barely be distinguished in the image as separate (Figure 2.10). Two points or two lines are involved for a dark-white-dark pattern to be visible, and resolution is commonly expressed in millimeters, or in line pairs per mm. Similarly with digital, resolution can be indicated either as pixel or voxel dimensions (mm) or pixel pairs per mm (mm^{-1}). So a short answer is that tiny details in the object being observed can be resolved and incorporated into an image only if the voxels in the body are roughly half the size of the details of interest or smaller.

But insufficient resolution is not the only trouble that arises when voxel dimensions Δx and Δy are too large. Because of a phenomenon called *aliasing*, digital images can sometimes display "wrap around" artifacts (Figure 6.9a). Aliasing can be explained in terms of the so-called *Nyquist sampling theorem*, which reveals just how frequently samples should be taken when scanning an image, as in Figure 6.7d. The cause of the problem is easy to see by carrying out a little experiment (Figure 6.9b).

Suppose we are scanning something whose value changes sinusoidally and fairly rapidly along a line, as with the light, solid gray curve. Our objective is in two parts: first, we sample the curve at some frequency, shown as the small shaded circles in the figure. Then we give the raw data to a first year resident, telling him only that it's some sort of sine curve, and that his job is to try to reconstruct the original curve from the sample data. He begins by selecting a large number of medium-frequency sine curves of different amplitudes and, after many sleepless nights, he stumbles on one very much like the original. Success! But being a very conscientious clinician, he keeps going, and eventually finds another, the longer-wavelength curve in red dashes.

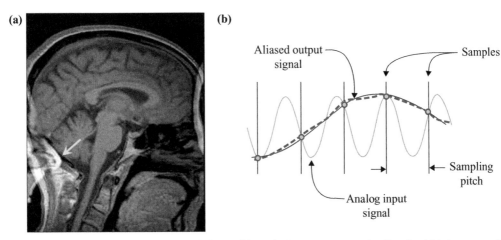

(a)   **(b)**

Aliased output signal — Samples

Analog input signal

Sampling pitch

Figure 6.9 Sampling, the Nyquist theorem, and aliasing. **(a)** An aliasing or wrap-around artifact, in which the nose to the left is wrapped around from the front of the patient. A clear case of sticking one's nose where it doesn't belong. **(b)** The wave is sampled (shaded circles) at a frequency that is only $^3/_4$ times that of the original, higher-frequency gray line. The dashed curve reconstructed from the sampled data seems to be a normal sine wave, and it fits the sampled data, but it is totally misleading, and would introduce aliasing into the original image of interest. Photo reproduced from Zhuo J, Gullapalli RP, AAPM/RSNA physics tutorial for residents: MR artifacts, safety, and quality control. *Radiographics* 2006;**26**:275–97, with permission of the Radiological Society of North America (RSNA).

Uh oh. Two curves fit the data, and there is no way of telling, from the data alone, which one is correct.

If, however, the sampling had occurred somewhat faster, at more than twice the frequency of the original one scanned (i.e., following the Nyquist prescription), no problems or confusion could ever arise, and he can reproduce the original sine curve unambiguously from the data. The point: if you under-sample or, equivalently, if the pixels are too large relative to the object being imaged, you can end up with your nose out of joint.

More determinants of image quality: gray scale and windowing

In addition to adequate resolution, there must also be enough distinct gray levels available to avoid the abrupt changes apparent in Figure 6.8c; indeed, the steps between levels should be somewhat less than what can be distinguished visually. To achieve the fineness of possible shading of Figure 6.8a, say, 256 levels of gray are employed, with a pixel-value of 0 corresponding to pitch black on the display, and 255 to pure white. Since $256 = 2^8$, the full range can be represented by the set of possible discrete sequences of 8 bits, and the *image depth* is said to be 8 bits or 1 byte *deep*.

A *liquid crystal display*'s (*LCD*) gray scale is typically 8 bits deep – that is, an eight-bit number is used to identify each of 256 possible gray-scale values. Little is gained visually by making the separation of gray levels correspond to a difference much smaller than the 50–100 shades that the eye can distinguish, or than the amplitudes of the random fluctuations in intensity that may occur as noise. Thus, the eye and the inherent imaging and elec-

tronic noise level imposes a natural lower bound on the useful brightness level step-size. At the other extreme, too small a number of gray scale levels can give rise to artifacts, such as the false appearance of sharp edges in Figure 6.8c.

The levels of gray on the display should be set so as to span and reflect the range of parameter values for the tissues being imaged. (This corresponds to the physical attribute of interest, such as the X-ray attenuation coefficients, or T1- or T2-value, or gamma-ray emission rate.) Suppose, for example, that a T1 examination initially yielded Figure 6.8d. Another setting of the gray scale might well be preferable. Fortunately, imaging machines provide a quick way, known as *windowing* (also *contrast enhancement, contrast stretching*, and *gray-level mapping*) to manipulate the gray scale to improve image appearance (Figure 6.8e). By adjusting the *window level* and *window width* so that the average value if T1 throughout brain tissue is a good deal less bright, one can arrive at Figure 6.8a.

Number of bytes per image: matrix dimensions and gray-scale depth

In determining memory, archiving, and data transmission capabilities and requirements for a computer imaging system, it is essential to be aware both of the number of bytes each image entails and how many images will be produced in a patient study. Typical achievable resolutions for the principal digital modalities, in terms of the length of the side of a square voxel, along with pixel matrix dimensions, and gray-scale bit-depths are shown in Table 6.1, and the information content (total number of Mbytes per image) for some of the principal modalities. These are steadily improving, and

Table 6.1 How many bytes are required to capture a patient study? Typical pixel and matrix sizes and bit depths, along with Mbytes per images (before compression), as of 2012.

	Voxel (mm)	Matrix	Bit depth	Mbytes/image
CR/DR	0.2	2000 × 2500	12	10
Digital mammography	0.05	4800 × 6000	16	60
MSCT	0.5	512 × 512	16	0.5
Planar nuclear medicine	7	128 × 128	16	0.03
PET	5	128 × 128	16	0.03
MRI	1	512 × 512	12	0.5
US	0.4	512 × 512	8	0.3

individual systems may differ significantly from these numbers.

The number of bytes required to *address* any particular pixel depends on the total number of pixels. If an image is to be presented on a 128 × 128 (= 2^7 × 2^7) matrix for a planar nuclear medicine study, for example, the pixel values (intensity and color) have to be specified at 16 384 (about 16k) pixel sites: the *x*-coordinate of every pixel can be expressed here as a 1-byte binary number, and so also for the *y*-coordinate, so that every individual pixel site can be addressed with a single 2-byte word. Suppose here that any pixel assumes a value between 0 and 255, and can be expressed as a single byte. But we can cleverly adopt a coding convention in which pixels are numbered in a fashion known to all, so that addresses do not have to be expressed explicitly; then we only need to list the pixel values. If an 8-bit image-depth suffices, complete information about an image is conveyed as a set of 16k (one for each address) 1-byte words

Let's tie all this together with simple case of transmitting a 12-bit-deep digitized radiograph from NYC to LA. Suppose the laser beam of the digitizer has a diameter of about 0.2 mm so, to be safe, we shall plan on pixels that are a little finer than that, such as 0.1 mm on a side. The film FOV is 20 × 30 cm^2, so the rows of the matrix contain (200 mm/0.1 mm) = 2000 pixels, and the column is 3000 pixels high (Figure 6.6), for a total of 6 megapixels (6 × 10^6). The ordering of the addresses has been predefined, so they need not be transmitted, just the pixel value data. For pixel values that are 12 bits deep, you might anticipate the need for 2 full bytes per pixel. But a neat trick allows us to reduce this: let's arrange for the data in two pixels (12 × 2 bits) to be inserted into 3 bytes (8 × 3), rather than 4 – in effect, needing only $1^1/_2$ bytes, not two, to code each pixel. So the total information content in a complete image is (6 × 10^6 pixels/image) × ($1^1/_2$ bytes/pixel) = 9 Mbytes/image. If a transmission system has a relatively slow data transfer rate capacity of 5 MByte/s, say, our radiograph arrives on the west coast a little under 2 seconds after we press the Send button.

Image compression

It should be apparent, when all is said and done, that it can become expensive and time consuming to store or transmit large volumes of data. A qite simple way to compres written English somewhat, for example, would be to replace an *ss* with a single *s*, and to eliminate a *u* after a *q*. (You have to make special allowances for Iraq.) Efficient *image compression* techniques, going by such eso-

teric names as discrete cosine transform and fractal compression, are a good deal more complex, but in a few moments of computer time they can reduce the number of bits required to represent an image by an order of magnitude or more. The reverse process, of restoration of an image to its perfect or near-perfect original form, is known as *decompression*.

It is possible, for example, to establish a convention for listing the picture addresses – and the associated picture values – in a specified order that is well understood by everyone in the loop, as already discussed. In that case, the addresses themselves do not have to be stored or transmitted, and a single file of the pixel values alone, in the same order, will carry complete information.

Another simple one: suppose we are using a 10-bit gray scale (yes, it may require 2 bytes per pixel, even though 6 bits are wasted), with possible pixel-values running between 0 and 1023. The computer discovers that, in some image, pixels at the six consecutive addresses 283 through 288 happen to have the same gray level, namely, "5", as seen in Table 6.2a. (Such values might correspond to background, say, outside the tissues.) We could store this information as it is. Alternatively, we could compress the file by removing the particular pixel-value "1023" from the regular gray scale, reserving it to serve

Table 6.2 Data compression. (**a**) Original set of pixel address and pixel value data (running from 0 to 1023). (**b**) A simple form of loss-less compression: flag the first "5" with a special pixel-value, namely "1023," and then remove all the fives in the string until a different pixel value appears.

(a)		(b)	
Address	*Value*	*Address*	*Value*
281	620	281	620
282	623	282	623
283	5	283	*1023* – 5
284	5	289	614
285	5	290	612
286	5		
287	5		
288	5		
289	614		
290	612		

only as a *flag* and *command*: 1023 tells the computer to drop and delete all the addresses and values after the first "5", but start up again only when a different pixel-value appears (in this case "614") (Table 6.2b).

This is an example of perfect *noiseless* or *lossless* encoding. It may be possible to obtain more compression with "noisy" methods, in which there is some loss of information and degradation of image quality, but such methods can be adopted only if images, after they are decompressed and redisplayed, remain clinically adequate.

Reconstruction

Computers, and the digital representation of images, are absolutely essential for CT, MRI, and PET. Their images are not obtained directly, as with X-ray film, but are mathematically reconstructed out of thousands of separate measurements. Without the ability to orchestrate these measurements, and then to manipulate the results numerically, performing millions of computations in seconds, such imaging simply would not be possible. Image reconstruction is a critically important topic, and we shall discuss various forms of it in some detail in the chapters on CT, nuclear medicine, and MRI.

Digital image processing: enhancing tissue contrast, SNR, edge sharpness, etc.

In addition to windowing, one can *process* a digital image in other ways that can significantly enhance its appearance and/or its utility. Parts or all of the image can be blown up in size or minified, or transformed from a positive to a negative. The computer can draw a narrow line where the shades of gray change abruptly to artificially enhance the sharpness of a border or *segment* (delineate) an organ, and that may help the eye to distinguish clinically relevant patterns. Digital filters can reduce some kinds of visual noise, compensate for certain inherent inadequacies of the imaging system, and in other ways improve perceived image quality. Such image processing can make the difference between a clinical study that is definitive and one that contributes little.

With MRI, multi-slice CT, SPECT, and PET, three-dimensional image reconstruction and display are commonly available, which increases the possibilities for image manipulation many-fold: one can rotate a 3D image to optimize the view, stretch it in various ways, view any plane in it from any perspective, "surgically" cut blocks out of it, and so on.

Likewise, a series of still images obtained at different times can be run in rapid sequence, to yield a cine effect. Watching a beating heart rotate freely in space is visually dazzling, and may be of clinical value. Also, information from different technologies can be combined to produce a single composite; PET or SPECT fused with CT or MRI can yield images that are highly sensitive and specific in their detection of pathologies, and at the same time bring in enough resolution to reveal exactly where the defects are — a synergy in which the whole may far exceed the sum of the parts.

We shall describe briefly two image enhancement processes that are widely used, those for smoothing and edge enhancement.

Smoothing

Random-appearing fluctuations in a temporal signal or in the pixel values in a region may actually have an underlying structure that can be examined through sophisticated statistical analysis, and may sometimes be of clinical interest. In general, however, it is beneficial just to reduce or remove noise with some sort of *digital smoothing filter*.

Suppose some analog temporal voltage signal is sampled every tenth of a second, and is seen to vary significantly between samples because of noise (Figure 6.10a). Assume, moreover, that previous studies have already established that any meaningful clinical changes occur on a scale at least ten times longer. The rapid jumps up and down are just noise, and visually distracting, so it is helpful to perform an elementary form of *moving average* to smooth them out somewhat. At every sample, the signal value is replaced by the average of it with the three that preceded it, say, and the three that follow; then on to the next sample point, and repeat. The random ups and downs will average out, but the long-term trends, suggested by the dotted line, should remain.

In some situations, alternatively, it is possible to sample the full output of a device with multiple runs of the same study, and

(a)

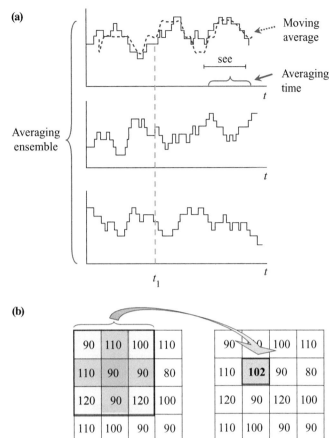

Figure 6.10 Averaging out random noise over time or space. **(a)** The *temporal* signal at the top is being smoothed by generating a *moving average*, where the signal at some instant is averaged with the raw data points near it, and then replaced by the average. Then on to the next sampling instant. Alternatively, if several identical signals are obtained either in sequence or parallel, but always with the same starting point, then the data can undergo an *ensemble average*, one instant at a time, as indicated by the vertical dashed line. The repeated real signals add, but the randomly changing noise cancels out. **(b)** Uniform *spatial* averaging, in which the voxel in the center of each possible nine-voxel square is replaced with an average of it and its eight neighbors; the pixel value highlighted here, originally 90, is thus replaced with [90 + (110 + 110 + 90 + 90) + (90 + 100 + 120 + 120)]/9 = 102. Alternatively, with a 4-2-1 weighted smoothing, the central pixel might receive a weight of 4, a face-neighbor a weight of 2, and a corner 1, and the central voxel is superseded $\{4 \times 90 + 2 \times (110 + 110 + 90 + 90) + 1 \times (90 + 100 + 120 + 120)\}/\{4 \times (1) + 2 \times (4) + 1 \times (4)\} = 99$.

with all operational parameters identical and with a common "start" event. The first run is sampled every tenth of a second after the start event, the data are stored, and the second run begins, is sampled again, etc. A *temporal ensemble average* averages the values obtained from all the runs at exactly the same time, as indicated by the vertical dashed line in Figure 6.10a, and then moves on to the next sample time and repeats. Meaningful data will simply add, but random noise fluctuations are equally likely to be positive or negative, and will partially cancel out. The result may, or may not, be very close to that of the moving average and, if not, more information may be needed before deciding on which approach, if either, to trust.

Suppose that in a nuclear medicine study, the gray-level value of a pixel is the count of detected gamma-rays coming from the corresponding part of the body. Even with an apparently uniform spatial distribution of radionuclide, there will be some naturally occurring variations in the numbers of counts in adjacent voxels, as described by Poisson statistics; this is so purely because radioactive decay, photon-detector interaction,

etc., are stochastic processes, by nature. With one very simple *spatial smoothing* algorithm, a spatial counterpart to the temporal moving average just introduced, the value n_1 for a pixel is replaced with a simple average, n_1', of it and the pixel values at the surrounding eight pixels, according to the prescription: $n_1' = (n_1 + n_2 + \cdots + n_8 + n_9)/9$, and $n_1, \ldots, n_9$ are the original of counts in the nine (Figure 6.10b). The computer then does the same for pixel 2, and so on. This spatial blurring does represent a real loss of information, in particular of pixel-sized detail, but the resulting smoother image may nonetheless be clinically more meaningful visually. (This procedure, and a number of other forms of image manipulation, are carried out relatively easily by means of a mathematical technique known as *convolution.*) Other algorithms can smooth images in more subtle ways, or subtract the average background from throughout the image, etc.

As noted in Chapter 2, in another form of image averaging, MR clinical images are commonly obtained two at a time with the parameters unchanged, and it is a spatial ensemble average of the pair, pixel by pixel, that the physician sees. This improves the signal-to-noise ratio by a factor of $\sqrt{2}$.

Sharpening

Rather than smoothing things out, it may benefit a study to accentuate and draw attention to edges and lines in it. It's a bit like sculpture. Michelangelo was once asked, legend has it, how he created his marvelous *David*, who guards the Piazza della Signoria in Florence. "Easy," he said, "just take a block of granite and cut away everything that doesn't look like David." (Actually, it sounds better in Italian.) We'll do pretty much the same thing here: to obtain something sharp, just take away the stuff that isn't sharp. Or, in slightly more technical lingo, you bolster the relative presence of the high-frequency spatial components of the image by, in effect, canceling out and thereby removing the lower-frequency parts.

To carry this out in practice, create a digital copy of the original image (Figure 6.11a), and then deliberately blur it a little

(Figure 6.11b). A simple way to do that is to replace the value for every pixel with an average of the values for that pixel and its nearest neighbors, as just described. The change is so slight that you couldn't tell the difference by eye, but the sharpness has definitely been lowered. Now, by subtracting the blurry copy from what we started out with pixel by pixel, we end up with the very crisp Figure 6.11b. To provide a bit of anatomical landmarking and make this more visually familiar, we can even add back a little of the original. The improvement in the sharpened image may not bowl you over, but it might be just enough to reveal some important fine-detail features that were previously hidden.

Finally, there is always the danger that the wrong kind of image processing might lead the viewer to see things that are not really present, or to inadvertently eliminate features that are. A smoothing or sharpening program might eliminate a rough surface when it actually is rough, for example, or create a sharp edge where there should be a gradation. In other words, while improving some aspect of an image, you may inadvertently mask an even more important one. So it is a good idea to learn about the subtle quirks of the processing tools you employ – and *caveat emptor*!

Computer networks: PACS, RIS, and the Internet

Modern medical facilities, like everything else, are going digital. Computer-based *hospital information systems* (*HIS*) are helping patients to register rapidly and end up in the correct place at the proper time. This lets a hospital assign beds and nurses with relatively little confusion, and it streamlines the coding and billing process.

A *radiology information system* (*RIS*), in addition, ensures that those carrying out a study and the physician reading the results have a clear understanding of precisely what is being done, and how, along with other needed patient information (general medical records, dictated notes, graphs of clinical parameters, medication records, discharge summaries, operative reports, lab reports, pathology images, electrocardiogram tracings, pulmonary function testing, etc., as appropriate).

The images themselves can be manipulated and processed in various ways under the control of a PACS (Figure 0.2 and Figure 6.12a). Ideally,

(a)

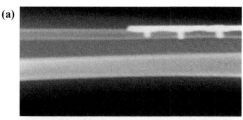

(b)

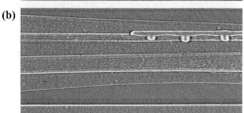

Figure 6.11 Edge enhancement to sharpen up the appearance of the image of a long bone. **(a)** A digital radiograph has been copied, and the copy deliberately blurred a small amount; you could not visually tell it from the original. **(b)** The computer subtracts the blurred version from the unblurred, pixel by pixel, thereby removing the visual information that is not much affected by the blurring – which means, in effect, the more slowly-changing parts of the image, where there are no sharp edges. Left behind is an artificial image of the *changes* that *do* occur, in which the edges and sharp features stand out.

(a)

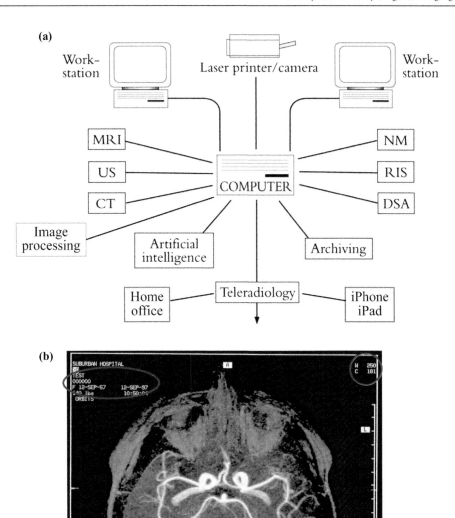

(b)

Figure 6.12 PACS. (a) A modern hospital's picture archiving and communications system consists of input from CT, MRI, nuclear medicine, PET, etc., units, an optical film scanner, artificial intelligence capability, long-distance image communications (teleradiology) links, remote workstations, and perhaps much else. Many systems provide two levels of viewing. For radiologists within an imaging department, viewing stations have specialized, high-resolution monitors that are optimized and QA'd for radiographic interpretation. There is also a web-based PACS interface for outside physicians to review images on standard workstations. (b) The parts of a PACS talk with one another easily because virtually all manufacturers have adopted an international networking protocol known as the Digital Imaging and Communications in Medicine (DICOM) system, designed specifically for handling image information. This MRI image displays standardized clinical and administrative "header" information in the DICOM format (see http://medical.nema.org). Photo courtesy of Mohsen Gharib, Suburban Hospital, Bethesda, MD.

the PACS is incorporated with the RIS, HIS, and electronic medical record systems as part of an integrated, seamless health care environment. That way, the EMR and other relevant clinical information about a patient can be rapidly available wherever the network infrastructure allows, greatly enhancing the diagnostic value of the images themselves. A PACS allows digitized images from all modalities to be stored inexpensively, retrieved and displayed at any system workstation in seconds, and transmitted to and from critical care units, outpatient clinics, classrooms, and offices – and even, late at night, to physicians' homes or to a Board-certified, wide-awake diagnostician in India, hard at work while we sleep (teleradiology). Emergency departments, for example, order and view significant numbers of images (plain X-rays, CT, US), for example, and PACS retrieval of old studies for comparison is much faster, more efficient, and less likely prone to error or failure than manual searches.

PACS had a difficult birthing, because they were not radiologist-friendly and were often unreliable. The industry has cleaned up its act, however, and a PACS is now a central performer in the operation of any modern, large imaging center. Since the prices have dropped considerably for small systems, even rural stand-alone facilities recognize that a PACS would not only improve radiologist quality of life considerably, but even be cost-effective as well.

The essential technology of PACS has matured and, as an important part of that, a standardized system of electrical signals and hardware has been constructed and widely accepted to allow for the connectivity of all kinds of imaging devices, database management systems, and computer networks. The Digital Imaging and Communication in Medicine (DICOM) standard, established in the mid-1980s and updated frequently, was devised to facilitate the interfacing of devices (regardless of manufacturer or model) for the acquisition, communication, and archiving of image information. DICOM specifies the syntax and semantics of data-file formats, directory structures, commands involved in data management, and much else. Some of this is visible in the headers of DICOM-based clinical images (Figure 6.12b) (http://medical.nema.org). A separate

protocol, HL7, does the same for RIS and HIS clinical and administrative data.

The advantages to placing all patient-related information into web-based interoperable data sets that link physicians, hospital medical records, and laboratories may seem self-evident. For many clinics and medical centers, however, the idea remains a remote dream. The health care industry invests only a few percent of its gross revenues in information technology, compared with other information-intensive industries. And some older clinical information technology systems cannot readily connect with one another. An investment in a PACS and other information infrastructure offers great payoffs, both to the patient and to the facility; but it is necessary to acquire a system powerful enough to do the job adequately, and to pay for training or hiring of technical support personnel.

In 2011, the FDA cleared the use of iPhone, iPod touch, and iPad, including zoom, windowing, and other capabilities for remote and mobile diagnostic viewing of CT, MRI, PET, and SPECT. While some physicians and others have concerns about various kinds of possible misuse, this approval is suggestive of a new wave of web- and other-based applications.

Image analysis and interpretation: computer-assisted detection

"Intelligent" computer programs are becoming ever more capable of detecting irregularities in images and, in a few cases, even interpreting them. The science of computer-based *artificial intelligence*, which attempts to mimic the processes by which the brain inputs information, processes it, and learns from it, is still in its embryonic stage. Yet computer-based *neural networks* and other *deep-learning* expert systems are already augmenting certain roles of the physician as diagnostician. CAD pattern-recognition systems already act as second readers in many mammography departments, and they can do so for hours on end without being distracted by phone calls from sick kids at home, and without growing the least bit bleary-eyed or grumpy. The computer is not about to displace the diagnostic physician anytime soon, but it will continue to bring major, rapid changes to medical imaging — indeed, to all aspects of the practice of medicine.

Computers excel at analytic jobs that involve memory, logic, repetitively following directions, and applying simple if-then tests, as in playing chess or calculating, well, just about anything. But even the most clever of them have a much harder time with the ordinary, elementary human activities of everyday life that require conscious intuition, judgment, and simple common sense, where there are no obvious rules. And to a large extent, they lack the kinds of learned visual skills that allow a radiologist to distinguish a liver with a small abscess from one that's normal but just looks irregular.

Considerable progress has already been made in computer recognition of patterns in one-dimension. Human speech, for example, may be viewed as a signal that is a function of only one variable, time, and highly accurate speech-processing programs are already available. Similarly, programs have been written that can analyze electrocardiograms (which also are one-dimensional images) with success rates comparable to those of skilled cardiologists; these routinely scan Halter signals for cardiac abnormalities.

The application of computer analysis to general two-dimensional radiological images is orders of magnitude more difficult, however, and will be much slower in coming. It is not hard to imagine how a computer might locate a point in a two-dimensional mathematical area: it would sweep a vertical line horizontally until it makes contact, and then would repeat with a horizontal line moving upward. Likewise it could find the two ends of a straight line, or even the shape, size, and orientation of an oval, rectangle, or other regular form, by comparison with shapes it has already "learned." But a search for clinically significant spatial patterns in two or three dimensions is far more challenging, and has to be sensitive to much more subtle and complex aspects of the image. The intricacy of many of the clinically significant variations in detail and contrast, together with the degrading effects of statistical noise and overlapping tissues, along with the great range in normal and abnormal patterns occurring among different individuals, makes the general problem of automated diagnosis highly demanding. But while CAD is still in its infancy, programs that search for spatial patterns characteristic of certain pathologic conditions in mammograms, chest films, virtual colonoscopy, ultrasonograms of the liver, etc., are already finding widespread acceptance (Figure 6.13).

The designers of medical expert systems intend that they be able to accumulate the body of knowledge required of physicians, and then to some extent mimic their actual thought processes in decision-making. The algorithms are meant to consider the implications of the evidence at hand, weigh the probability of correctness of each possible explanation, perhaps demand more information to reduce the range of possibilities, and generally propose and test hypotheses. Neural networks, programs that use feedback information from humans to "learn" decision rules from their own mistakes (without "understanding" the reasons for them) are highly promising for this kind of effort. We know next to nothing about how the intelligence of a human really works (or even that of a nematode, for that matter), and the "intelligence" we develop for machines is most likely to be quite different from our own – after all, an airplane doesn't flap its wings. In any case, computerized medical diagnosis, treatment decision-making, and medical informatics are highly promising fields, and it is to be expected that they will grow to reach higher-hanging fruit.

In a related effort, the relatively young discipline of *biomedical informatics* is beginning to provide tools to search for, identify, retrieve, integrate, analyze, model, display, store, communicate, and manipulate all this information. Biomedical informatics is perhaps best known for its role in untangling the vast quantities of data coming from work on the genome. Another area of considerable interest is the need to find and display the few clinically essential visual items contained within an overabundance of imaging data from hundreds, perhaps more, of CT or MRI sections per patient (with numerous such patients each day). A physician clearly cannot examine them all individually (despite the chance that a critical sign may lurk faintly in one of them), so researchers have to continue to develop ways

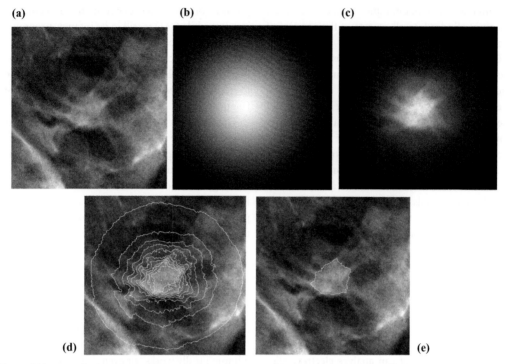

Figure 6.13 Example of a segmentation method that incorporates the knowledge that breast lesions tend to be relatively circular in shape; it uses mathematical techniques to suppress potential overlapping normal structures. (**a**) A mammographic lesion on a breast tomosynthesis slice (**b**) is multiplied by a two-dimensional Gaussian function. (**c**) The resulting modified image (**d**) demonstrates suppression of the overlapping tissues, allowing for the more circular candidate contours, and (**e**) the resulting lesion segmentation. Courtesy of Mary Ellen Giger and Ingrid Reiser, The University of Chicago. See also Kupinski MA, Giger ML, Automated seeded lesion segmentation on digital mammograms. *IEEE Trans Med Imaging* 1998;**17**:510–17; Reiser I, Nishikawa RM, Giger ML, *et al.*, Computerized detection of mass lesions in digital breast tomosynthesis images using two- and three dimensional radial gradient index segmentation. *Technol Cancer Res T* 2004;**3**:437–41.

to search effectively through the various sorts of databases, which are growing in number, size, and complexity.

This business is discussed further at the end of Chapter 13.

Computer and computer-network security

We shall conclude our discussion of computers on a note of caution. Any computer, or network of interlinked computers, is a system for processing and sharing information, and to a large extent it is built on trust. It is regrettable, but to be expected, not only that systems experience inadvertent failures, but also that some misguided souls may take pleasure or seek benefit in intentionally causing disruptions.

It is essential to put in place measures to maintain a system's *availability* (in which those with a legitimate need for it have access to it), *confidentiality* (so that those who don't, don't), and *integrity* (so that no unauthorized changes are made in programs or data). Computer security is now primarily the domain of specialists, but there are common-sense things we all can do to reduce hazards to ourselves and others. In particular, the Three Golden Rules of computer security are:

Restrict access: restrict access, both electronic and personal, to your computer and network. Only the most trusted of people and information should be let in. The easiest way of introducing problems is to accept bad files from flash drives, etc., or from emails and the web. And complex, long passwords and such are but minor nuisances compared with the havoc that the malicious hacker can wreak. Often you will receive messages claiming to be from your computer system administrator and asking for your password; don't give it out, *ever*, except directly to your system administrator whom you know personally.

Counteract infection: there are programs to protect almost completely against viruses, worms, phish, etc. Take full advantage of them and keep all your means of protection (antivirus programs, backups, password changes) up-to-date. If your system does come down with a virus, immediate use of a virus removal program may be able to remedy, or at least contain, the problem.

Backup: back up and lock up important files on a second computer, flash drive, CD, etc., routinely, and keep them safe somewhere else; the number of layers and frequency of backup needed depends on how valuable and rapidly changing your files are. Make certain that if the place burns down (which it won't, but it might), or if someone steals or messes with your PC (which could happen, even to you!), you still have the essential stuff.

Practice the computer equivalent of safe sex. First, abstain if you can. Don't open suspicious email or attachments, and don't enter any outside program into your system unless you definitely need it and you're 99.7% sure about the reliability of its source. Obtain the programs that you do require from reputable vendors or colleagues who are unlikely to be carriers. Borrowed or inexpensive pirated software packages, in particular, are poor and perhaps catastrophic investments.

And whenever in doubt, don't be shy about getting professional help.

Liquid crystal displays and other digital displays

At the end of an imaging train are, of course, the display and the observer.

In the beginning was the cathode ray tube (CRT) display, where a narrow beam of electrons of variable intensity swept across the face of a fluorescent screen. It's extinct, vanished, gone forever, and not missed, along with computer monitor and TV vacuum tubes. For reasons of image quality, weight, size, the low voltage, ruggedness, energy efficiency, and cost-effectiveness, flat-panel display technology has pushed them out of the clinic and out of mind.

One way to generate an image on a solid-state display is to produce a uniform field of white *backlight*, and cover it with an array of individually regulated microscopic shutters and color filters that can control the amounts and shades of light let through at each pixel. *Liquid crystal displays* (LCD) with several million pixels are of this type. In earlier LCDs, "cold cathode" fluorescent lamps provided the white background, but more recently silicon-base *light emitting diodes* (LED) have taken over: they require less power and generate less heat, they contain no toxic mercury, and, although their brightness does diminish slowly over time, they have longer lifetimes. LCDs currently account for something like 99% of all flat-panel displays produced, employed in virtually all laptops. It would take us pretty far off track to explain how they work, but that may not matter anyway, since there are several other technologies nudging forward, and a few years from now another may have taken over.

Some of these take the other approach of creating images out of actively generating millions of individual, unrelated pinpoints of light; for example, an array of microscopic LEDs that produce pixel-sized spots of light and modulate their intensity and color, as also does the *organic light emitting diode* (OLED). Also under development are *plasma*, *field emission*, and *quantum dot* displays and others. Chances are pretty good that whatever you're looking at in a decade, it won't be an LCD.

Meanwhile: true three-dimensional viewing is a reality. The reader may have seen stereoscopic drawings and movies in which two slightly different perspectives of an object were presented in blue and red; when one wore special glasses with one red and one blue lens, the spears and arrows really did fly right out of the screen, giving a definite sense of depth. Viewers on opposite sides of the theater see essentially the same thing, however, unlike the full three-dimensionality one enjoys in a live performance.

Likewise, stereoscopic radiography, which involved obtaining images from two neighboring locations and then viewing them simultaneously through prism-lens glasses, conveys a sense of depth. This approach has been updated with electro-optical glasses in which the lenses themselves can display slightly different electronic images for the two eyes – the images can be made to be perceived as fully three-dimensional, and they can be of value in virtual reality applications such as surgical planning or virtual endoscopy.

With *holographic* displays, the viewer will not even need special glasses, but still will view an object in three dimensions, from all angles, long after it is no longer present. Such displays are in the early stages of development, and it is apparent to the authors that should they come to fruition, they will have (like CT) a revolutionary impact on the way physicians view the body.

The writing is clearly on the wall-mounted, thin-panel liquid crystal and/or holographic display. May as well get ready for it.

The joy of digital

It should be apparent that a great deal of the work in an imaging group, other than dealing with patients and actually reading the images, is becoming digital, and that the trend is likely to accelerate. This is inevitable largely because it is so clinically beneficial and cost-effective.

Back in the old days, to make a screen-film radiograph, one selected the kVp and mA-s based on tables and past experience, and expected the result to be neither under- nor overexposed. But the processes of image acquisition, processing, storage, communication, and display were all interlinked, determined once and for all by the technique factors, and attempts to improve any of these aspects could have a negative impact on the others.

With a digital image receptor, on the other hand, these are separate and independent operations, and we can take unrelated steps to optimize each individually (Box 6.2). A digital image receptor has a latitude hundreds times wider than that of film; no image will be overexposed, and underexposure is unlikely – although the noise level may be unacceptably high with too few photons. In addition, while the contrast and latitude are inversely related for film, they are unconnected for digital, and each can be adjusted on its own.

Box 6.2   Benefits of digital imaging.

Image acquisition, processing, display unlinked:
  each can be optimized separately
Image receptors of broad latitude:
  linear characteristic curve, no toe, plateau
  contrast adjustable, independent of latitude
Image processing highly flexible
  windowing, noise reduction (e.g., smoothing), contrast/edge enhancement, etc.
Images managed through a PACS
  immediate archiving (storage, retrieval)
  communications (local, teleradiology)
  artificial intelligence (CAD)
  databases for statistical analysis

After a film is shot and developed, there are no ways to improve its appearance or its clinical utility. With digital, acquisition is just the beginning. The image can be manipulated electronically to improve its contrast, through windowing or by other means, to sharpen up its edges, and to eliminate some of the noise. And the nature of the displayed image can be altered through panning, zooming, cropping, rotation, and so on with the touch of a button. Likewise, one can follow in real-time and record a changing process, such as the flow of a bolus of contrast agent along a blood vessel, and immediately replay or freeze any moment of it.

And once in a PACS, an image can enjoy all the advantages of any centralized digital system: immediate and loss-less archiving, with rapid retrieval; electronic communications, whether local or over long distances; data compression for storage or transmission; connection to research databases and to artificial intelligence programs such as CAD for other sorts of analysis – and much else!

Image processing, management, communication, and analysis in the clinic will doubtless continue to improve significantly in the near future. Not only do the technologies continue to develop, but also powerful hardware and software tools produced for the military, the intelligence community, the entertainment industry, the space program, and the basic sciences are being transferred into the medical imaging research laboratories and clinics. Likewise, extending routine computation into the realm of the Internet, having access to virtually infinite amounts of cloud memory, etc., are likely to change everything. It is not obvious where these developments will be steering the field, but one thing is for sure – they will keep on evolving rapidly, and persist in surprising us.

A final comment on the importance of overall quality and efficiency of patient care even in a digital department. Imaging is a central service component in health-care management, but the competition among providers of imaging services is stiff, and referring clinicians do shop around. They demand reliable diagnosis, of course, but they also want simple, easy, and secure processes for ordering procedures and for receiving results, with shorter turnaround times. Same-day service is often achievable for most patients, with a little extra effort and planning; and it certainly not only improves patient care, but it also makes a great impression on referring physicians. A clinician should almost never have to wait more than a few days to be able to pass imaging results on to the patient and discuss them.

Similarly, 3-D visualization capability matters for some surgeons, as do calibration markers. Other specialties have their own wish lists, which a hustling imaging group can go out of its way to try to satisfy.

The point is simple, yet easily overlooked. Even a fully digital imaging center has to be well and conscientiously managed, in ways that take full advantage of all the speed and communications capability of the high technology. Computers alone don't bring about high quality and productivity; efficiencies don't materialize automatically just because of the new PACS. Hence the absolute necessity of sensitive, strong and positive leadership that is constantly striving to improve, and willing to listen carefully to feedback from the customers. A major part of the job is to find out what your patients and referring physicians want, and give it to them.

CHAPTER 7

Digital Planar Imaging

Replacing Film and Image Intensifiers with Solid State, Electronic Image Receptors

Nearly all advanced imaging centers are moving toward, or have finished, going digital and filmless. This transition has been made possible largely by the remarkable successes of physicists and electrical engineers in inventing and developing transistors, integrated circuits, and microchips. These devices have led, in one essential application, to the creation of ever faster and more powerful computers. But the evolution of microchips in a different direction, as actual optical and ionizing radiation sensors, is a driver of the ongoing sea change in imaging. This has had a particularly profound effect on planar X-ray imaging – radiography and fluoroscopy.

Digital planar imaging modalities

Over the past decade, image intensifier-based image receptors (IRs) and, even more so, screens and films, have largely had to step aside, and make way for the IRs of *computed radiography* (*CR*), *digital radiography* (*DR*), and *digital fluoroscopy* (*DF*) (Fig-

ure 7.1). A common progression, in clinics that are considering making the transition, is to start out by replacing traditional screen-film cassettes and chemical developers with their immediate digital counterparts, CR cassettes with their rather slow electro-optical readers. The initial costs for this approach are relatively low, so nervous newcomers can acquire a taste for the joys of digital without sensing too much risk in the change-over.

Then, after they have become true believers, they move on to the much faster and more flexible DR and DF systems. DR and DF came into being with the creation of an IR built around a huge (life-sized) semiconductor chip, the *active matrix flat panel imager* (AMFPI), which transforms the spatial pattern of X-rays emerging from the patient into a digital signal. With a great deal of guidance and help from the businesses that gave the world solid-state optical cameras, liquid crystal displays (LCD), and vast arrays of transistor circuits on chips, manufacturers can now produce AMFPIs for DR and DF at acceptable costs.

Medical Imaging: Essentials for Physicians, First Edition. Anthony B. Wolbarst, Patrizio Capasso and Andrew R. Wyant.
© 2013 John Wiley & Sons, Inc. Published 2013 by John Wiley & Sons, Inc.

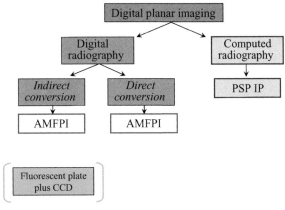

Figure 7.1 There are two major families of modern digital planar modalities: digital radiography (DR) and digital fluoroscopy (DF), in the one, and computed radiography (CR) in the other. DR and DF both make use of solid state, pixelated *active matrix flat-panel imagers* (AMFPI), and these are of two distinct kinds. *Indirect detection* digital radiography (iDR) employs a thin phosphor screen first to convert X-ray photons into light, as with a screen-film system; the light is then detected by an immediately adjacent array of millions of tiny optical sensors, one per pixel. (There are also non-AMFPI indirect conversion methods in which X-ray photons expose a fluorescent screen, which, in turn, is watched by a charge-coupled device (CCD) or some other form of electronic optical camera.) With a *direct detection* AMFPI system (dDR), an X-ray striking the photoconductive material of a pixel results in a detectable pulse of electric current through it. CR does not employ an AMFPI: an exposure excites pixel-sized regions of its *photo-stimulable phosphor* (PSP) *imaging plate* (IP) by amounts proportional to the air dose level there – then, in its separate electronic CR reader, a laser beam scans the plate in a raster pattern, stimulating it to release this stored energy as light of another color, which is recorded much as with a screen digitizer.

Film suffers a number of disadvantages, among the most demanding of which is that the user has only one chance, at the time of the exposure, to achieve good image quality. There is nothing to be done to make things better after the fact (Table 7.1). With CR and DR, on the other hand, it is possible to optimize separately image acquisition, image processing, and display. First one selects the X-ray machine technique factor settings at values that yield the greatest differences in attenuation of the beam by the various tissues, hence subject contrast; in doing this there is almost no worry about

Table 7.1 Attributes of screen-film and digital imaging systems.

Attribute	Screen-film	Digital / electronic
Acquire/display/store	Film sole medium	Optimize separately
post-processing	∼ none	contrast; edge; noise; . . .
image transport	manual	PACS/teleradiology
image storage	film	PACS/DVD, tape, etc.
Image receptor	H&D curve	Linear
latitude	40:1	1000:1
contrast	film Γ, OD	window; modify H&D
contrast/latitude	tradeoff	independent
spatial resolution	≤ 20 lp/mm	≥ 50 μm pixels
noise	grain, mottle	low, quantum limited
resolution/dose	screen tradeoff	∼independent
Image dynamics	Cine	DF with DR (*not* CR)
Dose	Generally low	Possibly lower
Cost	Film/processor	CR cassettes; DR high

over- or under-exposures, apart from patient-dose considerations. Then, one can independently introduce image-processing programs to enhance contrast or bring out edges, to reduce noise, or even to electronically change the shape of the effective characteristic curve. Thereafter, the operator can window the gray scale and other display parameters for the most visually useful image. In addition, digital imaging makes accessible the full range of invaluable image storage, communications, and artificial intelligence features that computers allow. And DR and DF, in particular, can provide images that are often of better quality than film, taken incomparably faster, and sometimes of lower patient dose.

Indirect detection with a fluorescent screen and a CCD

Perhaps the simplest digital planar image receptor, just one step beyond screen-film, is a fluorescent screen observed by a *charge-coupled device* (*CCD*) electronic optical camera (Figure 7.2). The mirror keeps the CCD out of the direct path of the X-rays, which would stimulate it as well, giving rise to excess noise. A number of variations on the theme have appeared over the years, fiber-optic or other connection between the screen and camera, and scanning slits of radiation, but few of them are still in service. This is similar to how analog fluoroscopy operates.

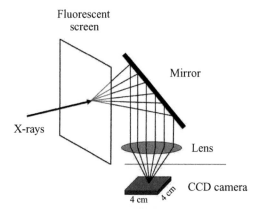

Figure 7.2 A simple imaging device, reminiscent of the kind Roentgen introduced, in which a fluorescent screen is observed by an electronic optical camera.

Computed radiography

Computed radiography (CR), which has been around since the mid-1980s, is the natural digital successor to traditional screen-film radiography. It works somewhat like radiography, but replaces the fluorescent screen plus photographic film combination with a special *photostimulable phosphor* (*PSP*) plate, also known as an *imaging plate* (*IP*) (Figure 7.3a). The IP is commonly housed in a CR cassette that protects it from both light and touch. Cassettes are manufactured in the sizes of standard radiography, to facilitate and encourage the adoption of CR by allowing the continued use of much of the radiographic equipment already in place. The only items to be replaced when switching to CR are the cassette and the automatic IP developer.

The active ingredient of the imaging plate is a heavy-metal phosphor, such as barium fluorohalide, lightly doped with europium, as with $BaF_xCl_yI_z[Eu]$. The dopant gives rise to *traps*, irregularities that can loosely hold electrons that have wandered by, but normally nearly all these traps are empty. X-irradiation releases photoelectrons in the material, and these are immediately excited into and populate the traps; the number of them that end up holding electrons in a small region of the IP is directly proportional to the amount of dose deposited there. It is energetically favorable for these newly trapped electrons to stay in place, moreover, until they are somehow activated with the input of additional energy and thereby released.

After a CR X-ray exposure, the imaging plate is not developed chemically, as is done with film. Instead, its spatial information is extracted within a *CR reader*, where a monochromatic laser beam (typically red or near infrared) scans it in a raster pattern (Figure 7.3b). Resolution is limited by the diameter of the laser beam and by the distance of light diffusion within the IP to about 100–200 microns, or 5 lp/mm. Meanwhile, a photodetector, such as a photomultiplier tube (PMT), continuously monitors the amount of fluorescent light of a different color (blue, green, ultraviolet) emitted from the IP surface because of the laser-light stimulus; an optical filter passes only this fluorescent light, and rejects the red. The brightness of the stimulated blue-light emission coming from any point on the IP is proportional to the amount of X-ray energy that transited the patient and struck there. Through the raster scanning pattern, a two-dimensional spatial pattern of light emission is transformed into a corresponding one-dimensional temporal electrical signal from the photodetector. The computer keeps track of the time, to monitor the address of the pixel being stimulated at any instant, and the intensity of blue light emitted, the pixel value.

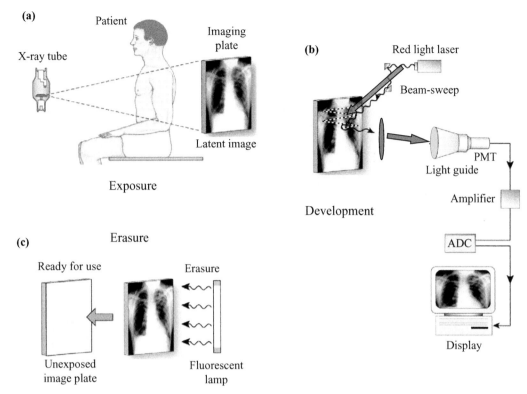

Figure 7.3 Computed radiography (CR). The (**a**) exposure, (**b**) electro-optical "development," and (**c**) optical erasure of the imaging plate (IP) during CR.

After completion of the readout, the IP is bathed in intense white light, which clears all the traps and refreshes the IP for its next exposure (Figure 7.3c).

With some stimulated luminescence CR systems, the imaging plate is moved into place for exposure, laser-read following exposure, and erased in preparation for the next image, all automatically and under computer control, rather than by hand. Readout might take half a minute or less, so development of about 100 IPs per hour is possible.

Figure 7.4a presents two of the numerous different effective characteristic curves that a typical commercial CR system might store, available for selection by the operator. The output of the PSP is itself directly proportional to X-ray intensity, and curve **A** describes the linear relationship between display brightness at a point and the output of the image receptor there. This particular choice of characteristic curve is responsible for image **A** of Figure 7.4b. If radiologists were raised examining radiographs that looked like this, all would be fine, but such is not the case – they are accustomed, rather, to images created with the characteristic curve **B** of Figure 7.4a, with the familiar toe and shoulder of film, that yields image **B** in Figure 7.4b.

Preferences may shift over time, as viewers explore the various possibilities but, for now, CR and DR images resemble old-fashioned film because we force them to.

Finally, image QA for CR, as described in [1], for example, is more sophisticated than that for screen-film.

A few vendors have devised specialized, clever CR devices that fit certain niche applications well. But the greatest promise for the CR industry is probably among developing countries, and in particular China. CR and a rudimentary, low-cost PACS can transform a fairly primitive and isolated facility into one that produces state of the art images and that is connected with the rest of the world, all at reasonable cost.

Digital radiography with an active matrix flat panel imager

CR remains less expensive, but solid-state, flat-panel DR and DF devices underlie the new

(a)

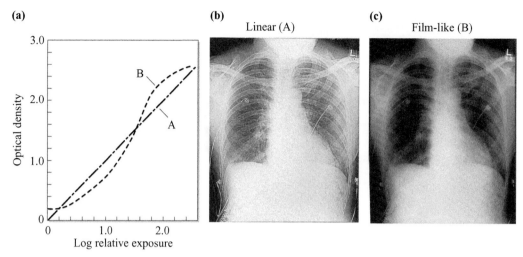

(b) Linear (A)

(c) Film-like (B)

Figure 7.4 Characteristic curves in CR. (a) Two characteristic curves stored in a CR system and available for creating diagnostic images. Curve **A** is linear, as are the dose response properties of the IP itself, and (b) gives rise to the image marked "linear." CR and DR images are almost always presented using a characteristic curve like **B**, however, that resembles that of standard radiographic film.

generation of planar X-ray imaging. The advantages of their AMFPI are many-fold.

Active matrix flat panel imager

Flat-panel detector IRs are relatively thin and light. Unlike CR cassettes, which are readily interchangeable, AMFPIs for DR and DF are usually permanent fixtures (although some are interchangeable). They allow for immediate reading, with no need for a development step, and they are convenient to operate. For digital fluoroscopy, an AMFPI with a 30 × 40 cm^2 active area and 50 cm diagonal replaces not only a 40-cm diameter image intensifier tube, but also the attached CCD (or other) electronic optical camera, the 35-mm cine camera, etc., yet it takes up only 15% of the volume. The result is much improved access to the patient in interventional procedures. Mounting a 40-cm II on a mobile C-arm would be impractical, but a flat panel even with a larger active area is significantly easier to manipulate.

An AMFPI consists typically of four to twelve million pixels (as of 2013), each 70–150 microns on a side, that detect and report on local X-ray intensity independently of one another, with a bit depth of 12 or 16 bits (Figure 7.5a,b). The resolution of an array of 100 μm pixels, for example, would correspond to that of a screen-film combination that could accommodate 10 lines per millimeter, or 5 lp/mm; the associated Nyquist frequency would be 5 cycles/mm.

Each pixel contains a region that is sensitive to the X-irradiation, and the fraction of that area, relative to that of the entire pixel, called the *filling factor* (f_p), which can range from 40% to 70% and up (Figure 7.5c). There is also a small region that contains a *thin film transistor* (TFT) complex, the origin of the word "active," along with a capacitor for charge (the surrogate for detected dose) storage. The pixel communicates with the computer by means of the solid-state equivalent of wires; quite remarkably, a 1000 × 2000 array of pixels does not require 4 000 000 attachments to operate, two for each pixel, but rather only several thousand, because of clever electrical engineering.

There are two significantly different families of AMFPI. They create images through either *indirect* or *direct detection* of patterns of X-ray energy into electronic signals, and support *indirect detection digital radiography* (*iDR*) and *direct detection digital radiography* (*dDR*), respectively. Both are widely used.

For iDR, dDR, and DF, sensitivity can be gained, at the expense of resolution, with pixel binning. Reading out a 2 × 2 neighborhood block of pixels as one square super-pixel is easily done by summing the signals from the four adjacent pixels. The

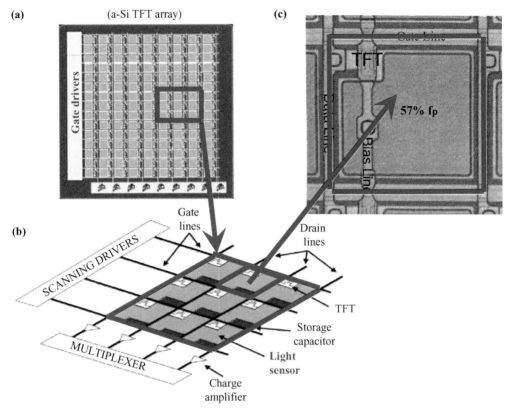

(a) (a-Si TFT array)

(b)

(c)

Gate lines

Drain lines

TFT

Storage capacitor

Light sensor

Charge amplifier

Figure 7.5 The array of pixels of an *active matrix flat panel imager* (*AMFPI*). **(a)** Overhead view of a small fraction of an AMFPI. **(b)** Close up of a few pixels of an *indirect detection digital radiography* (*iDR*) AMFPI, with its optically sensitive area and overlying film of translucent, luminescent material; amorphous silicon (a-Si) thin film transistor (TFT) complex; charge storage capacitor; and attachment "wires," called "gate" and "drain lines." **(c)** This AMFPI has a fill factor, the relative area of pixel that is actually sensitive to ionizing radiation, of 57%.

super-pixel will see four times as many X-ray photons, and have twice the signal-to-noise ratio (SNR). Also, the maximum digital data-read rate from a panel is often limited; binning trades spatial resolution for reduced matrix size, which allows higher frame rates. A 1024 × 1024 AMFPI capable of 7.5 frames per second, for example, can also be read out as 512 × 512 super-pixels at 30 fps.

Manufacturing silicon chips involves extraordinary control and precision, and things do not always come out perfectly, or stay that way. Fortunately, it is often possible to correct, or at least accommodate, small mistakes. A pixel simply may not perform; in that case, it is almost always possible to replace the value for this *dead pixel* with the average of its neighbors. Such is not the case, however, if the defunct pixel happens to affect adversely all the others in its row or column. Likewise, there may be some *dark noise* or *dark current* present even when there is no exposure. But electronic circuits can counteract this by subtracting it, pixel by pixel, from the measured

pixel values determined when the X-ray beam *is* on. Since the gain or degree of amplification may differ among the pixels, the electronics can be adjusted also for uniformity of response during a uniform exposure.

Indirect detection digital radiography

As with a screen-film cassette, *indirect detection DR* (*iDR*) involves a two-step process, in which X-ray energy is first transformed into visible light by a phosphor, and then the resultant optical image is captured with an array of millions of pixel-sized light-sensitive photodiodes (Figures 7.6).

An iDR AMFPI is manufactured in two steps. Working backwards, the vendor first purchases or produces in-house the so-called *glass*, the thin layer (supported on a rigid substrate) of semiconductor within which is embedded a repetitive, periodic array of millions of independent, pixel-size photodiodes

(a)

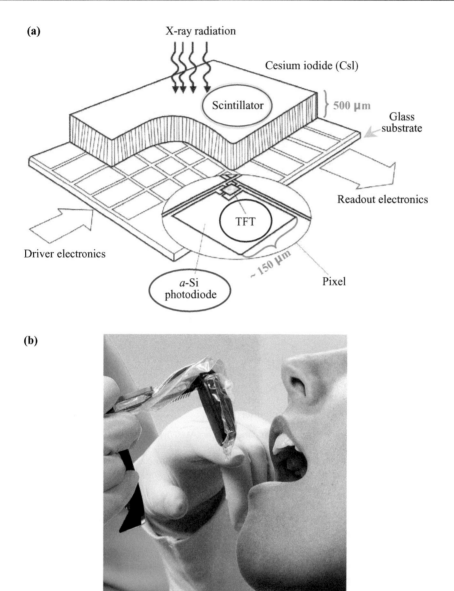

Figure 7.6 iDR image receptors. **(a)** An iDR AMFPI, like that of Figure 7.5, consists of a continuous thin sheet of scintillator material, such as structured CsI, lying on an array of independent, pixels; the pixel hardware consists of a light-sensing amorphous-silicon (a-Si) photodiode and the associated thin-film-transistor circuit that manages the data it obtains. **(b)** This Gendex GXS-700 iDR IR is a bite-wing used in dentistry, capable of 20 lp/mm resolution. Courtesy of Gendex Dental Systems.

and the associated pixel-size *thin film transistor (TFT)* circuit that services each. The photodiodes themselves are made of *amorphous* silicon (*a-Si*), a glassy material that lacks the periodic regularity of atom or molecule placement found in a crystal (Figure 7.7).

A continuous, uniform CsI layer is then added, such as by heating the phosphor under high vacuum and causing it to evaporate and then deposit directly onto the glass. Like a film screen, the fluorescent layer must be efficient at absorbing X-ray photons in the diagnostic range, yet transparent to the visible photons produced. Most commonly found is thallium-doped cesium iodide, the same phosphor as the input screen of an image intensifier; this is produced in "structured" form of long, thin (5–10 microns in diameter) needles lying perpendicular

(a)   (b)

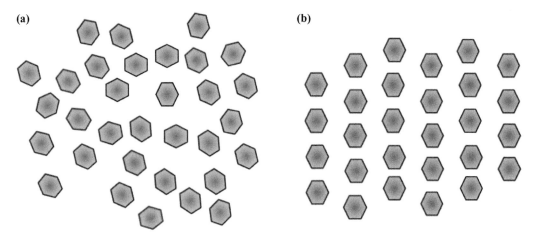

Figure 7.7 Amorphous and crystalline solid phases of the same material can have radically different electrical, physical, and other properties. (**a**) The structure of an amorphous solid, such as glass or amorphous silicon (*a*-Si), would closely resemble a snapshot of the liquid phase of the same material, (**b**) while that of a crystal displays a precise order and symmetry. Both light-sensitive *a*-Si and the X-ray photoconducting ingredient in dDR, amorphous selenium (*a*-Se), find applications in AMFPIs.

to the AMFPI; this cuts down on light scatter and resultant image blur, yielding better resolution. Gadolinium oxysulfide (GOS), which is employed widely in modern rare earth radiography screens, is easier to manufacture and therefore less costly.

The scintillations from the phosphor do not disappear instantaneously; the level of light falls off exponentially, rather, with a half-life that depends on the type of phosphor, and it can be as slow as milliseconds. This may cause a faint afterglow or *ghosting* to remain longer than one would like. Likewise, some *lag* may appear in digital fluoroscopy if the object being imaged is moving so fast that light from previous frames stays visible.

Direct detection digital radiography

The image receptor for *a direct detection* AMFPI (*dDR*) system is entirely electronic, bypassing the intermediate step of converting X-ray energy to light. X-rays impinge on a 1 mm thick plate of a *photo-conducting* semiconductor material such as *amorphous selenium* (*a*-Se) ("photo-" here refers to X-ray photons) (Figures 7.8). (A number of other materials are being explored, like PbI_2, PbO, TlBr, and Gd-compounds, but none so far has yet achieved the commercial success of *a*-Se.) An electrode, a thin veneer of metal, coats one side of the entire selenium plate, and a matrix of pixel-sized electrically independent electrodes covers the other. A high voltage (10 kV) is applied between the com-

mon electrode and each pixel-electrode separately. Every time an X-ray photon strikes the *a*-Se layer, electrons are briefly liberated, and a pulse of current is swept through it by the high voltage, and this is detected by the adjacent pixel-electrode and associated TFT circuit.

For each pixel, charge accumulates on the capacitor in its TFT circuit during the exposure (such as for 0.1 ms), after which the total charge captured is sent off to an analog-to-digital converter (ADC) and from there to the computer. The greater the number of X-ray photons that strike a pixel during that time, and the more the charge buildup, the higher the electric voltage pulse signal sent to the ADC and computer.

Finally, comparisons between iDR and dDR depend strongly on who you talk with. It is generally agreed that because of light diffusion even within structured CsI, dDR has the potential for finer resolution, since there is little signal charge spread (unlike light) to adjacent pixels. dDR devices are also inherently somewhat more sensitive, and can perform with lower patient exposure. But the technology of manufacturing large plates for dDR is more demanding, hence more costly. As a result of this tradeoff, standard DR AMFPIs are commonly iDR with CsI, while the smaller mammographic plates are of both types.

(a)   **(b)**

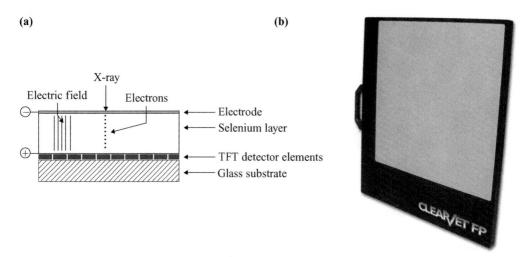

Figure 7.8 Direct detection digital radiography image receptors. (**a**) The X-ray photosensitive material of a dDR IR is a continuous thin layer of photoconductive material, most commonly amorphous selenium (*a*-Se). A coat of metal on the outer face of the *a*-Se serves as a common electrode, while electrically isolated pixel-size electrodes on the other side connect to individual TFT circuits. (**b**) Most modalities of radiology have veterinarian applications as well, even MRI for equine extremities. This *a*-Se IR, designed for small-animal X-ray studies, is 17 inches on a side, and provides up to 16 megapixel images and 4.6 line pair per millimeter resolution. Courtesy of ClearVet™ Digital Radiography Systems (www.ClearVetDigital.com).

Digital mammography

More than half of all women are screened for breast cancer, and this has contributed to a decline in the mortality rate by a third over the past two decades.

At present, there are some 12 000 mammography units in the US, and the vast majority of new ones are digital. Like their screen-film predecessors, DM systems must have contrast capabilities sufficiently high to detect the presence of malignancies, the resolution to categorize microcalcifications, and at the same time the ability to operate at very low dose. To displace the screen-film gold standard, moreover, DM has to do all of this better, faster, and eventually cheaper.

Full field digital mammography

Because its requirements for low X-ray energy, high resolution, and low-dose are somewhat different from those of conventional DR, *full field digital mammography* (*FFDM*) needs specialized flat-panel detectors. Both CsI-based iDR and *a*-Se dDR AMF-PIs have been adapted to mammography, and the vendors of each vociferously proclaim its virtues. Pixels are typically between 0.7 and 1 micron in dimensions, and matrices range up to 25 Mpixels,

with a depth typically of 12 or 14 bits. Four images are taken for screening two breasts, so each patient needs (4 images/study) × (2 bytes/image) × (4 to 25 MPixels/image) = 30–200 MBytes of data.

FFDM AMFPI tolerates a wide range of exposures, and experiences virtually no over- or under-exposures More to the point, clinical studies have shown that DM yields more early defects and fewer false-positives than film. There is also immediate correction of positioning errors when they occur, and considerably faster overall throughput. It is generally agreed that DM images are better for women with radiographically denser breasts (less adipose, more connective tissue), which makes it more difficult to adequately diagnose early disease. In such patients, where breast adenocarcinoma has a tendency of being more aggressive, such an increase in diagnostic sensitivity may have a dramatic impact on patient overall survival [2].

In addition, the smart software of *computer-aided diagnosis* (CAD) (Chapter 6) can search for abnormalities in a DM image, such as calcifications and spiculated masses. CAD algorithms are more effective if the data come directly from a DR, rather than being degraded in the intermediary step of digitizing a film mammogram. At present, these systems acting alone experience too many false positives, so they are used primarily as an aid to the interpreting physician, providing an independent second opinion. They can raise flags to identify suspicious regions overlooked by the reader on initial viewing. And they *will* improve over time.

A downside of FFDM is its initial cost of up to one-half million dollars, whereas that of an SF unit might be a quarter of that. But there can be long-term and operational cost advantages – patient throughput increases, and also today's Medicare reimbursement rates are currently higher for digital, so the financial difference becomes less of an issue.

The Mammography Quality Standards Act (MQSA) and program establish a limit of 3.0 mGy (300 mrad) per image to the radio-sensitive glandular tissue of a breast compressed to 4.2 cm and composed half and half of glandular and adipose tissues (Figure 4.25). With a risk/dose estimate provided by Report V of the BEIR (Biological Effects of Ionizing Radiation) committee of the National Academy of Sciences and an assumed typical mean breast glandular dose of 4 mGy from a two-view per breast bilateral mammogram, one can estimate that annual mammography of 100 000 women for 10 consecutive years beginning at age 40 will result in eight or fewer radiogenic breast cancer deaths during their lifetimes. Mortality is reduced by a factor of a quarter with biennial screening: the odds clearly favor those who undergo it.

In sum, it is estimated that there is a benefit-to-risk ratio of about 50 lives saved per life lost, and 120 years of life saved per year of life lost. Thus, the theoretical radiation risk from screening mammography is extremely small compared with the established benefit from this life-saving procedure. It should be borne in mind, however, that this sort of analysis is built ultimately upon the fundamental linear no-threshold *assumption*, that stochastic radiogenic risk is directly proportional to dose even at the low exposures of mammography. But as discussed in Chapter 5, this is a reasonable assertion supported by considerable radiobiological evidence, and the great majority of radiation scientists are willing to accept it in the making of radiation-protection policy – but still, it is an assumption, not proven fact.

All of this having been said, it should be noted that several recent meta-studies have renewed concerns about the number of patient treatments that arise from false-positive mammography readings. The benefit-risk debate is not settled – especially when coupled with uncertainties about the the LN-T assumption. The best strategy, we feel, is to follow closely the most recent recommendations of the American College of Radiology (ACR), and bear the opinions of other responsible bodies in mind, with an eye on new technical developments. One of the most important of these may be the integration of FFDM with digital tomosynthesis, discussed below.

Other breast imaging modalities

Mammography, whether screen-film or digital, remains the first line of defense against breast cancer, and it catches 80–90% of neoplasms in asymptomatic women. But it is not flawless, and as many as 20% of breast cancers occur in patients with normal screening mammograms. In addition, 5–10% of those detected are so-called "interval cancers," found between normal screening examinations. A significant number of women have very dense breasts, moreover, and the sensitivity of mammography is lower for this group. And of the mammograms called positive on the basis of microcalcifications, many are found not to be cancerous under biopsy. So the search continues for complementary, and perhaps alternative, ways to identify breast cancer at an early stage (Figure 1.1).

Abnormalities are more easily identified in the fatty, less dense breasts of older women (Figure 4.20). Since detection rates are lower for younger women, some of these at high risk for breast cancer are being screened with MRI. MRI can discern some tissue differences in early breast cancer for lesions smaller than 1 cm, and it has high sensitivity for invasive disease. Although expensive, MRI can be of particular advantage with subpopulations of dense-breast, high-risk women who are premenopausal, or who have a strong family history of the disease, or have previously had the disease. Special MRI instrumentation and software have been devised that are dedicated to breast studies, and the ACR requires special certification for them.

Ultrasound is useful, after a breast mass is found by physical or mammographic examination, because it can frequently discriminate between solid masses and cysts; and thereafter it can often provide imaging guidance during cyst aspiration, fine needle and core biopsy, etc. Because ultrasound (like MRI) does not involve ionizing radiation, and because the breast tissues of young females appear to be more susceptible to radiogenic breast cancer, it may be selected as the primary modality for teenaged girls and young women who have palpable breast lumps. A development known as the automated breast ultrasound system (ABUS) has recently been approved by the FDA, and it should make the success of the modality less reliant on the experience and training of the operator. Time will tell whether or not it is widely accepted.

One promising area of therapy research, incidentally, is on MR-guided, focused-high-power (as opposed to diagnostic) ultrasound tumor ablation.

Finally, with reimbursement available for some kinds of breast examination, PET is also carving out a niche for itself. This will probably grow if PET is approved for the evaluation of breast masses before biopsy.

Digital fluoroscopy and digital subtraction angiography

Digital fluoroscopy with an AMFPI operates much as conventional fluoroscopy with an image intensifier tube and CCD camera does. Because of its considerably greater cost, however, it is found primarily where its potential for superior performance can make significant differences clinically (Figure 7.9). *Digital subtraction angiography* (DSA), in particular, is a DF application that serves splendidly in imaging arteries and veins in exquisite detail – nothing else shows up on the screen *but* the arteries and veins and a little background landmarking.

Image quality with an AMFPI tends to be better than that with an II tube. With II-based imaging, there are a number of stages in the signal conversion chain, discussed in connection with Figure 4.26, and each of these steps is subject to losses, distortion, noise, and inefficiencies. By comparison, flat panels have a very direct and short signal-conversion path, with essentially no distortions, and the result is a flat, uniform, image of film-like quality from edge-to-edge.

Temporal DSA

Suppose an obstruction in a carotid artery is suspected. A conventional non-subtraction angiographic approach begins with threading a guidewire and catheter percutaneously into the femoral artery, up along the aorta, and into the carotid, to a point upstream from the region of interest, all under fluoroscopy. Iodine-based contrast agent is injected. The result will be an image, captured on cine or in memory, of the vessels that contain the contrast material, superimposed on an irrelevant background of patterns caused by soft tissues and bones. The background gives rise to visual interference, and the evidence of the blockage may be lost in all the confusion. Since the procedure is invasive, and can cause complications that may be clinically significant, it is of utmost importance to obtain the most precise images with the highest diagnostic potential on the first attempt.

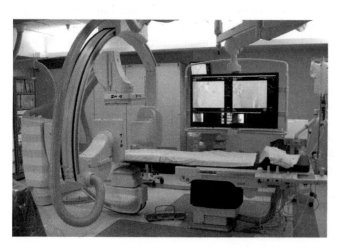

Figure 7.9 A modern angiographic system. There are two X-ray tubes, to the right and below, and two corresponding large (30 × 40 cm) AMFPI image receptors in this biplane angiographic system. The two sub-systems are mounted independently, and capable of a wide variety of independent beam orientations. This allows a series of orthogonal images, typically AP and lateral, to be obtained virtually simultaneously, and from optimal vantage points. Courtesy of Jie Zhang.

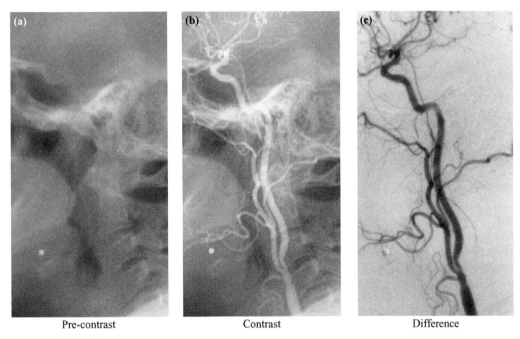

| | | |
| Pre-contrast | Contrast | Difference |

Figure 7.10 Temporal digital subtraction angiography images are made before and after contrast medium fills the blood vessels of interest, and the two images are subtracted from one another, pixel-by-pixel. For this DSA study, a narrow catheter is threaded into a femoral artery, up the aorta, and into the common carotid artery. Images are obtained both **(a)** before and **(b)** immediately after a bolus of iodine-based contrast agent is injected through the tip of the catheter into the vessel. **(c)** Aligning the two pictures and subtracting the before image from the after, point by point, yields a difference image that highlights those areas where a change has occurred, revealing the vessels that have just filled with the iodine. It may help with interpretation to reintroduce some faint background anatomic landmarks.

With *temporal* or time-difference DSA, the catheter is again first guided into its proper position. Once there, the system captures a pre-contrast *mask image* of the region of interest, which is digitized and shipped off to computer memory (Figure 7.10a). Contrast agent is then injected and multiple separate *angio images* obtained (Figure 7.10b). Aligning the mask and an angio image carefully, the computer subtracts the one from the other pixel by pixel, and displays the difference between the two as a new image in its own right. This third *difference image* highlights those (and only those) places where the first and second differ, in particular where blood vessels contain contrast agent (Figure 7.10c). All the uninteresting background patterns are eliminated, leaving behind a remarkably clear, high-contrast view of blood vessels alone. It may help with interpretation to reintroduce some faint background anatomic landmarks.

Since it is in digital form, a DSA image can be windowed and, in other ways, computer-processed to enhance its clinical utility, and the physician can view the results immediately, or continuously in real time. Because of the improved contrast, it may be possible to image with less contrast agent; for an arterial injection, a relatively small amount of contrast agent can be introduced through a finer catheter, at less patient discomfort and risk (e.g., from arterial spasm or damage, from the effect of iodine on the kidneys, or from stroke).

Patient motion is a potential source of image degradation with mask subtraction. The injection of iodine contrast agent may elicit a swallowing reflex, for example, or peristalsis can be significant. Even with small motions, misregistration of the mask and angio images gives rise to a difference image that displays a characteristic form of visual noise (Figure 7.11a). If the entire region of interest moves or rotates rigidly between exposures, then re-registration of the two images can readily eliminate the problem (Figure 7.11b). Through *pixel shifting*, the images are intentionally displaced

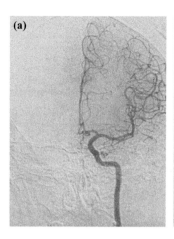
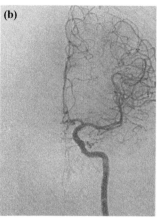

Figure 7.11 Image registration. (a) Even a small amount of mis-registration of the contrast and mask images in DSA, often because of patient motion, gives rise to characteristic visual noise. Analogous problems arise in attempting to register SPECT and PET studies with CT to create so-called *fusion* studies, and with other forms of multi-modality imaging. (b) It is possible to improve registration manually or semi-automatically. This can involve rigid translation and/or rotation of one image relative to the other, or even stretching or twisting, either in-plane or not.

relative to one another until the presence of streaks and other noise in the difference image is minimized. This can be performed manually, but now one image is normally moved relative to the other automatically until the two are superimposed in the best way, with the fewest wrinkles. Software is becoming adept, moreover, in salvaging a situation in which only parts of the patient in the field of view stretch or twist, moving more than others, or when movements occur that are not in-plane.

Time-interval difference subtraction is a variation on this theme. Suppose images A, B, C,..., are obtained at equally spaced times post-injection. A is subtracted from B to produce the first difference image, B from C to form the second, and so on. This may also allow the identification of certain pathologic vascular conditions from irregularities in the advance of the contrast agent over time.

In DSA, CT, MRI, or other studies that require rapid administration of a contrast agent, incidentally, it is necessary to inject a considerable amount of somewhat viscous fluid through a thin catheter into a vein or artery. If this is done too slowly, the contrast density may be inadequate, and a repeat needed. Too high a flow rate resulting from excessive pressure, on the other hand, may cause injury to the vessel, even its rupture. A modern contrast-injector typically employs an electromechanical motor to drive the syringe. A microprocessor establishes precise control over pressure, flow rate, and volume of fluid delivered, and synchronizes the injection with the activation of the imaging device. Safety is a serious concern, and sensors and switches are built in to prevent accidental premature or overpressure injections; to terminate when the syringe

is empty; to prevent the inadvertent injection of air, which could produce an embolus; to cut off the flow of contrast medium back into the syringe or into nearby tissues; and to perform other worthy tasks.

Dual-energy DSA

Dual-energy subtraction is an alternative to temporal subtraction DSA. The attenuation coefficient of soft tissue decreases relatively gently with increasing energy in the region of 33 keV, but iodine exhibits an absorption edge there (Figure 4.23b). Two images, one created with monochromatic 32 keV photons (just below the absorption K-edge of iodine) and another at 34 keV photons would display significant differences where contrast agent is present. In practice, one could switch rapidly back and forth between bremsstrahlung beams with quite different kVp settings while maintaining a nearly constant exposure rate, but the basic idea is the same. This can usually be performed fast enough to eliminate motion effects. Alternatively, or in addition, one can employ detectors that have some ability to distinguish between photon energies.

More generally, the total X-ray attenuation coefficient depends on the photoelectric and the Compton components together as $\mu = \mu_{PA} + \mu_{CS}$ (Equation 3.3c). The photoelectric part is a function of the atomic number and the effective energy as $\mu_{PA} \sim Z^3/(hf)^3$ (Equation 3.3b), while μ_{CS} is nearly independent of both (Equation 3.3a), in effect a constant and therefore irrelevant here. This suggests that by measuring the relative intensities of a beam passing through the same voxel but at two different energies, $I(E_1)/I_0 \sim Z^3/E_1^3$ and $I(E_2)/I_0 \sim Z^3/E_2^3$, it should be possible to subtract the two and obtain

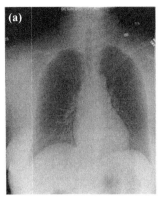 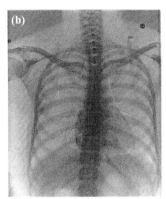

Figure 7.12 Dual-energy DSA. The energy dependences of the linear attenuation coefficients of soft tissue and bone differ substantially. By creating a pair of images with significantly different bremsstrahlung spectra, it is therefore possible to extract enough information from the two to make possible display primarily of either soft tissue or bone. Courtesy of RC Gilkeson and University Hospitals of Cleveland.

Soft tissue image   Bone image

the average value of Z, that is, information on the chemical makeup of the tissue. One can thus adjust chest studies so that either rib or soft tissue shadows are almost entirely removed in the difference image (Figure 7.12). A similar approach is becoming widely used in dual-energy CT. Doing all this in practice is more complicated, of course, but you get the general idea.

Digital tomosynthesis: planar imaging in three dimensions

"Conventional" tomography images a planar section of the body, as does CT, but it acquires information in a totally different way: it removes the shadows from over- and underlying tissues by blurring them out with intentional, specific motions. What remains unblurred is an image primarily of tissues in the plane of interest. Screen-film tomosynthesis is somewhat easier to describe than the digital variety, but the end result is much the same, so we'll go there first.

An X-ray tube and a film cassette move in opposite directions within fixed parallel planes (Figure 7.13a). The *focal plane* within the patient, which is to be imaged, also lies parallel to these two. The planes of motion of the tube and of the cassette are attached to one another by means of a lever pivoted at a fulcrum point *in the focal plane*, so that their motions are tightly linked, in accord with the dimensions of the similar triangles AS'S'' and AA'A'' – that is, by the unchanging distance of the desired image plane from each of the other two.

Consider a point, A, on a plane *midway* (for simplicity here) between the other two, and let it serve

as the fulcrum. If the tube is displaced during an exposure by the amount S'S'' (green arrow), then the *image of point* A (red) shifts the same distance as the tube, but in the opposite direction. But since the cassette position is linked to that of the tube, the film (blue) will move exactly the same distance during an exposure as the shadow of point A, resulting in a sharp image there. So, too, for any other spot on the image plane. As a result, the entire image of the tissues in the focal plane will be fully in focus at the cassette!

The image of the point B above the image plane, however, has different similar triangles; it travels farther (blue plus yellow) than the film (blue) during the shift, and the difference (yellow) is the extent of blur. The amount of blur will increase with its distance above or below the focal plane. It's all simple geometry.

One can reduce the thickness of the section of body in focus by increasing the distance through which the X-ray tube and cassette travel during the exposure. And to image a plane higher in the body, just lower the patient. This flexibility enables the radiologist to scroll through different planes imaging specific structures along not only the x- and y-axes, but also the z-axis.

To examine another tissue slice, you could shift the focal plane by elevating or lowering the patient. Alternatively, you could displace the cassette a small distance up or down while causing it to move at exactly the same linear velocity as before; it will be traveling a bit too fast and far to focus the previous focal plane, which contains the fulcrum – but it will be moving in just the right manner to bring into focus another plane of tissue, one lying slightly above or below the fulcrum.

(a)

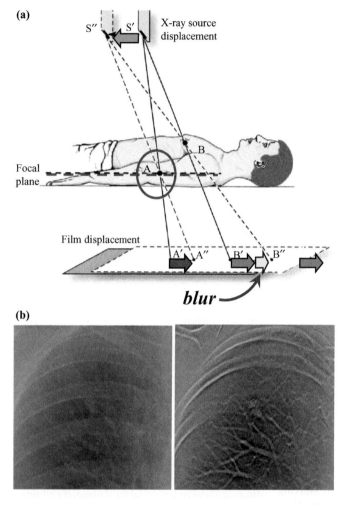

(b)

Figure 7.13 Digital tomosynthesis. (a) The geometry of conventional tomography. (b) PA DR and digital tomosynthesis images of the same region of the right upper lung; tomography revealed a 6 mm nodule that was rather obscured in the PA image by overlying rib structure. The slice was acquired from 71 projections over a 20° scan, and assembled by way of matrix inversion tomosynthesis (MITS) reconstruction. Total exposure was estimated to be 1–2 times that for a single screen-film lateral radiograph. Courtesy of Devon Godfrey, HP McAdams, and James Dobbins, Duke University School of Medicine.

With *digital planar tomography*, a single set of typically 15 separate, discrete images (rather than a single continuous film exposure) are acquired with the X-ray tube taking 1° steps along an arc, but with the long and wide flat-panel detector held immobile. This takes about four seconds and, in breast imaging, altogether deposits about the same dose as a mammogram. It is then possible to manipulate the data in a computer in a manner similar to that of CT to reconstruct images from numerous different planes. This is known as *digital tomosynthesis*, and it is much more powerful and flexible than the film type.

Tomography and digital tomosynthesis can often extract features that are obscured by other tissues in radiography and DR (Figure 7.13b). While not as revealing as CT, there are many clinical situations where it is called upon routinely because it can be diagnostically definitive at very much lower cost and patient dose.

References

1 AAPM. *Acceptance Testing and Quality Control of Photostimulable Storage Phosphor Imaging Systems*, AAPM report no. 93, 2006. Available at www.aapm.org/pubs/reports/RPT_93.pdf. Accessed October 24, 2012.

2 Hendrick RE, Pisano ED, Averbukh A, *et al.* Comparison of acquisition parameters and breast dose in digital mammography and screen-film mammography in the American College of Radiology Imaging Network Digital Mammographic Imaging Screening Trial. *AJR Am J Roentgenol* 2010;**194**:362–9.

CHAPTER 8

Computed Tomography

*Superior Contrast in Three-Dimensional
X-Ray Attenuation Maps*

With film radiography, CR, DR, and conventional and digital fluoroscopy, information from throughout a three-dimensional body is projected and flattened onto a two-dimensional plane. In the process, subtle irregularities can become lost in the interplay of image patterns created by overlapping tissue structures. Within the lung, for example, soft-tissue lesions are easily obscured by the strong variations in X-ray beam attenuation caused by the ribs and by the convoluted shapes of the larger air spaces. Similarly, most photons entering the head are absorbed or scattered by cranial bone, rendering difficult the imaging of the gray and white matter within.

Medical Imaging: Essentials for Physicians, First Edition. Anthony B. Wolbarst, Patrizio Capasso and Andrew R. Wyant.
© 2013 John Wiley & Sons, Inc. Published 2013 by John Wiley & Sons, Inc.

Digital subtraction angiography (DSA), as discussed in the previous chapter, can circumvent this problem in the study of arteries and veins by subtracting "before" and "after" images. The problem is that while the approach performs beautifully in the study of blood vessels and in a few other special situations, it isn't much help elsewhere where structures and materials remain static.

Tomosynthesis employs another tack, blurring out all planes except for the one of interest. While low in dose, relatively inexpensive, and with in-plane resolution of down to 1 mm or less, the z-directional sharpness was typically an order of magnitude lower, which makes it inadequate in some applications.

Computed tomography pursues a strategy radically different from these to achieve essentially the same end – the removal of extraneous but visually competing patterns – and it displays the data commonly in the form of multiple transverse, thin, non-overlapping planar tissue slices, each with exquisite contrast and good resolution. Modern machines typically produce 64 or fewer images of adjacent, parallel slices per rotation of the gantry, making possible both slice and smooth three-dimensional display, with thickness and in-plane resolution down to $1/2$ mm or less. The gantry can rotate in $1/3$ second, and can cover an adult torso in one breath-hold. The only major downside is the unnecessarily high patient doses to be found at some centers, but even that problem seems soluble.

Computed tomography maps out X-ray attenuation in two and three dimensions

Imagine that you can, without causing too much discomfort or mess, temporarily excise a pancake-thin cross-sectional tissue slice from a patient's body for study (Figure 8.1). You might put the slab on a film or CR cassette, and briefly turn on an overhead X-ray tube. Anywhere in the resulting image, the optical density of the developed film is determined by, and reflects, the attenuation properties of the materials within the thin slab that was lying above it. The contrast among soft tissues would be good enough for you to distinguish virtually all the organs from one another, unlike the case of an ordinary AP or lateral radiograph. The resolution would be sharp, and the noise level low.

For various technical and ethical reasons, this approach is unlikely to find widespread clinical acceptance. Fortunately, CT opens a back door to the same place. A CT picture of the same section, back in the intact patient, would look almost exactly like the image of Figure 8.1. It, too, would show how the rate of attenuation of X-rays by tissues varies from voxel to voxel.

CT takes a more indirect approach. It first makes thousands of *transverse* X-ray transmission measurements of the region of interest, with the X-ray tube and X-ray detector(s) situated on opposite sides of the body, facing one another and circling about it. The computer then performs a

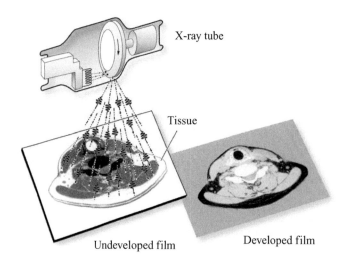

X-ray tube

Tissue

Undeveloped film   Developed film

Figure 8.1 The image created with an X-ray beam directed normal to a pancake-thin transverse slice of tissue lying on a sheet of film. CT can produce a nearly identical image, but from thousands of external measurements, from numerous angles, of the attenuation of X-ray "rays" passing transversely (i.e., from the sides) completely through the body.

tremendous number of sophisticated computations to calculate what the insides of the patient must be like so as to yield the measured set of transmission data.

Earlier we presented the scenario of a parent who suspects that his kid has swallowed some objects (Figure 0.1). One film does not provide an unequivocal answer. With an X-ray film taken from a second angle, however, it is now possible to make sense of the *set* of pictures. By integrating separate pieces of two-dimensional information obtained from several perspectives, one can imagine a three-dimensional picture that is much more revealing than what can be learned from any single view alone.

That, in essence, is how CT works. It creates, digitizes, and stores in a computer the X-ray "shadows" obtained from a large number of different viewpoints around the patient. The computer then works backwards from these data to mathematically *reconstruct* the spatial distribution of the materials (or, more precisely, the spatial distribution of the X-ray attenuation properties of the materials) that are responsible for this particular set of hundreds of images.

As with other X-ray imaging modalities, much of what reaches the image receptor is scatter radiation. CT employs beam collimators at the detectors to reduce scatter (somewhat like a grid), and another trick from standard radiography, as well: it uses a relatively thin fan-beam of radiation. Instead of irradiating a large rectangle of tissue, as with screen-film or DR, earlier CTs exposed a slice of tissue only a centimeter or less tall. Even modern multi-slice scanners commonly produce a diverging *cone beam* tall enough to cover a segment of the patient only from 4 to 16 cm thick.

A moving or fixed ring of hundreds of small, independent radiation detectors senses how much radiant energy from any part of the fan beam makes it through and emerges from the far side of the patient (Figure 8.2). Because the exposed section is thin, little scatter radiation arises, and nearly all that is produced ends up heading randomly away from the plane of the detectors.

Thus CT chops the body into thin, transverse slices of anatomy, in effect, and views each one separately from the side, but from multiple positions and angles, acquiring enough data to recon-

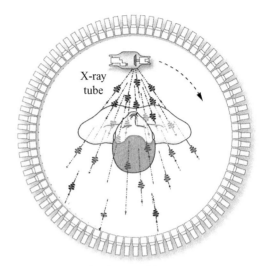

Fixed array of detectors

Figure 8.2 With this so-called "fourth-generation" scanner, the X-ray fan beam is wide enough to cut completely across the patient from any angle, but the irradiated slice may be only millimeters or so tall. The X-ray tube moves along a circular path around the patient, always pointing inward, and a fixed single ring of hundreds of small detectors sense the intensity of every "ray" emerging from the body.

struct slice-images. The necessary mathematical manipulations are complex, and must be carried out on a fast computer, but the general concept is simple.

CT maps the linear attenuation coefficient throughout a transverse (axial) slice of tissue...

Let us return to the question of what it is, exactly, that a CT image reveals.

As has been noted before on numerous occasions, the tendency of a tissue (or other material) to remove X-ray energy from a beam is quantified in terms of the linear attenuation coefficient, μ, which may be defined as the spatial rate of attenuation that the beam experiences in traversing a very small piece of material (Equation 3.1b). If the intensity of a particular X-ray beam is diminished by 2.5% in passing through 0.1 centimeter of a certain tissue, for example, then $\mu = (0.025/0.1 \text{ cm}) = 0.25 \text{ cm}^{-1}$. The greater μ is for a tissue, the more rapidly the beam is absorbed and scattered in it; the value of μ, in turn, depends on the tissue density and effective atomic number (as well as on the average photon energy for the beam). Thus, by mapping out spatial variations in the attenuation coefficient throughout each segment, resulting from differences in tissue density and chemical makeup, CT provides an image of the anatomy. And that, of course, is exactly what an ordinary radiograph does, only not slice by slice, and not with the X-ray beam entering from a direction perpendicular to the plane of clinical interest.

Imagine a thin transverse portion of a human body is to be partitioned by means of an imaginary grid into a matrix of voxels, each a millimeter or less on a side, but as high as the slice is thick (Figure 8.3). The grid size is commonly expressed in terms of the numbers, $\mathcal{N}_x$ and $\mathcal{N}_y$, of voxels in each dimension, as was discussed in Chapters 6 and 7. A 512×512 matrix, which is typical for CT, contains about a quarter million of them in one slice. Voxels may be 0.3–0.7 mm on a side, give or take, and from 0.4 to 10 mm or so in depth (that is, the thickness of the slice of tissue irradiated and/or imaged). In the x-dimension, the matrix size, $\mathcal{N}_x$, the in-plane dimension of a voxel, Δ_x, and the dimension of the field of view, FOV_x, are related as $FOV_x = \mathcal{N}_x \times \Delta_x$ (Equation 6.1).

The CT image of a tissue slice is a voxel-by-voxel map of the values of the tissue X-ray attenuation coefficient throughout it. Image *reconstruction* involves back-calculating, from the results of thousands of radiation transmission measurements on a transverse section of tissue, to determine the linear attenuation coefficient associated with every voxel. The computed map of the attenuation rates is then displayed as a mosaic of pixels of various shades of gray, also 512×512, arranged so that regions of greater attenuation coefficient appear lighter, as in radiography.

... And displays it as a matrix of Hounsfield numbers

The attenuation coefficient of any material depends on beam energy. CT uses relatively high-energy X-rays (80–140 kVp, with an effective energy of 40–80 keV. These interact with soft tissues by means of both the photoelectric and the Compton effects, but the *contrast* in a CT image of soft-tissue structures depends primarily, apart from tissue density influences, on the photoelectric effect alone (as is also the case for planar imaging).

The energy dependence of the attenuation coefficients normally is not of direct clinical interest, and it simplifies matters to remove it by normalizing the tissue *CT number* relative to that of water. The CT number of a tissue at a point is defined in terms of the linear attenuation coefficient there, $\mu(x,y)$ as

$$\text{CT number (HU)} = 1000\{[\mu(x,y) - \mu_{H_2O}]/\mu_{H_2O}\}, \quad (8.1)$$

where μ_{H_2O} is the linear attenuation coefficient of water at the effective energy of the beam. The value 1000 has been selected as the convention, and CT numbers are then expressed in *Hounsfield units* (H or HU).

Display consists of a map of pixel values that indicate relative (to water), rather than absolute, linear attenuation coefficients. Pure water is chosen as the reference material mainly because it comprises 80–90% of soft-tissue mass. The gentle variation of μ_{H_2O} with photon energy is very similar to that for soft tissues, moreover, and while taking the quotient does not cancel out the energy dependence of

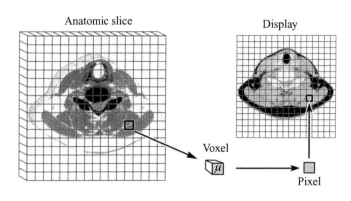

Figure 8.3 This transverse slice of tissues has been partitioned into voxels by means of a hypothetical 512×512 matrix. CT evaluates the linear attenuation coefficient, μ, of every voxel. Then the Hounsfield unit (HU) equivalent for each, obtained from Equation 8.1, determines the gray-scale value for its corresponding pixel in the display.

Table 8.1 Representative approximate Hounsfield unit (HU) values for various materials, as defined in Equation 8.1, for an X-ray beam in the range 80–140 kVp, where CT normally operates. Listed HU values from different sources are often not in close agreement.

Tissue	CT number (HU)
Dense bone	1000 +
White matter	46
Gray matter	43
Blood clot	75–80
Acute hemorrhage	60–110
Blood	40–60
Liver	40–60
Kidney	30
Muscle	10–40
Water	**0**
Lung	~ −700
Air	−1000

the CT number completely, it does remove a great deal of it. In addition, water is a convenient and absolutely reproducible material for use in machine calibration, and so CT numbers of a tissue should differ little from one scanner to another.

1 H represents a 0.1% difference in linear attenuation coefficient from that of water. Typical approximate values of CT numbers, in Hounsfield units, appear in Table 8.1 The CT number of water is 0 HU, as demanded by the definition of an HU, and that of air (for which the linear attenuation coefficient is nearly 0) is −1000 HU. Reported values for cortical bone vary widely, but typically are in the neighborhood of +1000 to +2000.

Computed tomography is widely used to examine soft tissues which, apart from lung, do not differ much from one another in CT number. When imaging such tissues, it is therefore desirable that most of the gray scale variation of the display, from black to white, should correspond to this rather narrow range of CT values. As discussed in Chapter 6, the display window level can be set by the technologist so that the middle of the gray scale corresponds to the middle of the CT number range for the region of interest, and the window width is adjusted to cover that range adequately. The chest, for example, contains air-filled lungs, bone, and mediastinal soft tissues, materials that differ substantially in density and chemical makeup, so the optimal window level

and width will vary greatly, depending on what one is evaluating (Figure 8.4).

At the 1972 Annual Congress of the British Institute of Radiology, the British firm EMI (Electrical and Musical Industries), Ltd., stunned the radiological community with the unveiling of a novel clinical imaging technology. The EMI device came into being primarily through the efforts of one person, Godfrey Hounsfield, and for their respective contributions to this work, Hounsfield and Allan Cormack shared the 1979 Nobel Prize for Physiology or Medicine. (Cormack, a South African nuclear physicist, had produced a working table-top CT apparatus and published in 1963 – but made the mistake of doing so in a physics journal, rather than medical; alas, there is no Cormack unit.) Also deserving of a note of appreciation are John, Paul, George, and Ringo; it was largely through the enormous influx of cash from the Beatles' recordings that EMI was able to support the development of Hounsfield's machine.

The ray-projection/ray-sum measures the total attenuation along the ray

We move now from what CT numbers mean to how they are obtained.

The X-ray tube and the signal detector of the earliest commercial CT machine, the EMI head scanner, now called a *first-generation* device, are mounted on a gantry. Their positions were fixed relative to one another, but they were allowed both linear and rotational motion relative to the patient. The beam was collimated so as to irradiate a region of tissue, at any instant, only several millimeters wide and a centimeter or so high. Such a beam is called a *ray*.

In each slice-scan, the tube/detector assembly (and the narrowly collimated X-ray beam) were swept together laterally across the patient's head, cutting out a transverse plane (Figure 1.12c). The gantry was then rotated through 1° about the patient, and the beam swept again. This procedure was repeated 180 times. The tube was turned off during gantry rotation, but left on continuously while the transmitted beam intensity (hence attenuation) was sampled 160 times (along adjacent and parallel but separate rays) during each transverse sweep. The $180 \times 160 = 28\,800$ ray measurements for a single transverse section provided more than

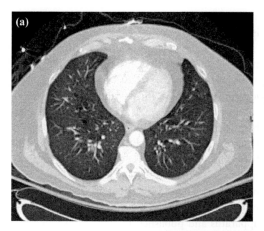
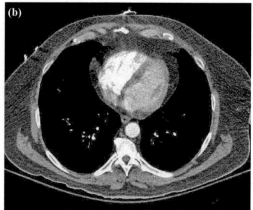
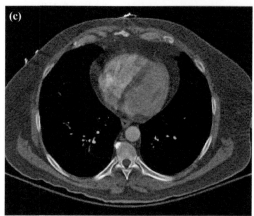

Figure 8.4 All three of these images were obtained during a single enhanced (with iodine-based contrast medium) scan of a patient, through computer controlled post-processing, without any additional radiation to the patient. To consider the patient's chest completely, each organ must be viewed properly with its own window level and width settings. (a) Within the air-filled lungs, of primary diagnostic interest are the soft tissue and vascular components of the sponge-like pulmonary tissue; healthy lung tissue consists typically of about ⅔ air. The viewer will be searching for any architectural distortion that may be caused by scarring, or by the presence of a mass or infiltrate. In this case, a wide window of 1300 HU was used with a center value much lower than for most soft tissues. (b) By re-windowing the same axial image, we can also fully evaluate the mediastinum, containing intravascular iodinated contrast media. The contrast agent gives additional optical density to the blood within the arteries, veins, and cardiac chambers, and it can also enable better visualization of adjacent tissues as well. Since we are evaluating radiologically similar structures, the window is narrow, 335 HU, with a center slightly higher than that of water, 35 HU. (c) To evaluate bone at the level of the spine and ribs, the same image is windowed in a way to pick up differences between cortical and cancellous bone, or between the cortex and bone marrow. Here, the window is set to 1600 HU with a center at 360 HU.

enough information to allow the reconstruction of a 160×160-pixel matrix of values of the attenuation coefficient.

Suppose that a collimated beam is 1 mm wide and 10 mm high, cutting out a 1 cm thick slice of tissue. We shall mathematically partition the tissue into voxels of comparable dimensions (square and 1 mm on a side, say, and 10 mm deep) and give them

addresses according to an embedded hypothetical (x,y) coordinate system. The ray that happens to lie parallel to the x-axis and at $y = 7$ mm is singled out in Figure 8.5a.

How much attenuation does the horizontal ray at $y = 7$ of Figure 8.5a, say, suffer in traversing the patient? It enters the body at the voxel with address $(x,y) = (5,7)$, and passes

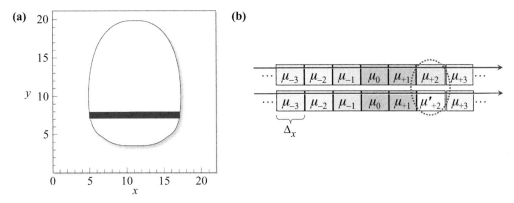

Figure 8.5 Creating CT contrast. (a) The horizontal geometric "ray" of a very narrow X-ray beam lying at $y = 7$ in the patient's body along the x-axis; a corresponding band of color could be laid down, or *back-projected*, along a corresponding horizontal line at $y = 7$ on the display. (b) These two horizontal rays pass through adjacent rows of tissue voxels, all of length Δx, that happen to be equivalent in content at every point except the ones at the $x = +2$ position. While a radiograph with X-rays passing through the entirety of both rows may not pick up the difference, CT considers the attenuation in each voxel separately, and would much more likely do so.

also through voxels at addresses $(6,7)$, $(7,7)$, $(8,7)$,... $(17,7)$, where the linear attenuation coefficients are $\mu(x,y) = \mu(5,7)$ mm^{-1}, $\mu(6,7)$ mm^{-1}, $\mu(7,7)$ mm^{-1},..., respectively. In the first voxel lying within the body, the ray is attenuated by the amount $e^{-\{\mu(5,7)\Delta x\}}$. It is further diminished by a factor of $e^{-\{\mu(6,7)\Delta x\}}$ in the second. Since $e^{\alpha} \times e^{\beta} = e^{\alpha+\beta}$, the net attenuation in the first two voxels is $e^{-\{\mu(5,7)\Delta x\}} \times e^{-\{\mu(6,7)\Delta x\}} = e^{-\{\mu(5,7)\Delta x\} + \{\mu(6,7)\Delta x\}} = e^{-[\mu(5,7) + \mu(6,7)]\Delta x}$, since the voxels are all the same size. The total cumulative attenuation of the ray along the entire length of its path in tissue is obtained by continuing this process in the same fashion. With "sigma" notation indicating the addition of a series of terms, this becomes $I/I_0 = e^{-\sum \mu(x,7)\Delta x}$, where the sum is taken over all the discrete values of x.

It is awkward to work with exponentials, so one takes the logarithm of both sides of this and defines a *ray-sum* or *ray-projection*, p, as $p(7) \equiv -\ln I/I_0 = \sum \mu(x,7)\Delta x$ along the ray-path, so that $I/I_0 = e^{-p}$. More generally,

$$p(y) \equiv -\ln I/I_0 = \sum \mu(x,y)\Delta x \quad (8.2)$$

Things get messier when the X-ray beam is not aligned along the x- or y-axis, but the basic idea is the same.

CT contrast is much better than that of radiography, because it eliminates the overlap of confusing patterns from over- and underlying planes of tissue that are not of interest. Also it can significantly lower the amount of scatter noise present, since

the thickness of the volume of tissue being irradiated, hence causing Compton interactions, is so much less.

There is another reason as well, that has to do with happenings within the tomographic slice itself. Suppose the X-ray tube points from left to right, and two adjacent ray-projections within a tissue plane have identical attenuation coefficients except at one point (Figure 8.5b), With some arbitrarily voxel labeled the 0th, say, then all the other voxels are paired up with the same voxel values *except* for the two at the $x = +2$ position. For the creation of a radiograph, two parallel ray-projections pass through all the voxels of the two rows, and they differ only because of unequal attenuation at the $x = 2$ voxel site. The overall ray-projections will be nearly the same, with a *relative* difference of a fraction of a percent, or so. CT, on the other hand, focuses on each of the two $x = +2$ voxels individually, and their pixel values will differ by the ratio (μ'_{+2}/μ_{+2}), which can be high if the voxels contain radiologically dissimilar materials.

The eye can (barely) distinguish a small region of pixels that differs from background by 5 HU Such a 0.5% difference is readily apparent with CT, but corresponds to a change that is a factor of 10 times too slight to be seen in a radiographic film. On the other hand, the best resolution achievable with CT is something like a third of a millimeter, which is several times poorer than with film or DR. That is why one may select CT when good contrast among soft tissues is important but the finest detail is not.

Image reconstruction

We have been talking of calculating the ray-sum from knowledge of the values of $\mu(x,y)$ along a path (Equation 8.2). In practice, it is the converse process that is needed: one measures the ray-sums, by means of the radiation detector, for each of a large number of rays, and then computes, by means of a *reconstruction algorithm*, the set of $\mu(x,y)$ values that would give rise to the measured set of ray-sums.

In the example of Figure 8.5a, the process begins with a measurement of the ray-sum for the ray at $y = 1$. The beam then steps up to $y = 2$, and the new ray-sum is acquired. A *complete set* of such ray-sums at any particular gantry angle is called a *projection* or *profile*, as opposed to a ray-projection or ray-sum along a single geometric ray. In the case of the EMI scanner and Figure 8.5a, the first projection might consist of the set of separate ray-sums for the 160 rays running parallel to the *x*-axis. The production of a single-slice image involved the measurement of such 180 profiles, one for each of 180 gantry angles separated by one degree. The image will be reconstructed by extracting the attenuation coefficients for all voxels from the $160 \times 180 = 28\ 800$ resulting ray-sums; this reconstruction would involve manipulation of and solving 28 800 equations of the form of Equation 8.2, in effect, each with a unique, measured, and stored value of p. In effect, CT obtains a large number of pieces of one-dimensional information about the contents of the body, along the geometric rays, and then transforms that into a two-dimensional visual image on the display.

Several mathematical reconstruction methods have been devised for translating a set of CT attenuation measurements into a pixel map from a sufficiently large set of projections, $\{p(r,\varphi)\}$. Among them are the *algebraic, iterative, two-dimensional Fourier*, and *filtered back-projection* approaches. All of these involve the same basic two-step approach: First, *data acquisition* and *pre-conditioning*: the CT device acquires a *set* of attenuation/transmission profiles for a slice of tissue as the tube alternately shifts across and then rotates about a central axis. Then the computer carries out a number of steps for air dose calibration, reference normalization, and corrections for beam-hardening, bad channels, scatter, afterglow (of the detectors), cross-talk correction, etc.

Then the computer carries out *axial* (i.e., in the *transverse* plane) *slice reconstruction*: with a mathematical *algorithm* (a recipe for performing a calculation), it converts the transmission profiles into an *estimate* of the spatial distribution of the values of the attenuation coefficients in all the voxels of the slice.

The two general categories currently used in CT (and elsewhere) are *filtered back-projection* reconstruction and *iterative*, discussed below. But perhaps the easiest to visualize, although no longer used in commercial CTs, is known as the *algebraic reconstruction technique* (ART). ART harnesses a lot of simple algebra to solve a huge set of linear equations, each of the form of Equation 8.2, that correspond to the complete set of 180 projections. Let's work through an especially simple example.

Algebraic reconstruction: obtaining the $\mu(x,y)$ map from a complete set of profiles

Suppose we are imaging a body slice that consists of four voxels of unit dimension, $\Delta x = \Delta y = 1$. To simplify the notation, we shall label the voxels 1 through 4 and the rays A through F, as indicated in Figure 8.6a.

The ray-sum for horizontal ray A is related to the attenuation coefficients in the voxels through which it passes as $p(A) = (\mu_1 \times \Delta x) + (\mu_2 \times \Delta x) = (\mu_1 + \mu_2)$. Suppose that, in our example, $p(A)$ is measured by the CT machine to be of magnitude 12, so that

$$p(A) = \mu_1 + \mu_2 = 12. \qquad (8.3a)$$

Similarly, three other ray measurements yield

$$p(B) = \mu_3 + \mu_4 = 16, \qquad (8.3b)$$
$$p(C) = \mu_2 + \mu_3 = 24, \qquad (8.3c)$$
$$p(F) = \mu_2 + \mu_4 = 8. \qquad (8.3d)$$

This quartet of linear equations in four unknowns, μ_1 through μ_4, is easy to solve with elementary algebra. Subtracting Equation 8.3b from 8.3c leads to $\mu_2 - \mu_4 = 8$, and adding this to Equation 8.3d immediately gives $\mu_2 = 8$. Continuing in this fashion provides all four attenuation coefficients (Figure 8.6b), which can be translated immediately into Hounsfield units.

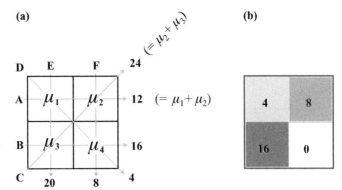

Figure 8.6 Algebraic reconstruction is conceptually simple, but computationally slow. **(a)** Measured projections for this 2 × 2 example, and **(b)** (don't peek!) the solution.

We have just created a genuine, 100% real CT image from a set of transmission measurements supplied by the scanner! This algebraic reconstruction technique, known also as *matrix inversion* after the mathematical tool normally involved, is not optimal, but it does work. It becomes extremely cumbersome and time consuming, however, when the number of voxels grows large. Major complications arise, moreover, when the linear equations are not all mutually consistent; such a situation might arise, for example, if a patient moves slightly in the midst of a measurement.

Still, it was long hoped that ART could be speeded up considerably by coupling it with a powerful mathematical technique known as the fast Fourier algorithm (FFA), which actually is central to other approaches to reconstruction. But this unification effort was severely hampered by, among other problems, lack of a suitable acronym.

Iterative reconstruction

Other approaches to the general reconstruction problem have been explored, and the ones found to work best fall into two general categories, the iterative and the analytic.

A number of iterative approaches have been developed for SPECT and PET, but they are finding increasing application in CT as well — largely because they can accommodate statistical methods that reduce the impact of random noise, and also of internal inconsistencies in a dataset arising from patient motion, etc. An iterative reconstruction might begin with a good image, already generated by the fast analytic filtered back-projection approach – a big head-start – and continue on to fine-tune things. Iteration produces, for the slice being reconstructed, a sequence of improving images, each of which is a refinement over its predecessor and closer to the real thing.

Iteration starts off with an earlier slice-image or an educated guess of pixel values based on the raw CT data. In the first iteration, the algorithm then (i) computes a complete set of *re-projected* ray-sums calculated from the entries in the initial, trial $\mu(x,y)$ matrix; then (ii) compares these newly computed ray-sums with the ray-sums originally measured; and (iii) following specific "correction" rules, calls upon a *correction loop* to adjust the previous matrix of pixel-values accordingly. The new set of μ' values should be closer to reality than was the original set of matrix values. (iv) In the second iteration, the algorithm re-projects the ray-sums obtained from the revised pixel matrix, compares the newer values with the original ray measurement data, makes the correction again, and thereby obtains yet a better approximate map of the $\mu(x,y)$ values. (v) Repeat this feedback loop procedure until the calculated pixel map no longer changes much between further iterations.

To impart a sense of how it works, let's go through another very simple, four-voxel example. Four real projections have been *measured*, as with $p(A) = 3$, etc. (Figure 8.7a). We begin by generating a preliminary estimate of what the values of the set of four values of μ_i, $i = 1, 2, 3$, and 4 might be close to. With these, we compute what four new, artificial pseudo-projections, $p'(A)$, etc., would be close to. These contrived projection-values will naturally differ from the real measured ones, and we shall ascertain by how much.

First, the upper *horizontal* projection was originally *measured* to have the value $p(A) = 3$. This suggests that reasonable initial trial guesses for μ_1 and μ_2 might be 1.5 each, sharing $p(A)$ equally between them. Likewise for the second row, $p(B) = 4$, and we'll choose $\mu_3 = \mu_4 = 2$ (Figure 8.7b).

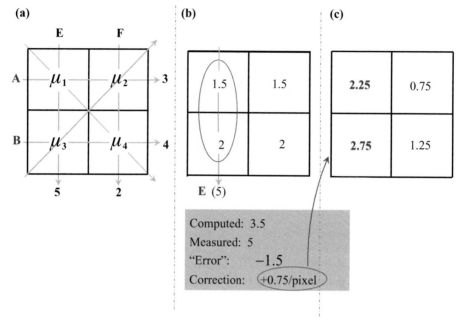

Figure 8.7 Iterative reconstruction (a) for a different four-voxel example. (b) As a first step, half the *measured* value (3) is assigned to each of the two cells of the top row, and similarly for the second. With these initial trial μ values, the left column projection is now *computed* to be 3.5. This is 1.5 less than the measured projection for column E (5), so (c) one half that "error" is selected to "correct" (i.e., +0.75 is added) the cells in that column. Likewise for the column to the right. In this particularly simple case, a single iteration solves the problem.

Now we *calculate* the two *vertical* pseudo-projections with these assumed trial attenuation coefficients: $p'(E) = 3.5$, and the same for $p'(F)$. But these two vertical profiles were independently *measured* to be $p(E) = 5$ and $p(F) = 2$, respectively, so we need somehow to make a correction for the difference between our current estimate and measured reality. Consider $p'(E)$ first. It is less than the measured $p(E)$ by the *difference* amount $[p'(E) - p(E)] = [3.5 - 5] = -1.5$. That is, our calculation is in "error," at this point, by that amount. Now our correction algorithm comes into play to modify the current μ_i values, and to partially overcome that error. The correction algorithm that we choose says to reverse one half the error amount in both pixels; so with an error of -1.5, we compensate by adding the amount $+0.75$ to the current μ_1 and μ_3, resulting in $\mu_1' = (1.5 + 0.75) = 2.25$ and $\mu_3' = 2.75$, as in Figure 8.7c.

For the F column, the error is $[p'(F) - p(F)] = [3.5 - 2] = +1.5$, so the correction is -0.75, leading to the second column in Figure 8.7c.

Based on the differences for the four pairs, the correction algorithm has adjusted the four initial trail μ_i values so that their four replacements, the set $\{\mu'_i\}$, will generate another round of pseudo-projections – and presumably these will agree better

with the measured projection (which they will, if the algorithm is any good).

And then you *iterate* this exercise again and again until the contrived projections change only a little from round to round. In this example, the entries in Figure 8.7c already agree with the measured projections after only one iteration, and there is no need to continue.

Filtered back-projection reconstruction is much faster

Analytic algorithms are faster than the iterative ones for CT, and they suffice for nearly all purposes. The two most commonly employed analytic methods are Fourier reconstruction and filtered back-projection. The two are related, and are based on the mathematical Radon transform, published in 1917, which describes a way to determine what's within something by studying what passes through it. Filtered back-projection (which actually does use the FFA!) has the advantage that calculations can begin after a single profile is obtained, rather than having to wait for completion of all profile measurements on a slice. It is, indeed, the primary reconstruction technique currently used in commercial CT machines.

The mathematical details of *filtered back-projection* are somewhat complex, but the basic notion is quite simple. The approach employs a modification of the *simple back-projection* method, so we will start by describing that. And it is easiest to talk about a scanner of Hounsfield's original design, with a tall, narrow X-ray beam, one slice high and one voxel wide, that moves laterally across the body and then rotates a degree or so around it and scans again.

Let us first examine the simplest of all possible patients, one who is transparent to X-rays everywhere except at one voxel-sized bone sliver at an unknown location (Figure 8.8a). Our objective is to find and display the position of this single, radio-opaque voxel. Back-projection does this by repeating many times a simple three-step procedure with the X-ray beam aligned with some fixed orientation; the beam angle is then changed, and the repetitive three-step procedure is carried out again. Typically, 180 or more different angles of the beam are required to generate an image, but for locating a single opaque voxel, 2 will suffice.

We start by obtaining the first profile, in this case by orienting the X-ray beam horizontally, parallel to the x-axis of the coordinate system, and positioning it low, so that it passes through the row of (empty) voxels at $y = 1$ (Figure 8.8a). At the same time, we define a corresponding pixel coordinate system on the display, such as a piece of graph paper. With this first beam angle, we repeatedly carry out this three-step procedure:

Step 1: Measure the transmission and ray-sum along the ray, which is to say, the attenuation of the narrow X-ray beam by the phantom.

Step 2: Back-project (paint) a narrow stripe, one pixel wide and parallel to the x-axis, at the corresponding level on the display. The brightness of the stripe is to be proportional to the ray-projection of the X-ray beam; that is, to the amount of attenuation of the X-ray beam along this path through the phantom, as determined in step 1; and the greater the amount of beam attenuation, the whiter the stripe to be laid down. Where there is no attenuation, the stripe is made black.

Step 3: Move the X-ray beam one voxel-width upward, and the line on the display one pixel up, and return to step 1; that is, after the completion of the first cycle, move the X-ray beam to $y = 2$ in the phantom and the paint brush to $y = 2$ on the graph paper, and carry out the three steps again.

For this first (fully horizontal) orientation of the X-ray beam, repeat the procedure 160 times, so

Figure 8.8 Unfiltered back-projection for a patient with one radio-opaque voxel. (**a**) Stepping or sweeping the horizontal beam upward allows detection of the dark voxel at $y = 7$ (see Figure 8.5a). (**b**) A horizontal stripe one unit wide is painted at the corresponding height in the display. (**c**) The voxel is completely localized with a sweep of a vertically-oriented beam along the x-axis, and painting the corresponding vertical stripe on the display. (**d**) Additional sweeps darken the background, but much more so the cross-fire region of the dense voxel.

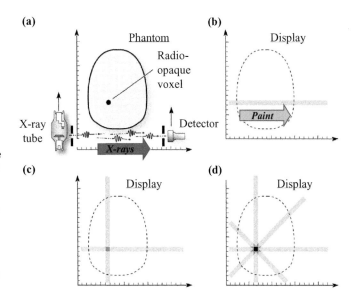

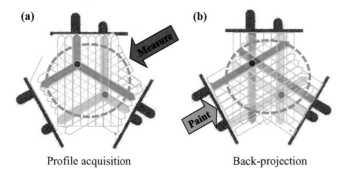

(a) **(b)**

Profile acquisition   Back-projection

Figure 8.9 Projections and unfiltered back-projection for two tissue voxels, one with twice the attenuation coefficient of the other. (a) After measuring a projection along a geometric ray, (b) paint a corresponding stripe, in the display, whose brightness increases with the total beam attenuation. Where X-rays are attenuated more, paint a brighter stripe. Sweeping along only y- and x-axes does not suffice to identify the two voxels unequivocally, but a third will finish the job.

that the entire phantom (along with some empty space, at the bottom and top) has been traversed. Again, in the first and second steps, you carry out the attenuation measurement on the phantom and then back-project on display; in the third, shift one voxel position upward in the phantom, and one pixel up on the display. Repeat the process until the entire phantom is covered for this orientation of the X-ray beam. With our example of the single radio-opaque voxel, the profile of beam attenuation across the phantom will be reflected on the display as a single, narrow stripe at $y = 7$ (Figure 8.8b).

Rotate the X-ray beam and the display line through an appropriate angle, perhaps 1° in reality (but 90° for this little exercise) and walk through the whole process again, this time stepping the (now vertically-oriented) profile 160 times from left to right. A new (vertical) stripe will intersect the horizontal stripe only at the pixel in the image that corresponds to the opaque voxel (Figure 8.8c). (The computer does not actually create an image one stripe at a time, but its memory does keep track of where the stripes should be, and displays on a monitor the overall image they collectively generate.)

Thus, two X-ray beam alignments are enough to locate unambiguously a single point opacity. The part of the display that represents the region of high CT number, moreover, is twice as bright as elsewhere along the individual back-projection slices. Back-projecting at a number of additional gantry angles enhances this difference, so that eventually the back-projections blur out and are not too noticeable, except where they intersect (Figure 8.8d).

But one pixel does not an image make. Let's try this again on the considerably more challenging patient with two partially opaque voxels, the atten-

uation in one of them being twice that in the other. Back-projections obtained from two perpendicular profiles intersect at four places (Figure 8.9), and there is no way to tell which two of them are "real." A third scan resolves the issue, however, since back-projections from all three angles will all overlap at only two places. Expansion of this argument leads to the conclusion that enough back-projection profiles can generate a map of local X-ray attenuation for any real slice of tissues.

Image quality can be significantly enhanced by incorporating a suitable mathematical *filter* or *kernel* into the back-projection calculation. A filter, in effect, replaces the single back-projected stripe (about one pixel wide) with a narrow bundle of several adjacent narrower stripes that have different, cleverly selected levels of darkness. Some of them are even of negative brightness, in the sense that they subtract from other bundles, coming in at other angles, wherever they may overlap. This is somewhat analogous to the destructive interference of waves. Adding a good filter to back-projection renders the stripes vanishingly faint everywhere except where they intersect. This doesn't just happen by chance, incidentally; there is a firm mathematical basis for the approach, as discussed in the Appendix to this chapter, although some trial and error does enter into the act for fine adjustments.

Both simple and filtered back-projection begin with the formation of a sufficiently complete set of projections (Figure 8.10a). Non-filtered back-projection entails simply the laying down of uniform stripes (Figure 8.10b). For filtered back-projection, a stripe is made to vary across its width, as indicated in Figure 8.10c, with the result that the reconstructed figure much more closely resembles what is in the body. A variety of kernels have

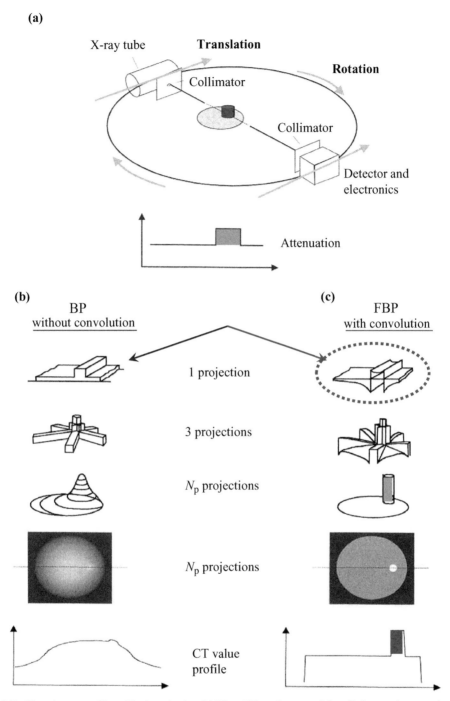

Figure 8.10 Filtered versus unfiltered back-projection. (a) When CT imaging an upright cylinder near isocenter (on the line about which the gantry rotates), each projection will be a rectangle of twice the width at the detectors. (b) Simple superpositioning of back-projections results in a blurred image. (c) When a *filter* is convolved with each projection before back-projection, nearly all the mess vanishes.

been developed to improve the display of soft tissue contrast, for high-resolution studies, etc. Acting on the raw data with the kernel involves the mathematical process of *convolution*, because of which Europeans tend to call filtered back-projection *convolution back-projection*. This business may sound somewhat complicated, but the whole filtered back-projection image reconstruction process can be accomplished with surprisingly few lines of computer code.

The basis for filtered back-projection is sketched, for those mathematically inclined, in the Appendix to this chapter.

Seven generations of CT scanners

CT scanners have been evolving continuously since the early 1970s. A few of the changes, however, have been sufficiently radical to distinguish what are known currently as the seven generations of CT devices, where the last two incorporate helical motion and multi-slice capability. New machines are nearly all of the helical, multi-slice variety.

First and second generations: sweep across patient, then rotate tube and detectors, and repeat

The first commercial CT scanner was built by Hounsfield to image the head, and its general design and operation have been sketched earlier. In such a *first-generation* scanner, a single X-ray tube and collimator produced a 1-cm-tall, narrow beam, with two adjacent sodium iodide signal detectors monitored the intensity transmitted through the patient (Figure 8.11a). The tube and detector were mounted rigidly on opposite ends of the same supporting gantry, so as to rotate about the central isocenter line with their positions fixed relative to one another. The beam always pointed directly into the detector with the patient's head in between, but the tube and detector, in tandem, could undergo both linear and rotational motion relative to the patient. With the sweep-then-rotate procedure described above, the system made 180 × 160 separate X-ray projection measurements for one or two thin slices of tissue, a process that took 4 minutes per slice.

The *second-generation* machine underwent translate-rotate motion like the first, but with a fan-shaped beam narrowly diverging over 10° and

pointing at a linear array of separate detectors (Figure 8.11b). The great advantage was the considerably shorter scan time, under 20 seconds.

Third generation: rotate tube and detector array

Since Hounsfield's day, CT image quality has improved phenomenally, and the imaging and reconstruction time has dropped to practically nothing. The introduction of the *third-generation* scanner in 1976 eliminated the need for the slow linear motions of the X-ray tube and radiation detectors across the patient (Figure 8.11c). The fan-beam is wide enough to completely cover the patient, cutting an arc of about 60°, and the linear array typically of 500 to 800 separate detectors is spread out so as to intercept the entire fan. The gantry rotates the tube and the detector array together about the isocenter in a single, smooth 360° swing, obtaining 500–1000 views along the way. While the earlier scanners employed parallel X-ray beams, the beams of third- and higher-generation devices diverge significantly as fans wide enough to cover the patient, requiring more complex and powerful reconstruction techniques.

Fourth and fifth generations: rotate tube, or just the beam

The *fourth-generation* machine has a *stationary* ring of as many as 5000 small, closely spaced detectors completely circumscribing the patient, and only the tube moves (Figure 8.11d). While the detector array of a third-generation machine extends only for an arc of 60°, that of a fourth-generation machine requires (other things being equal) six times as many detector elements, and detectors and their associated electronics are not cheap. It is largely for this reason that seventh-generation multi-slice CTs, which typically have 64 rings of detectors, are of third-generation geometry. Both third- and fourth-generation single-slice machines were highly successful, and neither has revealed itself to be of unequivocally superior design.

The virtue of the *fifth-generation* (known also as *electron beam tomography*) machine, built by the Imatron Corporation and subsequently taken over by Siemens and GE, is its ultra-high speed, invaluable for cardiac studies. The array of detectors is fixed, but here not even the X-ray tube moves. The

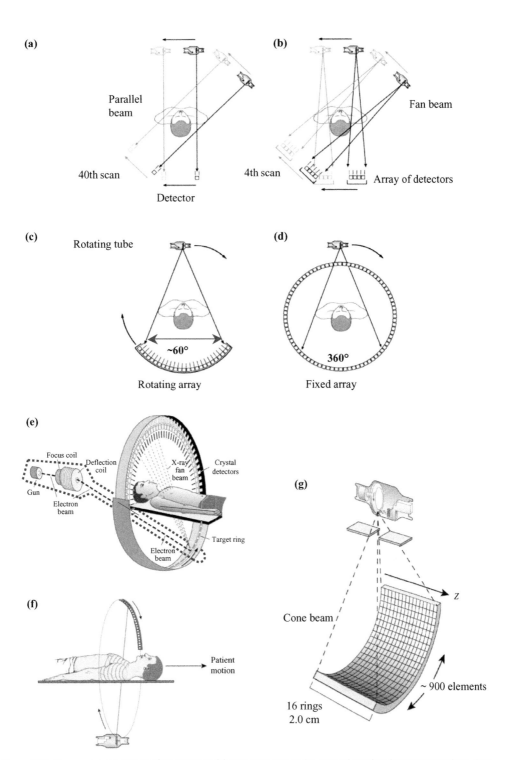

Figure 8.11 The seven generations of CT scanners. (**a**) First generation: the original EMI head scanner: translate, then rotate the linked tube/pencil beam and the detector, and repeat 180 times. (**b**) Second generation: translate-rotate with a fan-beam and bank of detectors; much faster; the fan is 10 (rather than 1) degrees wide, so only 1/10 as many scan angles are needed. (**c**) Third generation: rotating tube and rotating ~60°-detector assembly. (**d**) Fourth generation: rotating tube and fixed 360° ring of detectors. (**e**) Fifth generation: electron-beam tomography CT, great while it dominated, but driven nearly extinct by seventh-generation devices. (**f**) Sixth generation: helical/spiral, in which the table moves smoothly forward as the gantry rotates continuously; made possible by slip-ring technology. (**g**) Seventh generation: helical multi-slice CT typically obtains 64 slices (but currently up to 320) with each rotation of the gantry. Built upon third-generation design and used in either sequential/axial or helical/spiral mode.

X-ray "tube" is quite different from the standard design: its envelope (red dashed line in Figure 8.11e) is shaped as a double-walled, evacuated half-funnel, the wide-open end of which half-surrounds the patient. An electron gun creates an electron beam that travels along parallel to and between the pair of walls of the funnel, and is swept along a curved tungsten-strip target (green dashed line) that half circumscribes the body. The electron beam and focal spot, swing half-way around the patient in 50 milliseconds. This was fast enough to freeze the motions of the heart and, with a number of such images taken in sequence, could produce a smooth cine of the entire cardiac cycle.

The fifth generation machine was complex and of very large size, the electronics were somewhat noisy, and it was cost-effective only with a steady flow of cardiac patients. Still, due to the speed of data acquisition, motion artifacts such as those caused by cardiac and bowel movements disappeared. Multi-slice, helical scanners can now do practically any kind of heart study, and are otherwise enormously flexible, and have largely displaced the fifth-generation – which was in its day, though, quite a marvel!

Sixth generation: helical/spiral

Virtually all new scanners are both helical and multi-slice, but it is easier to discuss these two attributes separately.

Before there was helical, so-called *axial* (also *sequential*, or *stop-and-shoot mode*) scanners acquired data within one transverse plane of tissue at a time. The tube and detectors on the gantry rotated once about an immobile table. The table was then advanced by a small increment in the longitudinal, *z*-direction, and then the tube was rotated back again, rewinding the electrical cables and coolant hoses – and so on and on, each time producing data on a different flat plane of tissue. *Helical* or *spiral mode* scanners, introduced in the late 1980s, could be of either third- or fourth-generation configuration; that is, with either rotating or fixed detectors (Figure 8.11f). But in either case, they differ from the pre-helical designs in several ways: they provide a method of rapid volume imaging, a development that has been pushed forward even more with multi-slice devices; the table and the gantry both move continuously and

smoothly throughout all of data acquisition, which makes possible much faster scanning; the tube follows a cork-screw path, from the table's perspective, so there are no natural transverse planes of data; it is necessary to produce them artificially, rather, through interpolation of the data that are available; and it was necessary to develop special ways to get high-voltage electric power to the rotating X-ray tube and, for third-generation machines, electrical signals from the rotating detectors.

Let's start with the last of these. Power to and data from third- and fourth-generation axial designs can be carried directly on permanent cables – but that limits operation to a single gantry revolution each way. The essential new component that makes the helical approach possible is the *slip ring*, fixed on the rotating gantry, and the conducting brushes of silver or carbon fiber that rub against the rings and connect the gantry to the stationary world (Figure 8.12a,b). A scanner requires a half dozen or so rings to supply low-voltage a.c. power to both the high-voltage d.c. generator and the tube-cooling system mounted on the gantry, and for the transmission of data and control signals. Each slip ring must be electrically insulated from everything else, of course, and the brushes must ensure noiseless electrical contact.

Relative to the slowly advancing patient, the tube traces out a continuous spiral path, so that each detector acquires data at discrete points lying along a helix around the patient, rather than on a circle on a single plane as in axial scanning. There are no display planes that are created with complete, consistent data obtained from single transverse planes of data, so it is therefore necessary to interpolate the data mathematically, and project them onto hypothetical transverse planes for reconstruction and display in a planar format. The linear interpolation in the *z*-direction involves the pairs of helical data points, at every gantry angle, that straddle the reconstruction plane being created, and calculation of their weighted average (Figure 8.12c). A series of sections can be reconstructed from the data, moreover, with any desired spacing between the presented images.

The *pitch* is an adjustable determinant and measure of the closeness together of the coils of the helix, relative to how much of the body is being imaged at any instant (i.e., the width of the collimator

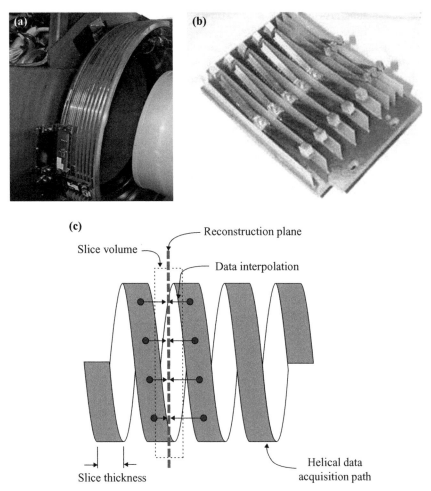

Figure 8.12 Slip-rings are essential for helical and helical multi-slice imaging. a) Electrically isolated strips of metal on the gantry ring surrounding the patient. The heavier ones convey relatively low-voltage a.c. to power the high-voltage, d.c. X-ray tube generator, mounted on the gantry, and the others convey control information and signals. (**b**) Fixed, non-rotating carbon or silver brushes make low-noise contact with the revolving rings. (**c**) Helical scanning with a *pitch* of 2; the imaginary reconstruction plane utilizes suitably weighted averages of data from the two partial spirals on either side of it.

opening in the *z*-direction). It is conventionally defined as

$$\text{Pitch} = \frac{\text{table } z\text{-travel/360}° \text{ rotation (mm)}.}{\text{beam width in } z\text{-direction (mm)}} \quad (8.4)$$

With a pitch of 1, the table moves one beam-width forward as the beam rotates through 360°, like a ribbon or trail of spray paint wrapped on a round dowel, with neither gaps nor overlaps. When the pitch is less than 1, the helices are more tightly packed and overlapping; and the pitch is greater than 1 if they are stretched out, with gaps between. Typical pitches range from 0.7 to 2. Higher pitch means both increased speed and lower dose, but slice noise and resolution tend to worsen.

Seventh generation: helical multi-slice

Until the arrival of multi-slice *seventh generation* scanners a decade after helical, there was only one row, or ring, or belt of detectors lying along the circumference of a single circle, and it was exposed (through the patient) by a thin, fan-beam of X-rays. The great virtue of a multi-slice device (MSCT), also known as a multi-detector-ring (MDCT) or multi-row scanner, is that it can acquire multiple slice-images simultaneously, in either axial or helical mode. It can thus provide much shorter data acquisition times, or thinner slices, or longer scanned volumes in the same time, and any of these can have obvious benefits.

Creating the seventh-generation CT involved exchanging the one rotating partial ring (a 60° arc) of small detectors of a third-generation single-slice device with a set of multiple adjacent, parallel clones of the detector ring array (Figure 8.11g). The single belt of detectors of the single-slice machine is replaced with multiple adjacent such belts; equivalently, each detector of the single ring is replaced with a row of them, lined up along the patient and the z-direction. The first MSCT, coming on the scene in 1998, could acquire four slices, with slice width down to 1 mm; modern devices can produce 64 or more slices each 0.6 mm thick. Devices with over 300 rings have been built, but there appears to be general agreement that 64 are clinically adequate (although for cardiac and perfusion studies, wider is better).

Multi-row CT scanners employ classic third-generation scan geometry, largely because the detectors are expensive, and a fourth-generation machine (in which the detectors completely encircle the machine) would have five or six times more of them. The detector arrays come in various sizes and configurations, depending on the vendor. Machines now boast sub-millimeter slice-thicknesses, and truly isotropic, cubic voxels, of equal length in all three dimensions; this makes possible full three-dimensional *multiplanar reformatting* (MPR), from near-transverse data acquisition to coronal or sagittal (or other) display.

To accommodate the much greater length (along z) of the matrix of detectors, the X-ray tube and collimators no longer generate a thin transverse fan beam; rather, they must produce a pyramidal *cone beam*, rectangular in cross-section; the beam may have to be up to 8 cm long along the patient at the rings of detectors on the far side of the patient, so as to expose the outermost of them (the ones farthest from the beam's central axis.)

The reconstruction process is similar to that of single-row helical scanning, except that now there are data from multiple detector rows. The majority of manufacturers employ *filter interpolation*: for each projection angle, it uses all the data points that fall within a fixed distance along the z-direction, called the filter width, of the image plane being reconstructed. This width is determined and set automatically through operator-selection of the desired slice thickness, and it is independent of the pitch. Unlike the situation for single-row scanners, this generally results in more than two data points being used for interpolating the projection data at each angle. The projection data can be reconstructed for various slice thicknesses and increments (pitches), depending on the machine design.

The numbers and dimensions of detectors and slices, and the numbers of *channels* of communication between the ring of detectors and the information processor can be confusing, and it is critical to define them clearly for establishing protocols and carrying out QA. Individual detectors are small, commonly a millimeter or so in dimensions (Figure 8.13a). These minute, separate detectors are packaged together in blocks; here the blocks are eight on a side, shown along with parts of nearest neighbors, all lying along eight rings that circumscribe the patient. You might expect that each detector would communicate directly with the computer for reconstruction, but this is often not so — the number of available channels of communication, N, may be less than the number of individual radiation sensors, so some information that would otherwise be obtainable from a set of detectors cannot be collected. In such cases, two (or more) detectors can be *binned*, in effect becoming a single detector of twice the area and sensitivity, and $\sqrt{2}$ times the SNR. We are not getting something for nothing here, of course: what is gained in noise reduction is lost in resolution. This same choice arises in selecting kVp (in particular, to account for patient size), mA-s/rotation, pitch, channel width and binning, and other dose-related factors.

Devices are being marketed that can capture several hundred slices at a time. For multi-row detectors with a large z-direction beam collimation, the conventional filtered back-projection algorithm for image reconstruction is inadequate: as the number of detector rows and tube collimation width increase, so also does the cone beam angle, inducing artifacts. Mathematically and computationally complex algorithms, going by names like *weighted hyperplane reconstruction*, *advanced single-slice rebinning*, and *adaptive multiple plane reconstruction*, are steps toward a general solution, and cone-beam image reconstruction algorithms remain an area of active research.

Technology and image quality

Although the image quality issues for CT will be familiar from discussion of radiographic and fluoroscopic systems, some of the tradeoffs required, and problems that arise, are new. But as with radiography and fluoroscopy, the five most desirable

(a)

$\longrightarrow$ *z* $\longrightarrow$

4 × 1.25-mm
channels

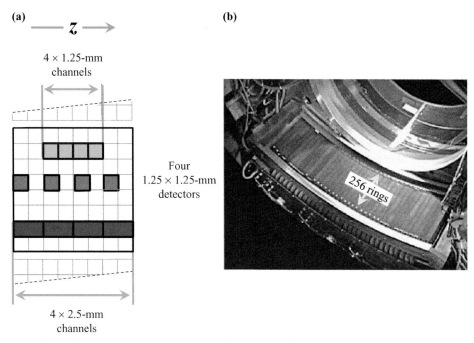

(b)

Four
1.25 × 1.25-mm
detectors

256 rings

4 × 2.5-mm
channels

Figure 8.13 The number of detector elements may exceed the number of electrical channels of communication between the detector assembly and the computer. (**a**) This is an eight-slice machine; there are hundreds of short rows surrounding the patient each parallel to the z-axis and with eight detectors, but there happen, in this case, to be only four channels for each row. Here are three possible ways of extracting the data; are there others? (**b**) A detector assembly with 256 (a huge number!) partial rings going around the patient (i.e., 256 detectors per row) and 912 detectors on each ring. Reproduced from T Flohr, B Schmidt, Advances in CT. In: Wolbarst AB, Capasso P, Godfrey DJ, *et al.* (eds), *Advances in Medical Physics*, vol. 4. Madison WI: Medical Physics Publishing, 2012, fig. 4-2. Courtesy of Dr. DS Mori, National Institute of Radiological Sciences (NIRS), Chiba, Japan.

attributes of CT images are strong tissue contrast, low noise, fine resolution, no artifacts, and low dose.

X-ray tubes and detectors

Tubes

CT typically uses a small focal spot, down to 0.5 mm. The anode-cathode axis is aligned along the patient, perpendicular to the plane of the patient slice being irradiated, eliminating complications from the heel effect. More filtering is employed than with radiography because of problems introduced into the reconstruction calculations by beam hardening within the body. A *bow-tie beam filter*, "scooped out" toward the middle, provides a crude form of tissue compensation that makes the intensity and the hardness of the beam emerging from the (somewhat oval-shaped) patient's head or body more uniform.

In part to reduce the arcing of electrical sparks among moving parts, it is common practice to hold the anode and bearings at ground potential, with the cathode at a high negative voltage; with other X-ray technologies, the cathode and anode are nor-

mally maintained at equal but opposite potentials, equally far below and above ground. It adds to the engineering challenge that the rapidly rotating anode, of several kilograms mass, is swung around the gantry every $\frac{1}{3}$ second, making it feel ten or more times more massive to the bearings.

Nearly all CT scanners generate X-rays continuously, at 80, 100, or 120 kVp with currents up to 800 mA. It is especially important that the selected values for these technique factors be held highly stable during a scan, since variations would lead to data inconsistencies, which can be problematic for reconstruction algorithms. The power that must be dissipated as heat greatly exceeds anything that a normal radiographic source has to deal with by a factor of up to ten, and for seconds, rather than tens of milliseconds. Several approaches have been developed to address heat stress. The tube is oil-cooled with a heat exchanger also on the gantry and, so as not to exceed its heat capacity, a cooling period between scans or sets of scans may be required. The anode is larger (16 cm in diameter) than for a standard tube (10 cm), it has heat-radiating *fins* on its back side, and there is a ring-shaped *aperture* near the focal spot to prevent electrons ejected inadvertently from the *anode* from crashing back into it.

The Siemens Straton CT X-ray tube takes a radically new and clever approach to keeping its cool. The anode is built into, and serves as, one end of the tube, and it is the entire tube that rotates, supported mechanically at both its front and back on external bearings (Figure 8.14). The electron beam from the cathode is bent sharply downward by a magnetic field (pointing into the page), and strikes the target at two possible adjacent *flying focal spots*; wobbling the magnetic field slightly several thousand times a second produces two different beams, in effect, thereby doubling the number of slice images that can be produced, a technique known as *double-z sampling*. Cold oil, in direct contact with the back side of the anode, largely eliminates the problem of overheating. Associated with the Straton tube are a number of electronic sensors for operational parameters such as oil temperature and pressure, filament current, and tube current that can give early warning indications of potential tube failure from cooling problems, high voltage breakdown, vacuum loss, loss of focal spot stability, etc. This advance notice is particularly advantageous in busy departments where machine downtime for a day or two is both inconvenient for patients and quite costly.

Detectors

Commercial scanners currently employ *indirect detection*, with ceramic scintillators plus silicon photodiode detectors. Primary design considerations are detector efficiency, a short response time (no afterglow), stability of operation, low dependence of detector response on X-ray energy (to reduce the effects of beam hardening), and cost. Gadolinium oxide and oxysulfide, and other rare-earth ceramic scintillating materials with trace dopants have replaced sodium iodide and cesium fluoride (and, before that, high-pressure xenon gas) because of their greater detection efficiencies (from higher Z) and much shorter fluorescence decay times.

Another approach is to adapt to CT the flat-panel area detectors of DR, but with smaller pixel matrices, which would make it possible to cover the entire heart, the brain, or the kidneys in a single axial rotation, and with $1/4$-millimeter resolution. Active matrix flat panel imaging (AMFPI) indirect

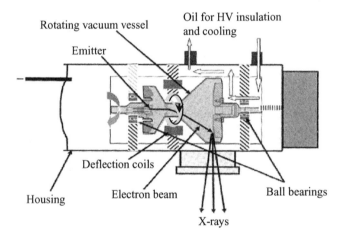

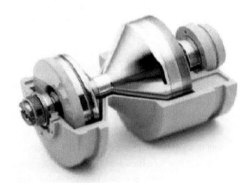

Figure 8.14 The entire Siemens "Straton" X-ray tube rotates on bearings at either end. The back side of the anode serves also as one end of the tube, and its external surface is in direct contact with circulating cold oil. A magnet bends the electron beam from the cathode downward, enabling the full benefits of a rotating anode; it also wobbles the focal spot back and forth between two adjacent points on the target at high frequency, in effect doubling the number of imaging slices. Courtesy of Siemens Medical Solutions USA, Inc.

detection devices designed around CsI-aSi technology, for example, are under active research, and prototype flat-panel detector CTs have been built. The principal problem is the (relatively) slow readout from the panels: while 100 frames per second is fine for DF to follow the flow of contrast media through vessels, it would be far too slow for the rapidly rotating IR of CT, and would require a significant slowdown of gantry revolution speed.

There is also considerable interest in a direct detection scheme that operates somewhat like direct DR (dDR) planar X-ray imaging, called *direct photon-counting*. A semiconductor such as cadmium-zinc-telluride (CZT) forms electron-hole pairs when struck by a high-energy photon, and these are swept by a high electric field to the opposing electrodes, creating a charge pulse.

Contrast and scan noise

The level of visual noise depends on several factors, including the slice thickness desired, the in-plane resolution required (hence the pixel size) and, of course the dose imparted to the patient. These can always be balanced against one another in such a way that noise is not a limiting problem – but some of it will always be present.

When you scan a homogeneous water phantom, not all the pixels will exhibit a CT number of exactly 0 Hounsfield units. There will be a small spread, rather, in the relative numbers of pixels exhibiting different CT numbers near zero (Figure 8.15). Images from modern scanners are primarily quantum limited, in the sense that the most significant contribution to noise is due to such Poisson fluctuations in the number of X-ray photons passing through tissue and eventually striking and triggering the detectors.

If we double the dose deposited in a slice during a measurement, or double the thickness of the slice (either of which will double the number of photons reaching the detector), the signal-to-noise SNR $= \mu^{1/2}$ will improve by a factor of $\sqrt{2} = 1.4$ (Equations 4.4). Relative noise declines as dose goes up, as $D^{-1/2}$, simply because of the decrease in the number of photons involved, and this poses a fundamental, statistically based limit on image quality.

Noise is introduced into CT images in a number of other ways, as well. Electronic noise arises spontaneously in the preamplifiers of the X-ray detectors, and this will be amplified along with the true signal by the rest of the electronic circuitry. Information is lost also in the process of digitizing the continuous electrical signals coming out of the preamplifiers. And the SNR is reduced further through approximations made in the mathematical reconstruction and application of the convolution kernel; scanners allow the selection of the filter for a particular study from a range of them that influence the appearance of

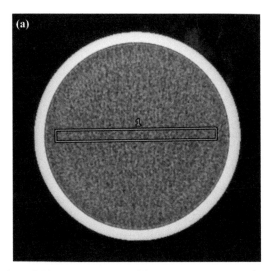
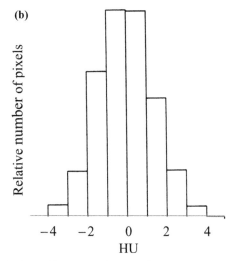

Figure 8.15 Assessing CT noise. (**a**) From a narrow rectangular region imaged in a water phantom. This image is quite noisy because the selected mA-s per revolution was low. (**b**) Relative numbers of pixels with HU values near 0 are displayed in a histogram. For the Poisson component of the noise, the standard deviation, a measure of the width of the distribution and a gauge of noise, is numerically equal to the square root of the mean – which is *not* 0!

the image in various ways, and those yielding sharper images tend to be noisier. It is necessary to hold down the level of noise, but other important objectives of CT are to make the scan time short and to keep the patient dose low, both of which may themselves diminish the SNR.

Resolution

The resolving power of CT must be considered from two perspectives: resolution within each transverse plane and resolution in the direction perpendicular to those planes, along the z-axis. Both depend on a number of factors, including some obvious ones: focal spot size and penumbra, detector element width and length, binning, field of view, patient size, numbers of views, pitch, nature of the interpolation, the reconstruction kernel, the presence of scatter or other noise, patient dose, and patient motion.

A cause of reduction of resolution unique to CT is differential magnification. If part of an organ is away from the axis of rotation of the gantry, then its image will be most magnified when the X-ray tube is closest to it, and least for the tube 180° away. As the gantry swings around, its position will appear to vary laterally (Figure 8.16), and the incompatibility of the data sets will affect the reconstruction

algorithm, resulting in blur. A way to minimize the impact of this problem is to position the region of interest, to the extent possible, on the axis of rotation.

Within a plane, a high-contrast resolution of 0.4 mm is normally achievable, with commercial manufacturers' claims ranging down to 0.25 mm. It is limited by detector aperture size, the image spatial sampling rate, the tube focal spot size, and imperfections in the reconstruction algorithm (including, for filtered back-projection, the mathematical filter), and is considerably poorer than that of conventional radiography. The displayed resolution is intimately linked, of course, with the achievable pixel size. The dimension of a pixel should be about a half of the system's required in-plane resolution, or less, to make full diagnostic use of its inherent capabilities. Thus with a 512 × 512-pixel matrix, a system may be able to display a 25 × 25-cm^2 region of interest at 0.5-mm resolution and 2 lp/mm.

The attenuation of the intensity of a ray by a voxel depends on an average of the radiological properties of all the tissues in it, so increasing slice thickness or voxel area has the effect of assessing the attenuation coefficient over a longer volume. If one voxel contains several quite different materials, such as fat and bone, the Hounsfield unit of the voxel may be an average of them, and representative of none, an artifact known as the *partial volume effect*. Even a speck of high-atomic-number,

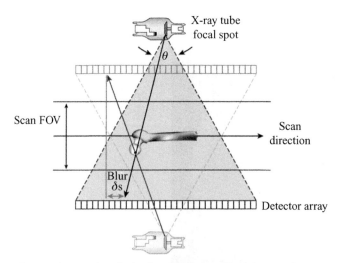

Figure 8.16 Blur arises when an object, such as the border of the femoral head, is not at the isocenter. Its distances from the tube's focal spot, and from the detectors, therefore depend on the table position and the gantry angle. The image's raw data can go through electronic post-processing, however, to reduce the blur, with no additional radiation to the patient. This blur, and the optical parallax effect associated with the divergence of the beam at its edges, are the main reasons why the area of interest should always be at or near the center of the field of view. Reproduced from Flohr T, Cody D, McCollough C, Computed tomography. In: AB Wolbarst, Zamenhof RG, Hendee WR, *et al.* (eds), *Advances in Medical Physics*, vol. 1. Madison, WI: Medical Physics Publishing, 2006, fig. 3-14.

high-density material within a voxel can significantly bias the calculated average CT number of the corresponding pixel. It is this partial volume effect that causes small calcifications, which might well be invisible in radiography, not only to show up clearly in CT, but even to appear significantly larger (pixel sized) than they really are. Other partial volume effects can also cause clinical confusion, as well, so when in doubt, one can select smaller pixels and/or thinner slices.

Slice thicknesses of less than 1 mm can be obtained, with slices taken every 1 to 10 mm; if coronal and sagittal plane views are constructed out of many transverse slices, slice thickness is what limits longitudinal resolution. Modern CT machines can, like MRI scanners, generate isotropic voxels and pixels, in which the sub-millimeter resolution is the same in all three dimensions.

Connecting contrast, resolution, slice thickness, patient size, and dose

The doses delivered in a single CT slice tend to be in the range 1–6 cGy at skin surface, and to fall off somewhat in the middle of the head or body. While not excessive, this is considerably greater than one generally finds with most other imaging techniques, and often considerably higher than it needs to be. There is a major concern among patients, physicians, and the vendors to find ways to reduce CT doses by a factor of two or so, especially for children. But, as with just about everything else in imaging, it seems, there must be tradeoffs.

The average dose required for an object to be barely detectable in a slice, D_{det}, is interconnected with a number of the other imaging parameters, and we shall present without proof a simple, approximate, semi-empirical guide relating them:

$$D_{det} R^2 h \, e^{-p}/(SNR)^2 = \text{constant}. \qquad (8.5)$$

where R is the in-plane resolution in millimeters, comparable to the pixel size, and h is slice thickness, so that $R^2 h$ is roughly the voxel volume. The signal-to-noise ratio (SNR) is a primary determinant of the amount of contrast available (and/or required) for detection of a pattern in an image. And, with p serving as a typical ray-sum for the patient, then e^{-p} is a direct measure of patient size.

Equation 8.5 suggests that to reduce the level of noise by a factor of 2 while keeping the resolution and slice thickness the same, it is necessary to increase the dose fourfold. So also, when passing from the head to the body, resolution and/or signal-to-noise would have to be sacrificed to maintain the same skin exposure and slice thickness. Likewise, to

improve the in-plane resolution by a factor of 2 with no increase in dose or loss of possible contrast, one could switch from a slice thickness of 2 mm to one of 16 mm, assuming no problematic loss of resolution because of partial volume or other effects.

Image post-processing

A tomographic approach like CT, MRI, SPECT, or PET allows creation of truly three-dimensional images; adoption of a full *3D platform*, as well, provides a variety of tools with which to manipulate and display them. One can rotate a 3D rendering for a surface or interior view, carve away and discard parts that are in the way or just not of interest, enhance certain aspects of their appearance, and much more, as discussed in Chapter 6.

Such *multi-planar volumetric reconstruction* (*MPVR*) and *multi-planar reformation* or *reformatting* (*MPR*) preserve anatomic distances and characteristics accurately, making possible precise 3D measurements. (Note that the meaning of "reconstruction" in this context is quite different from that in "FBP reconstruction", etc.) MPR, the simpler of these, stacks together adjacent transverse images (Figure 1.13a), and from that assemblage generates sagittal, coronal, and other thin planes, or even radiograph-like views (e.g., for radiotherapy treatment planning purposes).

Surface rendering allows the viewer to see the overall surface of a three-dimensional structure, by cutting away over- or outer-lying tissues at boundaries where the attenuation coefficient changes abruptly (Figure 1.14c). In many situations the distinctions between tissues is clear enough for this *segmentation* process to be carried out automatically. This is of particular interest for individual bones, which may be taken apart at the level of joints since the tissues between them have much lower HU values.

Maximum intensity projection (MIP) post-processing provides a planar transmission view, like that of an ordinary X-ray, with a somewhat unnatural but useful quality that helps with certain visualization tasks. Imagine a body partitioned into a 3D matrix of cubic voxels, with an associated 2D matrix of pixels directly above it, for a vertical view. Let us establish a regular array of hypothetical parallel geometric "rays" passing downward through the body, one starting out in each pixel. The MIP steps along every such ray, passing through the numerous voxels it skewers, and selects out the one with the highest HU value; it uses only that voxel (rather than the sum over all those along the ray) to set the gray-scale value of the corresponding pixel. It is used commonly with PET and magnetic resonance angiography (MRA), and increasingly so with CT. MIP is used effectively for the vascular system with a bolus intravenous injection of iodinated contrast medium (Figure 8.17). The downside is that by choosing the maximum density value, minute variations that could be seen with standard volume imaging and might be of clinical interest are lost.

Contrast enhancement

Today's high-speed multi-slice scanners can reveal much more than just anatomic information. A computer-controlled power injector enables the examiner not only to observe flow pattern through different vessels at the level of an organ, but also to follow the time-dependent *perfusion* of the tissue. Now that scanners can acquire full information on a region in under 10 seconds, we can obtain images of a structure or organ at different *phases* of enhancement by the contrast medium, simply by rapidly repeating CT acquisitions. It is possible to image an organ or tissue as the contrast arrives within the feeding artery, as it progressively enhances the organ's parenchyma, and as it leaves. Such *enhancement* and *wash-out* patterns can be pathognomonic in the diagnosis of numerous disease processes.

Overall *enhancement*, the increase in optical density due to the presence of iodine, depends on the total amount of iodine injected (measured in milligrams of iodine) and on the concentration of iodine within the injected contrast solution. Although the two are intimately interconnected, each primarily affects a separate portion of a dynamic CT examination. When evaluating the early *arterial phase*, the objective is to fully opacify the luminal components, to highlight the arteries and the distribution of smaller vessels within an organ (Figures 8.18a, Figure 8.19a,b). Since the blood in these vessels is a suspension of cells in liquid plasma, this phase will primarily be affected by the iodine concentration within them; and that, in turn, is largely controlled by the initial concentration of the contrast medium and by the rate of injection. Power injectors can administer the con-

trast at rates of about 5 mL/s, with iodine contrast agent at concentrations of 320–370 mg/mL. This gives adequate opacification of vessels for diagnostic CT-angiography (CTA) studies.

Contrast enhancement in the subsequent *parenchymal phase*, on the other hand, depends on numerous factors, including focal neovascularization and vascular dilatation; disruption of flow patterns through these vessels; and irregularities in vessel wall permeability that enable the contrast medium to pass into the extracellular perivascular space (Figure 8.18b,c, Figure 8.19c). Here, the primary factor affecting the degree of parenchymal enhancement will be the total quantity of iodine administered. This is strongly affected by the total volume of contrast injected, but not by the rate of injection. Specific protocols will then enable optimal visualization of target organs and tissues during different times of enhancement, to improve the diagnostic quality of the examination. These protocols will not only control the slice thickness and pitch of the acquisition but also the type of contrast, rate of injection, and timing of the acquisition.

Similarly, other imaging modalities are using multi-phase acquisitions to provide functional information along with the more basic anatomic details. Fast MRI sequences employ gadolinium compounds as enhancement agents, and bone SPECT scintigraphic studies can be evaluated during early vascular and tissue phases, demonstrating increased local blood flow and abnormal vessel wall permeability, observed with inflammatory or infectious processes such as osteitis.

Cardiac CT

Cardiac CT is technically challenging, and there are variations from site to site in how it is carried out. Rather than attempting to cover the field, even lightly, instead we shall consider briefly how a few of the standard cardiac CT and *calcium scoring* procedures are commonly performed.

When a patient presents with acute typical chest pain with positive EKG changes and/or positive enzymes (troponin or CK-MB), indications of advanced coronary artery disease and impending or evolving infarction, he or she will go directly to coronary angiography for intervention with stents or angioplasty (PTCA) (see the Appendix to Chapter 1). In a modern clinic, cardiac catheterization

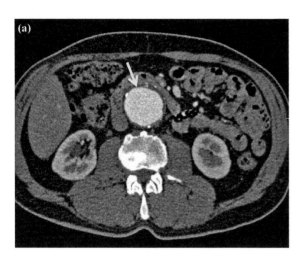
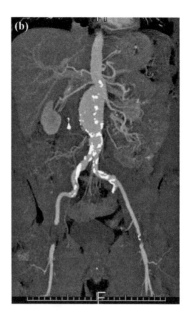
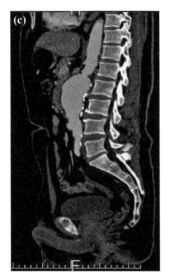
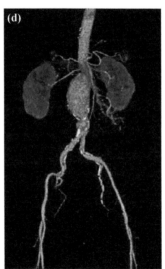
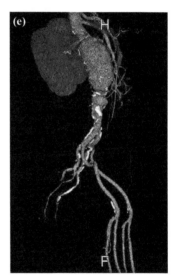

Figure 8.17 A patient presented with abdominal pain. Physical examination demonstrated the presence of a palpable abdominal mass that was pulsatile, suggesting an abdominal aortic aneurysm (AAA). Iodinated contrast medium, injected into a peripheral vein in bolus fashion, opacified the intravascular compartment, and a spiral CT acquisition of the abdomen and pelvis was performed. (**a**) An axial image of the abdomen through the AAA revealed the markedly enlarged, fusiform abdominal aorta (arrow). (**b**) Several modes of 3D presentation are particularly helpful for visualizing the entire abdominal aorta, and they can assist in planning some surgical or endovascular intervention. Here MIP provides a clear view of the lumen of the aorta in the coronal plane, and of the mural calcifications (in white) of the abdominal aorta associated with atheromatous changes. A thick plane of reconstruction has led to a more three-dimensional rendition of the vessel. (**c**) This view of the AAA was created by digitally manipulating a stack of closely spaced axial/transverse slices created from the spiral run data and then viewing from a sagittal perspective. All structures appear as they did in the initial axial images but with a different viewpoint. With isotropic voxels, any measurements will be as precise as in the original axial reconstructions. (**d**) Coronal and (**e**) sagittal (or any other) views of a three-dimensional surface rendering of the AAA reveal the overall external configuration of the lumen of the abdominal aorta and of other areas of enhancement. The kidneys appear in darker red; such color shading can represent different degrees of enhancement or optical density.

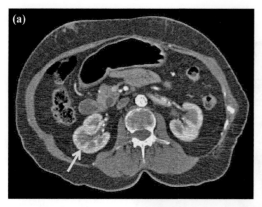
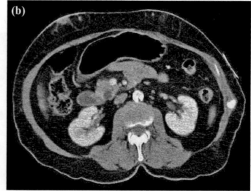
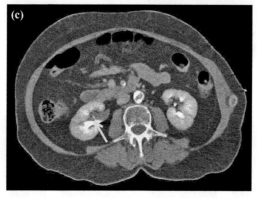

Figure 8.18 Spiral contrast-enhanced CT at the level of the kidneys. The overall enhancement pattern of the renal parenchyma and the actual excretion of the iodinated contrast medium into the renal pelvis and ureters provides functional information. (**a**) In the early *arterial phase*, the contrast follows the arterial blood supply to the kidneys, and enhancement appears immediately in the periphery of the renal cortex, the area containing the glomeruli (arrow). (**b**) In the *parenchymal phase* some 20 seconds later, the remainder of the renal parenchyma also enhances, resulting in a homogeneous density throughout. There is still no significant excretion of the iodinated contrast medium. (**c**) In an image performed 1 to 2 minutes after its injection, the contrast is pooling within the proximal renal excretory tracts (arrow).

is carried out with biplanar digital fluoroscopy, where two views at right angles can be shown simultaneously (Figure 7.9). A pair of perpendicularly aligned X-ray tubes face into two independent AMFPI image receptors. With rapid intermittent pulsing of the two tubes, a bolus of contrast agent flowing into and through a coronary artery can be followed. The motion of the bolus can be freeze-framed or played continuously in slow motion, but it is generally agreed that diastole images are best suited for the assessment of stenosis. This is so partly because much less motion blur arises during relaxation of the myocardium; also, as the heart muscle relaxes, there is less extrinsic compression of the coronary arteries, allowing for more coronary blood flow.

The common complaint of acute chest pain in a patient with low-to-moderate risk factors for coronary artery disease, but with no personal history of heart disease and no abnormal EKG findings or enzyme elevations, poses something of a diagnostic dilemma. Current management usually consists at least of admission for observation with a 24-hour rule-out with serial EKGs and enzyme levels.

With equivocal results, discharge could be premature, but going straight to cardiac catheterization might be overly zealous. This patient would be an excellent candidate, rather, for non-invasive *CT cardiac angiography* (CTA) to evaluate coronary anatomy (Figures 8.20).

Chest CT and CTA can also be combined for the "triple-rule-out" of coronary syndrome,

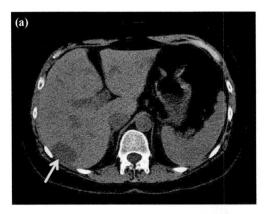
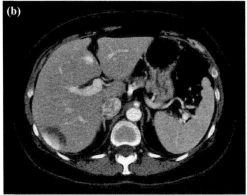
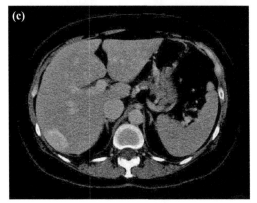

Figure 8.19 Spiral multi-phase CT examination of the liver, in an attempt to complete the evaluation of a lesion seen on a routine ultrasound study. Certain lesions can present typical enhancement patterns under CT that enable a specific diagnosis without need for further studies or for intervention such as a biopsy. (**a**) Initial non-contrast CT demonstrating the liver parenchyma with the presence of a hypodense lesion of the posterior portion of the right lobe (arrow). (**b**) Early in the *arterial phase*, as the contrast bolus first arrives to the liver, there is peripheral enhancement with pooling at the level of the lesion. (**c**) In the *parenchymal phase* or, in this case, the *portal venous phase*, performed about 45–60 seconds after administration of contrast agent, it has extended centrally into the lesion (in centripetal fashion) and now fills all of it homogeneously. This phase occurs after the contrast has gone through the bowel and opacifies the mesenteric veins that drain into the portal vein. The portal venous phase is observed specifically in the liver and represents a type of parenchymal phase, where the contrast uniformly fills the hepatic parenchyma from both arterial and venous directions. The displayed enhancement pattern is typical of a hemangioma, a benign lesion commonly found in the liver that has no significant chance of degenerating or of causing symptoms in the near future. This CT study enabled the radiologist to give a high enough degree of diagnostic certainty to obviate the need for further analysis.

pulmonary embolus, and aortic disease such as dissections and aneurysms by simply performing two separate spiral CT acquisitions during a single examination. The clinical efficacy and ultimate utility of such a triple rule-out is a hot topic of debate in clinical circles. It may offer an expedient modality in clinically ambiguous situations of chest pain, but there is significant potential for overuse and diagnostic overreliance on such a test. The amount of contrast required is significant, the radiation expo-

sure risk must be considered, and the information available from a triple rule-out must be viewed with judicious foresight, rather than from a stance of convenience.

Calcium scoring (assessing the amount of soft and calcified plaque lining the aorta and/or the coronary arteries) can also be performed as a stand-alone CT procedure or combined with other studies such as CTA. The CT-based calcium score is most useful as an outpatient screening test for cardiac disease

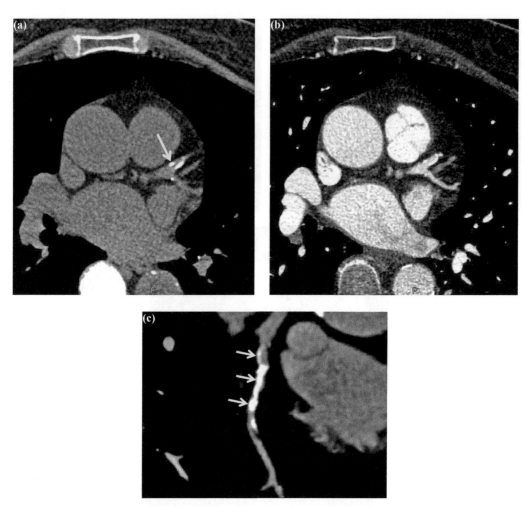

Figure 8.20 Many patients presenting with symptoms compatible with cardiac angina do not have to undergo selective coronary arteriography, with its relatively high risk to the individual and cost. Instead, the patient may undergo CT coronary angiography. With the heart rate decreased pharmacologically, if needed, spiral CT acquisition can be gated (synchronized) to the heart rhythm, which makes it possible to obtain "frozen" views of cardiac structures. This can give very precise images of an enhanced coronary artery lumen, in which vessel wall anomalies such as plaques and extra-vascular anatomic changes can be clearly visualized – something that is often not possible during angiographic examinations. (a) Conventional axial image of the heart during a gated CT study without contrast enhancement, revealing the coronary arteries and the presence of calcified plaques at the level of the left anterior descending (LAD) coronary artery (arrow). (b) After the peripheral intravenous administration of a bolus of iodinated contrast media, the same images are obtained with isotropic voxels for optimal 3D display of the same coronary arteries. (c) With post-processing, the LAD coronary artery can be flattened into a 2D plane (curved planar reformatting), so that its entire length can be analyzed in a single plane of view. This image displays the length of extension of the calcified atheromatous plaque, starting at the origin of the LAD (arrows).

in patients with risk factors but who present with only vague symptomatology. No CT iodine-based contrast agent is employed.

With the gantry rotating through 360° every $\frac{1}{3}$ second, but with a need to acquire data over only 180°, it is possible for a multi-slice machine to gather enough data for a reconstruction in $\frac{1}{6}$ second = 167 ms with a single X-ray source. A state-of-the-art *dual-source* cardiac CT device, like a high-end cardiac catheterization system, employs two identical X-ray sources, aligned at right angles to one another. Two (non-identical, for reasons of space) banks of 64 partial-belts of detectors on opposite sides of the gantry face them. With the two sources rapidly pulsing intermittently and both generating data, the time needed is only $\frac{1}{3} \times \frac{1}{2} \times \frac{1}{2} = \frac{1}{12}$ second = 80 ms. With this short period of data collection gated with an electrocardiogram, and for a sufficiently slow heart rate, the system can virtually freeze cardiac motion over a good part of the heart, and cover the entire heart in one breath-hold. This is possible around the time of diastole even with fairly high heart rates. The sub-millimeter spatial resolution, moreover, is sufficient to examine small and complex structures such as small calcified and non-calcified plaques in the coronary arteries.

A dual-source system can also be used for a totally different purpose, to provide information on the chemical makeup of tissues being imaged, not only on their anatomy. The two tubes might pulse rapidly, but each at a different kVp, and the detectors might be of a type that can resolve energies. The topic of dual- (or multiple-) energy imaging in general was discussed in Chapter 7.

Cardiac imaging is generally *electrocardiogram-gated*, and this is carried out in two ways, the retrospective and the prospective, for different applications. *Retrospective* ECG-gated CT scans are commonly helical, with the X-ray tube left on throughout the period of gantry rotation. The R-wave provides timing for stitching together parts of the composite image with proper phasing. *Prospective* scanning is typically sequential axial, with the table advancing a short distance while the beam is off, during every other heartbeat. The tube is on only for a relatively short time, beginning after some offset time following the R-wave. There is therefore less patient dose and, since no spiral interpolation is required, the images may be clearer. There are variations on these themes, such as *multi-segment* scanning, which can achieve much shorter temporal resolution by imaging the same segment multiple times while varying the timing.

For a study of the cardiothoracic anatomy of a non-obese patient over 45 with normal and regular heart-rate, the complete examination might consist of a calcium scoring study first, and then the CTA. The CTA is typically prospective sequential at 120 kVp and 150 mA-s per rotation, with contrast agent and a breath-hold. The top 4 cm of the heart (the standard width of the fan-beam at isocenter for a 64-slice machine) are scanned first. The ECG-gating system starts its timer at the R-wave, and ensures that the beams fire only over an 80 ms interval at diastole. The table then shifts 4 cm along the z-axis during the next heartbeat, and is ready to scan again, 4 cm lower, over the next cycle.

For obese patients or those with fast or irregular heartbeat, ECG-gated retrospective spiral scanning is preferable, despite the somewhat higher dose. The X-ray tube is left on continuously as the table moves, and the ECG's R-wave provides the timing necessary for data manipulation

While CTA may not fully replace cardiac catheterization in the near future, it is highly effective at determining the absence of coronary artery disease, although not so much so at confirming its presence. It is a test with a negative predictive value over 90%, so a negative result is a good sign of a need to look elsewhere for possible causes of chest symptoms. A positive result, however, may call for a cardiac catheterization follow-up study with planned intervention.

Patient- and machine-caused artifacts

CT images display various kinds of characteristic artifacts, and several of them have already been mentioned, like the partial volume effect and the blur from differential magnification (Figure 8.16). Artifacts can arise because of issues related to the patient or to the machinery.

Patient-related artifacts
Aberrations arise at the interfaces of materials of significantly different radiological properties within the body. Surgical clips and other metallic objects, in particular, will lead to *star artifacts* (Figure 1.12d and 8.21a), as may pockets of bowel gas.

The direction of entry of X-rays into an object can have a significant effect on its apparent dimensions, as with this dependence of cranial wall thickness on axial position of the transverse slice (Figures 8.21b).

Patient motion may be somewhat controllable (breathing, coughing, squirming) or totally involuntary (cardiac and GI tract). Either way, motion during a scan can lead to loss of resolution and sometimes to streak artifacts (Figure 8.21c,), as the reconstruction algorithm tries to assemble an image

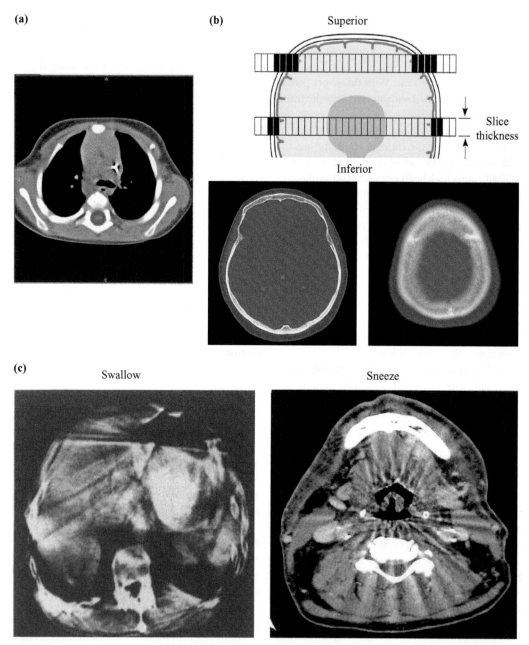

Figure 8.21 CT artifacts. (**a**) A central line catheter made of or containing high-Z (atomic number) materials, causing a high number of photoelectric events to take place. The reconstruction algorithm may have difficulties at the resulting abrupt spatial disconnects in attenuation coefficient at a tissue interface, giving rise to star artifacts, sometimes also occurring adjacent to areas of signal void, such as from a gas pocket. (**b**) The skull appears to thicken as transverse slices are taken in increasingly superior positions. (**c**) Motion artifacts from a swallow and a sneeze come about because data obtained at slightly different times during a scan are mutually inconsistent. (**d**) These streaks are caused by differential hardening of the beam as it progresses through different amounts of high-density and high-Z materials (bone) at different angles, again giving rise to incompatibilities in the data obtained at different beam angles. (**e**) A defective detector in a scanner of third-generation design, such as in any multi-slice helical device, will generate in a characteristic dark ring centered on the gantry's axis of rotation. Modified from Cody *et al.* [2], figs 4-3 and 4-13.

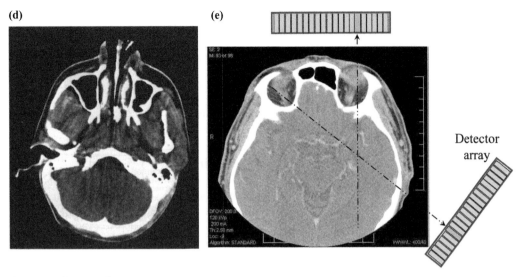

Figure 8.21 *(Continued)*

out of inconsistent data. Problems may be caused by respiration or even peristalsis, when there is bowel gas. Solutions include instructing the patients to hold their breath and remain still, the application of immobilization devices, antiperistaltic drugs, and sedation, but most important of all has been the advent of faster scanners. In addition, there are cardiac and respiratory gating systems that allow the X-ray tube to fire only when the motion is acceptably small.

Machine artifacts

An X-ray beam is polychromatic. Even after filtering, the remaining lower-energy photons interact with matter as a beam enters tissue, and are attenuated more readily than are those of higher energies. As the beam penetrates further, the effective attenuation coefficient for a tissue continues to decrease because of this *beam hardening*, so that its value depends somewhat on its position in the body (Figure 8.21f). This effect can easily lead to 10-HU non-uniformities in the image of even a homogeneous tissue, and it can be especially troublesome in the head because of the high calcium content of the skull. Thick copper beam filters and mathematical beam-hardening corrections of the data (based on measured beam hardening in phantoms) can greatly reduce the impact of such artifacts.

One problem with third-generation scanners, hence with multi-slice machines (which are built with a third-generation architecture), is *ring artifacts* (Figure 8.21g). When the response of one detector differs significantly from those of the others, either because it became defective or just drifted slowly, all the ray-sums that it picks up will be irregularly large or small. The effect of this detector imbalance on an image is the appearance of a ring artifact, whose diameter depends on the position of the detector in the array. It was partly to remedy this nuisance that the fourth-generation scanner was designed.

Finally, image quality is generally excellent with multi-row scanners, and artifacts appear rarely, especially in helical scan mode. But when the device is operating in axial mode, if the detectors are partitioned into K bins/channels and one of them is somehow defective, then a characteristic artifact may arise – and it will repeat in every Kth slice in the series of images (i.e., every 8th image for 8-channel scanning).

Dose and QA

Determination of doses is of central importance in CT for two reasons. CT is the largest medical contributor of collective dose to the patient population, so dose to the patient must be as low as reasonably achievable, both to avoid deterministic health effects completely and to minimize the risk of stochastic harm. At the same time, irradiation of the image receptor (hence dose to the patient) must be sufficient for the formation of a diagnostically adequate result. It can be difficult to achieve an optimal balance in this tradeoff for any modality, or even to know how to carry it out. This is especially true with CT, where assessing and reporting doses is a complex matter and, in any case, doses tend to be relatively high, especially to children, and often unnecessarily so.

Many imaging physicians make a serious attempt to select optimal study- and patient-specific protocols — those sets of operational settings and parameters that will provide adequate images but minimize the overall dose and risk. But CT invariably results in very non-uniform irradiation of a variety of organs with different radiosensitivities, so what, exactly, does "overall" dose mean?

The closest thing we have to an answer at present is the *effective dose* (ED) of Equations 5.4. ED = $\Sigma w_T D_T$, where D_T is the local tissue dose, w_T is a stochastic risk-weighting factor that accounts for the relative radiosensitivity of tissue T, and the sigma indicates summation over T. The overall risk from a CT exposure may then be estimated from $Risk = 0.05 \; (\text{Sv}^{-1}) \times ED \; (\text{Sv})$. Bear in mind that built into the ED is the important fundamental LN-T assumption, that stochastic risk in each voxel is linearly proportional to the gamma- and/or X-ray dose. It is because of the adoption of this ED formalism (which uses sieverts rather than grays, because general radiation safety must sometimes account also for irradiation by high-LET particles), incidentally, that clinical CT doses are commonly expressed in terms of the numerically equivalent (for gamma- and X-rays) units of Sv.

ED is pretty much the only game in town for radiogenic stochastic risk assessment, for now. Some CT machines display a crude estimate of ED, which they arrive at through a three-part computation. First, they calculate a so-called *CT dose index* (CTDI) for the given technique factors chosen for the current patient, where the CTDI is a *patient-independent* measure of machine output for the given set of technique factors, etc. They then multiply this number by the length of the region irradiated, L, to obtain a *dose-length product* (DLP).

And finally, another conversion factor, κ obtained from Monte Carlo (numerical, statistical) calculations based on a generic patient, transforms the DLP into an estimate of ED.

$$ED = CTDI_{vol}(\text{kVp, etc.}) \times L \times \kappa. \quad (8.6a)$$

The first link in this somewhat rusty chain is the CTDI:

CT dose index

The CTDI is an index of the *X-ray output* of a CT machine. Earlier on, the *multiple scan average dose (MSAD)* was defined to be the average dose within a specially designed, plastic phantom resulting from multiple adjacent axial exposures. Carrying out the measurements was laborious, and the CTDI was invented to give the same result with a single axial slice. This is all a little technical in the details, so we'll present a simplified sketch here. It is described fully by the American College of Radiology (ACR), which demands its application in a certification process that is becoming required for radiology departments, imaging centers, and others to obtain reimbursement.

The starting point is the dose profile from a single narrow axial (transverse, non-helical) study of the FDA-designed CTDI phantom, which is an acrylic cylinder 15 cm long (Figure 8.22). The head and body phantoms are 16 cm and 32 cm in diameter, respectively, and both contain 5 longitudinal holes for a calibrated 100-mm-long "pencil" ion chamber — one in the center and four others 90° apart near the periphery.

The distribution of dose being deposited in the phantom at any instant depends on the beam angle (Figure 8.23a), but the *dose profile* describes the dose averaged along the central axis from a full rotation of the gantry (Figure 8.23b). One might have expected the CT profile to be rectangular, but two factors combine to reduce it to a bell-shape. The finite size of the focal spot causes a small amount of penumbra blurring at the edges of the primary beam, but usually far more important is Compton scatter within the phantom or patient. With 10 adjacent 10 mm scans, or 1 that is 100 mm wide, or 10 helical rotations of a 10 mm beam with a pitch of 1, the amount of primary, unscattered beam is the same as for a single slice, but the overall scatter radiation piles up and grows with scan width (Figure 8.23c).

Near the center of a band of slices, the dose is fairly uniform, with a little ripple, and its average value is the MSAD (Figure 8.23d). Because of the scatter contributions from the other slices, the MSAD can be considerably greater than the peak

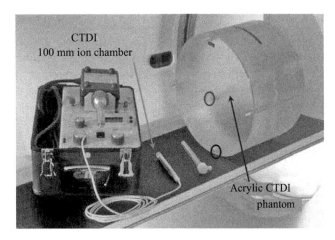

Figure 8.22 CTDI dosimetry. A 100-mm pencil ion chamber attached to its electrometer, along with the standard CTDI head phantom; the central and one of the four peripheral ion-chamber holes are indicated. Reproduced from TG Flohr, DD Cody, CH McCullough, Computed tomography. In: Wolbarst AB, Zamenhof RG, Hendee WR (eds), *Advances in Medical Physics*, vol. 1. Madison WI: Medical Physics Publishing, 2006, fig. 3-34.

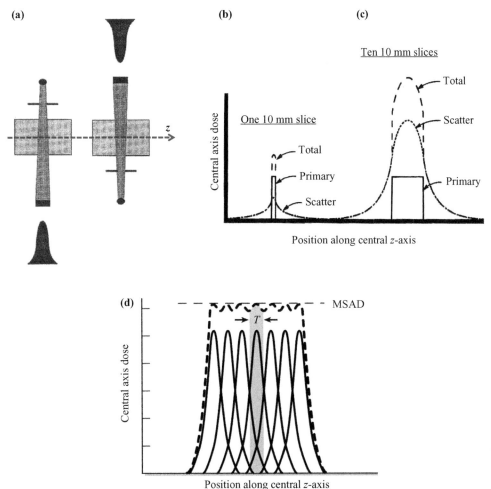

Figure 8.23 The slice sensitivity profile. (a) The point spread function (Figure 4.14a), in effect, of a single non-helical slice plane perpendicular to the central axis of rotation is made up of contributions from all gantry angles, two of which are shown. (b) The dose from the primary, unscattered beam is the same for a single 10 mm slice as for (c) 10 contiguous 10-mm slices. Because of overlap of the scatter component, however, the total dose in the central portion of a multi-slice scan is considerably higher. (d) The *multiple scan average dose* (*MSAD*) from seven (in this case) adjacent scans each of width T (not to be confused with T = tissue), or from seven rotations of a helical scan with pitch = 1.

dose from one alone. FDA staff developed the CTDI method as a quick way to obtain essentially the same information as the more cumbersome MSAD (21 CFR 1020.33).

When exposed to a single, narrow-beam 360° scan of width W mm within the CTDI phantom, the dose along the ion chamber varies as $D(z)$. The FDA defined the $CTDI_{100}$ as the integral dose recorded by the chamber over its entire 100 mm length,

$$CTDI_{100} = \int D(z)dz \Big/ 100. \qquad (8.6b)$$

which it showed to be essentially the same as the MSAD. FDA also demonstrated that the $CTDI_{100}$ can be *measured* (quite a different thing!) simply as

$$CTDI_{100} = k_{cal} \times Q_{meas} \times (100/W), \qquad (8.6c)$$

where Q_{meas} is the charge accumulated by the ion chamber for one rotation, and k_{cal} is its charge-to-dose calibration factor (which itself must be re-assessed periodically at a regional calibration center). The effect of the width of the beam is removed, and the measurement is normalized, by the factor of W in the denominator. The ion chamber is calibrated to provide an output dose in *air*, incidentally, not in the acrylic phantom. When considering people, yet another conversion factor is needed.

$CTDI_{100}$ is measured with the ion chamber in the central hole and in one or more of the peripheral ones. A weighted average of these readings defines $CTDI_w$. Another modification accounts for pitch in a real clinical helical scan, leading to the final CTDI result, $CTDI_{vol}$.

The $CTDI_{vol}$ does not, however, reflect the total ionizing energy deposited into the scan volume which, ultimately, is what is presumed to correlate with stochastic risk. Its value

remains unchanged whether 1 cm or 100 cm of patient anatomy is exposed. To better represent the overall risk for a real clinical study, the dose can be integrated along the scan length to compute the *dose-length product* (*DLP*), approximated as the product DLP (mSv-cm) = $CTDI_{vol}$ (mSv) × length (cm).

Based on Monte Carlo statistical calculations, the ACR and others devised a procedure to transform the DLP into a crude estimate of effective dose; in practice, this involves simply multiplying the DPL by one of two constants, $\kappa = 0.002$ for the head and 0.015 for the abdomen: $ED = \kappa$ DLP. The method of conversion from DLP to ED (Equation 8.6a), is clearly adopted for convenience and extreme simplicity, not for accuracy.

Problem: a patient with a very large but healthy liver, say, might require a scan twice as long as normal; and with normal technique factors, the CTDI calculation for effective dose would result in twice the amount as for someone with a small liver. This is the opposite of what Equations 5.4 suggest, however, namely that with the same D_T, any liver taken to the same dose contributes the same amount to the ED.

Typical values for the calculated effective doses of many CT protocols are 1–2 mSv for a head examination, 5–7 mSv for the chest, and 8–11 mSv for the abdomen or pelvis (Tables 8.2 and 5.4). The $CTDI_{vol}$ for a scan is a poor measure of patient dose, but does offer a reproducible measure of device output, and it may be useful in the inter-comparison and improvement of CT parameter-setting protocols. Also, it is central to the ACR CT accreditation process, which is concerned primarily with machine output. The table also shows the ACR's pass-fail levels for measurements on the CTDI phantom.

Table 8.2 Representative $CTDI_{vol}$ values for common CT protocols, at 120 kVp, pitch = 1, and representative values of mA-s per revolution. ACR has listed pass-fail limits for three of them. The length and $CTDI_{vol}$ together give the dose-length product (DPL) which, in turn, leads to a crude estimate of the effective dose. The pediatric patient is 5 years old.

	mA-s rotation^{-1}	$CTDI_{vol}$ (mGy)	ACR[a] pass (mGy)	L (cm)	ED[b] (mSv)
Head	350	60	<80	10	1–2
Chest	140	10	–	30	5–7
(chest X-ray)					(0.01)
Abdomen	150	12	<30	30–35	5–7
Pediatric abdomen (5 yr)	90		<25	20–25	
Pelvis	160	20	–	20–25	3–4
Coronary artery Ca score	150	10	–	–	1–5
Coronary CTA	380	20–30	–	8–13	5–15

[a] ACR: www.acr.org/Quality-Safety/accreditation/CT

[b] AAPM Report 96: www.aapm.org/pubs/reports.

Many new CT scanners display the CTDI on the operator console for the scan of a real patient, presumably as a radiation protection measure. This might be viewed as something of a red herring, however, since the CTDI does not involve any measurements of patient dimensions or anatomy, which strongly influence any dose distribution. Once again: the CTDI for a given set of techniques factors is a measure only of *dose to the CTDI phantom*, not to a human. That is, it is a measure primarily of *machine output*, and definitely not of *patient dose*, unless, of course, the patient is 15 cm long and made of plastic. Over time, this inconsistency hopefully will be resolved [1].

Dose reduction strategies, especially for children

Reduction of CT doses, especially for children, has been one of the hottest topics of discussion in imaging for several years, and appropriately so. The growing realization that clinically adequate images can be obtained with much lower than current exposure levels is driving the development of improved technologies and the re-examination of long-accepted protocols, and it is even helping to modify physician and technologist behavior in a positive manner. And all of these good things are happening with little increase in cost or time.

Much of the improvement is occurring because of a growing *awareness* of the need for it, and of what can be done to make things better. Programs like Image Gently (www.pedrad.org/associations/5364/ig) (Figure 5.7b), established by the ACR, the American Association of Physicists in Medicine (AAPM) and others, and recommendations by the FDA (www.fda.gov/medical devices/safety/alertsandnotices/ucm185898.htm), are helping to make physicians aware of reports that as many as 30% of CT examinations of children are medically not necessary, or could be carried out with modalities with no ionizing radiation (US, MRI) or much less (DR). Partly in response to these efforts, some physicians are ordering fewer of them; they are reducing the numbers of non-essential multi-phase studies, moreover, which involve multiple images within one exam. Likewise, they are making efforts not to scan outside of the region of interest, and not to generate redundant information from overlapping scans. And perhaps most important, they are ensuring that the scanning parameters used are appropriate for kids.

Many CT *protocols* for specific types of studies are site- and even physician-specific, and clearly not all of them can be optimal, especially for imaging neonates and children. An effective way for a facility to reduce dose is to undertake a comprehensive comparison of its own protocols, and to consider those employed at other facilities for the same machine type. Dose reductions of up to 50%, still with adequate image quality, have been reported simply from a change of kVp. With conscious support from the radiographers, one can try to go beyond that with a little trial and error: Reduce the mA-s/rotation for a study by perhaps 10% and, if everyone is still satisfied with the images, do it again – another example of iteration.

The moral of this story, if you will forgive a little preaching, is four-fold:

If another diagnostic modality can obtain the needed information without exposing the young patient and the staff to ionizing radiation or incurring excessive cost or delay, then select it.

Consider the overall clinical impact of a study. If the information from a CT procedure is not likely to change the patient treatment or follow-up significantly, no matter what it might demonstrate, then do not perform it.

If you do image with CT, fit the scanning parameters to the patient's body shape, size, and even age. Also, be willing to tolerate images that may have some degree of noise so long as the study can deliver all of what is needed.

Encourage your organization to re-appraise the benefit-dose tradeoff of the current scanning protocols.

The Radiological Society of North America (RSNA), ACR, AAPM and other national organizations have recently begun actively collaborating in re-examining the numerous and inter-dependent scanning parameters (kVp, mA-s/rotation, pitch, slice thickness, etc.) for specific studies and body types, and they have already made available several suggested new protocols (www.aapm.org/pubs/CTProtocols). This is the start of what will be a work-in-progress for a considerable time, but one already of great value. In the meanwhile, *technique charts* have been published listing ways to modify current operator settings for adults so as to make them suitable for children of different ages and/or weights — which is fine as long as the adult protocols were good in the first place.

CT vendors now incorporate various forms of *automatic exposure control* circuits, similar in concept to the AECs in screen-film and digital radiography. A system begins typically with a preliminary low-dose *scout* view along the patient with the gantry (and tube) angle fixed. It then might employ this information, and/or various assumptions about body shape and contents, to modulate X-ray tube current (mA) at any instant to maintain, say, a *constant noise* level (Figure 8.24). That is, as the gantry rotates and/or as the table moves, the tube current modulation circuit continuously varies the instantaneous mA in real time in an attempt to achieve acceptable, nearly uniform SNR. Tube current is increased when the beam is passing laterally through the shoulders or pelvis, for example: less radiation passes through there, and the beam intensity must be increased to maintain adequate average exposure of the detectors. There are variations on this theme, such as some involving control of the kVp, others to reduce exposure of the female breast, etc. Another possibility is to sculpt the edge of the beam at the end of the region of clinical interest, cutting down on *over-ranging*, the irradiation of tissues outside it.

Available on some of the newer CT units, *fluoroscopic CT* offers quite different an approach to dose reduction, by adopting a current (mA) that is much lower than normal as the gantry rotates. The interventionalist can use fluoroscopic CT to guide and follow the progression of a biopsy needle or of a drainage catheter in real-time, or perform other procedures that do not require highest image quality, but with significantly reduced dose (Figure 8.25).

Finally, there may be benefit for the radiology information system (RIS) to search a patient's electronic record to track and display the prior cumulative dose. This should have no effect if a new study is clinically called for, but it would provide a regular reminder to think again about the need for another exam.

Quality assurance

Despite its obvious importance, there is not a great deal of guidance available on CT QA [2].

Vendors commonly will provide a handbook of recommended QA activities and, if under contract,

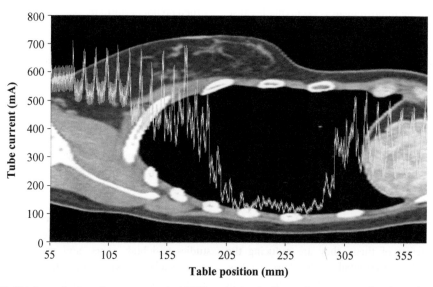

Figure 8.24 This form of automatic exposure control (AEC) modulates the X-ray tube current continually, as the tube circles the patient and as the table moves forward, in an effort to maintain a uniform signal-to-noise ratio throughout. Reproduced from Michael F McNitt-Gray. CT doses. In: Wolbarst AB, Mossman KL, Hendee WR (eds), *Advances in Medical Physics*, vol. 2. Madison, WI: Medical Physics Publishing, 2008, fig. 5-2.

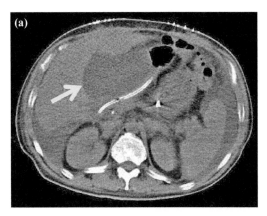
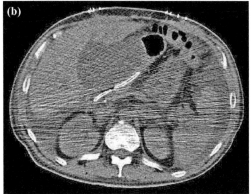
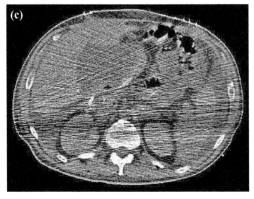

Figure 8.25 Fluoroscopic CT. (**a**) An unenhanced CT acquisition of the abdomen at the level of the liver, performed with a conventional spiral CT at 200 mA-s per rotation. A complex fluid collection in the more posterior portion of the left lobe of the liver has an overall optical density lower than that of the hepatic parenchyma, and thus appears a darker shade of gray (arrow). This requires percutaneous drainage, which was performed under fluoro-CT guidance. (**b,c**) Fluoro-CT images at the same level at 85 and 50 mA-s respectively; lower exposures and the resulting greater noise will lead to a progressively more granular appearance. If the image degradation is too great, the contours of the target lesion become difficult to delineate; this can lead to longer fluoro-CT acquisition times that increase the dose deposition to levels that are even higher than those from conventional CT.

they also carry out routine preventative maintenance. PM engineers are very knowledgeable about keeping the scanner running, and capable of reviving it when it needs a little tender care, but they are generally not trained in assessing image quality or dealing with dose and radiation safety issues.

Most daily, weekly, and monthly QA activities are commonly undertaken by CT technologists, while semi-annual and annual QA is the domain of a qualified medical physicist who has had specialized training and also experience on the machine. The entire QA program and remediation actions are typically the responsibility of the chief physicist, who reports directly to the chief physician of the imaging department.

QA for CT equipment in the United States is regulated primarily by state governments. A few states, including Minnesota, New Jersey, and New York, have written detailed state-specific guidelines and regulations for QA testing. Similarly, the Conference of [state] Radiation Control Program Directors (CRCPD) has prepared a set of Suggested State Regulations for the Control of Radiation (SSRCR). In addition, several national and international organizations offer general QA guidelines, including the AAPM, the European Commission, and the British Institute of Physics and Engineering in Medicine (IPEM).

It is the ACR CT Accreditation Program requirements, however, that now serve as the gold QA standard (www.acr.org/Quality-Safety/accreditation/CT). For reimbursement, some (and soon all) facilities must undergo formal and extensive accreditation testing of the equipment for CT, mammography, MRI, nuclear medicine and PET, ultrasound, breast MRI, breast US, and stereotactic breast biopsy (with more programs coming). Because of its importance, here we shall discuss CT QA in the ACR context.

ACR accreditation every three years

The American College of Radiology has set up an accreditation program for CT and other modalities that involves the evaluation not only of the individual imaging machines at a facility, but also of all interpreting physicians, medical physicists, and technologists working with it, as was discussed in Chapter 5. It is the device that is accredited, not the entire facility, and re-accreditation is required every three years.

Preliminary paperwork to be submitted for a device covers the training, qualifications, experience, and Continuing Medical Education of staff who use it; numbers and types of protocols; the site's

physician peer-review program; results of the site's appropriateness/outcomes analysis; and a copy of the detailed routine QA manual, along with records of the results, and for the set of medical physicist's annual QA assessments. ACR does not specify details of a QA program.

There are three general categories of actual tests of a machine dealing, respectively, with sample clinical images, measurements on the highly specialized ACR CT phantom, and dose assessments with the CTDI phantom.

The first of these three requires the submission of a set of *clinical images* of various types with details of the protocols that are used routinely at the facility. These are examined by experienced radiologists who offer their services to support the ACR in this important effort. As often as not, failure to receive accreditation comes either from not following the detailed instructions precisely or from simply not making sufficient effort to do it right.

The second category of tests involves measurements on a specially designed *ACR CT phantom* (Figure 8.26). (A much simpler, water-filled phantom is adequate for most routine QA.) The

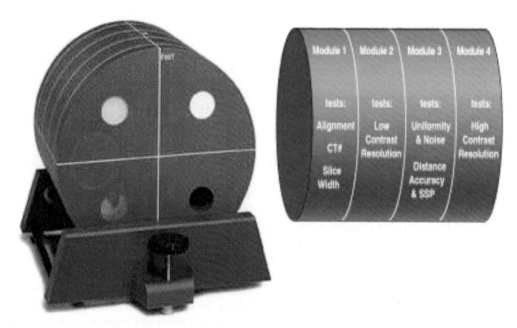

Figure 8.26 The ACR CT accreditation phantom is far more complex than what is needed for most routine QA. Its four modules serve as test materials for assessment of linearity of CT number with attenuation coefficient; patient and table positioning; slice thickness; a contrast-resolution study at low contrast; image noise and uniformity around the field of view; and high-contrast resolution. Courtesy of the Gammex Corporation.

phantom consists of four modules, which together allow for assessment of: the average HU value for pure water for a range of machine operational settings; linearity of CT number with the attenuation coefficients of a number of materials within; image uniformity and Poisson noise throughout the field of view; low-contrast resolution by way of a contrast-detail test device like that of Figure 2.15; and high-contrast resolution down to 0.4 lp/mm (which is virtually never achievable with current machines).

The third category of tests (as revised in 2008) calls for CTDI measurements for three distinct protocols. The adult head, with the small CTDI phantom, should yield a reading below the pass/fail criterion of 80 mGy (Table 8.2). For the adult abdomen protocol with the large phantom, $CTDI_{vol}$ has to be below 30 mGy. The pediatric abdomen, also with the small phantom but with the site's standard pediatric setting, must be below 25 mGy. At present there is no pediatric head phantom, and no ACR pass/fail criterion.

The ACR recognizes that parts of this are complex, and that some of their directions and instructions are not particularly perspicuous. Fortunately, the ACR staff generally go far out of their way in being helpful in resolving difficulties.

Appendix: mathematical basis of filtered back-projection

A variety of reconstruction algorithms have found application in CT, digital tomosynthesis, SPECT, PET, and elsewhere over the years. This appendix describes the one currently used most widely for CT.

It simplifies matters to approach some of them with the translate-rotate, pencil-beam geometry of Hounsfield's original first-generation machine. An X-ray tube and a radiation detector are linked rigidly together so that the detector always faces the beam; the tube and collimator produce a narrow "pencil" beam, and as the tube-collimator-detector assembly moves laterally across the body, it traces out and observes a thin slice of tissue, defining an *x-y* plane. For one *scan profile*, the system makes transmission measurements along 160 or so parallel *scan lines* or *projections*; it then rotates through an angle of perhaps one degree and repeats the process, rotates again, etc. (Figure 8.27). After viewing through 180 angles, the dataset obtained from the $180 \times 160 = 28\,800$ independent measurements is processed to *reconstruct* the unique attenuation matrix $\mu(x,y)$ for the specific spatial distribution of attenuating materials within the body that gave rise to the data.

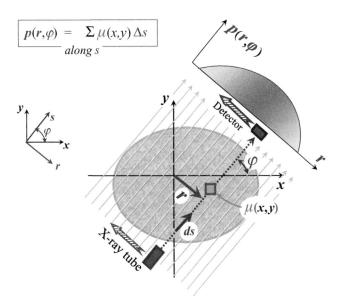

Figure 8.27 Pencil beam geometry for first-generation scanner.

The x-y coordinate system is fixed in the body. It is suitable, however, to label each of the 28 800 separate and independent projections as $p(r, \varphi)$, where φ is the angle for the projection, relative to the x-axis, and r is its perpendicular distance from the origin of the x-y coordinate system. It is an easy exercise to show that the line along which the projection is made can be expressed as

$$r = x\cos\varphi + y\sin\varphi, \qquad (8.7)$$

where the line lies along the s-direction. Thus while $\mu(x,y)$ is expressed in a conventional orthonormal coordinate system, the projections will be presented in a polar system, and we will need to hop back and forth between the two.

Each projection involves the measurement of X-ray attenuation along a single straight line through the body, defined by its r and φ, and heading in the direction of the vector ds:

$$\int e^{-\mu(x,y)\mathrm{d}s}. \qquad (8.8a)$$

It simplifies matters to take the negative of the logarithm, focusing on the exponent alone:

$$p(r, \varphi) \equiv \int \mu(x,y)\mathrm{d}s. \qquad (8.8b)$$

A more modest version of this, with attenuation along the x-axis, appeared as Equation 8.2.

The plane of tissue being viewed is partitioned into a matrix of voxels, the position of each labeled as (x,y), and the integral for a projection is replaced with a discrete summation,

$$p(r, \varphi) = \sum \mu(x,y)\Delta s. \qquad (8.8c)$$

The sum includes contributions only from the small subset of the voxels through which the (r,φ) line happens to pass. For values of φ other than integer multiples of $\pi/2$, Δs will cross voxels at an angle, so it is necessary to account for partial volume effects in the summation.

The Radon transform

There is a mathematical operator that we shall designate $\mathscr{R}$, known as the *Radon transform*, after the German mathematician who in 1917 successfully addressed the question of how to determine the structure of the interior of a body from a set of projections through it, as measured from outside.

As in Equations 8.3, $\mathscr{R}$ models the geometry (not the physics) of the projection process, in the sense that

$$\boldsymbol{p} = \mathscr{R}\mu. \qquad (8.9a)$$

This is of the same general form as Equation 8.8c, but more compact. In matrix form,

$$p_{\mathrm{j}} = \sum \mathscr{R}(r, \varphi)_{\mathrm{ij}}\mu_{\mathrm{i}}, \qquad (8.9b)$$

where $\mathscr{R}_{\mathrm{ij}}$ represents the contribution of the ith voxel to the jth projection. That is, $\mathscr{R}(r,\varphi)$ selects out those (and only those) voxels that lie along the line defined by (r,φ), namely Equation 8.7, for inclusion in a summation.

Our objective then is to solve the *inverse* problem,

$$\mu = \mathscr{R}^{-1}p, \qquad (8.10)$$

and obtain $\mu(x,y)$ from a sufficiently large set of projection data, $\{p(r,\varphi)\}$. The *algebraic* and *iterative* reconstruction approaches to this task were sketched earlier in the chapter, along with mention of *back-projection* (BP) and *filtered back-projection* (FBP). Here we describe the last of these in more detail, but we begin with the *exact solution*; it is not used in practice, but it is revealing.

The exact solution, $\mu_{\mathrm{exact}}(x,y)$

Let's begin by seeing what our target, an exact solution, $\mu_{\mathrm{exact}}(x,y)$, might look like.

Recall that a simple, one-dimensional function periodic in space can be represented by a Fourier sum of sine terms of the appropriate frequencies, phases, amplitudes (Figure 4.10b). *Spatial* frequency, k, is expressed in units of cycles per mm, or mm^{-1}, and if the spatial period of the pattern of interest is x_0, then the *fundamental frequency* is defined as $k_0 = 1/x_0$. The Fourier expansion for an odd (as opposed to an even) spatial square wave of fundamental frequency k_0, for example, and *harmonics* $k = n \times k_0$ for integer n, is well known to be of the form (see Figures 4.10 and 4.12)

$$S(x) = 2/\pi[\pi/4 + \sin 2\pi k_0 x \\ + {}^1\!/_3\sin 6\pi k_0 x + \cdots.], \qquad (8.11)$$

We can imagine the values of k as defining points along the k-axis in a one-dimensional k-space. The greater k is, the higher the spatial frequency of the Fourier component, and the shorter its wavelength.

The weighting factor preceding each sine term is the amplitude of its contribution to the whole so that, in effect, the equation reveals the spatial frequency spectrum of the pattern.

Three generalizations reconfigure this Fourier sum into something more powerful and flexible. First, we can replace the trig functions of Equation 8.11 with their exponential counterparts, where

$$e^{2\pi \, i k \, x} = \cos 2\pi k x + i \sin 2\pi k x. \quad (8.12)$$

This expression may not be intuitively obvious, but it can be demonstrated by taking the Taylor expansion of both sides.

Also, by extending the set of discrete k-values into a continuum, and replacing the sum with an integral over spatial frequency, the approach of Fourier integrals becomes applicable to non-periodic functions, as well.

Finally, to expand into two or three dimensions, it is necessary only to morph the term $(k_0 x)$ into the vector dot product of vectors $\underline{x} = (x,y)$ and $\underline{k} = (k_x, k_y)$.

The exact solution to the reconstruction problem, $\mu_{\text{exact}}(\underline{x})$, can be represented as an equivalent Fourier integral of multiple spatial waves, as

$$\mu_{\text{exact}}(\underline{x}) = \int\int M_{\text{exact}}(\underline{k}) e^{+2\pi i (k_x x + k_y y)} dk_x \, dk_y.$$
$$(8.13a)$$

The values of the coefficients $M_{\text{exact}}(\underline{k})$ provide the prescription for adding together the right frequencies and amplitudes of spatial waves in real 2D space so as to end up with $\mu_{\text{exact}}(\underline{x})$. The only problem is that unfortunately, we do not know them yet; indeed, our primary task is to find $M_{\text{exact}}(\underline{k})$, for use in this equation!

To proceed, we shall replace $M_{\text{exact}}(\underline{k})$ with something we *can* find, by taking advantage of a useful relationship known as the *central* (or *Fourier*) *slice theorem*. Equation 8.13a happens to be already of the form of an (inverse) Fourier transform (FT), which suggests taking *its* inverse:

$$M(\underline{k}) = \int\int \mu(\underline{x}) e^{-2\pi i \underline{k} \cdot \underline{x}} \, dx \, dy; \quad (8.14a)$$

$M(\underline{k})$ is just the FT of $\mu(\underline{x})$. Let us rotate from the current (x,y) coordinate system to a new orthogonal system with r- and s-axes, also indicated in Figure 8.27. The magnitude of $\underline{k}$ does not change under

the rotation, and is $k = (k_x^2 + k_y^2)^{1/2}$. Equation 8.14a becomes

$$M(\underline{k}) = \int \left[\int \mu(\underline{x}) ds \right] e^{-2\pi i k r} dr$$
$$= \int p(r, \varphi) e^{-2\pi i k r} dr, \quad (8.14b)$$
$$= P(k, \varphi).$$

The second line follows from the definition of a projection (Equation 8.8b), and the third is a recognition that the second line happens to be equivalent to the one-dimensional FT, $P(k,\varphi)$, of $p(r,\varphi)$ with respect to r. This proves the *central axis theorem*, which states that

$$M(k_x, k_y) = P(k, \varphi); \quad (8.14c)$$

it says that the Fourier transform of μ is equal to the Fourier transform of the projection p taken at the same angle. This has largely solved the problem of finding the $M_{\text{exact}}(\underline{k})$-coefficients for application in Equation 8.13a.

Given a sufficiently large set of measured projections, $p(r,\varphi)$, two of which are shown in Figure 8.28a, one can take the FT with respect to r of each of them, thereby generating $P(k,\varphi)$ (Figure 8.28b). Application of the central slice theorem allows us to replace $M(k,\varphi)$ in Equation 8.13a with this $P(k,\varphi)$; it has to be reconfigured as $M(k_x, k_y)$, through numerical interpolation (Figure 8.28c), and the equation becomes

$$\mu_{\text{exact}}(\underline{x}) = \int\int P(k, \varphi) e^{+2\pi \underline{k} \cdot \underline{x}} \, dk_x \, dk_y, \quad (8.13b)$$

which amounts to a final FT back to $\mu(\underline{x})$, which is what we want (Figure 8.28d).

To sum this up: we FT the measured numerical data set $\{p(r,\varphi)\}$ to obtain $P(k,\varphi)$. With the aid of the central slice theorem, we replace $M(k,\varphi)$ of Equation 8.13a with the measured $P(k,\varphi)$, yielding Equation 8.13b. $\mu(x,\varphi)$ drops out with this final reverse FT back to real space.

It will soon prove opportune to express this exact solution equivalently but in polar coordinates:

$$\mu_{\text{exact}}(\underline{x}) = \int\int P(k, \varphi) e^{2\pi i k(x \cos \varphi + y \sin \varphi)} |k| dk \, d\varphi.$$
$$(8.13c)$$

where the $|k|$, the 'absolute value' of k, happened to come along with this last change of variables.

(a)

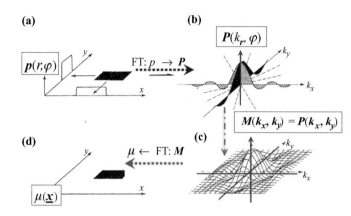

(b)

$P(k_r, \varphi)$

$FT: p \to P$

$M(k_x, k_y) = P(k_x, k_y)$

(c)

(d)

$\mu \leftarrow FT: M$

$\mu(\underline{x})$

Figure 8.28 Exact Fourier reconstruction: obtaining $\mu_{\text{exact}}(x,y)$ from $p(r,\varphi)$ data. **(a)** Acquisition of $p(\underline{x})$ projections. **(b)** Fourier transform of projection data into $P(k_r,\varphi)$. **(c)** Application of central slice theorem, followed by interpolation into (k_x,k_y) coordinate system, yielding $M(k_x,k_y)$. **(d)** Reverse transformation back to real-space, giving $\mu(x,y)$. Modified from RA Brooks, G di Chiro. Principles of computer assisted tomography (CAT) in radiographic and radioisotope imaging. *Phys Med Biol* 1976;**21**:689–732.

This two-dimensional Fourier reconstruction is aesthetically pleasing, and one might have hoped it to be the end of the story, but it is computationally problematic. It accumulates many small numerical approximation errors that skew the results and lead to image artifacts. It does, however, suggest another path, filtered back-projection, that is more reliable. How this works will become clear as we compare plain vanilla, *un*filtered BP with this exact solution just found.

Unfiltered back-projection

FBP starts off with simple, unfiltered BP, and modifies it so as to bring it close to the same exact solution that we just found with the two-dimensional Fourier approach.

The projection $p(r,\varphi)$ of Equations 8.8 and Figure 8.9a lies along a straight line (Equation 8.7). The integral grows as it acquires many little contributions, each of magnitude $\mu(\underline{x})ds$, along its path, and the requirement that the projection include only those voxels that lie along the line appears as

$$p(r, \varphi) = \int \mu(x, y)\delta(x \cos \varphi + y \sin \varphi)dx \, dy,$$

$$(8.15)$$

an explicit expression of the Radon transform. The Dirac delta function, δ, is constructed and defined to be infinitesimally narrow and infinitely high, and $\int g(x) \, \delta(x - x_0) \, dx = g(x_0)$.

In actually reconstructing the map of $\mu_{\text{BP}}(x,y)$ from the projection data, on the other hand, the BP algorithm paints narrow-width stripes along

$r = (x \cos \varphi + y \sin \varphi)$, one for each combination of r and φ, but selecting only lines that pass through the points (x,y) (Figure 8.27). The brightness of a back-projected stripe is made to be proportional to the magnitude, p, of the corresponding original projection. The uniform line painted by the single stripe passing through (x,y) at angle φ may be expressed as $p(r,\varphi) = p(x \cos \varphi + y \sin \varphi, \varphi)$.

To assess $\mu_{\text{BP}}(x,y)$, we simply ombine the effects at (x,y) for all the stripes together that pass through it,

$$\mu_{\text{BP}}(x, y) = \int p(x \cos \varphi + y \sin \varphi, \varphi)d\varphi,$$

$$(8.16a)$$

where each contribution is weighted according to its profile-value. This is just a representation of what is

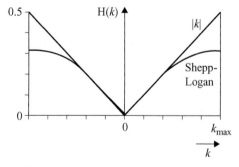

Figure 8.29 Convolution kernels. From the above discussion, one might favor a filter of the shape of $H(k) = |k|$, somehow truncated at high values of k, but others perform better in specific tasks.

going on in Figure 8.27. In terms of its FT, $p(r,\varphi) = \int P(k,\varphi)e^{2\pi i k r}dk$, so Equation 8.16a becomes

$$\mu_{BP}(x,y) = \iint P(k, \varphi)e^{2\pi i k(x\cos\varphi + y\sin\varphi)}dk\, d\varphi.$$

$$(8.16b)$$

We finish off BP by multiplying and dividing by $|k|$:

$$\mu_{BP}(\underline{x}) = \iint \{P(k, \varphi)/|k|\}e^{2\pi i k(x\cos\varphi + y\sin\varphi)}$$
$$\times |k|dk\, d\varphi. \quad (8.16c)$$

The reason for that critical and probably unexpected final step will become clear immediately.

Filtered back-projection

Let us repeat here Equation 8.13c, the exact solution in polar coordinates,

$$\mu_{exact}(\underline{x}) = \iint P(k, \varphi)e^{2\pi i k(x\cos\varphi + y\sin\varphi)}|k|dk\, d\varphi.$$

$$(8.13c)$$

Comparison of this form of $\mu_{exact}(\underline{x})$ with the approximate $\mu_{BP}(\underline{x})$ of Equation 8.16c reveals that they are exactly the same *apart from the factor of* $|\underline{k}|$ *in the denominator of the integral for* $\mu_{BP}(\underline{x})$! In other words, the amplitudes of the Fourier components of the BP integral are being driven down at large k by the factor of $1/|\underline{k}|$; that is, for the higher spatial frequency, shorter wavelength contributions to the image. This mishandling of short-wavelength contributions to the image means the introduction of blur. Putting it a different way, the two big problems with ordinary BP are that it back-paints a stripe that is uniform across its width, and that it lays down only positive values of darkness, so it cannot subtract out the effects of over-painting parts of the image. That results in a blurring.

This difficulty does not arise in the exact solution of Equation 8.13c, which suggests that the BP approach can be made exact simply by forcing a factor of $|\underline{k}|$, known as a *ramp filter*, into the integrand for $\mu_{BP}(\underline{x})$. With *filtered* BP, one modulates

Table 8.3 The choice of kernel affects not only the resolution and the general appearance of a FBP image, but also the level of noise in it.

Kernel/filter	Noise σ (HU)
Standard	5
Soft (obese)	4
Lung	20
Bone	20
Detail	7
Edge	35

the degree of "brightness" of the stripe in accord with the dictates of the product of the projection data and the filter together, in effect, rather than of the data alone, as in BP.

This method of bringing FBP about most commonly is by way of *convolving* the projection data with a *convolution kernel*, in effect the filter, because of which FBP is known also as *convolution reconstruction*. For obvious computational reasons $|\underline{k}|$ cannot be allowed to grow indefinitely – nor does it need to, given the instrumental limits on in-plane resolution – so a real filter is made to curve downward and eventually drop to zero above a suitably high cut-off spatial frequency $|\underline{k}_{max}|$, and short associated wavelength (Figure 8.29). Various kernels that differ somewhat from this truncated ramp have been designed for particular clinical applications, such as lung or detail imaging. These filters/kernels differ not only in their impact on the appearance of detail, however, but also in the amount of noise they bring along with it (Table 8.3), and it is necessary to consider both issues in the clinic.

References

1 Wolbarst AB, Hendee WR. An approach to assessing stochastic radiogenic risk in medical imaging. *Med Phys* 2011;**38**:6654–58.
2 Cody DD, Stevens DM, Rong J. CT quality control. In: Wolbarst AB, Mossman KL, Hendee WR (eds), *Advances in Medical Physics*, vol. **2**. Madison, WI: Medical Physics Publishing, 2008.

CHAPTER 9

Nuclear Medicine

Contrast from Differential Uptake of a
Radiopharmaceutical by Tissues

There are three critical components to a nuclear medicine (NM) study: (i) a pharmacologic agent that is taken up preferentially by some organ or other biologic compartment of interest; (ii) a radionuclide that can be attached to the agent and produces photons (gamma-rays or 511 keV annihilation photons) of sufficient energy to escape the body; and (iii) a device to detect or image these high-energy photons.

An NM examination reveals information on the physiologic status of a certain specific tissue or organ, primarily, rather than on anatomic detail. It is of relatively low spatial resolution, and indicates only the rough shape and size of the tissue under consideration. But if a portion of the organ fails to take up the radiopharmaceutical, or is missing, or is obscured by overlying abnormal tissues, the corresponding region of the image normally appears

Medical Imaging: Essentials for Physicians, First Edition. Anthony B. Wolbarst, Patrizio Capasso and Andrew R. Wyant.
© 2013 John Wiley & Sons, Inc. Published 2013 by John Wiley & Sons, Inc.

dark. Likewise, any part of the organ that takes up more radiopharmaceutical than normal, or fails to wash it out properly, will glow especially brightly on the display, and perhaps remain longer on it. Thus the radiopharmaceutical acts somewhat like an X-ray or MRI contrast agent, but a NM image provides information primarily on physiology and pathology: increased or reduced local uptake, or atypical wash-in or wash-out rates in dynamic studies, may point to an abnormality.

A quality essential to a radiopharmaceutical is its tissue-specificity: different radiopharmaceuticals tend to go to different tissues or lesions. Iodine concentrates almost entirely in thyroid tissue, for example, and there is little visual interference in a thyroid study from take-up of the agent by other tissues. NM studies are also extremely sensitive; the amount of radiopharmaceutical required may be millions of times less, by weight, than the contrast agents for other sorts of imaging.

An X-ray beam *transmission* study, as in DR, DSA, CT, etc., involves only one, single fundamental phenomenon, tissue-specific, *differential attenuation* of the photons through photoelectric and Compton interactions. With the *emission* imaging of NM, SPECT, and PET, however, there are two: of primary concern is the tissue-specific *differential concentration* of radiopharmaceutical and subsequent *differential emission* of gamma-rays. But secondary to this are the subsequent non-productive and sometimes misleading *absorption* and *scatter* of gamma-rays by overlying tissues, and even by the organ itself. Virtually all PET and many SPECT studies in modern facilities are superimposed on and combined with corresponding CT images. This *fusion* process not only makes possible *attenuation corrections* that greatly improve the image quality of PET and SPECT images, but also can provide a valuable high-resolution depiction of underlying *anatomic landmarks* on them.

Unstable atomic nuclei: radioactivity

Gravitational and electromagnetic interactions are responsible for all the familiar, commonplace processes of life. Virtually all the chemical, electrical, thermal, mechanical, ordinary magnetic, and other everyday properties of molecules, gases, liquids, and solids are determined by the arrangement of the electron cloud bound to each of its atoms. That, in turn, depends only on the nuclear charge for it, hence on the number of protons in it (i.e., the atomic number, Z), and the resulting configuration of the Z (for a neutral atom) electrons orbiting it.

The properties of a nucleus itself, by contrast, are determined primarily by the two other fundamental forces, the strong and weak nuclear forces, which have effect only within nuclei. The behavior of a nucleus, in particular whether is radioactive or stable (critical in NM, SPECT, and PET), and whether or not it has a nuclear magnetic moment (for MRI, it must), depends not only on its element type and Z, but also on the number of *neutrons* it holds, N (Figure 1.15a). Both protons and neutrons are known as *nucleons*.

There are several notation schemes designed to label nuclei, but a common one starts with the chemical symbol, such as C for carbon; adds the *atomic number* (redundant but sometimes helpful) after (or before) as a subscript; and ends up with a superscript of the total number of nucleons: C_6^{12} (Figure 9.1). The isotope also appears as C-12 and ^{12}C. The *atomic mass* for a pure isotope is close to the total number of nucleons, $(Z + N)$. Since we've been tossing around the term *isotope* so unabashedly, it might be a good idea to define it: two nuclear types of the same element, with the same Z but with different numbers of neutrons, are said to be different *isotopes* of the element (Figure 1.15a). If

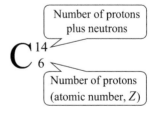

Figure 9.1 One of several common forms of isotope notation and terminology. *Isotopes* of an *element* have the same atomic number, Z, and therefore have nearly identical electrical resistivity, bulk magnetism, thermal conductivity, and other everyday properties. They differ, however, in the number of neutrons, N, in the nucleus, which has just as much impact on nuclear characteristics as does Z. As indicated in Figure 1.15a, ordinary C-12 is stable, but the carbon isotope C-14 is radioactive and, with a half-life of 5730 years, is widely used to date biological artifacts less than about 25 000 years old.

radioactive, a nucleus is also called a *radioisotope*, a *radionuclide*, and a *nuclide* (not to be confused with the nucleotide, from a different sort of nucleus.)

Stable and unstable nuclei

An atomic nucleus is held together by the attractive strong nuclear force between nucleons: proton–proton, neutron-neutron, and proton-neutron. This force is extremely powerful, as its name implies, but it extends for just a short distance, little more than the diameter of a proton or neutron, $\sim 10^{-15}$ meters. So at any instant, a nucleon is pulling only on those others that happen to be directly adjacent. Also present within the nucleus are the electric forces among the protons, which tend to shove one another (hence the entire nucleus) apart. As opposed to the strong nuclear force, the electric field of a proton falls off slowly over a long distance, with the familiar inverse-square form (Figure 2.23); indeed, the combined electric field of the Z protons extends far beyond the nucleus, and is what binds its electrons to it.

The weak interaction does little to hold the nucleus together, but it does instigate a certain subclass of nuclear transition known as beta decay. Physicists have found that the electromagnetic and the weak interactions are two faces of the so-called electro-weak force, just as Maxwell and Einstein demonstrated that electric and magnetic forces are different but intertwined aspects of electromagnetism.

The balance between the attractive strong nuclear forces, the electric repulsion among the protons, and input from the weak interaction determines whether a particular nuclide will be stable or radioactive. Of the 2800 or so different naturally occurring and man-made nuclides, or distinct combinations of protons and neutrons (with several still being added every year), only for 255 of them, indicated by the line of stability in Figure 9.2, does the interplay of the three forces result in a stable nuclear balance. The common isotopes of hydrogen, carbon, nitrogen, oxygen, sulfur, phosphorus, silicon, iron, and the other elements that comprise us and our planet are stable.

The other nuclei come into being with an unsuitable N/Z ratio, being too proton- or neutron-rich, and with too much energy, rendering them unstable. Every element, even hydrogen, has one or more

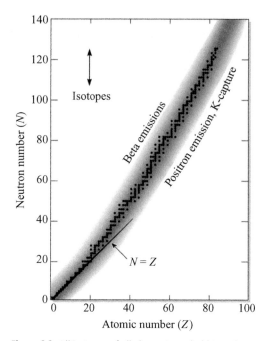

Figure 9.2 All isotopes of all elements are held together, at least temporarily, by the strong nuclear force. Of the 2800 known nuclear forms, about a tenth of them are stable (or have half-lives too long to be measured) and form a *line of stability*, indicated by the black dots, in this chart of atomic number and neutron number. The various isotopes of an element, whether stable or not, lie along a vertical line. For the lightest elements, the number of neutrons tends to be about the same as the number of protons, $N \sim Z$. The N/Z ratio for high-Z elements increases to about 1.6. An unstable nucleus with too high or too low an N/Z ratio will try to move toward the line of stability through radioactive decay.

radioactive isotopes, and for any element of atomic number 84 or above, every isotope is radioactive. All radioactive nuclei emit alpha (the nuclei of helium atoms) or beta (negatively or positively charged electrons) particles, and subsequently gamma-rays. The gamma-rays and positrons (positive beta particles) are what make standard NM, SPECT, and PET possible. Alpha and negative beta particles generally take no constructive part in imaging, but they can be important for clinical laboratory testing and for radiation therapy.

A glance at Figure 9.2 reveals that a nucleus with Z protons also contains typically between Z neutrons, for the lighter elements, and $1.6 \times Z$ neutrons, for the heavy ones. (Ordinary hydrogen, H-1, with no neutrons, is the sole, and important, exception to the rule.) For a small nucleus, the short-range strong nuclear force among neighboring nucleons may be sufficient to hold the nucleus intact. But as Z grows larger, and as the long-range inter-proton electric forces become more pronounced, a few extra squirts of nuclear glue are required, along with a bit more separation between the protons, and this is provided by the neutrons, resulting in a higher N/Z ratio.

Modes of radioactive decay

Like the electron cloud of an atom, a nucleus can exist in a number of quantized energy states. The lowest of these is called the *ground state*, and the ones lying above it are said to be excited, the same as for the states of the electrons surrounding an atom. An excited nucleus can often get rid of excess energy directly and easily by emitting mass, or energy, or both.

Radionuclei are by definition unstable, which is to say that they cannot already be in their lowest-energy, stable ground states. An unstable nucleus will continually vibrate, contort, and churn away in attempts to rectify its nuclear discomfort, and sooner or later, it will undergo spontaneous radioactive decay. (Nothing is "decaying" in the ordinary sense of the word; the term refers loosely to the decline over time in the number of radioactive nuclei in a sample that still have not yet undergone such a transformation.) There are a number of ways that nuclei in excited states can move in that direction (Figure 9.3). We shall skip over two of them briefly, the release of an alpha particle or of a beta particle, and then turn to the two that are of importance in imaging: gamma-ray and positron emission.

Alpha emissions

Some heavy radionuclides contain too much positive charge for comfort, and attempt to improve their situation by getting rid of some of it through *alpha* emission. Although not used in clinical imaging, alpha particles play important roles in medical research, particularly in radiobiology. An alpha particle, indicated as α or α^{++}, is a tightly bound, doubly charged highly stable cluster of two protons and two neutrons; once free of the nucleus, an alpha particle is indistinguishable from the nucleus of the normal helium atom, He_2^{4++}, fully ionized and stripped of

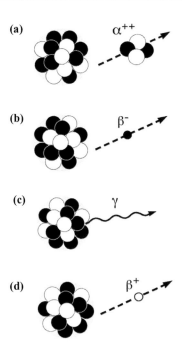

Figure 9.3 Common modes of nuclear decay. (a) Some heavy nuclei emit alpha particles, which are identical to the nuclei of ordinary helium, He_2^4. (b) With the emission of a beta particle (an electron, but of nuclear origin), the atomic number increases by one, and the number of neutrons decreases by one. (c) An excited nucleus may give up excess energy by emitting a gamma-ray photon. Gamma emission normally occurs subsequent to alpha, beta, and positron events. (d) A nucleus can reduce its atomic number (and net positive charge) by one by emitting a positron, which is the anti-particle of the electron, in effect a positively charged electron.

its two electrons (Figure 9.3a). Following alpha emission, the resulting daughter radionuclide will contain two fewer protons, as well as two fewer neutrons, than the parent – that is, it will be of a new element type, with a different (lower) Z. Shades of the Philosopher's Stone! The daughter (sorry – that's the standard terminology) normally finds itself highly excited, as well, and will often lose much of its energy through the subsequent emission of a beta or another alpha particle and/or gamma-rays.

An alpha event involves the emission of electrical charge from a radionucleus, altering its Z-value and element type. This disrupts not only the nucleus, but also the atom's orbital electrons: the daughter nucleus will contain two fewer protons, and so the parent's electron cloud will have to release two of its orbital electrons to retain electrical neutrality; the cloud then readjusts, and settles down into the somewhat different electronic configuration characteristic of the daughter atom. This part of the process is a purely atomic phenomenon, however, rather than a nuclear one, and it may well be accompanied by the emission of one or more characteristic X-ray photons from the electron cloud (as opposed to gamma-rays from the nucleus).

Beta emissions

Beta particles are formally of two sorts, ordinary negative electrons or their positively charged anti-particles, the positrons. We shall follow popular custom and consider "beta particle" to refer only to a negative electron of nuclear origin, and write it either as β^- or as e^- (Figure 9.3b).

Beta particles (negatively charged) tend to be ejected by radionuclides of lower Z in which *the* N/Z ratio happens to be too high. Strontium-90, iodine-131, and cesium-137 are familiar examples of beta emitters; while they play practically no role in medical imaging, they are widely encountered as tracers in laboratory studies and as environmental contaminants. Explaining the mechanism of beta emission could get involved, so let's just blame it all on the weak nuclear force and move on.

The archetypal beta event is that for a free neutron. With a half-life of about 15 minutes, a solitary, isolated neutron transforms into a proton, a beta, and an antineutrino, $\underline{v}$, as $n_0^1 \rightarrow p_1^1 + e^- + \underline{v}$. The total charge on the left and the right are the same, in agreement with the fundamental law of conservation of charge. The *antineutrino* is a virtually undetectable waif associated with weak interaction events; it conveys energy, but carries no electric charge, and it exits the scene at just under the speed of light.

The same thing happens, in effect, within a beta-emitting nucleus. One should not think of a beta particle as an electron that had been rattling around a bit too long inside a neutron, or even the whole nucleus. There are no electrons zipping here and there anxious to escape, any more than there is an omelet waiting to emerge from an egg. A nuclear event takes place, rather, in which a neutron briefly metamorphoses into a proton, an electron, and an antineutrino; the electron and antineutrino streak away long before the process has time to reverse itself, and they leave behind a nucleus excited and with one more proton and one fewer neutron than it had before.

Once ejected from the nucleus, the beta particle behaves like any other high-velocity charged particle, and can ionize the matter through which it happens to pass, which is why betas can pose a radiation hazard. Most beta decays are followed immediately by the de-excitation of the daughter nucleus with the emission of a gamma-ray(s), and possibly with further events.

Gamma-ray emissions and metastable states

Alpha and beta emission both alter the numbers of protons and neutrons present in a nucleus, hence bringing about a complete makeover in the resulting daughter nucleus. The new nucleus, moreover, is not only of a different element, but also almost always resides in an energetically excited state. This daughter nucleus can usually drop immediately into a state of lower energy through the emission of a gamma-ray photon (Figure 9.3c). Indeed, alpha and beta events are usually followed almost instantaneously (typically in much less than a millisecond) by the release of a gamma-ray. That is, unlike alpha or beta events, a gamma emission does not occur just out of the blue; it follows some other nuclear transformation, rather, that happens to leave the resulting nucleus in an excited state. Because this involves a transition between a specific pair of well-defined nuclear energy levels of the same element, a gamma spectrum consists of sharply monochromatic, discrete lines (Figure 9.4a).

A gamma-ray photon differs from an X-ray only in that it originates from a *nuclear* transition, rather than from an atomic orbital *electron* transition (which produces a "characteristic X-ray") or a bremsstrahlung collision. Gamma-rays from radionuclides generally tend to have more energy than diagnostic X-ray photons, but they are much less energetic than some of the X-ray photons produced by radiotherapy linear accelerators (up to 25 MeV). In any case, it is where they come from, not their energy, that distinguishes gamma-rays from X-rays. And, like X-rays, gamma-rays can be imaged, by a suitable image receptor.

For a few radionuclides, the daughter nucleus remains in an excited state for a significant time following a beta emission (i.e., seconds, hours, or more) before a gamma-ray is given off. This may occur because a standard transition to a lower energy level is blocked ("forbidden"), for this particular nuclide for some odd quantum mechanical reason, and it must find a back door out, which usually takes much longer. Such a nuclide is said to be *metastable*, and is distinguished with an "m" following the atomic mass. Indeed, one might be inclined to view a metastable nuclide simply as a radionuclide in its own right that emits only gamma-rays. The classical example of this is technetium-99m, the

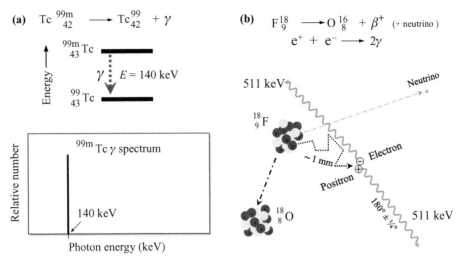

Figure 9.4 Gamma- and positron-emission nuclear processes are the ones of importance in medical imaging. (**a**) The energy level diagram and the most clinically relevant part of the (discrete) gamma spectrum for metastable technetium-99m, which de-excites most notably by emitting a 140-keV gamma-ray. Following an alpha or beta transition, and certain others, a daughter nucleus almost always emits a gamma photon within nanoseconds as it drops into a more stable nuclear state. In the case of Tc-99m, however, the decay process does not occur immediately, but rather with a half-life of 6 hours, and is said to be *metastable*. (**b**) Positron decay and annihilation. Within a nucleus, a proton undergoes the transformation $p_1^1 \rightarrow n_0^1 + e^+ + \upsilon$, in effect; also called a positive beta particle, the positron is sometimes written as β^+. The newly created, massive neutron remains within the nucleus, while the light positron escapes, along with the neutrino. The positron meanders for a millimeter or two through tissue, ionizing thousands of molecules along its path and slowing down, until it collides with an atomic electron. From this explosive interaction emerges a pair of 511 keV *annihilation photons* (some folks agonize over whether to call them gamma-rays, but they're really quite different in origin) heading off in opposite directions, to within $1/4°$ or so. The spectrum of the annihilation photons is a single, monochromatic peak at 511 keV (the amount of energy equivalent to the rest mass of an electron or positron).

main workhorse of a nuclear medicine department, apart from PET, and it decays as

$$Tc_{43}^{99m} \rightarrow Tc_{43}^{99} + \gamma. \qquad (9.1a)$$

The daughter nucleus (Tc-99) has the same numbers of protons and neutrons as the parent, but lower energy and other different nuclear properties (such as a much longer half-life.).

A saline solution of the nuclide can be extracted daily from a *Tc-generator* from a local commercial radiopharmacy that continues to provide daily in the clinic for about one week. Its gammas have an ideal energy, 140 keV, which is sufficient to escape the body but low enough for a high probability of undergoing photoelectric interactions with the IR. The 6-hour half-life allows for preparation of the radiopharmaceutical and then concentration within an organ, and the patient becomes non-radioactive soon after completion of the study. It

also has, as we shall see, a host of other admirable qualities.

Positron emission and PET

A few lighter nuclei with too much positive charge emit a *positron*, the positively charged antiparticle of the electron (Figure 9.3d). It is of concern only to nuclear physicists, science-fiction buffs, and PET people – but to them, it is very important, indeed.

Carbon-11, nitrogen-13, and oxygen-15 are positron-emitters that can be incorporated into biochemicals for PET studies, but the nuclide adopted most commonly for that purpose, by far, is fluorine-18. As with standard beta emission, positron decay is brought about largely through the influence of the weak nuclear force. The overall positron emission reaction for fluorine-18 is (Figure 9.4b)

$$F_9^{18} \rightarrow O_8^{18} + e^+ + \upsilon. \qquad (9.1b)$$

Table 9.1 Some primordial, cosmogenic, and terrestrial naturally occurring radionuclides widely used in medicine and the sciences, along with some anthropogenic ones as well.

Radionuclide	Primary source	Half-life	Emissions (Mev)
H-3	Cosmogenic	12.3 yr (biol: 10 d)	β: 0.0186
C-14	Cosmogenic	5730 yr	β: 0.156
P-32	Activation	14.29 d	β: 1.71
K-40	Primordial	1.28×10^9 yr	β: 1.31
Co-60	Fission	5.27 yr	γ: 1.17, 1.33
Sr-90	Fission	28.8 yr	β: 0.546
Tc-99m	via Mo-99	6.0 h	γ: 0.140

In effect, a proton in the nucleus transforms into a neutron, which remains behind within the nucleus, while the associated positron and a *neutrino*, v, manage to escape it.

A newly minted positron enjoys a solitary, nasty, brutish, and short existence, but it does culminate in a rather spectacular final blaze of glory. For F-18, the maximum positron kinetic energy is 633 keV, enough for it to ionize atoms along a 1- or 2-mm-long, erratic track in tissue. It slows down rapidly and then latches onto an electron. The two spiral wildly toward one another with a fatal electric attraction and, upon contact, mutually annihilate, with the creation of a pair of 0.511 MeV *annihilation photons* that head off in nearly opposite directions, together contributing in creating a PET image.

Positron annihilation, incidentally, provides a perfect example of Einstein's prescription, $E = mc^2$, for keeping track of quantities of mass, m, and radiant energy, E, when either form is being converted into the other. The equation reveals that in the right units, a positron and electron together have an amount of mass that will lead to creation of a pair of annihilation photons of 0.511 MeV energy each. Indeed, it is commonly stated that the *rest mass* of an electron is 511 keV.

Production of radioactive materials: nuclear activation, nuclear decay, and fission products

Radionuclides are commonly viewed, for historical and regulatory reasons, as being either naturally occurring or man-made.

Naturally occurring radionuclides, moreover, are categorized as primordial, cosmogenic, and terrestrial. *Primordial* nuclides, such as potassium-40,

uranium-235, and uranium-238, have been in existence since their creation billions of years ago in supernovae (Table 9.1). Carbon-14 arises from the bombardment of stable atoms in the upper atmosphere by cosmic rays such as high-velocity protons, and is said to be *cosmogenic*. And light concentrations of uranium-238 are ubiquitous in soil and rocks and give rise, through the alpha and beta decay of its progeny, to an entire chain of *terrestrial* radioactive nuclides (Figure 9.5). One of the links, radium-226, is also present in soil everywhere, and it emits small amounts of gamma-rays; of far greater hazard is its daughter, the noble gas, alpha-emitter radon-222, that seeps in from soil and concentrates in basements, becoming a major health hazard.

By various means, humans also produce a broad range of radionuclides for medical, industrial, nuclear power, research, and other uses. *Neutron activation* and *nuclear fission*, both of which take place within a nuclear reactor, are the main mechanisms of anthropogenic nucleosynthesis. But small quantities of other nuclides, in particular most positron-emitters, come from *charged-particle activation*. And finally, several medical nuclides are produced in and extracted in the clinic from *generators*; as a longer-lived parent nuclide (itself generally anthropogenic, e.g., molybdenum-99, $t_{1/2} = 67$ hours) decays, for example, it releases a daughter (technetium-99m, 6 h) that may be extracted and made into part of a radiopharmaceutical.

Neutron activation

Neutron activation occurs when a stable or radioactive nucleus absorbs a free neutron that strikes it within a nuclear reactor. The new nucleus, now

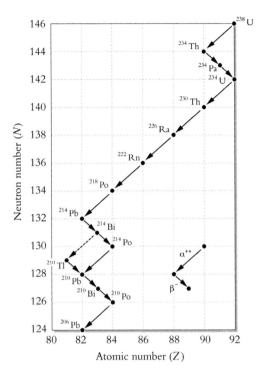

Figure 9.5 Decay chain. This particular radioactive series begins with the naturally occurring, long-lived (6.5 × 10⁹ year half-life) radionuclide uranium-238. In the first step, uranium-238 emits an alpha particle; the daughter thorium-234 has two fewer protons and two fewer neutrons. In the second step, thorium-234 emits a beta particle to become protactinium-234; the atomic number increases by one, but the total number of nucleons does not change. The series undergoes further alpha and beta decays down until it reaches the stable lead isotope Pb-206. There are two other such major, naturally occurring series, beginning with uranium-235 (half-life of 1.0 × 10⁹ years) and with thorium-232 (2 × 10¹⁰ years), and a fourth long chain that begins with a man-made radioisotope.

with one more neutron, will have radically different nuclear properties, and is almost certain to be radioactive. One medically important example of neutron activation involves the bombardment of non-radioactive molybdenum-98 with a high flux of neutrons, which leads to the formation of molybdenum-99 nuclei: $Mo_{42}^{98} + n_0^1 \rightarrow Mo_{42}^{99}$. The Mo_{42}^{99} nuclei come into being in an excited state; then, inside a *generator*, they undergo beta decay into technetium-99m, which can be captured and serve in imaging. Neutron activation also brings us phosphorus-32, chromium-51, strontium-89,

iodine-125, and fissile (fissionable) plutonium-239, and it can even induce fission itself of a few *fissile* radionuclei (e.g., U-235, Pu-238).

Fission products
Neutron activation of uranium-235 takes place only in a reactor or a nuclear explosion, as $U_{92}^{235} + n_0^1 \rightarrow U_{92}^{236*}$. It is a very special case of neutron activation, in which the daughter starts off in an unusually unstable, excited nuclear configuration, indicated by the asterisk. Rather than resolving its situation in a civilized fashion with an alpha or beta decay like U-238, the newly formed U-236* nucleus prefers to come undone, literally, by way of *nuclear fission*, instead: it splits into two large fission-product nuclei, one of which has somewhat more than half the mass of the original, and the other somewhat less (Figure 9.6a); both depart the scene with much kinetic energy and the release of a tremendous amount of radiant energy. (Recall that chemical reactions typically involve the transfer of a few eV per molecule, with the emission of visible light photons [2–3 eV each]; the fissioning of a nucleus is measured, rather, in *millions* of eV, or MeV, in the gamma-ray range.)

Of the many fission pathways a U-236* nucleus can take, the one producing the particular pair of *fission products* molybdenum-99 and tin-135 goes as $U_{92}^{236*} \rightarrow Mo_{42}^{99} + Sn_{50}^{135} + 2 n_0^1 + $ energy. Hundreds of radioisotopes of about 30 elements have been identified among fission products from U-235. Chemically separating Mo-99 from the others is a second way of obtaining that important radionuclide. While it is possible to obtain high concentrations of Mo-99 in that manner, the separation of it from other fission products is not perfect, and there will be some other radioactive contaminants that come along with. Iodine-131, xenon-133, and other medically valuable radionuclides are also extractable fission products.

Each fission event also produces several free neutrons that can themselves activate other neighboring U_{92}^{235} nuclei (Figure 9.6b); the number of fissionings taking place, and the number of neutrons flying about, will increase exponentially as 2, 4, 8, 16, 32 ... over time. With a sufficiently large *critical* mass (so that not too many neutrons escape through its surface) of highly enriched fissile material such as 90%-pure U-235, there results a *chain reaction* throughout it over the course of a microsecond

(a)

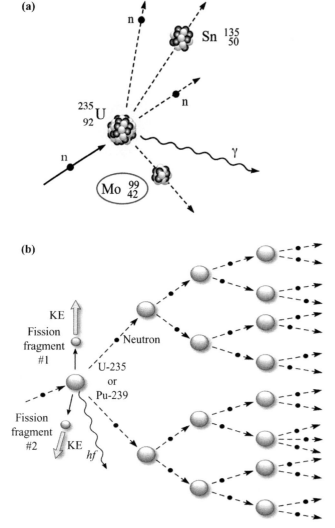

(b)

Figure 9.6 Nuclear fission. (a) If a fissile nucleus, such as one of U-235 or Pu-239, is neutron activated, it does not undergo normal radioactive decay. It fissions, rather, into two mid-sized fission-product nuclei. It also releases a great deal of radiant energy, and a few new free neutrons that can, in turn, go on to activate other fissile nuclei, and so on. (b) Nuclear chain reaction, which can be either slow and controlled or explosively fast.

that gives rise to a nuclear explosion. If the material is diluted, or of less than critical mass, an explosion is not possible, but the chain reaction can release heat at a slow, controllable, rate. This is typically put to work in a reactor boiling water, which drives steam turbines that power electrical generators.

Charged-particle activation

A charged-particle accelerator such as a *cyclotron* smashes high-velocity protons, helium nuclei, or other charged atomic particles into generally non-radioactive targets. Many of the resulting products have the high Z/N ratios favorable for positron emission, including fluorine-18, gallium-67, indium-111, and iodine-123.

Generators

Technetium-99m is routinely created on-site in a clinic in a molybdenum generator or "cow" (Figure 9.7a), or delivered daily from a nearby commercial radiopharmacy. Mo-99m itself can be obtained either from neutron activation of Mo-98 in a reactor or as a fission product from uranium fuel. It tends to adhere tightly to an alumina (Al_2O_3) or resin exchange column within a sterile chamber (Figure 9.7b), but the daughter technetium is chemically attached much less tightly than molybdenum to the column material, and can be eluted (washed) out of the cow with sterile saline solution.

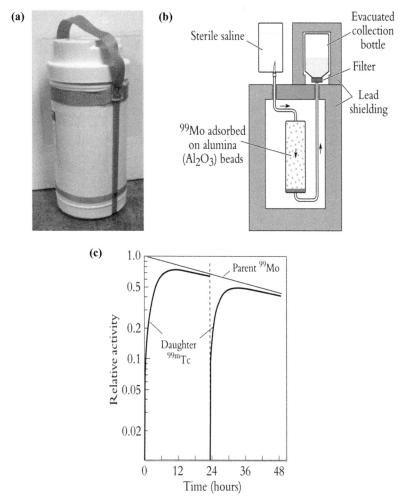

Figure 9.7 Radionuclide generators. (**a**) Tc-99m generator. Thanks to Walter Miller. Technetium-99m is eluted daily from this commercial molybdenum cow, or technetium generator, which is replaced weekly. (**b**) Mo-99 adsorbed strongly to the surfaces of beads of alumina undergoes beta decay with a 67-hour half-life. During elution with sterile saline, as shown here, daughter technetium-99m atoms, bound much less tightly to the beads than are their parent atoms, dissolve into solution and are flushed into the evacuated collection vial. (**c**) Within the generator, the activity of the Mo-99 parent is determined by how much was put there in the first place, and thereafter by its own 67-hour half-life; after the cow is milked, regrowth of the technetium is controlled by *its* 6-hour half-life.

Tc-99m regrows nearly to its previous activity over the course of a day, after which it is ready for another elution (Figure 9.7c). It is the rate of decay of the molybdenum that limits the useful lifetime of the cow. The elutant, which consists of nearly pure sodium pertechnetate in water and acts thereafter like a pure gamma-emitter, is then ready for combination with an agent by way of some simple radio-chemistry. The Tc-99m compound subsequently is injected into the body, and the nuclide decays with a 6-hour physical half-life. Generators are available also for krypton-81m, rubidium-82m, and the positron-emitters gallium-68 and rubidium-82.

A molybdenum-production mini-crisis is growing. With over 20 million NM procedures per year in the USA alone, and most of them employing technetium, only five reactors in the world produce the material, and none is in theUSA. All the active reactors are over 40 years old, and two are currently down for repairs [1].

Exponential decline in activity over time

The nuclei in any radioactively pure sample are undergoing nuclear transformations, which means that the number of those that have not yet done so by time t, the number of those un-decayed and still intact, $n(t)$, must be decreasing, from some initial value of $n(0)$ at $t = 0$; that is, the rate at which that number changes, dn/dt, is a negative number. It is proportional to the number of those remaining available to decay, moreover, so $dn/dt = -\lambda\, n(t)$, where the *transformation constant*, λ, is unique for each radionuclide; for stable nuclei, of course, $\lambda = 0$. Pretty straightforward, common-sense stuff, a matter of book-keeping rather than of any deep physics concepts. This differential equation will be familiar from the argument surrounding Equations 3.1, and here, too, the solution is the familiar:

$$n(t) = n(0)e^{-\lambda t}, \qquad (9.2a)$$

with a similar but slightly different interpretation.

The units of λ must be *probability per minute, per year*, etc., for the exponent to be unit-less and make sense – justifying its other name, the *decay rate*. The fact that λ is an invariant over time means that the probability of decay per unit of time of any individual nucleus is also constant. That is, a nucleus retains no memory of its history, is unaware of how long it has already been in existence, and is oblivious to its fellow travelers; it only knows that over the next instant, dt, its probability of decay is $\lambda\, dt$. This is quite different from things that *do* undergo aging, like populations of batteries and people, which do *not* fall off exponentially.

Amounts of most substances are measured in units of weight or volume, but a radioactive material is quantified in terms of *activity*. The activity $A(t)$ of a sample of radioactive material at time t is defined as the number of decay events occurring in it per unit time, $|dn/dt|$. (The "| ... |" makes dn/dt into a positive number, despite the fact that $n(t)$ is defined as the number of surviving radionuclei, so that dn is negative.) From the exponential form of $n(t)$, it appears that (Figure 9.8a)

$$A(t) \equiv |dn/dt| = \lambda n(t) = A(0)e^{-\lambda t}. \quad (9.2b)$$

Double the amount of radioactive material present in a sample, hence the number of active radionuclei, and you double the activity. While

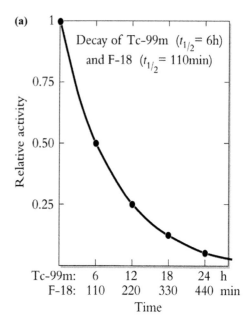

(a)

Decay of Tc-99m $(t_{1/2} = 6h)$ and F-18 $(t_{1/2} = 110\,min)$

| Tc-99m: | 6 | 12 | 18 | 24 | h |
| F-18: | 110 | 220 | 330 | 440 | min |

Time

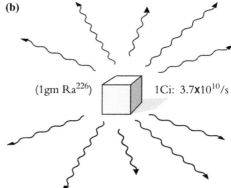

(b)

(1gm Ra^{226})   1Ci: 3.7×10^{10}/s

Figure 9.8 Activity. (a) Exponential decline in activity, $A(t)$, normalized to $A(0)$, of a sample of nuclide with the transformation rate, λ, or the half-life, $t_{1/2}$, characteristic of it, and unique to it. Here the time scales are adjusted to fit appropriately for either technetium-99m ($\lambda = 0.115$ h^{-1}, $t_{1/2} = 6$ h), or fluorine-18 ($\lambda = 0.0063$ min^{-1}, $t_{1/2} = 110$ min). The same decay pattern plots out as a straight line on a semi-log plot. λ and $t_{1/2}$ are related as $\lambda \times t_{1/2} = 0.693$. (b) The term "activity" refers to an important characteristic of any *sample* of radioactive material – the rate at which nuclear transformations are occurring within it. The activity of a sample depends on the specific radionuclide in it, in particular the half-life, and also on how many viable radionuclei are still in it at the moment: The more there remain in the sample, the greater the activity. For historical reasons, the standard unit of activity, the curie (Ci), was defined as that of a gram of natural radium, or 3.7×10^{10} events per second. The SI unit is the becquerel (Bq), which is 1 disintegration per second.

λ is a permanent, fixed parameter characteristic of any quantity of a particular radionuclide, $A(t)$ applies only to a *sample* of it, and it is continually decreasing exponentially over time.

Decay rates are often presented in terms of the *half-life*, $t_{1/2}$, the time it takes for the activity (also for the number of remaining particles) in a sample to fall to half its original value: $A(t_{1/2})/A(0) = 1/2$. This and Equation 9.2b lead immediately to the useful $\lambda \times t_{1/2} = 0.693$. So a large λ, indicating rapid decay, means a short $t_{1/2}$, and *vice versa*. The half-lives of the various radionuclides range from a small fraction of a microsecond up to billions of years — the primordial ones, like uranium-238, still exist in nature precisely because they decay so slowly.

The traditional unit of activity has long been the *curie*, where 1 Ci was defined as the activity of 1 g of radium, about 3.7×10^{10} disintegrations per second (dps) (Figure 9.8b). The newer SI unit is the Becquerel, or 1 dps, so 1 Ci $= 3.7 \times 10^{10}$ Bq. Appearing more commonly in NM are the millicurie (1 mCi $= 0.001$ Ci $= 37$ MBq) and the megabecquerel (MBq $= 10^6$ Bq $= 27$ μCi).

Example of radiopharmaceutical preparation: at 7:00 a.m., the NM technologist elutes the Mo generator and obtains 120 mCi of $Tc^{99m}O_4^-$ in 4 ml of saline. None is used during the day. What will the activity be at 7:00 p.m.? By the half-life method, $A(12$ h$) = 120$ mCi $\times 2^{-(12h)/(6h)} = 30$ mCi. Alternatively, given the tabulated value $\lambda = 0.115$/h, $A(12) = 120 \times e^{-(0.115 \times 12)} = 30$ mCi. Note that (6 h) $\times$ (0.115/h) = 0.693.

Radiopharmaceuticals: gamma- or positron-emitting radionuclei attached to organ-specific agents

Standard NM makes use of radiopharmaceuticals, special radioactive materials that display two key features:

An injected, inhaled, or ingested sample of such a material tends to be taken up preferentially by, and concentrate largely in, a particular biologic compartment, a specific organ or tissue.

From there, it emits gamma-rays or gives rise to 511 keV annihilation photons that can escape the body and be detected from outside it, thereby contributing to the creation of an image. Irregularities in the spatial uptake or deposition of the radiopharmaceutical within the compartment,

as revealed by the gamma/SPECT or PET camera, may thus provide information on patient physiology and pathology.

Desirable attributes of a radiopharmaceutical

A half dozen gamma-emitting (versus positron-emitting) radionuclides find routine use in a nuclear medicine department (Table 9.2). The most common one, by far, is technetium-99m, which is employed in three-quarters of all radionuclide imaging studies, largely so because its characteristics are so close to the ideal for imaging (Box 9.1).

Box 9.1   The virtues of Tc-99m.

Radionuclide properties

Emission	Monochromatic gamma
Particulates (α, β)	None
Energy	140 keV
Half-life	6 h
Toxicity	Non-toxic

Radionuclide production

Source	On-/off-site Tc-generator
Source duration	Replaced weekly
Cost	Low
Preparation	Elution, in minutes
Purity	<0.1% Mo-99, etc.

Radiopharmaceutical preparation

Availability	Kits
Preparation	Minutes
Binding to Tc-99m	Generally very stable
QA	ITLC, etc.
Specificity	Highly organ-specific
Sensitivity	Micrograms of tracer used

Tc-99m produces gamma-rays almost exclusively, no useless (but nonetheless dose-imparting) alphas and very few betas. Its complete decay scheme is complex, but only the 140-keV gamma-ray is of significance, and one may think of the entire process occurring within the patient as that of Equation 9.1a. The monochromatic gamma spectrum means that energy selection (energy windowing) by the image receptor can greatly cut out scatter and other photon noise. The energy of the gamma-ray photons is such that they will likely escape the body, but then be detected by the dense and thick sodium

Table 9.2 Several gamma-emitting radionuclides are in common use in gamma camera and SPECT imaging, but technetium-99m is the one most-frequently chosen, by far. Iodine-131 is a beta emitter, but is sometimes used for examination of the thyroid, rather than I-123, because of its relatively low cost. Thallium-201 finds application in cardiac stress studies, but Tc-99m deposits less dose.

Z	Nuclide	$t_{1/2}$	Gamma (keV)	Production
31	Gallium-67	79 h	92, 184, 296	Cyclotron
43	Techetium-99m	6 h	140	Generator
49	Indium-111	2.8 d	173, 247	Cyclotron
53	Iodine-123	13 h	159	Cyclotron
	Iodine-131[a]	8.1 d	364, 637	Fission
54	Xenon-133	5.3 d	81	Neutron activation
81	Thallium-201	73 h	70, 167	Cyclotron

[a]I-131 emits 610 keV β^-.

iodide scintillation crystal of the gamma camera. Its 6-hour half-life provides sufficient time for preparation of radiopharmaceuticals in the clinic, for physiologic uptake, distribution, and equilibration within the target biological compartment, and for the examination itself – but it is short enough for the gamma irradiation of the patient (and of those nearby) to diminish rapidly after the study is completed.

Tc-99m can be obtained every morning from an on-site generator or from a local commercial vendor and, with its 6-hour half-life, it remains available all day, if you start out with enough of it. It has convenient chemistry, and attaches easily and rapidly to a variety of agents, provided in commercially available kits (Figure 9.9a,b). You simply add radioisotope solution from the cow to the vial material from the kit, perhaps heat a bit, stir (don't shake), and mumble the requisite incantation. Then you load the right amount of it into a syringe, double-check its activity with a well counter (Figure 9.9b), inject it into the patient, and image after it has concentrated in the organ. If the prepared radionuclide or radiopharmaceutical is generated off-site, it must be transported to the clinic in accord with the stringent rules of the Department of Transportation (DOT) (Figure 9.9c), and checked again at the clinic before being administered to a patient.

The radionuclide, the agent, and the radiopharmaceutical combination must be non-toxic, of course, but this is rarely an issue since only trace amounts are administered; also, the binding between them must be adequately stable both *in vitro* (before administration) and *in vivo*.

A crucial characteristic of a good agent is that it be highly organ- or biological compartment-specific, preferably with a significant differential uptake between normal and pathologic tissues. There are a number of physiological processes by which agents distinguish among and concentrate in organs (Box 9.2).

Box 9.2 There are a number of biophysical and biochemical mechanisms by means of which specific agents tend to cause gamma- and positron-emitting nuclides to concentrate in particular biological compartments.

Compartmental filling	Xe-133 – lung ventilation
Capillary blockade	Tc-99m, MAA – lung perfusion
Active transport	I-123 – thyroid
Phagocytosis	Tc-99m colloid – liver
Exchange/diffusion	Tc-99m, pyrophosphates – bone
Metabolism	^{18}FDG – glucose analog (PET)
Antibody-antigen	Radio-labeled monoclonal antibody
Receptor binding	In-111 Octreotide

Pulmonary *ventilation* can be viewed through *compartment filling* of the lungs with, say, the noble gas xenon-133, or an aqueous suspension of pertechnetate (Figure 1.15c,d). Subsequent

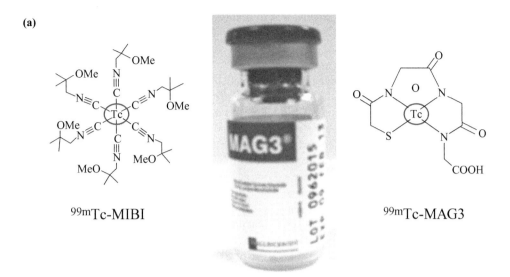

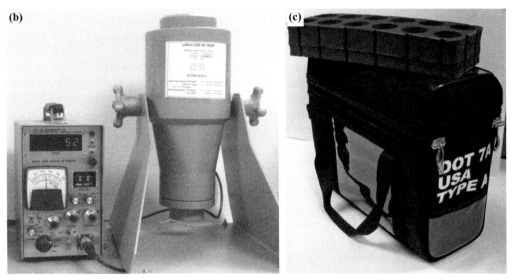

Figure 9.9 Radiopharmaceuticals. (**a**) A variety of organic and other "agents" serve to bring a gamma- or positron-emitting radionuclide to specific tissues or biological compartments; these include antibodies, glucose analogs, pyrophosphates, particulates such as macro-aggregate albumin (MAA), and gases. Many agents, such as sestamibi (MIBI) and mercapto acetyl triglycine (MAG3), come in prepared kits, and are combined chemically with Tc-99m eluted from a generator on-site or at a local radiopharmacy, or with other radionuclides. (**b**) The Nuclear Regulatory Commission (NRC) requires that trained personnel check the activities of radioactive materials in a well counter, both while a radiopharmaceutical is being prepared and loaded into syringes and before it is administered to a patient. (**c**) A carrying case for radioactive materials, approved by the Department of Transportation (DOT). Also, waste materials must be disposed of safely in special containers and according to federal regulations. Thanks to Walter Miller for the photos.

examination of the *perfusion* of the fine pulmonary vessels is made possible through a temporary *capillary blockade* of a small fraction of them with intravenously injected macroaggregated albumin tagged with technetium (Tc-99m—MAA). These microscopic lumps of protein, slightly larger than erythrocytes, break down soon thereafter, and are flushed out of the lung. Ventilation and perfusion studies are commonly performed together, and we shall return to them shortly.

In studies of the thyroid, radioactive iodine is brought into cells of the gland through *cellular active transport* by biochemical pumps in the cell walls. Reticuloendothelial cells recognize minute (0.1 mm), radio-labeled colloid particles as being foreign objects, and remove them from the bloodstream through *phagocytosis*, for imaging of the liver, spleen, and bone marrow. And so on.

Lately there has been much interest in certain monoclonal antibodies designed to bind to specific normal or diseased cells. For some agents of nuclear medicine, concentration in a tissue is determined by the tissue's overall physiologic status, by the general level of functioning of its parenchymal cells. Monoclonal antibodies, by contrast, can be disease-specific, and can provide more precise information on the nature of a disorder, as well as on its location.

Finally, a radiopharmaceutical may vanish in a *dynamic* gamma study much faster than its physical half-life might suggest. There are, in fact, two categories of its loss from the body: physical decay, parameterized by λ or λ_{phys}, and biological removal, often nearly exponential and at a rate λ_{biol}, which depends on physiological processes such as normal or excessive exhalation, urination, defecation, and perspiration. The simplest kind of biological compartment model assumes no continuing *inflow* of radiopharmaceutical, but it does permit the release of the activity remaining within it with a constant rate, λ_{biol}, so that $A(t)_{biol}(t) = A(0)e^{-\lambda_{biol}t}$. Physical and biological decay are mutually incompatible processes, in the sense that a radionucleus that undergoes a transformation cannot also be eliminated through washout, and vice versa. In establishing the overall rate of disappearance from a biological compartment, the two separate rates are then simply additive:

$$\lambda_{compart} = \lambda_{phys} + \lambda_{biol}. \qquad (9.3a)$$

Or, in terms of half-lives,

$$1/t_{1/2\,compart} = 1/t_{1/2\,phys} + 1/t_{1/2\,biol}. \qquad (9.3b)$$

Imaging radiopharmaceutical concentration with a gamma camera

With a few interesting exceptions, gamma-ray nuclear medicine imaging devices are comprised of a single scintillating crystal, normally one of sodium iodide doped with trace amounts of thallium to enhance its fluorescence characteristics, backed by an array of sensors of optical light. The intensity of a burst of light is proportional to the energy deposited in the detector, hence to that of the gamma-ray responsible for it. Gamma-ray energies are radioisotope-specific, which allows imaging instruments to select out and accept only scintillations from the imaging isotope. But ways had to be found to determine where in the crystal a scintillation occurred, and to relate that to the location of a decay in the body. The first successful approach to that problem was that of the rectilinear scanner.

Before gamma cameras

The rectilinear scanner is no longer seen in modern clinics, but its operation is easier to visualize than that of a gamma camera. Its front end (Figure 9.10a) is a *collimator*, a thick block of lead through which one or several narrow, straight, and parallel (or nearly so) channels are drilled. Only those relatively few gamma-rays that happen to be heading exactly along a channel can reach an otherwise shielded fluorescent crystal. A large single crystal of NaI doped with thallium is employed, rather than compacted polycrystalline material, so that light will not be lost through scattering or absorption at the grain boundaries. Pinpoint bursts of light travel from the NaI(Tl) along an optical coupling to a *photomultiplier tube* (PMT), which detects the light and generates a corresponding electrical pulse, the voltage of which is proportional to the intensity of the burst of light (Figure 9.10b). Care is taken to match the emission spectrum of the scintillation crystal, centered in the blue-green for NaI(Tl), to the sensitivity spectrum of the photocathode of the PMT.

The collimator/detector assembly was swept in a raster pattern, back and forth across the patient, while slowly moved down. In the early days, a pen was held over a sheet of paper and linked mechanically or electrically to the collimator/detector, and mimicked its path; every time a gamma-ray was detected, the pen tapped the paper. Later on, gamma-rays were indicated as points of light on an oscilloscope that was photographed throughout the study. Thus the density of ink dots anywhere on the paper (or points on film) indicated the rate at which

(a)

Amplifier, energy discriminator (PHA),
and pulse counter

Photomultiplier

Fluorescent crystal

Collimator

Recorder

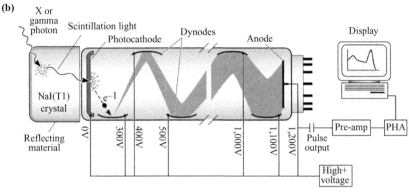

(b)

X or gamma photon

Scintillation light

Photocathode

Dynodes

Anode

Display

NaI(Tl) crystal

e^{-1}

Reflecting material

0V 300V 400V 500V 1,000V 1,100V 1,200V

Pulse output

Pre-amp — PHA

High+ voltage

(c)

Photomultiplier

Collimator

Detector output

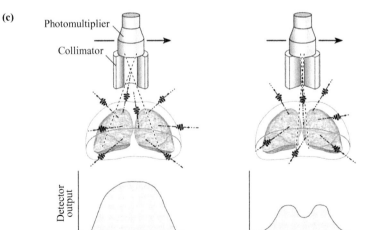

Figure 9.10 Mapping the spatial distribution within the body of a gamma-emitting radionuclide with a rectilinear scanner. (**a**) A scintillation detector consists of a collimator in front of a scintillating crystal attached optically to a photomultiplier tube (PMT). The *pulse height analyzer* (PHA) records the amplitude of each pulse, and passes on only those that correspond to the photopeak of the radionuclide, in which a photoelectric event deposits all the energy of the incident photon in the crystal. The two-dimensional scanning motions of the scintillation detector were mimicked by those of the recorder pen, and the density of points laid down on paper was proportional to the count rate sensed there by the detector. (**b**) In a PMT, scintillation light kicks out of the photocathode a number of electrons that is proportional to the intensity of the light burst. Each such electron dislodges a greater number of others at the next *dynode*, which is held at a higher voltage. The end result is a measurable voltage pulse, the size of which is proportional to the energy of the original X-ray photon. (**c**) A basic tradeoff for scanners, and gamma cameras, too: the wider the collimator channel(s), the greater the sensitivity of the instrument, but the lower its spatial resolving capability.

gamma-rays were emerging from the corresponding part of the body, hence of the concentration of radiopharmaceutical below the surface there.

Because of the relatively high density (3.7 g/cm^3) and effective atomic number ($Z_{eff} = 45$) of NaI, the intrinsic efficiency for capturing diagnostic energy X-rays and gamma-rays by means of the photoelectric effect is acceptably high. Thallium doping increases the crystal's conversion efficiency tenfold, so that as much as 25% of the gamma-ray energy imparted may be re-emitted from NaI[T1] as light photons. With the absorption of an X-ray or gamma-ray, the intensity of the resultant pulse of scintillation light (of mean wavelength 420 nm) rises for about 30 nanoseconds, and then decays exponentially with a characteristic time of 0.25 microseconds; this is short enough for many applications, but not necessarily for those that involve very high activities and require very fast detection of separate (i.e., non-overlapping) light pulses. Sodium iodide is hygroscopic (extracts water out of the air, and can dissolve in it), and the crystal must be protected from moisture. Some other crystals in use are $Bi_4Ge_3O_{12}$ (BGO), Gd_2SiO_5 (GSO), and Lu_2SiO_5 (LSO).

A photomultiplier tube is a vacuum tube that, when exposed to a very faint flash of visible light, generates a pulse of charge (Figure 9.10b). The process begins when several light photons eject a few electrons from the bi-alkali (K_2CsSb) metal photocathode, by means of the photoelectric effect. Typically, one electron is emitted for every 3–10 light photons incident. Each photoelectron is accelerated through 200 or 300 V toward the first *dynode*. On striking it, this first electron dislodges several new ones, each of which is then accelerated toward the second dynode, and so on. Typically there are 12–14 dynodes, each held 100 V more positive than the one before. For every photoelectron originally ejected from the photocathode, a million or so electrons eventually reach the final dynode, or anode, giving rise to a significant voltage pulse.

The intensity of a flash of scintillating light is proportional to the amount of energy from the gamma-ray that is actually deposited in the crystal – and that may be all (photoelectric event) or only some (Compton) of the incident energy. The number of photoelectrons kicked off the photocathode of the PMT, in turn, is proportional to the number of photons in the light burst. The magnitude of the voltage pulse coming out of the detector system is therefore proportional to the energy absorbed in the crystal. This is an essential observation.

There was a fundamental and important image quality tradeoff found with the rectilinear scanner, and it carries over to gamma cameras as well (Figure 9.10c). A larger-diameter collimator channel passes more gamma-rays, but provides less information about the precise location of their source. Thus an improvement in detector sensitivity obtained with larger-bore channels is paid for in loss of spatial resolution, and vice versa. The same situation exists with gamma cameras.

The photopeak and the Compton edge of a scintillation detector

Every gamma-ray interaction within the scintillation crystal gives rise to an electrical pulse at the output of the PMT. The initial event may be a photoelectric interaction, in which case the photon deposits *all* its energy in the crystal, resulting in a relatively bright burst of light and a highest-voltage pulse. For a Compton event in which the Compton scatter photon escapes the crystal, the pulse voltages will be lower. Either way, the pulse height (voltage) from the PMT is proportional to the energy actually deposited in the crystal and transformed to light.

It is the job of the *pulse height analyzer* (*PHA*), also called a *multi-channel analyzer*, to determine and graph the relative number of pulses versus their heights (voltages), and to then display the relative number of count versus energy deposited as a histogram. For photoelectric collisions, but only for them, the pulse height is proportional to the full energy of the original incident photon, and these give rise to the radionuclide's *photopeak* on the monitor. We can calibrate the energy scale simply by examining Tc-99m, and labeling the center of its photopeak "140 keV," as in Figure 9.11a. This x-axis scale is linear in energy and, once calibrated for a particular energy range, is valid for all photons and all radionuclides being examined.

It is almost always photopeak photons alone, corresponding to the complete absorption of the radionuclide's emitted gamma-ray, that are selected for NM imaging, with the rest rejected through energy windowing. Below the photopeak appears the *Compton plateau*, produced almost entirely by Compton scatter electrons released in the crystal; the highest energy of the plateau defines the *Compton edge*.

Photon 1 in Figure 9.11b deposits all its energy within the NaI[T1] crystal in a single photoelectric event. Photon 4 does so as well, but only after creating a Compton scatter photon that itself is subsequently fully absorbed. Both of these contribute to

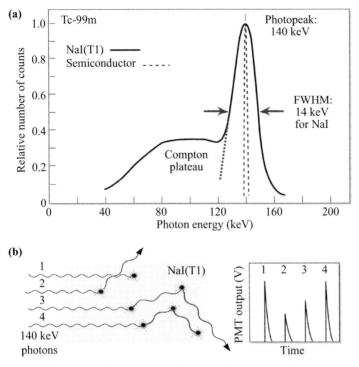

(a)

(b)

Figure 9.11 A scintillation detector can determine the energies of high-energy photons, but even a monochromatic source may produce a complex (rather than a single peak) spectrum. **(a)** The solid line indicates the energy spectrum (from the calibrated pulse height analyzer) of Tc-99m in NaI[Tl], displaying the *photopeak* at 140 keV. The *Compton plateau* lies at lower energies, and the *Compton edge* at the top of the plateau. The dashed peak is the photopeak of the same radionuclide obtained with a germanium semiconductor detector. The full width at half-maximum (FWHM) of the peak from germanium is about 20 times narrower than that from sodium iodide. **(b)** Four 140-keV photons strike a scintillation detector in sequence. The amplitudes of the voltage pulses are assessed by the PHA, which keeps track of the numbers of them arriving with various energies (voltage pulse amplitudes), and displays this information as, in this case, the spectrum of Tc-99m in NaI[T1].

the photopeak. Some of the energy of photons 2 and 3 escapes the crystal as Compton scatter, however, and the PMT output pulses are of correspondingly lower voltage. For some nuclides and detector materials, there can be considerably more structure than seen in this spectrum.

One might expect a narrowly peaked pulse height spectrum for NaI[Tl], but it is somewhat broad, and its *full width at half maximum* (*FWHM*) is about 14 keV. It is useful to define the relative *energy resolution* for the photopeak as $E_{res} = FWHM/E_{photopeak}$. $E_{res} = 14$ keV/140 keV = 10% for Tc-99m in NaI[Tl], as indicated by the solid curve in Figure 9.11a. The photopeak width depends on the gamma energy of the radionuclide, but even more so on the detector material. When obtained with a germanium (Ge) semiconductor diode detector, the peak

is nearly 20 times narrower, as with the dashed line in the figure. This has an interesting story, centered largely on Poisson statistics and the photon energy required to trigger the detector, but not for here. If semiconductor light-sensitive devices, such as avalanche photodiodes (APD) have begun replacing PMTs at the time of the next edition, we'll definitely address the issue then.

A PHA makes possible *energy windowing* (not the same as gray-scale windowing of the display in CT or DR), a powerful tool for noise reduction in nuclear imaging. The PHA selects only those pulses that lie sufficiently close to the center of the photopeak for counting and processing. That greatly reduces the effects of scatter radiation and, when several radionuclides are simultaneously present as happens for some studies, it lets the system respond

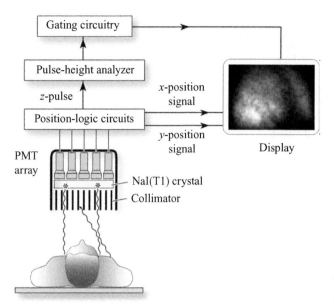

Figure 9.12 A modern gamma camera. The two-headed machine of Figure 1.16a can be used for standard planar imaging, for simultaneous AP and PA studies, or for SPECT. Each imaging head contains a *collimator*, a large-diameter, thin *single crystal* of NaI[Tl], and an *array* of *small PMTs*. When a gamma-ray from the body makes it along a collimator hole and strikes the crystal, the flash of scintillation light is seen by all the nearby PMTs. Their summed net voltage is checked against the energy window to confirm that it corresponds to the photopeak. The position of the flash is determined to within about 1 cm by the *position-location logic circuit*, and the brightness of the corresponding pixel on the display is incremented.

to the gamma-rays from only one of them at a time. It is common practice to set the width of the window equal to one or two times the FWHM, but the best choice depends on the application. The narrower the window, the more rejection there is of false counts from noise, but the less the sensitivity of the system. For gamma camera or SPECT imaging of Tc-99m, the window is commonly from 126 to 154 keV.

The gamma (Anger) camera

The rectilinear scanner brought about a novel and powerful way of examining the body, but there were fundamental limitations to it. Its detector had to move slowly enough across the body to obtain a statistically adequate reading of activity at each position, and this was extremely time-consuming. In addition, there was no way the system could follow rapid changes throughout an entire region over time. Dynamic imaging of the flow of a bolus of radioactive contrast agent throughout the vasculature, for example, was not an option. Both rapid data acquisition and the performance of dynamic studies call for the services of a gamma camera.

The gamma camera, also known as the Anger camera, was designed by Hal Anger in the late 1950s (Figures 1.15b and 1.16a). It is much more sensitive and efficient a device, cutting imaging time

considerably. And its ability to observe an entire anatomic region of interest continuously makes feasible the study of time-dependent phenomena, even the beating of a heart.

A gamma camera detects and images gamma-rays somewhat as an eye or optical camera images visible light (Figure 9.12). Unlike light or ultrasound, however, gamma-rays cannot readily be focused, so the role of the lens is played by the *collimator* at the front face of the gamma camera; and, like a lens, it projects from a three-dimensional object onto a two-dimensional surface on the monitor — just like planar X-ray imaging. A collimator is typically a thin lead plate through which pass hundreds of small-diameter channels (Figure 9.13a). A gamma-ray that does not travel along the straight and narrow is absorbed in the lead, as with a radiographic grid. Most common is the parallel-hole collimator, but there are also converging ones that produce magnified images, and the single-pinhole variety. Collimators are also classified according to the resolution they can provide or the photon energy; two of the commonest are the low-energy, all-purpose (LEAP) and the low-energy, high-resolution (LEHR) varieties.

Behind the collimator of a camera head resides a single NaI[Tl] crystal, some 25 cm (10 in) to 60 cm (24 in) across, and 1 cm ($^3/_8$ in) to 0.6 cm ($^1/_4$ in) thin (Figure 9.13b).

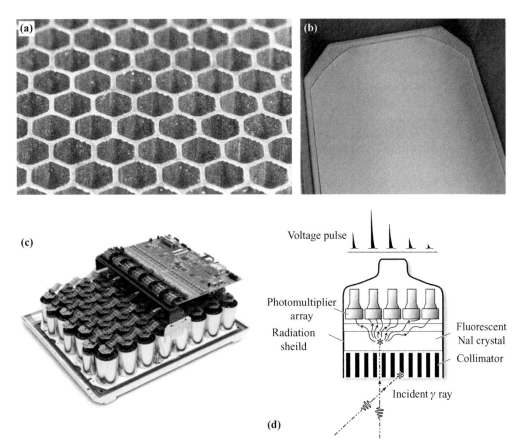

Figure 9.13 Behind the face of a gamma camera. (**a**) Blown-up view of the collimator, which performs the job of a lens of an optical imaging device. (**b**) Part of the large, thin sodium iodide scintillation crystal which is observed by (**c**) an array of up to 100 PMTs, each 5 cm or less in diameter, here seen from the back. Photo courtesy of Siemens Medical Solutions USA, Inc. (**d**) Because of the scintillation-location logic circuit, the image resolution is much better than 5 cm.

The scintillation crystal is observed by a close-packed honeycomb hexagonal array of 37, 61, 75, 91, or more small photomultiplier tubes, dozens of which will sense any nearby scintillation (Figure 9.13c). Together, they can lead to the determination of where within the crystal the gamma-ray struck. A burst of light elicits a voltage pulse in every one of the nearby PMTs, and the nearer a tube is to the site of the flash, the greater its apparent brightness and the larger the voltage pulse it generates (Figure 9.13d). The scintillation-location logic circuit knows the position of every PMT and, by comparing the voltage responses from all of them, it arrives at an estimate of where the flash occurred. A pinpoint of light then appears at the appropriate place on the display screen, and the several hundred thousand equally bright, fine-focused dots constitute a clinical image. Optically sensitive devices other than PMTs are being explored, such as solid-state avalanche photodiodes and silicon photomultipliers. It is even possible that the entire gamma camera may be displaced in the future by some sort of solid state flat panel imager.

Contrast, spatial resolution, sensitivity, and lesion detection

The achievable quality of an image, its contrast, noise level, resolution, and sensitivity, were introduced in Chapter 4. In nuclear medicine, they are determined largely by four separate factors: (i) the differential uptake of the radiopharmaceutical in various tissues; (ii) the amount of it administered and the duration of the study, hence the number of counts recorded; (iii) the extent of the attenuation and scattering of gamma-ray photons by overlying and adjacent tissues; and (iv) the characteristics of the equipment.

The *subject contrast* of a feature in a nuclear medicine image reflects only the first of these. It is commonly expressed as the relative difference in radionuclide concentrations, or specific activities, existing in a *lesion* or other irregularity and the background of *normal* tissues (Figure 4.18),

$$C_{subject} = (\text{Conc}_{les} - \text{Conc}_{back})/\text{Conc}_{back}, \quad (9.4a)$$

In some cases, the feature might appear as a "hot" spot, with higher uptake than in normal tissue, and in other as a "cold" spot.

The corresponding *image contrast* is the relative difference in the displayed number of counts, N, per unit area, A, of the object, in the region of interest:

$$C_{image} = [(N/A)_{les} - (N/A)_{back}]/(N/A)_{back}, \quad (9.4b)$$

seen earlier near Equation 4.4c. C_{image} is directly proportional to the administered activity, but the patient dose is, too.

Image quality tends to increase with the total number of counts – rapidly, at first, but then with diminishing returns. Patient throughput, on the other hand, declines with greater counting times. An average of the order of 1000 counts/cm^2 at the camera face is commonly held to represent a good balance of these factors.

As with radiography, scatter radiation degrades *contrast*, but energy windowing and the collimator both remove much of the Compton scatter radiation created within the patient. Nuclear medicine differs from radiography in that C_{image} is strongly influenced by the depth within the body of the organ being imaged, because of both the (undesirable) attenuation of gamma-rays by overlying tissues and the uptake of activity by other tissues (also unwanted), creating a form of background noise.

The *resolution* or resolving power of a gamma camera, R, is commonly taken to be the FWHM of the line spread function or the point spread function, $R =$ FWHM of PSF (Figure 9.14). Larger values of R, in centimeters (*not* in line pairs/cm!) indicate worse resolution. System resolution is determined by the finite size and separation of the holes pass-

ing through the collimator, by X-ray scatter and light diffusion within the NaI, and by imperfections of the PMT array and in the digital scintillation-localization circuit. The effects of these factors, and others, can be considered, quantified, and measured separately, and it can be revealing to generate the MTF(k) from a Fourier transform of the PSF(r) or LSF(x) (Equation 4.3b).

Resolution also depends strongly on depth of the emitting organ within the body, as can be seen from the LSF obtained at different source-to-image distances (SID). This is demonstrated directly in Figure 9.14b, where the SID is increased by moving the patient 10 cm away from the camera face.

The *sensitivity* of a gamma camera is also affected by both the collimator and the detector. The photopeak detection efficiency of the crystal/PMT system is nearly 100% for gamma-ray energies up to 100 keV. At higher energies, it depends strongly on crystal thickness.

Static and dynamic studies

Here is a sampler of some commonly found clinical examinations. In general, an abnormally dark area within the image of an organ may indicate missing tissue, or a failure to take up the radiopharmaceutical, or the presence of an overlying irregular structure or growth that attenuates emitted gamma-rays before they can reach the image receptor. A too-bright area, conversely, suggests that for some reason the corresponding tissue has accumulated an abnormally high concentration of the radiopharmaceutical.

Common static planar examinations
With some important exceptions, the radionuclide activities administered for most of these studies are in the range of 40–400 MBq (about 1–10 mCi).

Lung ventilation/perfusion (V/Q)
A middle-aged patient who leads a sedentary life presents with a leg that has become swollen and painful over the course of a day, followed that night by a sharp pain in the lower left side of the chest and the coughing up of blood. The electrocardiogram was normal, as was the chest X-ray, but arterial oxygen level was low, and a rub could be heard at the site of the pain. With a heart attack and pneumonia

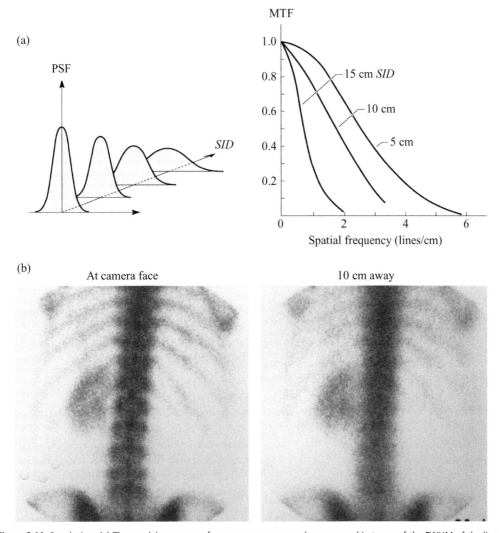

Figure 9.14 Resolution. **(a)** The resolving power of a gamma camera can be expressed in terms of the FWHM of the line spread function from a narrow tube containing radiopharmaceutical placed along the camera face and at a set of distances from it. The modulation transfer function (MTF) is even more informative. **(b)** Patient adjacent to the face of a gamma camera, and moved 10 cm away from it.

unlikely, signs pointed to an embolism plugging a major artery of the lung. Perhaps a thrombus formed in the leg, and a piece broke off and was swept through the heart and into the lung; there it lodged in a narrow pulmonary artery, blocking it off and creating a potentially life-threatening situation. A pulmonary embolism would cut off flow of blood to a region of the lung (perfusion), but air should still be able to reach it (ventilation). A finding by a pulmonary ventilation/perfusion, or V/Q, study that air could get to some region of lung where

blood could not go would strongly supports this diagnosis, as was seen in Figure 1.15. (In the old days, "Q" signified fluid flow.)

In the ventilation part of the study, the patient is seated close to the front of a gamma camera, and for minutes inhales either radioactive xenon-133 gas, with a photopeak at 80 keV (Xe-127, with a 203-keV gamma-ray, is better for imaging than Xe-133, but harder to come by), or aerosolized Tc-99m, while being imaged. The gas or aerosol enters the lungs and fills all parts that are not somehow

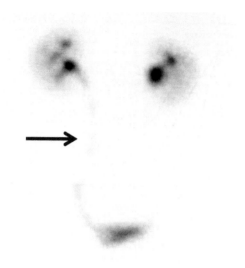

Figure 9.15 Anterior planar view from a Tc-99m MAG3 study of the kidneys. In this normal study performed during the excretory phase, one can observe both renal pelvises, which are symmetric, and the urinary bladder and the right ureter itself (arrow).

blocked off; a dark area in the image would indicate the inability of the radiopharmaceutical to get to a region that air normally occupies. This could be caused by a blockage of air passages, the presence of fluids, or the replacement of lung tissue with tumor or scar. But the ventilation scan of Figure 1.15c is normal. Both lungs appear clear, with xenon easily flowing in and out everywhere.

Xenon, a noble gas, tends to wash out quickly but, because it is radioactive and heavy, it must be disposed of carefully and in accord with regulations, as must other radioactive waste materials. When the much more readily available technetium aerosol is chosen, it must be of low activity, relative to that of the perfusion study to come, so that it does not generate a

ventilation-like background artifact; alternatively, it can be given time to decay away enough.

After the ventilation radiopharmaceutical is gone, lung perfusion is imaged. 100 MBq (3 mCi) of Tc-MAA is injected intravenously and the microscopic lumps become briefly lodged in about 0.1% of the pulmonary capillaries, a small but representative fraction of them. A cold area in the lower left lung reveals a region where the Tc-MAA (and blood) do not reach (Figure 1.15d). Thus the V/Q pair of isotope tests does find a portion of the lung that is ventilated but not perfused (called a mismatch), supporting the initial diagnosis of pulmonary emboli.

Kidneys

A MAG3 (mercapto-acetyl-triglycine with Tc-99m) scan can evaluate the excretion of the kidneys and the overall structure of the collecting systems (Figure 9.15). Injected into the peripheral venous system, ^{99m}Tc–MAG3 undergoes tubular secretion in the urinary outflow tract.

Cholecystitis

A hepatobiliary iminodiacetic acid (HIDA) scan with Tc-99m can be used for the diagnosis of acute cholecystitis (Figure 9.16). The radiopharmaceutical is taken up by hepatocytes and then rapidly excreted into the bile. Stagnation of the isotope within the gall bladder can be directly related to an obstructive process such as by a stone.

Hyperparathyroidism

In a patient suffering from primary hyperparathyroidism, a hyperfunctioning parathyroid gland

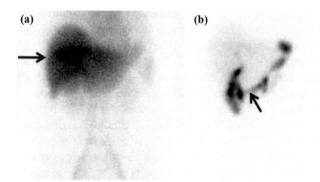

(a)   (b)

Figure 9.16 In this patient presenting with right upper quadrant pain, (a) a planar anterior view of the abdomen demonstrated hepatocytic uptake diffusely throughout the liver at 1 minute (arrow). (b) After 25 minutes, we observe a normal status, with the free passage of the isotope into the biliary tract and out into the GI tract (arrow).

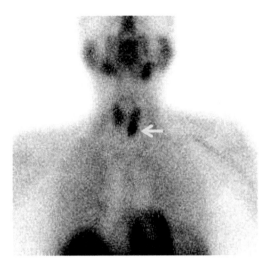

Figure 9.17 Here, excessive uptake of Tc-99m sestamibi by a parathyroid adenoma occurs at the level of the left lower pole of the thyroid gland (arrow).

produces excess parathyroid hormone, which causes bone resorption and ensuing hypercalcemia. The increased function may be due to a benign or malignant tumor or to diffuse hyperplasia. The four small parathyroid glands can usually be located in the neck or even in the mediastinum; it is imperative to know which gland is abnormal and where it is located for planning surgical resection (Figure 9.17).

Ewing sarcoma

Methylene-diphosphonate (MDP) labeled with Tc-99m is preferentially taken up by bone. Focal increased uptake of activity, or "hot spots," may indicate the presence of fractures or neoplastic processes with associated increased osteoblastic reparative function (Figure 9.18).

(a)   **(b)**

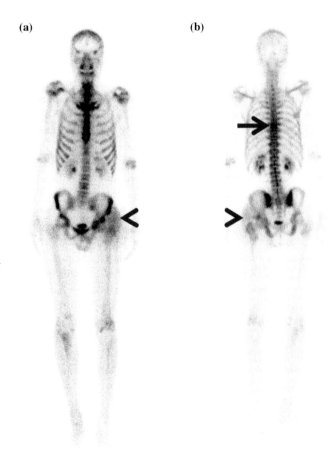

Figure 9.18 This planar whole body bone scan was made during the bony phase of the examination, 3 hours after intravenous administration of Tc-99m methylene diphosphonate. Seen in both the (a) anterior and (b) posterior views, the patient suffers from a Ewing sarcoma of the upper left thigh (arrowhead), and has a metastatic deposit involving the T4 vertebra. Both views are needed to avoid missing the vertebral lesion because of, when assessed from the anterior, the overlying normal sternal activity. The whole body was scanned by moving it slowly past the gamma camera heads, and keeping track of patient table and pixel position over time.

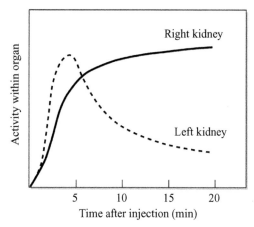

Figure 9.19 The activity of ^{123}I-Hippuran within each of a pair of kidneys is followed during radionuclide uptake and excretion. The shapes of their renogram curves indicates blockage of the right ureter, or some other malady.

These are but a few examples of the many static planar imaging procedures in common use.

Dynamic imaging

A renogram is a dynamic study in which it is the time development of radiopharmaceutical uptake and voiding that are of interest. Figure 9.19, for example, suggests that while the left kidney excretes Hippuran labeled with iodine-123 normally, there appears to be an obstruction preventing clearance from the right kidney.

With dynamic studies, of course, the system has to track the time variable. A modern gamma camera is attached to its own dedicated computer system, which has far more memory than any image capture or calculation process might require. The raw data from the camera consists of the x- and y-coordinates and the time, t, of every scintillation that the energy-windowing network accepts. This information can be stored in any of three formats, *list mode*, *static frame mode*, or *dynamic frame mode*, depending on how it will be used.

List mode data storage constitutes retention of all the raw data accumulated. The information from each and every scintillation event is held in its own memory location as a separate (x,y,t) data address (Figure 9.20a). Things can't get any more basic or complete than this.

With *static frame mode* imaging, for a non-dynamic study, the region of interest is partitioned into a matrix consisting typically of up to $512 \times 512 = 262$k voxels, each with its own (x,y) matrix address. Every gamma-ray event captured then simply increments the number of counts in the corresponding pixel by one, and its overall brightness increases accordingly (Figure 9.20b); the image is already in a form suitable for immediate display. Whole-body scanning employs a variant of static frame mode on which the patient's entire body is partitioned by way of, say, a 128×512 or a 256×1024 grid. The patient is moved past the gamma camera head at constant speed, and the computer links the addresses of scintillations to points fixed in the patient table, rather than to positions on the face of the gamma camera.

If one is examining a process that does not change appreciably during the course of the study, only a single frame is needed, and static frame mode image storage is adequate. But when it is the temporal changes themselves that are of interest, a sequence of frame images is obtained in *dynamic frame mode* of data acquisition, of which there are two general categories.

In the simplest version, the system counts into one frame for a preselected period, then closes out that frame and stores it, and begins immediately on a fresh one (Figure 9.20c). This procedure is continued until the study is finished. In a planar hepatic excretion study, for example, after being taken up by the liver, the radiopharmaceutical is secreted into the intestines via the bile duct and gall bladder. A region of interest (ROI) is selected (Figure 9.21), each frame accumulates counts for the same time interval, and activity within it is plotted as a function of time for quantitative analysis of liver function. This exemplifies the beauty of dynamic nuclear medicine: it allows the quantification of clinically relevant, time-dependent physiologic processes.

Breathing gives rise to a form of motion blurring, and it can somewhat degrade images of the affected organs. Several forms of respiratory *gating*, based on monitoring chest motion, are being devised to counteract that problem, and can lead to a noticeable improvement. The stretching of a belt around the chest can indicate the degree of inhalation and exhalation, as can monitoring the movement of laser bright dots on the skin, and gating directs the corresponding images to be recorded in separate frames.

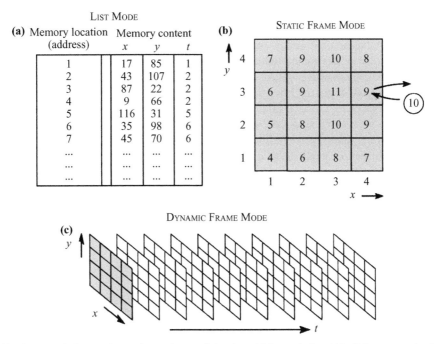

Figure 9.20 Three simple formats for storing nuclear medicine data: (a) list mode, in which all data are retained; (b) static frame mode, in which every event in a voxel increments its corresponding pixel count by one; and (c) dynamic frame mode, in which a matrix is filled for a specified period of time, and then a new one begins. A modification of the dynamic frame mode is applicable for imaging periodically changing objects, in particular the heart.

Nuclear cardiology I: EKG-gated planar blood pool studies

Nuclear cardiology offers a non-traumatic determination of whether portions of myocardium are ischemic or infracted, whether the coronary arteries supplying the muscles of the heart are too clogged to sustain it, and how well the heart is pumping blood to the rest of the body. For the evaluation of coronary artery disease, nuclear cardiology has largely become the instrument of choice,

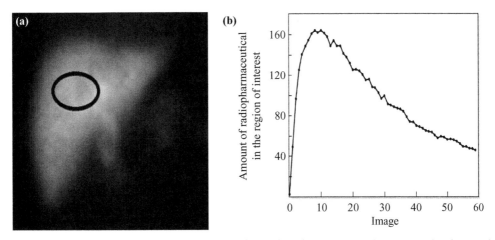

Figure 9.21 Planar, multi-frame dynamic liver scan, (a) one frame of which demonstrates the activity within the ROI. The patient is injected with a radiopharmaceutical that is taken up by the liver and (b) then secreted by it over time into the intestines.

with nearly 10 million procedures performed each year, about half of all NM examinations. ECG-gated SPECT, in particular, has become what is considered to be a state-of-the-art clinical technology, of particular value in the management of patients with ischemic heart disease and congestive heart failure.

There are two general types of nuclear cardiology imaging in common use. *Blood pool* studies, which may be performed with either planar imaging or SPECT, provide information about the pumping of blood by the heart, and may indicate coronary artery disease. *Cardiac perfusion stress* tests relate to the regional perfusion of the heart muscle itself, as in a myocardial infarct. They are normally carried out with SPECT, and to some extent with PET, and will be discussed in the next section on tomographic imaging

A normal gamma camera image of the heart would be blurred by its motion, so techniques have been devised to freeze that movement. A *multi-gated data acquisition* (MUGA) planar cardiac study employs a modification of the dynamic frame mode that exploits the periodic, repetitive nature of the heart's pumping. Working somewhat like a stroboscope, it stores separate images that correspond to different segments of the cardiac cycle in a set of 16 or more separate frames. Each frame is partitioned into a matrix, typically of $128 \times 128 = 16k$ pixels. The first frame is triggered open by the R-wave voltage spike once per heartbeat in the patient's electrocardiogram (ECG) signal, and accumulates counts for, say, 60 milliseconds. Any photopeak event in the first 60-thousandth of a second simply increases the level of brightness at the appropriate pixel in the first frame, as with any ordinary nuclear medicine image. After that, the second frame takes over, for the same length of time, then the third, and so on. This stepping procedure continues for all 16 frames, long enough to cover one heartbeat. Then the next ECG R-wave starts the whole business over again, back at the first frame (Special programs track and reject counts occurring during arrhythmias.) Although not too many counts are obtained during a single cycle, several hundred repetitions, each from a different heartbeat, result in cumulative frame images with adequate gamma-ray statistics, in which each frame gives an unblurred image. The frames can also be displayed in a rapid sequence, a loop that creates a most remarkable cine of a beating heart.

With erythrocytes or serum albumen labeled with technetium-99m, for example, a MUGA blood pool study can image the left and the right ventricular chambers through all phases of the cardiac cycle, of which the end-diastole and end-systole phases appear in Figure 9.22. Gated blood pool studies, typically with 8 or 16 images covering one heartbeat, can yield the ejection fraction for each ventricle. That, and regional wall motion and thickness, are important indicators of the heart's pumping efficiency and functional status. For the left ventricle, moreover, the ejection fraction and the wall motion can be assessed adequately if seen with MUGA planar images from three angles, with anterior, left anterior oblique (LAO), and near left lateral views.

Once an image has been produced, the computer can enhance its quality in various ways, such as by smoothing out naturally occurring, random fluctuations in the numbers of counts in pixels (Figure 6.10). In a dynamic study, the number of counts at each pixel address can also be averaged temporally, over several sequential frames. Spatial and temporal smoothing involve losses of high-frequency components of spatial and temporal information, respectively, but may nonetheless result in images more meaningful to the eye.

This is all straightforward when there is access to a SPECT machine, but much important clinical information can still be obtained when there is not one; indeed, even when a SPECT machine is at hand, a standard planar gamma camera is not uncommonly used instead, for reasons of time, throughput, cost/study, and count-statistics.

Tomographic nuclear imaging: SPECT and PET

Tomography has had as great an impact on nuclear studies as did CT on X-ray imaging. Indeed, cardiac SPECT is the most commonly performed nuclear medicine procedure in the US.

The two general families of three-dimensional nuclear imaging, single-photon emission computed tomography (SPECT) and positron emission tomography (PET), use radically dissimilar types of radionuclide emissions and correspondingly

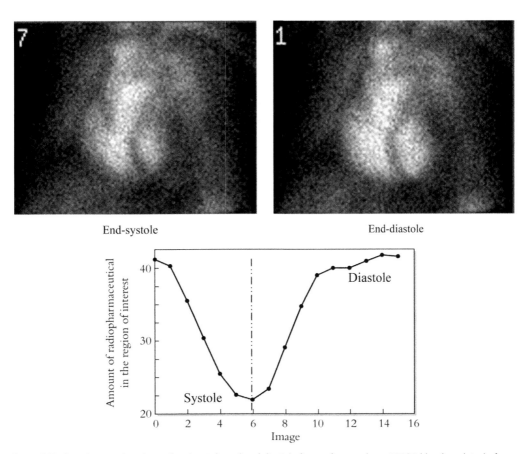

End-systole   End-diastole

Figure 9.22 Septal separation views of end-systole and end-diastole frames from a planar MUGA blood pool study, from a set of 16 images that cover the span of a heartbeat. A region of interest is drawn on each of the 16 to monitor the volume of the left ventricle, yielding a graph of the blood volume in the chamber over time. It indicates that for this patient, the *ejection fraction* is about 0.5. Courtesy of Mariusz Dymerski.

specialized technologies for image capture. They are, however, clinically somewhat complementary. PET may provide somewhat higher resolution and sensitivity and tap into a few metabolic pathways of medical importance, but it has fewer general applications (apart from oncology) at present, deposits more dose, and is generally more expensive.

SPECT and SPECT/CT

SPECT, the NM counterpart to X-ray (transmission) CT, came to the clinic in the early 1970s, along with CT, and it has remained largely unchanged since then. About a half of all SPECT studies are for coronary artery disease, and another quarter for bone, and most of the rest are in search of neoplasms. Not surprisingly, when considering the purchase of a new gamma camera for planar imaging,

growing numbers of nuclear medicine facilities are opting to spend a little more and get a SPECT system instead, which can carry out both planar and 3D studies. Half of new machines, moreover, are being bought with a CT device attached. (All new PET machines automatically come with CT.)

The principal clinical benefit is that while CT alone yields tomographic images of anatomy with high spatial and contrast resolution, SPECT gives tomographic images that are of lower resolution, but that reveal physiologic function. Spatial resolution ranges typically from 7 to 15 mm; a 128 × 128 matrix allows the display of higher resolution than does a 64 × 64, but at the price of lower SNR, because of the reduced number of counts per pixel.

Two or three fairly standard gamma camera heads, typically, each with its own collimator,

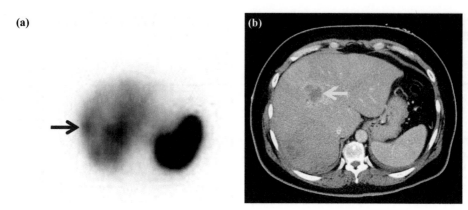

Figure 9.23 This patient suffers from a malignant carcinoid tumor with liver metastases. Pentetreotide is a diethylene-triamino-penta-acetic acid (DTPA) conjugate of octreotide, an analog of somatostatin, and indium-111 pentetreotide concentrate on somatostatin cell receptors. (a) Axial SPECT image of the liver, where focal areas of hyperactivity within the hepatic parenchyma indicate carcinoid metastases (arrow). (b) The associated contrast-enhanced axial CT image of the liver demonstrates the same lesions with peripheral contrast enhancement (arrow).

crystal, and PMT array, are mounted on a supporting gantry (Figure 1.16a). The gantry and camera heads rotate around the patient, and data are acquired at 32, 64, or 128 projection angles. The heads typically move in a circle, or on a body-contour orbit that allows closer approach to the patient at some angles, hence better overall resolution and SNR. The apparatus can also be employed for ordinary planar imaging, when appropriate, for faster throughput.

One advantage of a SPECT machine over a standard gamma camera is its higher contrast, just as with CT and DR. More obvious is its ability to enable the physician to visualize an organ in three dimensions, and in several quite different ways – as a set of individual tomographic slices, as with CT (Figures 9.23); or as a slice at any depth in the patient and seen from any angle (Figure 9.24); and as a solid object in three dimensions, to be viewed from any angle, or perhaps even while rotating.

The data are reconstructed into tomographic slices commonly by iterative methods (Chapter 8). Reconstruction computations are more complicated and susceptible to artifacts in SPECT than in CT, partly because far fewer quanta are detected. Also, the detected signal depends not only on the distribution of gamma-emitting material within the organ of interest (which is what is of primary

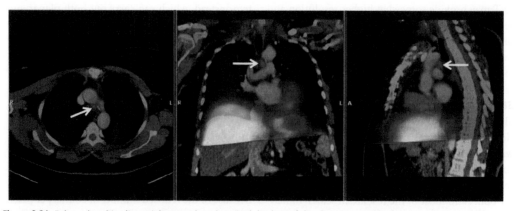

Figure 9.24 False-color, thin-slice axial, coronal, and sagittal displays of the chest, created by fusing separate Tc-99m sestamibi SPECT and unenhanced CT reconstructions. Hyperactivity is displayed in red and can be localized at the level of the mediastinum in the aortopulmonary window, just behind the ascending aorta (arrows).

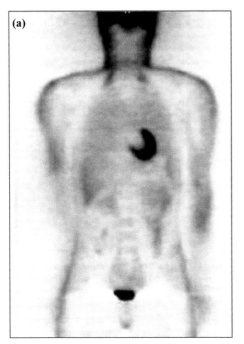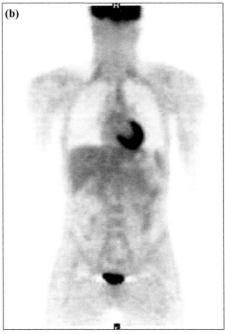

Figure 9.25 SPECT (**a**) without and (**b**) with application of self-attenuation correction.

clinical importance in nuclear medicine), but also on the absorption and scatter of photons by other nearby tissues (which does not help create the image; it just muddies the waters). Attenuation by other organs and tissues is, to the gamma camera, indistinguishable from a reduction in activity in the organ of concern, and gives rise to erroneous alterations in apparent contrast. This can be especially problematic for obese patients, or body builders, or even for women with large breasts. Algorithms that correct for tissue attenuation for both SPECT and PET have been developed and are continually being improved (Figure 9.25), as are others for scatter removal.

Some simple correction programs assume uniform attenuation, while others require input of attenuation coefficients throughout the region being examined; these can be obtained either from a CT device or from a CT-like study in which a small radionuclide source, attached to the SPECT machine and outside the body, provides photons for a transmission study. In the former case, it is also necessary to convert CT attenuation results obtained at 120 kVp (and of perhaps 70 keV average photon energy) for use in calculating attenuation of the significantly higher 140 keV of technetium, say. CT is fast, but registration of the SPECT and CT images may be demanding unless the two devices are adjacent and the same patient table serves both, as with PET/CT. Close registration is a critically important part of the process, as it is with DSA (Figure 7.11); while carried out manually in earlier days simply by eye-balling, now it is generally done semi-automatically.

Quality assurance and maintenance with SPECT are more demanding than with either planar gamma camera imaging or CT. It is especially important to confirm field uniformity, and the precise mechanical motion of the heads about the isocenter.

Nuclear cardiology II: cardiac perfusion SPECT stress test

A myocardium perfusion stress test involves the comparison of two gated-SPECT studies, one with the patient in the resting condition and the other after serious effort on a stationary bike or treadmill, or with pharmacological stress that simulates exercise (such as that from dipyridamole or dobutamine) (Figure 9.26). The resting image is good for

Rest

(a)

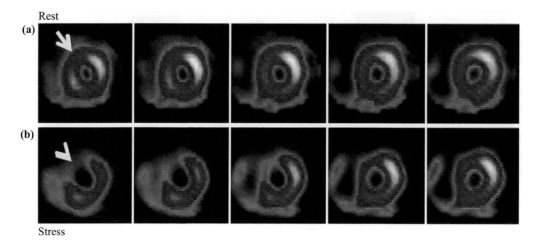

(b)

Stress

Figure 9.26 A SPECT myocardial perfusion test might consist of two parts, first with the patient at rest and then again, several hours later, immediately after heavy exercise. Here, a 71-year-old male patient with a history of anterior wall myocardial infarction was referred for evaluation of the extent of ischemia, infarct size, and reversibility. The test involves MUGA, a periodic dynamic-frame mode that cycles repeatedly through a set of several dozen frames in synchrony with the cardiac cycle, with the timing provided by the R-wave spikes of an electrocardiogram. A frame might collect data during each of 32 30-ms intervals, say, and then repeat this for many consecutive heartbeats. **(a)** For the resting phase study, 10 mCi of Tc-99m-mibi are administered, and the patient is imaged with a 15% energy window centered on the 140 keV photopeak. These sequential short axis views of a region of myocardium throughout the cardiac cycle show a small residual perfusion defect in the anteroseptal region (arrow), demonstrating almost complete reversibility. **(b)** Two hours later, 30 mCi of technetium-mibi (enough to overwhelm the remaining radionuclide from the previous study) is administered for the stress phase, demonstrating a large perfusion defect involving the anteroseptal wall (arrowhead). The patient was referred for catheter angiography with a suspected blockage in the left anterior descending artery in need of revascularization.

revealing permanent damage to the myocardium, while differences that materialize in the stress study may indicate coronary artery disease. Both studies are carried out in the gated mode. Images can be improved further by arranging for separate gating also for respiration motion.

In a typical 1-day procedure, Tc-99m-sestamibi (Tc-mibi) is injected intravenously while the patient is resting. Because it is lipophilic, sestamibi tends to accumulate in the myocardium according to blood flow, and "cold" regions indicate ischemic and infarcted tissues. With ECG gating and monitoring, the patient is imaged 15 minutes or so later and, afterwards, asked to wait several hours while the technetium decays away and washes out somewhat.

The patient is then stressed, either by exercise or through vasodilating drugs. After 10 to 20 minutes of exercise, at peak stress, he or she receives a second injection of three times the activity of the first injection.

Even when a coronary artery is 75–80% blocked, the heart muscle at rest may still provide itself with enough blood to continue functioning adequately as a pump. But when it is stressed, the myocardium demands considerably more oxygen-bearing blood. Those parts supplied by a partially obstructed vessel may suffer insufficient oxygenation, and complain by triggering angina. With a more severe occlusion of an artery, a myocardial infarction may have occurred, in which cardiac muscle cells have received so little blood (and oxygen) that they die. Either of these conditions may show up clearly on a SPECT myocardial perfusion test. Comparison of the stress and rest tests may indicate whether the area with reduced blood flow is ischemic but still alive, or infarcted and dead. In cases of ischemia, that part of the myocardium may regain adequate blood flow through intervention such as angioplasty or surgery.

Thallium-201 can also be used in one of the two parts of a cardiac stress test, rather than Tc-99m.

Thallium ions act physiologically much like potassium and seek to concentrate within muscle cells, but their uptake by myocardial cells can be significantly decreased by reduced blood flow. Its primary photon energies of 70 and 167 keV can readily be distinguished from that of technetium, and it can be counted separately from it through energy windowing, which can speed the study along considerably. But Tl-201 has a long (3-day) half-life and photons that are not too high in energy (because of which many of them do not escape the body), both of which mean that even a small activity can deposit a hefty dose

If the SPECT image is normal under stress, then the patient can go home greatly relieved. If there are indications of pathology only during stress but not at rest, then it is likely the myocardium itself has not been irreparably damaged, and so surgical or medical intervention may well be of benefit. A cold area of diminished image brightness that appears even at rest would be bad news, however, indicating a portion of myocardium damaged so severely and irreparably that the patient would not benefit from surgery or angioplasty. Still, a follow-up study with PET to evaluate tissue viability may suggest that the situation is not hopeless.

Positron emission tomography with ¹⁸FDG, and PET/CT and PET/MRI

PET is a subfield of nuclear medicine that has long been of considerable research value, initially to map local variations in the rate of glucose metabolism throughout the normal and abnormal brain during various kinds of cerebral activity. More recently, it has been finding important clinical applications in the detection and monitoring of tumors, in cardiology, and elsewhere. As with conventional NM or SPECT, PET involves the detection of high-energy photons. But PET differs notably in three important regards:

PET radionuclides emit *positrons*, not gammarays. When a positron-emitting radioisotope is injected into a patient, released positrons travel at high velocity through the tissue, rapidly losing energy in ionizing the atoms and molecules along their paths.

After passing through 0.2–1.5 mm, typically, depending on its initial kinetic energy, a positron has slowed down sufficiently to be able to single out some unsuspecting electron, with which it annihilates (Figures 9.3d and 9.4b). All their combined mass-energy is converted instantaneously into the form of a pair of 511 keV photons. These are of much higher energy than what is normally employed in nuclear medicine (70–200 keV), and are best termed *annihilation photons*.

The two leave the site of the collision in nearly opposite directions, $\pm\frac{1}{4}°$ (Figure 1.17a). Coincidence (i.e., simultaneous) detection of a sufficient number of *pairs* of 511 keV photons by corresponding pairs of detectors on opposite sides of the PET machine yields enough information for creation of a PET map of the uptake of the radioisotope of somewhat higher spatial resolution than planar NM or SPECT.

Some of the more important positron-emitting isotopes appear in Table 9.3. Almost all are created by bombarding stable nuclei with protons, deuterons (nuclei of hydrogen-2), or nuclei of

Table 9.3 Radionuclides employed for PET. While carbon-11 has a long enough half-life (20 minutes) for some imaginative and rapid biochemistry, nitrogen-13 and certainly oxygen-15 do not. The one of them utilized most widely clinically, by far, is fluorine-18.

Z	Nuclide	$t_{1/2}$	Production	$<x>$(mm in tissue)
6	Carbon-11	20.4 min	Cyclotron	0.3
7	Nitrogen-13	10 min	Cyclotron	0.4
8	Oxygen-15	2 min	Cyclotron	1.5
9	Fluorine-18	1.8 h	Cyclotron	0.2
29	Copper-64	12.7 h	Cyclotron	
31	Gallium-68	68 min	Cyclotron	1.9
37	Rubidium-82	1.3 min	Generator	2.6

helium-3 or He-4 in a cyclotron. Fluorine-18, for example, can be produced through targeting neon-20 gas with high-velocity deuterons, or more commonly an O-18 target in aqueous or gaseous form with protons.

One early reason for the interest in PET has been that the list of positron-emitting nuclei includes isotopes of carbon, nitrogen, oxygen, and other elements of particular biochemical relevance. These have been prepared for PET studies as gaseous oxygen, water, carbon monoxide, carbon dioxide, and ammonia. Water and molecular oxygen, for example, each containing one atom of oxygen-15, have been employed extensively to monitor blood flow and oxygen metabolism in the brain, heart, and tumors. Some positron-emitters have been incorporated into larger molecules such as sugars, amino acids, fatty acids, and even neurotransmitters, which trace more complex biochemical pathways. But the radiochemistry of positron-emitters is generally difficult, since they tend to have short half-lives (N-13, 10 min; O-15, 2 min), although C-11 (20 min) may be manageable. Most have therefore had to be produced locally, for many PET applications, in an on-site cyclotron. But gallium-68, which mimics iron and binds into transferrin, can be produced in generators. This and F-18 FDG are usually obtained commercially, and do not require an on-site cyclotron.

One particular combination of positron-emitting radionuclide plus agent largely dominates the field. Fluorine-18 can be substituted for hydrogen or hydroxyl in a number of biomolecules, with little change in their biochemistry. (A particularly attractive feature of F-18 is its half-life of nearly 2 hours, which provides enough time for its chemical incorporation into some complex biomolecules.) Since burning glucose is one of the principal ways in which the body produces energy, being able to monitor the rate of its metabolism is often of interest. Clinical PET makes such measurements almost exclusively with F-18 fluorodeoxyglucose (^{18}FDG or just FDG), a positron-emitting analog that is delivered to the cells in the same manner as ordinary glucose.

PET has proven invaluable in cardiac and brain imaging, but its most important clinical role is now in oncology. Cancer cells generally metabolize glucose at a higher rate than most normal tissue (Figure 1.17b). And while normal glucose is consumed by cells and then broken down, with the metabolic products (water, CO_2, etc.) rapidly eliminated, FDG behaves differently: the fluorine remains trapped in the cell for a good while, making it relatively easy to image tumors, in particular.

FDG studies are instrumental in the detection and monitoring of malignancies in the brain, head and neck, breast, lung, liver, colon, and other tissues. For many tumor-related applications, as in the staging of lung cancer, PET has better sensitivity and specificity than CT. PET is also finding an important role in monitoring the course of cancer therapy: it may take weeks or months before CT or MRI can reveal whether the size of a tumor is changing (one way or the other) following the onset of treatment. But the effects of radiation or drugs may be apparent much sooner through alterations in the tumor's metabolism; an early PET determination of therapy efficacy may help with treatment optimization, or indicate that another approach should be tried. Other F-18 radiopharmaceuticals are being explored, including fluoro α-methyl tyrosine (FMT) and fluoro-L-thymidine (FLT) for tumor cell proliferation imaging, and fluoromisonidazole (FMISO) for hypoxia imaging.

A PET imager differs from a SPECT machine in that when a positron annihilates within the patient, it has to detect *both* photons of the pair simultaneously, or else the event is not recorded. Several general types of PET cameras have been built, one of which makes use of a dozen or so adjacent rings of small, independent, solid scintillation detectors that circle the patient (Figure 1.17a), as with multi-slice CT. A ring might contain several hundred individual crystals of bismuth germanate (BGO), which has a higher sensitivity than NaI for detecting the high-energy 511 keV photons, or of lutetium silicate (LSO), or of other scintillation materials. There have also been designs of dual- or multi-head cameras built around NaI(Tl).

All designs share the common property that a coincidence circuit accepts only those events in which two opposing detectors (across from one another in either the same or neighboring rings) are struck by 511 keV photons at virtually the same time, to within 5 ns. PET cameras have no conventional collimators, but rather rely on coincidence detection as the sole means of emission localization:

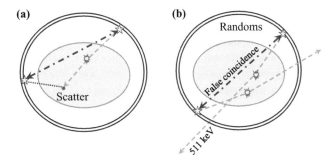

Figure 9.27 False PET coincidences. (**a**) Scatter and (**b**) random coincidences contribute a unique kind of noise to PET images.

as suggested by Figure 1.17a, the positron met its fate somewhere along the line joining the two detectors, which provides essentially the same locational information that a collimator does for a gamma camera. The absence of collimators is part of the reason why PET has much greater sensitivity than SPECT.

Resolution within a transverse plane of the patient is determined chiefly by the cross-sectional dimensions of the individual scintillation crystals facing the annihilation photons, a few millimeters. The ultimate achievable resolution is inherently limited to about 2 mm or so, however, because of positron travel within the patient before annihilation, and because the 511 keV photons are not emitted in exactly opposite directions, but these have negligible impact on clinical studies.

There are two major sources of image degradation unique to PET: *scatter* noise and *random* coincidences. Scatter noise arises when one of the annihilation photons undergoes a Compton scatter within the body, veers off in a new direction, and strikes a "wrong" detector (Figure 9.27a). With randoms, unrelated photons happen to hit two detector

crystals within an extremely short period of time, mimicking a coincidence event (Figure 9.27b). Scatter events are more frequent, since the two photons will always fit within the coincidence time window.

Every new PET scanner is now sold as part of a hybrid scanner with a CT attached, which serves two purposes. First, it makes possible attenuation corrections. The second driver is that PET is widely used to discover neoplasms, and radiotherapy and surgical treatment planning require the precise anatomic localization that CT can provide. Characteristic artifacts arise when the two images are misaligned, analogous to what occurs with the mask and contrast images in DSA (Figure 7.11).

As with SPECT, reconstruction is carried out commonly with iterative methods. For PET, too, reconstruction is complicated by the presence of attenuating tissues, but correcting for the problem is not quite so bad here. Photons that register in a particular pair of detectors must originate from some point almost exactly along the straight line connecting them (Figure 9.28a). The probability that one of the gamma-rays will travel through x_1 of radiologically uniform tissue, such as brain of attenuation coefficient μ, and then reach a detector is proportional to

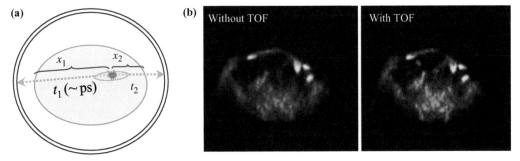

Figure 9.28 Time of flight (TOF) or "electronic collimating." For PET (**a**) the two detection events occur at slightly, but measurably, different times. The non-colinearity of the two photon paths is exaggerated here. (**b**) Improvement in PET lesion detectability with TOF.

$e^{-\mu x_1}$, and similarly for its partner photon. The likelihood, P_{coinc}, of a coincidence event, in which both photons arrive at their respective detectors without having been either absorbed or scattered in tissue, is therefore proportional to $(e^{-\mu x_1})(e^{-\mu x_2}) = e^{-\mu (x_1 + x_2)}$, where $(x_1 + x_2)$ is the length of the arc along x_1 and x_2. That is, the probability of a coincidence event depends on the total thickness $(x_1 + x_2)$ of the tissue along the line between the detectors, but not on the position of the positron-emitting nucleus along that line. This is a valuable simplification, not available with planar imaging or SPECT, that can help with the attenuation correction.

Time of flight (TOF) PET improves signal-to-noise by exploiting this notion more fully (Figure 9.28a). With c the speed of high-energy photons in tissue, the time required for one of the pair to travel the distance x_1 is $t_1 = x_1/c$, and likewise for the other. This leads to $x_1/x_2 = t_1/t_2$. So when one can measure t_1 and t_2 more precisely than is needed just for confirming coincidences, it is possible to determine better where the annihilation event occurred along the line between the two triggered detectors, a process sometimes called *electronic collimation*. At present, coincidence circuits can time pulses to about 500 picoseconds (1 ps $= 10^{-12}$ second). The amount of uncertainty in spatial position of the collision is therefore on the order of $(3 \times 10^{10}$ cm/s$)(300 \times 10^{-12}$ s$) = 10$ cm or less. This may seem like a lot, but it reduces the range of uncertainty down from 30 or so centimeters (Figure 9.28b), and the approach is bound to improve as faster scintillator crystals and electronics become available. The concept of TOF has been around for decades, but the technology has risen to the task only recently.

Cardiac PET with FDG may sometimes be better than cardiac SPECT in predicting the potential outcome of cardiac bypass surgery (Figure 9.29). PET reflects the actual metabolic activity (in particular, the rate of glucose consumption) of cardiac muscle after a heart attack. Some groups of heart muscle cells that are too damaged to take up thallium or Tc-mibi, and might previously have been considered beyond hope, may now be seen with PET still to be sufficiently functional to recover with the return of a good supply of oxygen – so PET offers a second chance to some patients who, before, would not have been viewed as potential surgical candidates.

Until the advent of *functional MRI* (*f*MRI) (Chapter 12), PET with FDG offered the only way to image the operation of the brain in different mental states (Figure 9.30a). Glucose (and FDG) can cross the blood-brain barrier, and is the primary energy source for the cranial neurons and neuroglia. This has led to much research in which areas of the normal brain light up when a subject is experiencing mental or physical stimuli, or is performing various mental/physical tasks. Similarly, abnormalities such as Parkinson's and Alzheimer's diseases, epilepsy, and schizophrenia are found to affect patterns of cerebral energy use. PET can even perform reasonably well in assessing when a person is speaking the truth or lying. While much of this work is in a basic research phase, there are a few important clinical applications in place, as in the investigation of epilepsy, of certain features of brain tumors, and of Alzheimer's disease. An exciting recent development has been the construction of a mobile PET scanner that fits on the head of a freely moving rat (Figure 9.30b).

Several technological developments helped draw PET out of the laboratory and into the clinical mainstream. PET has long been an exciting and productive research tool, but an expensive one: a standard PET/CT scanner has a sticker price of $2 million or more. But compared with the $1 million or so for plain vanilla multi-slice CT, PET-plus-CT no longer seems so excessive. Another cost problem with PET in the past was that the short half-lives of most positron-emitting radionuclides necessitated their production by means of a complex and pricey on-site cyclotron; then, too, there were the masters- or doctorate-level personnel required to operate and maintain the cyclotron and to perform the radiochemistry. With the rapid increase in the application of PET to cancer imaging, however, radiopharmacology companies are now producing FDG regionally for daily delivery; a hospital no longer has to operate a cyclotron or even do the chemistry.

Also, government agencies have now recognized the clinical value of PET, and have approved some PET procedures for reimbursement from health insurance programs.

The obvious next step is PET/MRI. A number of R&D groups are working on integrating the two modalities, one approach being to circle the patient, within the MR donut hole, with rings

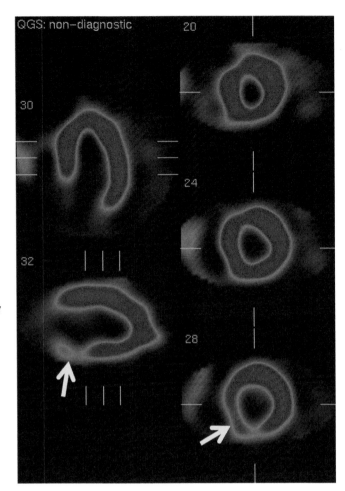

Figure 9.29 Cardiac PET can image not only functioning myocardium but also hibernating myocardium, which is largely dysfunctional but can return to near-normal performance following revascularization procedures. These images have been reconstructed in the horizontal long axis (top left), vertical long axis (bottom left), and short axis (right) to produce a virtual three-dimensional topography of heart function. We observe an ill-defined lack of activity in the infero-septal region (arrows) that could represent sequellae of frank ischemia and should be correlated clinically.

of small (non-magnetic) fluorescent crystals that send their scintillations to the outside world by way of fiber-optics. The considerable potential benefits will become clearer after we discuss MRI, with its capability of performing a vast and growing range of structural and functional studies. These come about largely through the introduction of whole dimensions of contrast creation that enable us to explore soft tissue systems in totally novel and unique ways. These include various forms of relaxation-time (T1

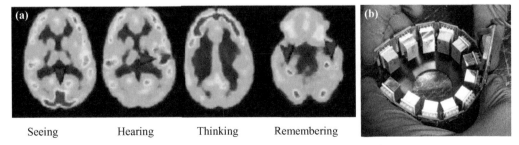

Figure 9.30 The first major use of PET was in the study of brain function. **(a)** Examples of changes occurring in transverse slices of the brain while the subject is carrying out various mental tasks. **(b)** A micro-PET image detector array, small and light enough to be worn by a conscious, freely moving rat. Courtesy of Paul Vaska. See also [2].

and T2) imaging, magnetic resonance spectroscopy (MRS) of neoplasms and other abnormal tissues, diffusion-tensor imaging (DTI) with its remarkable ability to track white-matter bundles, MR perfusion imaging, simultaneous PET and functional MRI (fMRI) studies of mental processes, and much else – and all without the radiation dose that is inevitable with CT. About the only major downside would be the greater expense, but MR costs continue to drop over time.

Quality assurance and radiation safety

As with the other modalities, it is essential to have comprehensive quality assurance and radiation safety programs in place, maintained, and with clear records. Nuclear medicine differs from the other modalities, however, in that the source of the radiation, the radiopharmaceutical, and the imaging device itself are disconnected, and can be considered separately.

Radiopharmaceutical QA and radiation safety

An important activity of a nuclear medicine facility is the maintenance of a rigorous quality assurance program for handling radiopharmaceuticals. It begins when a package first arrives at the clinic, with a survey for leakage of radioactive material, and carries through until the waste has been disposed of properly – and there is much in between.

Several specific tests must be carried out to demonstrate on-site that the radiopharmaceuticals are sufficiently pure. *Radiopharmaceutical purity* of a sample can be viewed as consisting of three aspects: the relative amount of radioactivity of the desired radionuclide (*radionuclide purity*); the fraction of total activity in the correct chemical form (*radiochemical purity*); and *chemical purity*. There are separate tests for all of these.

In addition, the activity of the material delivered to a department, or eluted from a generator and combined with an agent from a kit to prepare a radiopharmaceutical, or of anything to be administered to a patient, must be checked by means of a calibrated "well" dose calibrator (Figure 9.9b). Some well counters are built around ion chambers or Geiger counters; the scintillation detector can

count much more rapidly and discriminate among photons of different energies, and is commonly used also in survey meters as well as in gamma and PET cameras. The calibration of the dose calibrator itself at different gamma-ray energies must be checked routinely with sealed, long-lived calibration sources such as cobalt-57, cobalt-60, and cesium-137.

Many aspects of NM radiation safety are similar to those for diagnostic radiology (Figures 5.13 through 5.17, Table 5.4). The ultimate objective is to keep doses to staff and the public ALARA, and non-productive dose to the patient as well, and also well below any applicable legal limits. Time of exposure to radiation should therefore be minimized, and the distance and shielding from the source should be maximized, all within reason. Vials of radiopharmaceuticals and syringes, for example, should be kept within lead or lead-glass sheaths and behind lead bricks. Work areas should be covered with plastic-backed absorbent paper and always kept clean and neat. Areas where radionuclides are handled should be surveyed regularly with a sensitive contamination detector, such as a Geiger counter. Workers should wear coveralls and disposable gloves. There should be absolutely no consumption or storage of food or drink in the work area, and no smoking.

Regulating authorities, such as the NRC and the states in the United States, have spelled out detailed rules designed to ensure that the risk of radioactive contamination is minimized. There are prescribed procedures (in 10 CFR 20) for opening the boxes in which radionuclides are shipped; for storing the material before use; for disposing of that which is not employed (you cannot simply flush it down the drain!); for labeling work areas, samples, and waste; for educating and monitoring personnel; and for surveying work areas. And it is really, really necessary to keep accurate, comprehensive, intelligible records on all of this.

Most uptake and imaging studies involve the use of 1–10 millicuries (about 40–400 MBq) of radiopharmaceutical. But iodine-131 should be paid special attention: there have been incidents in which a patient in a clinic for diagnosis was inadvertently given a therapeutic dose, with severe consequences. The need for unflagging attention to QA and radiation safety procedures, and the importance of

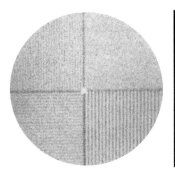 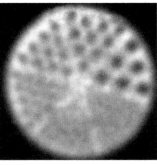

Figure 9.31 Two test phantoms, to be interposed between a uniform flood phantom and the camera face, that provide information on resolution and spatial linearity. Thanks to Walter Miller.

maintaining good ALARA techniques, cannot be overstated.

While most radionuclides employed for diagnosis emit gamma-rays in the 80–240 keV range, PET radiopharmaceuticals give off 511-keV photons. Once injected with fluorine-18, a patient becomes an unshielded source of highly penetrating radiation who can easily expose medical personnel or others for the better part of a day, so there should be an isolated, shielded waiting room for them. And the imaging suite requires more shielding than what is normal for X-rays.

Gamma camera QA

A nuclear medicine department must also have a procedure for routinely monitoring the performance of imaging equipment. Standard checks for a gamma camera and its computer system (some of which should be performed as often as daily) include tests of field uniformity, spatial resolution, spatial distortion, energy window peaking, background count, counting efficiency or sensitivity, and operation at high count rate. A typical QA program consists of, among other things, tests of:

The *sensitivities* of the individual PMTs. These may drift over time, which will lead to dark areas, distortions, and loss of linearity if not corrected. Modern gamma cameras have microprocessor circuits that adjust the PMTs automatically, and in other ways compensate for minor non-uniformities.

Energy window peaking, which involves centering the energy window on the photopeak of reference radionuclides of various energies and selecting the window width for optimal signal-to-noise for each.

Spatial resolution, which can be determined with a radio-opaque bar or other pattern placed between the camera and a flood phantom (Figure 9.31).

Imaging capability of the camera/computer combination when operating *at high count rate*. The total dead-time per pulse, typically less than 5 microseconds, depends on various electronic components of the system, some of which are paralyzable (are overwhelmed and freeze up at high count rates), others non-paralyzable. The system should be able to produce proper images at 75 000 counts per second or more.

ICRP/MIRD modeling of internal dose

We conclude the chapter with a very brief discussion of doses from radionuclides within the body. Sources of such doses are radionuclides occurring naturally in the body, such as potassium-40, and environmental contamination, potentially including that from the detonation of weapons, crises at nuclear power plants, dirty bombs, etc., as was discussed in Chapter 5. The other, with which we are concerned here, is diagnostic and therapeutic internal irradiation with radionuclides. Either way, dose assessment is more complicated than for the external exposures of X-ray imaging, and involves both physical and biological decay.

Following intake of a radionuclide, dose may be deposited over the course of days or longer. The duration of significant exposure from a biological compartment is determined primarily by the shorter of the physical and biological half-lives (Equation 9.3b). The total dose accumulated over a long time is then proportional to the total number of dose-depositing events taking place in the body, which is just the number of radionuclei administered in the first place, $n(0)$, diminished by the fraction that is washed out. The dose from complete physical decay (or over a specified period of time for radionuclides with long compartment half-lives) is known as the *committed dose*.

A good deal of modeling has been carried out of the inhalation, ingestion, injection, and transdermal routes of intake of various materials, and of the kinetics of the subsequent physiology. Much of the work on radionuclides has been undertaken by and for the ICRP and the *Medical Internal Radiation Dose (MIRD)* Committee of the Society of Nuclear Medicine. Researchers have mimicked the ventilation system of the average human body, for example, with a computational phantom of relative simple geometry but with a number of tissues of appropriate sizes, positions, and other properties. They then modeled this as a system of interconnected hypothetical biological compartments, among which radiopharmaceuticals can diffuse and flow and feed-back as they undergo decay. Tens or even hundreds of linked differential equations keep track of all this, and calculate the resultant concentrations in the various tissues. A separate set of computations then leads to the committed effective or organ doses. Some of the computations are done in a different manner, with statistical *Monte Carlo* algorithms, but exploring that would take us pretty far afield.

There are complications with these kinds of calculations. Many gamma-rays escape the targeted organ without interacting with it. (Otherwise,

radionuclides would not be very good for imaging!) Conversely, some radiopharmaceuticals go to untargeted tissues. Also, other decay products, such as Auger electrons, conversion electrons, and low-energy X-rays for technetium-99m, are deposited locally, and their energy must be accounted for. The task of critical importance is thus determining how much of the gamma-ray energy emitted from one piece of tissue will be absorbed in any other (or the same) piece.

Much information has been compiled in the simple and convenient form of the *source-to-target factor (S-factor)* tables. An S-factor, denoted $S(T \leftarrow S)$, reveals the dose deposited in a *Target* organ for each nuclear disintegration that takes place within the *Source* tissue. Assuming that the $n_{source} = n(0)$ radionuclei coming to the source organ (invariably somewhat less than the amount originally entered into the body) do eventually disintegrate there, then the total dose laid down in the target is calculated to be

$$D_{target} = S(T \leftarrow S) \times n_{source}, \quad (9.5a)$$

where

$$n_{source} = A_{source}(0) \times t_{1/2compart}/0.693. \quad (9.5b)$$

These two together give $D_{target} = A_{source}(0) \times t_{1/2 \, compart} \times S(T \leftarrow S)/0.693$. The tabulated value of $S(liver \leftarrow liver)$ for Tc-99m, for example, is 3.45×10^{-9} Gy/MBq-s.

From the S-factors, one can estimate doses from various nuclear medicine procedures (Table 9.4).

Table 9.4 Typical activities, effective doses, and critical-organ doses for a number of common nuclear medicine studies that employ technetium-99m.

Radiopharmaceutical	Radioactivity dosage		Effective dose (mSv)	Dose (critical organ) (mGy)	Critical organ
	mCi	MBq			
Pertechnetate	10	370	1.5	25	Stomach
Glucoheptonate	20	740	1.5	45	Bladder
Phosphate etc.	10	370	1	15	Bladder
Sulfur colloid	3	111	0.5	9	Liver
MA albumin	3	111	0.5	10	Lungs
DMSA	6	222	1	40	Kidneys
DTPA	20	740	1.2	35	Bladder
Red cells	20	740	4	4	Total body
Iron ascorbate	2	74	0.1	10	Kidneys

A recent entry in PET clinical dosimetry is the *standard uptake value* (SUV). Suppose that after administration of q (MBq/kg) activity of radionuclide per unit of body mass, the concentration, C, in the tissue of interest reaches A/m (kBq/ml). The SUV is defined as $(A/m)/q$ $(kBq/ml)_{organ}/(MBq/kg)_{administered}$. This reveals how much radiopharmaceutical concentrates in the tissue per unit of it given to the patient, after everything is normalized to account for his or her weight. Ideally, one could get the tissue concentration from a postadministration biopsy, but one can estimate it in various ways from an image. SUV finds particular use in comparing the functioning of tumors at different stages of treatment.

References

1 National Research Council. *Advancing Nuclear Medicine Through Innovation.* Washington, DC: National Academies Press, 2007.

2 Schulz D, Southekal S, Junnarkar SS, *et al.* Simultaneous assessment of rodent behavior and neurochemistry using a miniature positron emission tomograph. *Nat Methods* 2011;**8**(4):347–52.

CHAPTER 10

Diagnostic Ultrasound

Contrast from Differences in Tissue Elasticity or Density Across Boundaries

For all the other technologies described in this book, the radiation that interacts with body tissues is either ionizing (X- and gamma-ray) or radiofrequency (MRI) electromagnetic energy. With ultrasound, it consists of something quite different: high-frequency vibrational waves passing through tissues, typically in the 2–10 MHz range.

Medical ultrasound

Sound is the sensation that normally occurs when the tympanic membrane is perturbed sufficiently. Sound waves consist of periodic mechanical dis-turbances, repetitive phases of compression and rarefaction, that propagate through a medium such as air or water (Figure 10.1). For sound or ultrasound in air, water, or tissue, the wave travels along the direction of the back-and-forth motions of the medium (hereafter designated the *x*-direction), and is said to consist of *longitudinal* oscillations. In solid (but not fluid) media, a local disturbance can also involve motion perpendicular to the direction of propagation; such *transverse* or *shear* waves play little role in medical ultrasound imaging at the present time, apart from in *elastography*.

Medical Imaging: Essentials for Physicians, First Edition. Anthony B. Wolbarst, Patrizio Capasso and Andrew R. Wyant.
© 2013 John Wiley & Sons, Inc. Published 2013 by John Wiley & Sons, Inc.

1.0 MHz

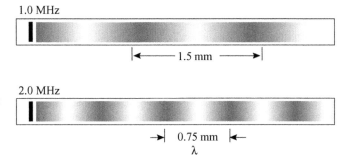

1.5 mm

2.0 MHz

0.75 mm
λ

Figure 10.1 The velocity, c, of ultrasound in a medium is nearly independent of its frequency, f. The wavelength, λ, and frequency are therefore nearly inversely proportional to one another.

Longitudinal US waves of frequency, f, and wavelength, λ, are subject to the familiar general relationship

$$f \times \lambda = c, \qquad (10.1)$$

seen earlier as Equation 2.1a. Unlike light waves in a prism, the velocity of propagation in a tissue, c, tends to be almost constant over a wide range of frequencies; the wavelength is therefore nearly inversely proportional to the frequency (Figure 10.1). In soft tissues, $c \sim 1540$ m/s, pretty much *independent* of f.

By Equation 10.1, US of 1 MHz frequency, which happens to be about as low as is routinely found in the clinic, has a wavelength of 1.5 mm in soft tissue; toward the other end of the standard clinical scale, at 10 MHz, the wavelength (which ultimately limits longitudinal resolution) is 0.15 mm = 150 microns.

Audible sounds involve oscillations in air or water in the range 20 Hz to 20 kHz. Clinical ultrasound involves much higher-frequency pulses, propagating through soft tissues and fluids. Frequencies commonly employed for medical imaging are 2.75, 3.5, 5, 7, and 10 MHz, but higher frequencies of 20 MHz, and sometimes much greater, find special applications. The specific frequency chosen for any particular examination is determined largely by optimizing the tradeoff between beam penetration and resolution requirements, as will be seen. Lower frequencies (below about 7 MHz) are generally used to examine deeper lying structures, like liver and kidneys, but in lower detail. US for more superficial structures, like muscles, tendons, testes, breast, eye, and neonatal brain, which require less beam penetration, operate at higher frequencies and, because λ is correspondingly shorter, can provide better resolution.

Like light and X-rays, medical ultrasound energy is absorbed and scattered by the tissues through which it passes. It also undergoes "specular" or mirror-like reflection at a sizable, smooth, and relatively flat interface between two tissues with different physical characteristics. The production of such echoes at organs, vessels, and other structures underlies image formation. Tissue attenuation is usually of limited clinical interest, but it must, and can, be taken properly into account by the US system. Refraction may also occur at an interface, but contributes only to image distortions.

Medical ultrasound works much like the SONAR used to detect submarines and schools of fish, sending out high-frequency sound and gaining information from the resulting echoes, as in Figures 1.18. And as with SONAR, the essential tasks are to produce precisely sculpted, high-frequency electrical pulses; transform them into localized bundles of high-frequency sound energy that radiate out from a *transducer* in a preordained direction; pick up the much fainter echoes, also by the transducer, and turn them back into electrical signals; process and analyze the echo signals, and extract and display the relevant information.

Ultrasound imaging is particularly useful in the study of soft tissues that are too similar radiologically (i.e., the X-ray attenuation coefficient values are too much alike) to provide adequate X-ray contrast. US is employed extensively for obstetric and gynecologic, cardiac, vascular, and general abdominal imaging. If a diagnostic question can be resolved by any of several modalities, then ultrasound may be the one of choice because the equipment is relatively inexpensive, compact, and portable, and does not generate ionizing radiation. If a mammogram indicates a localized irregularity in the breast, an

US study usually can distinguish rapidly, reliably, inexpensively, and safely whether it is a solid lesion or a fluid-filled cyst. Likewise, Doppler ultrasound can detect and monitor the flow (or lack thereof) of blood in the arteries and veins. And although the evidence-based information is not conclusive, it strongly suggests that the risks from the judicious use of ultrasound for diagnosis are extremely low.

When traversing a homogeneous material, such as the fluid within a cyst or large blood vessel, an ultrasound pulse simply penetrates to greater depths, and is attenuated smoothly in the process, but no echoes are produced: it thus appears uniformly blank (or black) on the monitor, with no internal structure. But if the beam passes through several different organs or dissimilar tissues, energy is reflected at interfaces between them. The *time* of return of an echo back to the surface of the body is proportional to the depth of the interface that produced it. The echo's *intensity* depends on the depth (because of attenuation), but also on the degree of difference in mechanical properties of the materials on the two sides of the interface.

The nature of an echo formed at a particular tissue interface depends strongly on its dimensions relative to the wavelength of the US (Figure 10.2a). If the interface is relatively large and flat, $Ð > λ$, as with the diaphragm or the outer surface of the liver, then significant specular reflection will occur. The echo depends also on the physical characteristics of the interface (gradual versus sharp changes, or smooth versus rough surface), on the geometry of the situation (the angle with which the beam strikes the interface).

Suppose inclusions, irregularities, and non-uniformities (hence interfaces) within a tissue are of dimensions $Ð$ that are much *smaller* than the wavelength of the sound, $Ð < λ$. Then the tissue will seem largely homogeneous and the image will be nearly anechoic Some sound energy undergoes isotropic (by equal amounts in all directions), diffuse scattering from the inclusions, like the scattering of long-wavelength ocean waves passing between the pilings of a pier. This may manifest as tissue *speckle*, or fine texture, the statistical analysis of which can sometimes be diagnostically informative (Figure 10.2b).

Between these two extremes, and more complex, are images of organs such as the kidneys, pancreas, spleen, and liver, which contain inclusions of intermediate size comparable to the wavelength

(a)

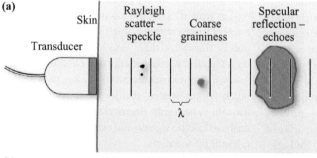

(b)

Figure 10.2 US reflections. **(a)** Flat objects of dimensions $Ð$ much larger than a wavelength can give "specular" or mirror-like echo images. **(b)** US "image" of a material containing only sub-resolution scatterers smaller than the US wavelength λ, where the amplitude of scatter power is proportional to $Ð^6/λ^4$. This *speckle* (an unfortunate name; it has nothing to do with specular reflection) pattern results from coherent summation of echoes from the scatterers, and does not reveal structure within the patient or phantom.

of the sound, $Đ \approx \lambda$. Rayleigh scattering at such inclusions manifests as grainy tissue image-texture, which may be of diagnostic value. (Same guy as in Rayleigh scattering of photons, but totally different phenomenon.) The nature of the texture can be of diagnostic value.

The US beam: MHz compressional waves in tissues

The middle C bar of a xylophone vibrates 261.6 times each second, for the equally tempered scale, and it creates local disturbances of the air around it primarily of this frequency. Also present are small-amplitude *harmonics*, vibrations occurring at integer multiples (i.e., 2 times, 3 times, etc.) of the base or fundamental frequency; the middle C of a xylophone is distinguishable from that of a piano entirely because of differences in their harmonic makeup.

As a wood or metal plate resonates, it acts like a piston or diaphragm, displacing the layer of air immediately next to it, and alternately increasing and reducing the pressure within that layer. This results in an unbalancing of the forces on the adjacent layer of air a very short time later, causing motion and compression and rarefaction there as well. This immediately thereafter pushes and pulls on the next layer of air, in effect, then the next, and so on. The disturbance radiates outward, along the direction of diaphragm motion, and eventually causes displacements of your eardrum, resulting in the perception of a sound. The harder the instrument was struck, the larger the amplitude of oscillations in air density and pressure reaching your tympanic membrane, and the greater the sensation. The same argument applies for US waves traveling through soft tissue.

Ultrasound waves

There are two simple and related ways to represent a longitudinal US wave traveling along the x-axis through a medium. In the first, imagine the longitudinal *displacement* of a voxel of tissue within the beam path as a function of time (Figure 10.3a); the magnitude of the displacement, X, is shown along the vertical axis in the graph but, in reality, the piece of tissue is oscillating back and forth along the x-axis. For nearly monochromatic sinusoidal oscillations, this may be expressed as $X(t) = X_0$

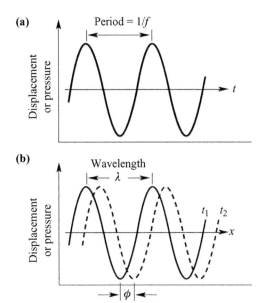

(a)

(b)

Figure 10.3 Representations of wave motion through an elastic medium. **(a)** At a fixed point in space, displacement of the medium and the local pressure vary sinusoidally as functions of time. **(b)** A traveling wave at two instants of time as a function of position in space, as might be produced by a pair of snapshots, one taken right after the other.

$\sin(2\pi ft)$. $X(t)$ is the displacement of the bit of tissue from its equilibrium position (or the pressure within it) at the instant t, and X_0 and f are the amplitude (maximum displacement) and frequency of the associated wave, respectively. For diagnostic ultrasound in soft tissue, the amplitude of the motion is typically less than 0.1 μm, one tenth of a micron. Since movement of the voxel to the left causes some compression both of itself and of the voxel on that side Figure 10.3a could just as easily illustrate the variation in the local pressure at the voxel within the medium.

Alternatively, Figure 10.3b shows two snapshots of a traveling wave, one taken immediately after the other. The shape in space of the wave at the first instant, at t_1, may be described as $X(x) = X_0 \sin(2\pi x/\lambda)$. The one shown a moment later differs from the first by a phase angle that is proportional to the time lapse between the two. Both waves, of course, are of wavelength λ.

Some kinds of vibrations, such as those of a piano string, form stationary or *standing* waves. Sound and ultrasound passing through air, water, or tissue, by contrast, are in the form of *traveling* waves. The waves of Figure 10.3b will oscillate up and down, but not flow to the left or right.

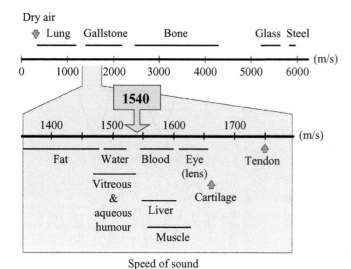

Figure 10.4 The velocity, c, of US in various materials. c for soft tissues tends to be near 1540 m/s, independent of f and λ.

The density and the elasticity or compressibility of a tissue will have a lot to do with the propagation of oscillations through it. In fact, apart from scattering and the frictional processes that cause attenuation of US energy, density and elasticity are *all* that's needed to tell the entire story. Nothing else is involved in the behavior of a spring, or a block of air, or voxel of tissue. The speed of propagation of the wave through the medium, in particular, is linked tightly to its density, ρ, and compressibility, K:

$$c = (K\rho)^{-1/2} \qquad (10.2)$$

The *speed* of US in *soft tissue* is about 1540 m/s and, again, it is practically *independent* of the US *frequency*. It is found, on the other hand, that the *speed of sound does depend* on the *medium* through which it is traveling (Figure 10.4, Table 10.1).

There is a good reason for the near constancy of c in a given material. It is easy to visualize a friction-free medium as consisting of small voxel-masses connected by perfect springs, with the speed of sound in it determined by its density and its compressibility. But the average density of a material is totally unrelated to the wavelength and frequency of any compressional wave passing through it, and

Table 10.1 Values of some ultrasound parameters for materials of interest in imaging: the speed of sound at imaging frequencies is determined solely by the density and elasticity of the medium, $c = 1/(K\rho)^{-1/2}$ (m/s). The acoustic impedance, $Z = (\rho/K)^{1/2} = \rho c$ (10^6 kg/m²-s), and the rate of attenuation at 1 MHz in dB/cm are both discussed in the text.

Material	$c = 1/(K\rho)^{-1/2}$ (m/s)	$Z = (\rho/K)^{1/2}$ (10^6 kg/m²-s)	dB/cm at 1 MHz
Soft tissue (mean)	1540	1.6	0.55
Muscle	1580	1.7	1
Heart	1580	1.6	0.5
Liver	1550	1.7	0.8
Brain	1550	1.5	0.6
Breast	1500	1.5	0.7
Fat	1450	1.4	0.5
Blood	1570	1.6	0.2
Water	1500	1.5	0.002
Bone	3500	5	10
PZT	4000	30	–
Air	330	0.0004	12

so also is its compressibility. As a result, the speed of propagation of sound in soft tissue varies by less than a few percent over the range of frequencies used in medical ultrasonography. The speed of *electromagnetic* radiation in a medium over the visible range, by contrast, may depend strongly on λ, which is why prisms and raindrops refract sunlight into their constituent colors.

The frequency spectrum of an ultrasound pulse

Clinical pulsed ultrasound differs from audio sound in another important way. Much of what you hear is made up of combinations of distinct, monochromatic tones that last for hundreds or thousands of cycles or more. The corresponding spectra therefore consist, at least briefly, of numbers of changing but fairly discrete frequencies. The disturbances used in pulsed ultrasound, by contrast, are 1–5 μs in duration and last only a few cycles (Figure 10.5a). As revealed by Fourier analysis (Figure 4.10b), the spectrum of ultrasound energy is continuous, spanning a range of frequencies (Figure 10.5b). Creating such a pulse requires superposing a set of waves of a band of frequencies, of *bandwidth* Δf, centered on the central frequency, f_0, of the pulse.

It is a fundamental characteristic of any kind of wave disturbance that its frequency bandwidth and its duration, Δt, are related approximately as $\Delta f \, \Delta t > \pi/2$. The shorter the pulse is, the greater the bandwidth of frequencies involved in producing it. Conversely, this is also the reason that a well-made bell with a clear, pure, nearly-monochromatic ($\Delta f \sim 0$) tone can peal out for a very long time. (This fundamental relationship, incidentally, underlies even Heisenberg's uncertainty principle, since there are wavelike aspects to moving electrons, photons, and other very small "particles.")

In imaging, determining the time of echo-reception must be precise, since it is the measure of the depth of an interface. This requires a short pulse again (Figure 10.5a), which, in turn, is comprised of a broad band of frequencies. As we shall see, for Doppler studies of blood flow it is shifts in frequency that are most critical, so Δf must be small, and the pulse must therefore be of longer duration.

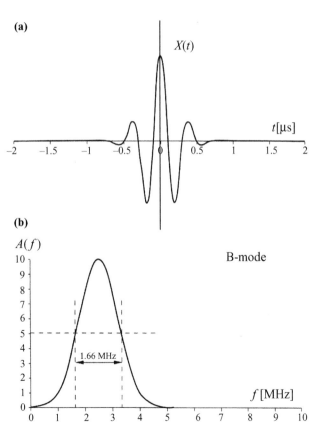

(a)

(b)

B-mode

1.66 MHz

Figure 10.5 US pulse. **(a)** For accurate placement of tissue boundaries or other objects, a pulse needs to be spatially short, which comes from allowing it to be only a few cycles long, or from selecting short wavelengths, or both. **(b)** According to Fourier theory, short pulses are made up of sine waves of a wide, continuous range of frequencies.

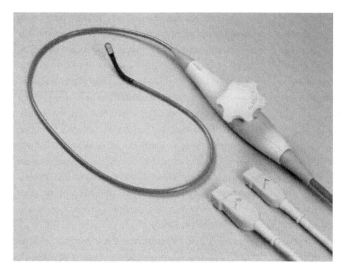

Figure 10.6 The transducer on the long stem contains two separate arrays of piezoelectric elements, for biplane (transverse and longitudinal viewing planes) transesophageal echocardiology. It can operate with center frequencies of 7.0, 5.0, and 3.5 MHz, providing a choice of three combinations of beam penetration and resolution. The lower two transducers, which are significantly smaller than standard adult size, are designed for neonates and pediatric patients, respectively. Caveat: transducers are delicate instruments, largely because the crystals are fragile, and it's a good idea not to drop them. They are also subject to heat damage.

Production of an ultrasound beam and detection of echoes with a transducer

The transducer is the pivotal component in a medical ultrasound system (Figure 10.6), and it performs two critical functions: it radiates ultrasound waves into the body, and then receives any reflected but attenuated echoes.

First, acting like a loudspeaker, it transforms strong voltage signals into pulses of mechanical vibrations of about the same frequency, duration, and waveform. With the transducer pressed firmly against the patient's body, the ultrasound energy enters at the skin and propagates inward along an *acoustic scan line* through soft tissues and fluids at 1540 m/s (Figure 10.7).

Shortly thereafter, the transducer performs its second critical task. Quiescent and now acting as microphones, the piezoelectric elements sense any reflected, much weaker echo-pulse US energy created at a tissue interface or object within the body, and transform it back into an electrical signal. A single ingoing pulse may be reflected at multiple interfaces among distinct organs at progressively greater depths, giving rise to multiple signals back at the transducer. The various returning signals are amplified and processed by the receiver, and are then sent to a computer, which keeps track of the beam direction, return times, and amplitudes. A thousandth of a second later, a new pulse is created by the transmitter and transducer and sent off through the body, perhaps in a slightly different direction, and the whole process begins anew.

Transducers have been designed both for general usage, commonly with a wide bandwidth and selectable multiple frequencies, and for special

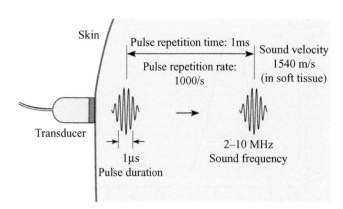

Figure 10.7 A typical US beam consists of 2- to 10-MHz pulses that are 1 microsecond (μs) short and repeated every 1 millisecond (ms). In soft tissue, ultrasound pulses travel at about 1540 m/s, with very little dependence on their frequency.

applications, such as OB/GYN, endovaginal obstetrics and gynecology, fetal echo imaging, and transesophageal echocardiology (Figure 10.7). Single-use, miniaturized (8 french, 10 french, and volume) ultrasound catheters have even been designed for intravenous and intracardiac imaging, for example, with steering in two planes. Applications include adult and pediatric ICE procedures for visualization of the left atrial appendage, pulmonary veins, and atrial septum.

Piezoelectric transducer elements

The heart of a modern transducer, the central component by means of which US carries out the two complementary duties of transmission and detection, is usually an array of one hundred or more thin and small ($^1/_2$ to 2 λ wide by several mm tall) wafers, called *crystals* or *elements* (even though they are neither) of a piezoelectric material (Figure 10.8a).

A piezoelectric (from the Greek piezo, meaning "to press") substance is one that deforms slightly when subjected to an electric field and, conversely, produces an electric voltage when it is compressed or bent, so it can both generate and detect mechanical vibrations. It is typically made up of polar molecules, each with a small, permanent excess of electron charge at one end and a deficiency at the other (Figure 10.8b). When an electric field is applied across the element, the molecules twist

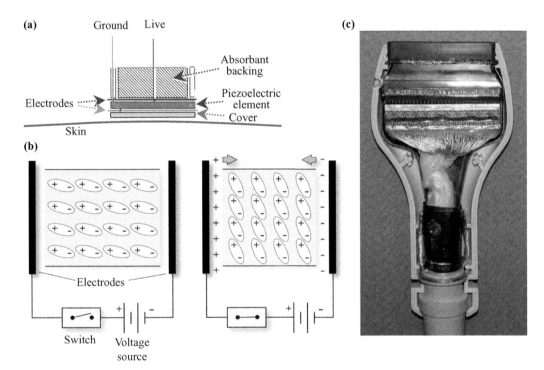

Figure 10.8 Piezoelectric transducer elements. (a) A single piezoelectric element in an array is sandwiched between a pair (live and ground) of electrodes. The backing material is designed to absorb nearly all ultrasound energy initially heading away from the patient, and the matching-layer cover plus coupling gel increase the amount of US that is conducted into and from the body. (b) One mechanism of piezoelectricity. When a voltage is applied across the element, the resulting realignment of the permanently polarized molecules leads to a change in element thickness. Conversely, mechanical stresses on the element cause re-alignment of the molecules and the generation of a voltage across it. (c) A multi-element transducer, behind the scenes. The active component is the plate of piezoelectric material at the top; coated on both sides with a thin conducting layer, the bottom of the plate has then been partitioned into hundreds of minute, electrically independent elements by way of cuts by a narrow-blade saw. Each electrode is wired separately to its own electrical circuit that feeds ultimately, through a cable, to the receiver and computer. Such a multi-element array can produce a wavefront parallel to the face of the transducer if its elements are excited simultaneously but, by firing them individually in carefully designed sequences, it is possible to produce a swept, focused beam. Courtesy of Siemens Medical Solutions USA, Inc.

around a little, trying to align along the field, and this results in small changes in its physical dimensions. Conversely, forcing a rotation of the molecules by compressing the piece alters the electric status quo within it, resulting in the emergence of a voltage across it.

The piezoelectric material most commonly employed in transducers is a "solid solution" ceramic called PZT, consisting of lead zirconate ($PbZrO_3$) and lead titanate ($PbTiO_3$). A rectangular block of the material mounted on a substrate is cut by a thin diamond or laser saw into hundreds or thousands of separate elements; a single silver or other metal covers the bottom of the block as a shared, common electrode, and each element is capped on the other side with its own electrode and wire contact (Figure 10.8a).

In the old days, when a transducer consisted of a single element, it was cut to such a size that it would resonate at a single frequency, because of which it was able to transmit considerable power. Modern multi-element transducers are less power efficient, but have a broad bandwidth. The elements are aligned side by side in the transducer but are electrically and mechanically isolated from one another, each attached to its own independent electronic system, which endows it with great beam-generating, steering, and focusing flexibility (Figure 10.8c). The transducer may be connected to hundreds of separate transmitter/detector circuits, all ultimately under the control of the computer. A single element and its associated individual electronics is referred to as a *channel*.

If only a single element in a one-dimensional array were excited, then the disturbance would radiate out through the nearby soft tissue as smooth, hemispherical wavelets (Figure 10.9a). Not very interesting. But when all the separate elements of the array fire simultaneously and with the same

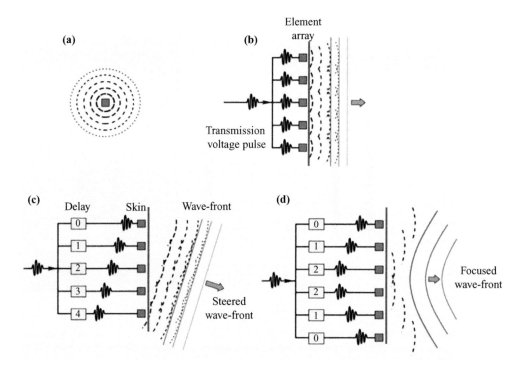

Figure 10.9 A modern transducer can steer and focus a narrow beam electronically by cleverly timing the emission of the pulses from an array of independent, piezoelectric elements. Then, wherever in the body the beam-line may be at any instant, and with whatever orientation, in B-mode the system displays a corresponding line on the monitor. (a) Hemispherical waves produced by the firing of a single element at the skin surface. (b) The flat-wave-front plane waves created when all the elements in a straight row or plane of closely spaced point sources are excited simultaneously and oscillate in phase. (c) Angling the beam by introducing the same delay between all pairs of adjacent elements; each element is triggered a short time after its neighbor to the left (above), and the resulting beam heads off at an angle to the right. By pulsing repeatedly while changing the delay between elements, the beam can be swept back and forth through a plane of tissue. (d) It can even be focused laterally within the tomographic slice, and the focal depth moved in and out.

amplitude, the result is a plane wave (Figure 10.9b). Each element will generate a separate wavelet, but a short distance away they will all combine to form a nearly flat wavefront that propagates outward and parallel to the array, an example of so-called Huygens interference. This can be understood by imagining the real, multi-element extended source as comprising multiple tiny adjacent point sources, the waves from which undergo complex constructive and destructive interference. Figures 2.3b shows this for only two such sources, while Figure 10.9b illustrates it for a row of them.

Creating a swept or stepped focused beam

Not only can the system produce a forward-heading plane wave, but also it can time the production of the electrical pulses sent to the elements of the array (hence the emission of US pulses from them) so as to deflect and focus the beam electronically. If adjacent elements are not fired together, but rather are staggered in rapid sequence, then the resulting wave front leaves the source at an angle (Figure 10.9c). Suppose that element 2 is excited a small fraction of a microsecond after element 1 (much less than the duration of an US pulse), and element 3 is delayed by the same amount after element 2, and so on. An unfocused plane wave will be produced that comes away from the array at an angle that depends on the amount of inter-element delay between excitations. After all the elements in the array have been excited, the computer can change the amount of the inter-element delay a little, so that the next wave front propagates out in a slightly different direction. By generating a sequence of such beams rapidly and systematically one after another, a *phased array* electronically *sweeps* the US beam back and forth.

The same general approach allows the electronic *focusing* of a beam within the plane of the topographic slice. This time, imagine that the two outermost elements, on either end of the array, are excited simultaneously (Figure 10.9d). After a brief delay, the two next-to-outermost elements are excited, and so on. With proper timing, the effect is like that of exciting a parabolic, focused wave front. Focusing or constricting the beam diameter, on the other hand, concentrates its intensity (by as much as a factor of 100) over the *focal region*, where the beam

is most narrowed, and the echoes produced there will be correspondingly stronger. Thus, focusing the beam energy partially overcomes the problem of weak echo signals. With a focused beam, moreover, beam width and lateral resolution may be of the order of a few millimeters.

The amounts of the delays between the excitations of adjacent elements determine the focal length. The operator can set the timing of these excitations so that the focal zone is stepped to a greater depth in tissue each time the beam makes a sweep. The system can then reconstruct an overall US image by retaining and using only the data obtained from near the focal depth, where the resolution and SNR will be best, and discarding the rest. It can thereby generate relatively high lateral-resolution composite B-mode images that extend far within the patient.

Sweeping the US beam, as just described, employs all the elements of an array in the creation of every beam, and adjusting the time delays between the excitation of adjacent elements to sweep it back and forth. This so-called *phased array* approach carves out a fan-shaped *sector* of tissue (Figure 10.10a).

A *linear array* employs a different strategy, activating only a small subset of the elements at a time. This generates a narrow beam but, immediately after the return of any echoes, it fires a partially overlapping parallel and adjacent subset (Figure 10.10b), with the multiple beams eventually covering a broad slice of tissue. It might begin by firing elements 1, 3, 5, 7, and 9 together, say, then elements 3, 5, 7, 9, and 11, and so on. This progression is designed to create a comb of independent, but partially overlapping, side-stepping parallel beams. A second series of beams can then be produced immediately thereafter, beginning with even-numbered elements 2 through 10, etc., interlacing among the first set. All the echo results can then be untangled.

In clinical practice, a linear array and higher frequency are often adopted for more superficial structures when more resolution and a clear view of the immediate sub-surface are needed. Phased array probes are used mostly for deeper structures and a broader view.

Meanwhile, either way, as the display line itself sweeps back and forth or steps to the side, for B-mode operation a line appears on the display,

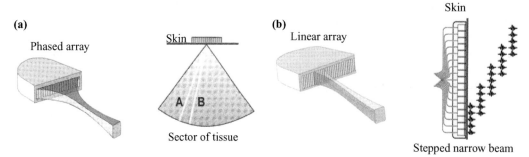

(a) Phased array   Skin   Sector of tissue   A   B

(b) Linear array   Skin   Stepped narrow beam

Figure 10.10 Two general approaches to moving the beam so as to cover a slice of tissues in B-mode. **(a)** Activating all the elements of a *phased array* for the creation of the narrow beam, and altering the time delay between elements so as to focus and sweep it back and forth within a *sector* slice of tissue. **(b)** With a *linear sequential array*, only a few elements fire at a time, and they do so simultaneously. As the subset of elements being activated steps across the array, several adjacent elements are, at each instant, producing a narrow tooth of a sideways-stepping comb beam.

continually following the beam, and bright spots on it indicate reflections. The deeper within the body that a tissue boundary occurs, the longer the echo signal takes to arrive back at the transducer, and the farther along the display line the spot will be from the starting place (at the location of the transducer); and the brighter a spot, the larger the amplitude of the associated echo signal, and the greater the tissue acoustic mismatch at the interface. So as the ultrasound beam cuts a thin plane through the body, the brightness-modulated lines generate a two-dimensional tomographic image.

The earliest electronically steerable transducers consisted of a single row of elements, and could image only a thin, two-dimensional slice of tissue. But a "1.5-dimensional" transducer, with a half dozen rows of independent elements, allows some electronic focusing in the third dimension. A fully 2D square array is capable of real, 3D imaging.

The Fresnel (near) zone of a beam

The beam coming from an infinitely wide transducer would be uniform both across the beam face and in depth, apart from attenuation. Real beams have structure. For one thing, they tend naturally to narrow for a while, and then fan out. An US wave with a planar wave front starts out with a cross-sectional area, D, comparable to that of the transducer. It displays wave interference pattern both in cross-section and along the central axis (Figure 10.11). The region over which the beam retains this general form but narrows is suitable for imaging, and is called the *Fresnel* or *near zone*.

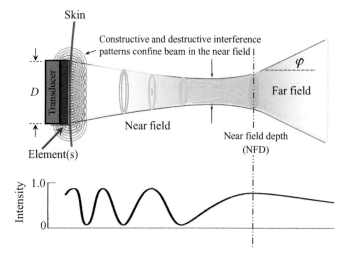

Skin

Constructive and destructive interference patterns confine beam in the near field

φ

Far field

D Transducer

Near field

Element(s)

Near field depth (NFD)

Intensity   1.0   0

Figure 10.11 Typical medical ultrasound beam from a single, disk-shaped element or from a planar array of tiny elements all fired simultaneously. The beam consists of the *Fresnel* or *near* (the source) and the far zone. The intensity across the beam face at several distances from the transducer shows wave interference effects, as does intensity measured along the central axis.

Transmission and attenuation of the beam within a homogeneous material

The *intensity*, *I*, of sound (like that of light or of an X-ray beam) refers to the *rate* at which energy is transferred through a *unit area*; that is, the power passing through it.

Attenuation of a monochromatic beam in a homogeneous medium

When a fairly monochromatic beam of ultrasound passes through homogeneous tissue, so that almost none of its energy is diverted into the creation of echoes, its intensity, $I(x)$, diminishes roughly exponentially with the distance traveled, x, as

$$I(x) = I(0)e^{-\mu_{US}x}, \qquad (10.3a)$$

as with Equation 3.1a. Some of the energy of the beam is absorbed by the tissue and transformed into heat, and some may scatter diffusely out of the beam from small irregularities. The net effect of these two processes is parameterized by the *ultrasound intensity attenuation coefficient*, μ_{US} (in units of cm^{-1}). We have chosen the same italic Greek *mu* (μ) here as for the X-ray linear attenuation coefficient because of the similarities between the two phenomena, even their units (cm^{-1}). The probes are totally different, of course, as are the interaction and attenuation mechanisms, but either way, the attenuation is exponential under idealized conditions, and the relevant coefficient can be expressed as $\mu = -(dI/I)/dx$, as in Equation 3.1b.

As with photons, there are two totally independent, mutually exclusive general categories of microscopic interactions of US radiation within a medium, namely absorption and scatter:

$$\mu_{US} = \mu_{abs} + \mu_{scat}, \qquad (10.3b)$$

directly analogous to $\mu_{X-ray} = \mu_{PA} + \mu_{CS}$ (Equation 3.3c). The *absorption* component describes friction-like processes that act at the molecular level and cause US mechanical vibrational energy to be lost as heat. *Scattering* occurs when the medium is not completely smooth and homogeneous; then US waves interact with irregularities of sizes comparable to their wavelength, as with ocean waves at the piers of a dock, and re-radiate their energy from these new small sources in all directions.

Because ultrasound imaging involves the processing of echoes that range widely in amplitude, it is convenient to adopt a logarithmic measure of sound power or intensity, the *decibel* (dB), as was done also for the optical density of Chapter 4. If the intensity of a pulse at one time or place is I_1, and that at another is I_2, the ratio of their intensities can be stated in decibels as

$$I_2/I_1 = 10^{dB/10}. \qquad (10.4a)$$

Again, this does not describe any physical process, but rather is just a convenient way to express a number, in this case a ratio, that can assume a broad scale of values. Equivalently, the ratio of I_2 relative to I_1 in dB is

$$dB = 10 \log_{10}(I_2/I_1). \qquad (10.4b)$$

To report a difference or change in sound or ultrasound *power* level in decibels, you take the base-10 logarithm of the ratio I_2/I_1 of the intensities involved, and multiply the logarithm by the number 10. If an echo is 0.01 as intense as the transmitted signal, for example, then the loss in intensity is $10 \log_{10} 0.01 = -20$ dB. Suppose I_2 is greater than I_1 by +30 dB; the ratio of their intensities is $10^{30/10} = 1000$.

The attenuation coefficient μ_{US} is a perfectly respectable parameter. But it is more convenient and common practice, instead, to characterize attenuation in the equivalent terms of decibels of intensity loss per centimeter of tissue (dB/cm) and the amount of tissue traversed, *x*. (You may wish to convince yourself that this is legitimate by relating dB/cm to the μ of Equation 10.4a.)

The rate of attenuation of ultrasound by homogeneous tissue, unlike its speed of propagation, *does* depend strongly on the frequency and wavelength (Figure 10.12a,b). The rate at which energy is dissipated depends on the viscosity, in effect, of the medium and on the natural time-dependent relaxation processes that allow it to settle back down to an equilibrium condition after the passage of a wave. For muscle, blood, and most soft tissues, the rate of energy attenuation, in decibels per centimeter, is found empirically to be approximately linear with frequency:

$$[dB/cm](f) \sim [dB/cm]_{1\,MHz} \times f. \qquad (10.3c)$$

A reference value for a material, $[dB/cm]_{1\,MHz}$, must be obtained at 1 MHz; and *f* is in MHz. $[dB/cm]_{1\,MHz}$ of soft tissue is 0.55 dB/cm (Table 10.1).

Figure 10.12c illustrates a fundamental tradeoff one has to make with US imaging. As the frequency of US pulses increases, the attenuation increases, and the beam falls off more rapidly with penetration through soft tissues. But the resolution

(a)

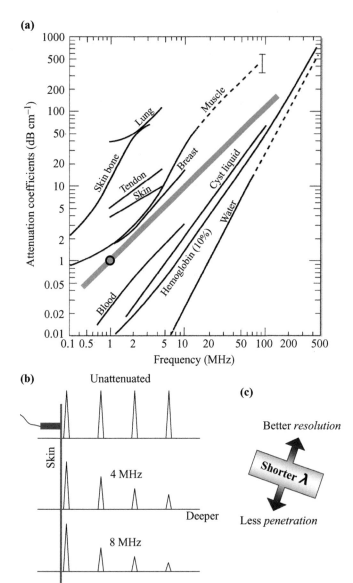

(b) Unattenuated

(c)

Better *resolution*

Shorter *λ*

Deeper

Less *penetration*

Figure 10.12 Exponential attenuation of US in a homogeneous material. (a) The attenuation coefficient (in dB/cm) for sound in a medium, unlike its velocity, *does* increase with the ultrasound frequency. The line indicating dB = [1 dB/cm (at 1 MHz)] × *f*, in orange, passes through the marked point (1 MHz, 1 dB/cm). (b) Sequence of pulses that are unattenuated in tissues, and; attenuated at the [dB/cm](*f*) rates for the frequencies 4 MHz, and 8 MHz, respectively. (c) A major tradeoff: the higher the frequency of the US, the shorter the wavelength so the better the resolution, but the greater the attenuation, so the lower the penetration of the beam into the body and the smaller the echo amplitudes. Shallower structures, such as muscles, testes, breast, and neonatal brain, commonly employ 7–10 MHz. For deeper organs such as liver and kidneys, 3 to 5 MHz. Modified from Webb, S. (ed.), *The Physics of Medical Imaging*, Philadelphia, PA: Adam Hilger, 1988, fig. 7.2 (part a).

capability of any wave-based modality is determined largely by its wavelength; it generally cannot see anything smaller than a single wavelength and, conversely, other things being equal (which they often are not), resolution tends to increase with *f*. So, here's one more imaging dilemma: we can see things with greater sharpness (high *f*), or we can probe deeper within the body (low *f*), but not do both at the same time. Ultimately, you have to choose one or the other, depending on the clinical situation.

Certain diseases can alter not only the average density and elasticity of a tissue, thereby affecting reflectivity at gross boundaries with other organs, but also its internal architecture and structure. This can affect its apparent "texture" in an US image, as with cirrhosis, and also affect the rate of attenuation within it, as with steatosis (Figure 10.13).

Time gain compensation

It has just been argued that the amplitude of a signal returning to the transducer depends not only on the

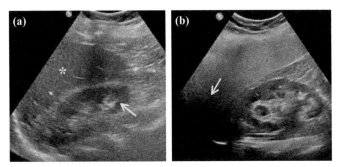

Figure 10.13 This liver provides a good example of how certain disease processes affect the attenuation of ultrasound waves. If the disease increases the number of reflecting interfaces per unit volume, US can readily reveal the tissue changes. With more reflections, less US power can penetrate deeper into the tissue, resulting in signal loss at greater depths. (**a**) Longitudinal view of the right lobe of a healthy liver. The liver parenchyma (asterix) is of similar echogenicity as the adjacent right kidney (arrow). The hepatic parenchyma can be visualized easily down to the deepest portion of the image. From US images of multiple parallel planes of tissue, it is found that the liver remains isoechoic throughout. (**b**) This patient suffers from significant steatosis. The liver detoxifies the body from certain medications, drugs, and alcohol, and a byproduct of their elimination is the deposition of fat within the cells of the liver parenchyma. Chronic exposure to these toxic substances, or simply obesity or a fat-laden diet, can cause the abnormal concentration of fat within the hepatocytes. The resulting steatosis is a common finding in developed nations, and the condition is curable as long as it does not lead to permanent scarring, such as with cirrhosis; on the other hand, it is intentionally induced in geese and ducks for the creation of the culinary delight *foie gras*. (Perhaps not such a delight for the geese.) The intra-cellular fat globules create more interfaces that reflect sound waves back toward the transducer, giving the tissue a brighter (hyperechogenic) and grainy appearance. Since the tissue reflects more echoes, moreover, the beam is attenuated more rapidly as it passes deeper into the body, reducing the ability to visualize its deeper regions (arrow) and thereby decreasing the overall diagnostic utility of the examination.

degree of reflection at the interface where the echo was created, but also on the extent to which the pulse was attenuated during its travels. By the time it returns to the transducer, in fact, an echo signal is typically 60 dB (a factor of 10^6) weaker in intensity than the original transmitted pulse, because of both attenuation and the losses that occur at tissue boundaries (from transmission through them, rather than a reflection there.) The various echoes that eventually reach the transducer after transmission of a single pulse may differ among themselves in intensity, moreover, by as much as 100 dB – a dynamic range of a factor of 10^{10} – which greatly exceeds the capabilities of a standard linear RF amplifier or pre-amp, or of any display.

One way to deal with this problem is to pass the signal through a *logarithmic amplifier*, which preferentially increases the gain for weaker signals for dynamic range control. Another powerful approach is to provide each channel's pre-amp with its own dedicated *time gain compensation* (TGC) circuit.

The deeper within the body that a reflection occurs, the weaker the echo will be because of attenuation, but also the

longer it takes the echo signal to arrive back at the transducer (Figure 10.14). TGC, also known as depth-gain compensation, is a signal processing method that makes use of the latter phenomenon to offset the former. For each pulse, it ramps up the *gain* (amount of amplification; that is, the volume control) of the pre-amplifier continuously during the time that the pulse is traveling into the body and its echoes are returning, in such a manner as to compensate for signal attenuation along the way. The deeper the tissue interface, and the later it is detected, the more it is amplified.

Noise suppression

Noise is as much of a problem with ultrasound as for the other modalities. *Clutter noise* arises from aftershocks occurring within either the patient or the transducer. Similarly, *speckle noise* is a wave interference effect that may be caused in an otherwise homogeneous medium by numerous particles too tiny to be seen individually (Figure 10.2b). Unintended off-axis *side-lobes* and *grating-lobes* (arising in array transducers from interference among the periodic spacing of the individual small piezoelectric elements) can give rise to false image signals. Additionally, some electronic noise in US images is created by the pre-amplifiers and other hardware.

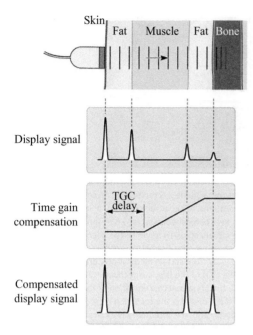

Figure 10.14 Time gain compensation (TGC) counteracts the attenuation of the US beam by continually increasing the level of amplification at the receiver throughout the time that the US pulse, and then its echo, are still traveling through tissue.

The signal-to-noise ratio decreases as the echo signal strength goes down, and turning up the gain increases the noise level as well as the signal. The SNR deteriorates with tissue interface depth in the body, limiting the amount of contrast that can be obtained, despite the efforts of the TGC. Tissue attenuation decreases with use of a lower frequency, and that may improve the SNR, as may increasing the focusing of the beam at the depth of interest. The chief problem with *noise*, of course, is that it *degrades* the *contrast-to-noise ratio* (CNR).

Of the several approaches that can give the CNR a boost, the simplest is noise-reject control, which simply filters out the weakest noise signals. The danger, of course, is the inadvertent rejection of weak real signals as well.

Reflection of the beam at an interface between materials with different acoustic impedances

What determines how strong an echo will be?

The intensity of a pulse of ultrasound passing through a *homogeneous* medium falls off nearly exponentially with the distance traveled, but no echoes are produced. The normal gall bladder of Figure 10.15a, for example, is *anechoic*, filled with non-viscous bile and containing no pathological calculi. At a different time (Figure 10.15b), the same bladder appeared to contain a thick sludge and numerous small inclusions, and the abnormally thick wall indicated significant inflammation, presumably arising from irritation caused by the sludge and indicating likely cholecyctitis.

Reflection, transmission, and the acoustic impedance, *Z*

To summarize: a reflection will occur at a smooth, flat, and large enough boundary between two tissues that have sufficiently different acoustic properties, and a part of the US energy will continue in the forward direction (Figure 10.16). Both the measured time until the return of the echo to the transducer and the amplitude of the echo signal contribute to creation of the image. The detection

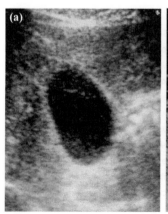
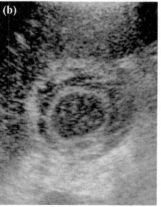

Figure 10.15 B-mode ultrasound of a gall bladder. **(a)** This normal bladder is filled with a thin fluid that produces no echoes, and the image of its interior is said to be *anechoic*. **(b)** The same bladder, before medical treatment, revealed no gallstones, but appears to contain heterogeneous echogenic sludge, the presence of which may be responsible for the abnormal thickness of the wall from inflammation (cholecystitis).

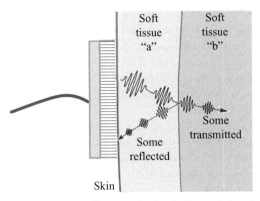

Figure 10.16 The reflection and refraction/transmission of US pulses at an interface between tissues of different density and/or elasticity; that is, of different acoustic impedance, Z.

time is proportional to the depth within the patient of the tissue interface. The intensity of the echo signal increases with the degree of physical mismatch between the two tissues in density and in elasticity (or, what is essentially the same thing, in compressibility). Echo signal strength depends also on the depth of the interface because of attenuation, and that causes the SNR and the contrast to suffer. US systems have time-gain compensation circuits to counteract much of that but, while they can jack contrast back up, they also amplify much of the noise as well, and can improve the contrast-to-noise ratio only somewhat.

Recall the analogy of Figure 1.18b. If you give one end of a long wire coil or a rope a hefty shake, a ripple will run along it. With the far end of this coil attached to a heavier or more rigid grade of coil, a smaller ripple will reflect at the juncture and head back toward you, while another wave, also smaller than the original, proceeds along the second coil. The same thing happens if the far end is attached to a *lighter*-weight coil, or a more springy one. But if the coil happens to interface smoothly with another one of exactly the same type, the ripple just keeps on going. The same thing occurs when ultrasound energy comes to a boundary surface between two materials, as opposed to when it just continues on through a homogeneous medium.

The amount of US reflection that occurs at an interface depends almost entirely on the differences in the elasticity and density of the media on the two sides of it. Audible sound behaves the same way. A submerged swimmer hears almost none of the poolside chatter because of the differences in density and compressibility between air and water, and practically no sound can cross the surface between them.

It is convenient to approach this issue in terms of a somewhat artificial construct known as the *acoustic impedance* of a substance, denoted Z (*not* to be confused with the atomic number) and defined as

$$Z = (\rho/K)^{1/2}, \qquad (10.5a)$$

the SI unit of which is the kg/m^2-s, called the *Rayl*. The only reason for inventing so unlikely a beast is that it leads directly to a simple and useful expression for the amounts of reflection and transmission at boundaries. One can also think of reflection as occurring where the velocity of the waves changes abruptly, in which case

$$Z = \rho c, \qquad (10.5b)$$

from Equation 10.2.

The reflection coefficient, R, which is the fraction of the energy or intensity of incoming ultrasound that bounces back from an interface, is determined by demanding simultaneous adherence to the laws both of conservation of energy and of momentum for waves. For normal incidence, R may be expressed in terms of the acoustic impedances of the materials on the two sides of it:

$$R = (Z_2 - Z_1)^2/(Z_2 + Z_1)^2. \qquad (10.5c)$$

The rest of the energy, of relative intensity $T = (1 - R)$, is transmitted across the interface and into the second tissue.

A material's density is clearly independent of the frequency of any ultrasound passing through it, and its compressibility as well – so Z and R, like the speed of sound, also vary hardly at all with f and λ.

The acoustic impedances of some materials are recorded in Table 10.1, and the amounts of energy transmission and reflection occurring at several important kinds of tissue interfaces, obtained from these values, appear in Table 10.2. For example, the density of fat is lower than that of other soft tissues, and its acoustic impedance is as well. The Z-values for muscle and fat are 1.7 and 1.4 MRayl,

Table 10.2 Fractions of intensity/power reflected (*R*) and transmitted (*T*) at some clinically important tissue interfaces.

Interface	R	T
Fat-muscle	0.01	0.99
Muscle-bone	0.23	0.77
Muscle-water	0.004	0.996
Water-air	0.999	0.001

respectively, and Equation 10.5c provides the prescription for the amount reflected, R: $R = (1.7 - 1.4)^2/(1.7 + 1.4)^2 = 0.01$, is small, and the rest of the incident energy, 0.99 of it, passes through. Still, this is enough to causes increased ultrasonic reflection with characteristic findings as are observed in the fatty infiltration of the liver, or *steatosis* (Figure 10.13b).

As would be expected from the large differences in density and compressibility, ultrasound energy does not pass readily across tissue-air or tissue-bone boundaries. US is therefore of little use in examining the lung or adult brain. For the abdomen, moreover, the strongest signals are often from the proximal walls of air bubbles in the GI tract. But ultrasound is employed widely in imaging both the anatomy and the physiology of other parts of the body.

Since soft tissues other than fat all have nearly the same density, variations in acoustic impedance among them are often due primarily to differences in their *elasticity*. The elasticity, in turn, is determined largely by the nature and amounts of the stroma of collagenous material in the connective tissue that binds the parenchymal cells of the tissue together. And pathological conditions that significantly alter the distribution of collagenous material within an organ (e.g., cirrhosis of the liver, some malignancies) may also give rise to diagnostically meaningful image patterns.

Structures containing fluid, such as the bladder, cysts, the common bile duct, and the aorta and other large blood vessels, may have no internal structures, and the ultrasound images of their interiors are fully or nearly blank. Blood is a suspension of reflecting cells and, with normal laminar flow, the biconcave erythrocytes tend to stack themselves like dishes; in this configuration they move with less resistance and with fewer reflecting surfaces

visible to the beam. But in a state of slow turbulent flow, as can be observed in aneurysms and around some venous valves, the cells will lose this alignment and create more reflecting interfaces. This is of importance in some situations because such turbulent flow patterns can lead to plaque genesis and thrombus deposition.

The lungs also appear largely empty, but for a different reason: the ultrasound energy is reflected every which way at the alveolar tissue-air interfaces, because of which all of it is rapidly attenuated out of existence.

The intensity of an echo coming back from a boundary between two tissues depends not only on the difference in their gross physical properties, but also on the size and flatness of the interface area. Sharp echoes will be produced at a sizable and relatively flat boundary between any two materials with significantly different Z-values (Figure 10.16), if any roughness on it is much finer than the US wavelength. And the angle at which the reflected wave leaves the boundary will be the same as the one with which it entered, as with a mirror, but normally the only echoes that matter are those reflected back toward the transducer.

The transmission of acoustic power into and from the body should be efficient, and at the same time extraneous echoes arising within the transducer itself must be prevented to the extent possible. These objectives can largely be achieved by minimizing the mismatches in acoustic impedance between the piezoelectric elements and the patient. This involves covering the front of the transducer with a matching layer of material, including a *coupling gel*, whose acoustic impedance is the geometric mean of those of the piezoelectric material and soft tissue.

Example: echoes from a bone embedded in soft tissue

We can consolidate all of this by working through a simple example. Suppose a flat bone is covered by 3 cm of muscle, which in turn is under 1 cm of fat (Figure 10.17). If a 1-MHz ultrasound beam of time-averaged intensity 0.05 W/cm^2 is directed in toward the bone, what will be the echo strength? Table 10.3, which you may wish to confirm, will help walk you through it.

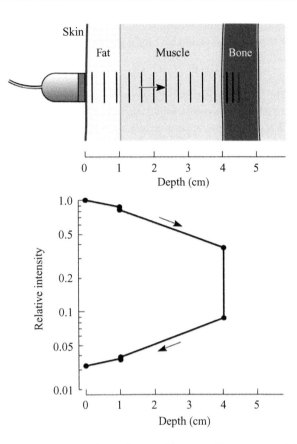

Figure 10.17 An US beam in sub-surface fat enters (creating a weak echo) and passes through muscle, then creates a second echo when reflected by bone. By the time it returns to the transducer, its intensity will have fallen to a few percent of its original value.

Imaging in 1 and 1 × 1 dimensions: A- and M-modes

Finally, to imaging. It has taken a good while to get here, largely because there was a lot of necessary background to cover first, as there was for general X-ray imaging in Chapters 3 and 4, but now we're ready to put the pieces together in an orderly fashion and proceed. Like any sensible physicians and scientists who desire to simplify matters as much as possible at first, we'll start off in one spatial dimension.

One-dimensional imaging: A-mode

US passing through homogeneous tissue at an average velocity v will travel in to a reflective boundary at depth $c \times t$ over the time interval t, where the average velocity is much the same for most soft-tissue materials, about 1540 m/s. If an echo is detected the

Table 10.3 Losses of intensity from attenuation (dB/cm), and corresponding transmission (T) through, homogeneous tissues; transmission (T) across tissue boundaries; and remaining intensity, for the example.

Tissue/interface	Distance (cm)	dB/cm	T	Remaining intensity
Skin surface	0	…	…	1
Fat	1	–0.5	0.89	0.89
Fat/muscle	…	…	0.99	0.88
Muscle	3	–1	0.50	0.44
Muscle/bone	…	…	0.23	0.10
Muscle	3	–1	0.50	0.05
Muscle/fat	…	…	0.99	0.05
Fat	1	–0.5	0.89	0.045

time t_{echo} after pulse transmission, then the interface that caused it would have to be at a depth of

$$\text{Depth} = \frac{1}{2}c\,t_{echo}. \qquad (10.6a)$$

The factor of $\frac{1}{2}$ arises because the sound has to complete both halves of a round trip before arriving back at the transducer. Equivalently, the echo return time increases by 13 μs for each centimeter of depth of a reflecting interface. If a pulse enters soft tissue and an echo appears 96 μs later, there must be a reflecting boundary at a depth of 7.4 cm.

The earliest, and conceptually simplest, form of US is A-mode, in which the *Amplitude* of the reflection from a tissue interface shows up as a voltage spike on the screen of an oscilloscope (Figure 10.18).

Creation of an A-mode display begins with the transmission of a pulse of US energy into the body. At the instant of transmission, a point of light begins sweeping horizontally across the screen of a monitor. If and when the transducer detects an echo signal, it generates a voltage spike that briefly deflects the spot of light upward. The position along the *x*-axis of the spike corresponds to the time of return of the echo, in accord with Equation 10.6a, hence to the depth of the responsible tissue interface. The amplitude of an echo pulse is determined both by

the mismatch in impedances of the two tissues at the interface and by the attenuation of the beam, although this is largely compensated for with TGC. More than one spike occurring along the *x*-axis indicates the presence of several reflecting surfaces at different depths.

A-mode display is still used for precise depth measurements such as of the fine structure of the eye, but A-mode displays no longer are found on conventional medical ultrasound machines.

Lateral and longitudinal resolution

In US, lateral resolution is determined by the width of the beam at the depth of interest (Figure 10.19a). If the beam can pass cleanly between two objects within the body without creating an echo, they can be resolved, and this leads to a definition of beam width and resolution capability.

Because of Huygens' principle, the width of the field from a large single element or from a flat array of multiple elements fired simultaneously tends to narrow naturally to a minimum at the near field depth, where the near field connects with the far field (Figure 10.11). Electronic focusing, moreover, can enhance that narrowing significantly (Figure 10.9d), so that *lateral resolution* is determined ultimately by the sizes and timing of the individual elements. Lateral resolutions of the order of a few millimeters are commonly achieved (Figure 10.19b).

The *axial resolution*, on the other hand, depends on the *wavelength* and the *pulse duration*, which is to say the length of the volume of tissue that will be covered by a single pulse. Two parallel surfaces can be resolved if the length of the incident pulse is so small that the resulting pair of echoes can be distinguished from one another. That occurs only if the separation is greater than half the pulse length (Figure 10.20a),

$$\text{axial resolution} = \frac{1}{2}\text{ pulse length.} \quad (10.6b)$$

If the surfaces are separated by *less* than half a pulse length, the echoes overlap and cannot be told apart (Figure 10.20b). The spatial pulse length, in turn, is determined by the number of cycles in the pulse, $(f\,\Delta t)$, where Δt the pulse duration, and by the wavelength, λ, so (Figure 10.20c)

$$\text{axial resolution} = (f\,\Delta t) \times \lambda = c\,\Delta t, \quad (10.6c)$$

Maximizing axial resolution calls for a brief pulse.

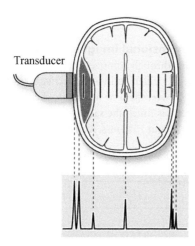

Figure 10.18 A-mode US provides one-dimensional (i.e., along the line of sight of the beam) information on anatomy. At the instant of pulse transmission, a point of light begins its horizontal sweep across the monitor screen, and any detected echo signal produces a spike on it, where the echo return time is proportional to the depth of the tissue interface.

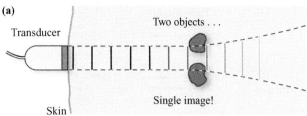

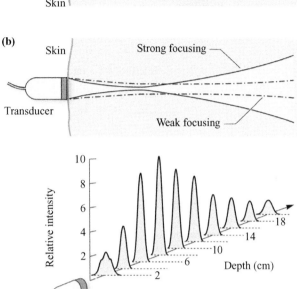

Figure 10.19 Lateral resolution. (a) An important reason to focus the beam: lateral resolution can be no better than the beam dimensions. (b) Two representations of how focusing reduces the cross-sectional area of a beam in the focal region and concentrates the sound energy there. The upper consists of iso-intensity lines (apart from attenuation effects) for both weak and strong focusing. The lower displays intensity profiles at various depths for a beam with an 8-cm-deep focus. Modified from National Council on Radiation Protection and Measurements (NCRP), *Biological Effects of Ultrasound: Mechanisms and Clinical Implications*, report no. 74. Bethesda, MD: NCRP, 1983, fig. 3.9.

The higher the center frequency, in general, the better are both the axial and the lateral resolution. But, again, most tissues attenuate US at a rate roughly proportional to the frequency (Equations 10.3c), so a short pulse created with short wavelengths means good resolution but rapid attenuation and poor beam penetration. The selection of frequency and transducer for a specific clinical study on a particular patient depends largely on this fundamental tradeoff (Figure 10.12c).

1 × 1-Dimensional imaging: M-mode

With A-mode, the transducer looks only along a single line through the body. The same is true for M-mode (for *Motion*; also called TM-mode, for *Time-Motion*), but two simple refinements allow the display of the motions of the tissues situated along that line.

As with A-mode, the dot of light on the display screen sweeps once along a line for each transmitted pulse of US. The light is bright enough to be visible only when an echo is being detected (it is suppressed the rest of the time), and its brightness increases with the strength of the echo signal. That is, a dot appears in M-mode where a spike would have occurred in A-mode, and it is the brightness of the spot that is modulated by an echo, rather than the amplitude of the spike.

M-mode display is commonly aligned with the beam entering vertically (Figure 10.21). Instead of retracing exactly over itself, as with A-mode, the vertical display line steps slightly to the right between consecutive pulses. Immobile structures give rise to straight, horizontal lines of closely spaced bright dots. Periodic motions of interfaces toward and from the transducer are readily revealed as quasi-horizontal wavy lines with repetitive vertical displacements. M-mode's most important applications are in cardiac studies, where irregular movement of the heart wall and of the mitral and tricuspid valves may indicate a diseased state.

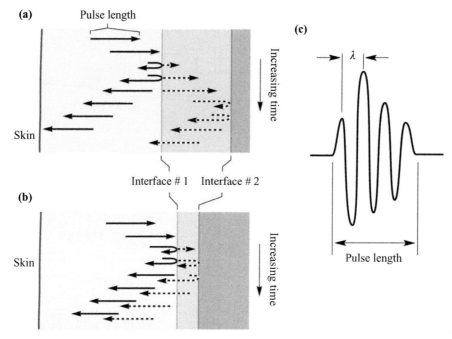

Figure 10.20 Axial (longitudinal) resolution and pulse length. Time increases in the downward direction. (**a**) Echoes from two surfaces do not overlap, and can be resolved, if the depths of the surfaces differ by more than half a pulse length, (**b**) but not if the surfaces are closer together than that. (**c**) Spatial pulse length is determined by the number of cycles, $f \Delta t$, and the wavelength, λ.

Imaging in two, three, and four dimensions: B-mode

B-mode may be thought of as an extension on the A-mode theme that incorporates two major refinements. Here, a spot of bright light tracing along a *scan line* on the display screen (as with M-mode) indicates an echo. And second, the scan line is swept or stepped throughout the tissue plane of interest, with each image comprised of one or a few hundred lines (Figure 10.10). Thus, like CT, B-mode imaging uses two dimensions of display plus

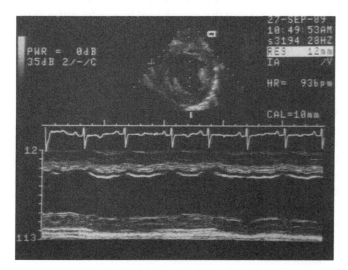

Figure 10.21 B-mode echocardiogram (parasternal short-axis view of the left ventricle). Below it is an M-mode image obtained along the single vertical grid of dots indicated in the B-mode image above it.

spatial variations in brightness of light to image a thin, quasi-two-dimensional slice of anatomy.

The transducer produces a pulse about 1 microsecond in duration, and then listens quietly for any echoes that might arrive over the next 200 μs or so, before transmitting the next pulse. The transducer may put out several thousand pulses (and scan lines) per second, but still manages to spend 99% of its time quiescent and acting as a receiver.

The thousands of scan lines the system initiates per second generate 30 or so image *frames* per second – fast enough to follow the operation of the heart valves throughout the cardiac cycle. As you might expect, there is an inverse relationship between the frame rate and lateral resolution: the resolution increases with the number of lines per frame (Figure 10.22a). But the same amount of time is required to create each line – so higher beam-line density makes possible better resolution, but with

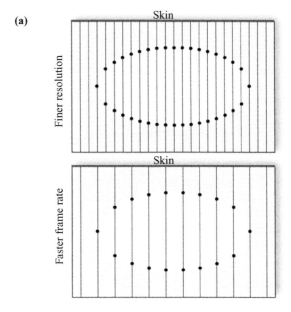

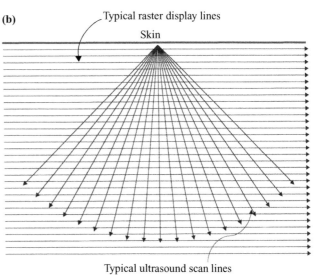

Figure 10.22 Display lines. **(a)** Linear array line pattern. Plausibility argument for the tradeoff between resolution and frame rate, as determined by scan line density: more lines in a frame means finer detail, but it takes longer to obtain them. **(b)** Loss of lateral resolution is proportional to depth with sector imaging.

more time per frame, hence lower frame rate. For sector imaging, there is also a simple relationship between depth in the body and lateral resolution, since the display lines diverge (Figure 10.22b).

B-mode started off as an essentially thin-plane modality. Created at first with only a single row of elements, the beam was commonly focused and flattened into one plane by means of a plastic acoustic lens. The transducer and lens could be rocked back and forth in the third dimension, however, either manually or by way of a mechanical "wobbler." After passing through "1.25D" and "1.5D" arrays that contained increasing numbers of rows of elements, we have now arrived at square, fully 2D element arrays that can produce 3D images completely electronically. One approach to using such a device is simply to have it rock the imaging plane back and forth automatically, obtaining several dozen planes per study. This is fine for examining a static condition, but several seconds per volume is far too slow for following some dynamic processes. There are tradeoffs that can be made, of course, involving some sacrifice of image quality. Combination of these with ECG gating currently allow the acquisition of images throughout the cardiac cycle that are adequate for the evaluation of valve performance, ejection fraction, etc.

B-mode hardware

Figure 10.23a outlines, in more detail than did Figure 1.18a, a modern B-mode US system with an 80 × 5 2D phased-array transducer. The circuit shown is for only one piezoelectric crystal of this multi-element array – there are 399 other channels that are identical to it, but separate from it.

Everything is timed and orchestrated by the computer. For a 400-element transducer, say, to create the first echo, the computer instructs the *transmit beam former* to create 400 voltage pulses at slightly different times, so as to bring about proper beam direction and focusing and send them into the 400 channels of the transmitter. After amplification, each high-voltage pulse passes through its dedicated transmit/receive (T/R) switch (shown here in the receive mode), which isolates and protects the sensitive signal reception equipment during transmission. From there, the pulse proceeds to its piezoelectric element, which generates an associated mechanical pulse.

Echo signal acquisition starts off like the inverse of transmission. The echo vibrations returning from a reflection point in the body are picked up by all the elements of the transducer at slightly different times, and the resulting voltage signals pass back through their T/R switches and on to their respective 400 low-noise logarithmic pre-amplifiers, samplers, digitizers, and TGC.

For transmission along the first scan line, delays were introduced in the firing of adjacent elements to steer and focus the beam. The *receiver beam former*, or *dynamic receiver refocusing* (DRR) circuit, introduces separate receive time delays to, in effect, re-focus the returning echo signals. The echo returning from transmission by a single element will be sensed by all 400 elements at slightly different times, in part because of the marginally different distances over which it had to travel to return from the reflection point. By inserting an appropriate extra delay to each, they can then be summed, in phase and "coherently," to create a single sharper scan line. A recent extension of this approach is for multiple return-beam formers to simultaneously generate a number of acoustic scan lines with a single pulse transmission. After passing through the DRR, the digitized echo signal enters the receiver, which processes it further.

The whole process is repeated to create and detect the second scan line pulse, sent off at a different angle or step position, and so on. One hundred such beam-lines, each generated with a pulse to every crystal, are typically required for a single image. In this final stage, the computer may carry out smoothing or other image processing, and make possible windowing of the display gray scale, color coding of images, etc.

Most US devices can fit onto a mobile cart that carries the main hardware, multiple transducers, connections with the radiology or cardiology department's PACS and RIS, etc. Coming onto the scene now, especially in the emergency department, intensive care units, and in rural, underserved areas, are laptop and even smaller units (Figure 10.23b). Another important ongoing development is that newer systems are becoming more operator-friendly, providing various forms of assistance in the clarification and interpretation of images; sometimes it is notoriously difficult for operators to extract the necessary clinical information from US images.

Applications of B-mode

Ultrasound is the only imaging modality employed routinely in obstetrics, because of its diagnostic value, low cost, rapid availability, and apparent safety. It confirms pregnancy and reveals the

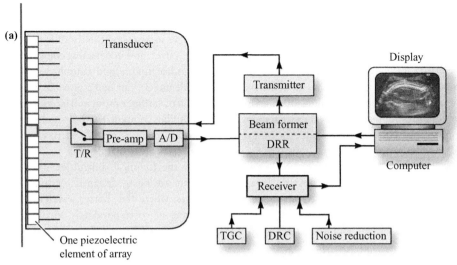

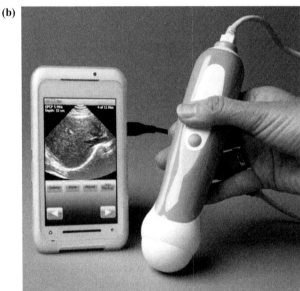

Figure 10.23 Schematic of a generic computer-controlled B-mode US system. (a) High-frequency electrical pulses generated by the transmitter are converted into mechanical vibrations by the piezoelectric elements of a transducer. Subsequently the transducer, acting as a microphone, picks up any echoes originating within the body and converts them into electrical signals, which are processed by the receiver and computer for display. A B-mode image is made up of lines of varying brightness. Each scan line corresponds to one pulse, to one beam direction in sector mode; a bright point along a line indicates an interface between dissimilar tissues. (b) B-mode transducer connected to a smartphone. Image courtesy of Mobisante, Inc. This compact MobiUS SP1 system is the first smartphone-based diagnostic device to be cleared by the FDA. Operating at 3.5–15 MHz and with a battery life of over 5 hours of scanning, it can acquire 480 × 480 pixel images, optimize them, and transfer them via phone, WiFi, or USB.

number of fetuses, and commonly the sex, as well. Early gestational ultrasound (6–10 weeks) is helpful in confirming implantation site (which confirms intrauterine location, ruling out ectopic) and viability (earliest heartbeat can be detected at 6 weeks). This type of US is usually done transvaginally for optimal visualization. Later studies, near 20 weeks of gestation, employ trans-abdominal scanning to search cardiac defects, spina bifida, microcephaly, hydrocephaly, limb deformities, irregularities of the placenta and umbilical cord, atypical fetal movement, and other fetal abnormalities, and guide the placement of the aspiration needle during amniocentesis.

Although not as suitable for routine breast cancer screening as mammography, US has nonetheless proven capable of differentiating fluid-filled cysts from solid masses found by physical examination or mammography. US is of especial value for young women or women with dense breast tissues, for whom X-ray may prove inadequate.

Ultrasound is the first-line modality in gynecologic evaluation of a pelvic mass. Transvaginal ultrasound is capable of discriminating many characteristics between benign and malignant ovarian masses: benign ovarian cysts are typically simple, thin-walled, anechoic, and smaller (<10 cm). Malignant cysts are typically larger than 10 cm in the pre-menopausal female, and malignancy is indicated by thick walls, internal septations, debris inside the fluid that demonstrates internal echoes, and multi-loculated pockets. Biopsy, of course, is necessary for confirmation. US characteristics of masses and cysts are prognostically useful for diagnosis and management, and valuable in guiding surgical approach. US is also useful in the diagnosis of fibroid uterine tumors and for measuring endometrial thickness in hyperplasia or malignancy.

US transducers have been designed for a variety of special purposes. Two that are used with neonates and small children, along with a transesophageal device for echocardiography, appeared in Figure 10.6b. Others include endovaginal probes for imaging the pelvis and fetus, endorectal for prostate and rectal wall, and intravascular (IVUS). Transducers have also been developed with attached needle assemblies for performing directly guided biopsies, as with endoscopy and bronchoscopy.

High-resolution, shallow-penetration (8–20 MHz) systems can reveal the thicknesses of the cornea and the lens, to detect intraocular tumors and foreign bodies (some of which may not show up with X-rays), to diagnose retinal detachment, and to guide lens selection for cataract surgery.

In assessing the functioning of the heart, real-time B-mode can map the spatial relations of its constituent parts in two dimensions and locate a valve or wall of interest; after that, an M-mode-like application can provide more precise information on the amplitudes and velocities of its motions. It is effective in assessing the condition and functioning of valves, and in detecting congenital heart disease, cardiac tumors, and a number of other cardiac problems. US can make possible an indirect calculation of cardiac output and ejection fraction. Doppler studies combined with B-mode can reveal various abnormalities in the arteries and veins, including cerebrovascular disease.

Despite the technical difficulties, miniaturized transducers are being designed for much higher frequencies, where the shorter wavelengths allow the imaging of correspondingly smaller objects. *Micro-machined Ultrasound Transducers* consisting of arrays of tens or hundreds of piezoelectric (pMUT) or capacitive (cMUT) elements on silicon chips only a few millimeters across are being built by way of semiconductor-chip manufacturing technologies. Such a transducer is small enough to fit within a narrow-gauge catheter and then into a coronary artery, looking either forward or laterally, and some can even be threaded into finer blood vessels. Vascular imaging is currently being performed in the 10–40 MHz range, and even higher frequencies are being explored (up to 100 MHz), with potential applications in ophthalmology, dermatology, and perhaps cellular-level imaging.

Tantalizingly, computer-based pattern recognition algorithms seem capable of determining certain pathologic conditions from statistical studies of tissue image textures. As with all other digital modalities, computer-aided diagnosis is bound to grow rapidly in ultrasound.

B-mode artifacts

B-mode suffers from a number of artifacts that can sometimes be confused with real parts of an image. Fortunately, they are well known to US operators and physicians, and usually they are easily recognizable.

Shadowing may occur distal to an object that reflects or attenuates strongly, such as a bone or gallstone, because there is less US energy left in the beam there to produce echoes (Figure 10.24a). Conversely, *enhancement* may occur on the far side of a fluid-filled bladder, cyst, or other organ that attenuates/reflects little, compared to its surroundings.

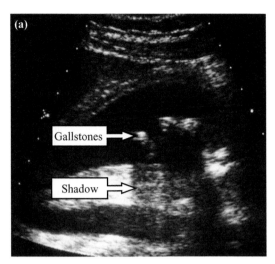 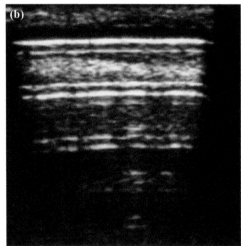

Figure 10.24 Several of the various artifacts that can arise in standard B-mode imaging. (**a**) Shadowing distal to a region of high reflection (in this case gallstones) or attenuation. (**b**) Reverberation of US between a flat reflecting object beneath the skin and the transducer gives the impression of reflecting surfaces at multiple depths.

Back-and-forth *reverberations* of US between two closely spaced, highly reflecting objects, such as metal fragments or small air pockets, or between a shallow reflective interface and the transducer surface, may manifest as a series of regularly spaced parallel lines (Figure 10.24b).

Because of *refraction*, images below a boundary between acoustically different tissues may not be exactly where they seem to be. Just as a swizzle stick bends where it enters a gin and tonic, the change of direction of an US beam path at the boundary may shift the apparent position of a reflecting object laterally (Figure 2.5d). Similarly, in a *speed artifact*, a region of atypically high or low US velocity may cause an apparent longitudinal displacement of a boundary beyond.

Artifacts caused by *grating-* and *side-lobes* to the side of the transmitted beam, coming from various kinds of wave interference effects arising at the transducer, may lead to the occurrence of pseudo-sludge in the image, which can resemble the real thing closely. Likewise, a *multi-path reflection* or *mirror* artifact may give rise to the appearance of livers, say, both above and below diaphragm.

Contrast agents and harmonic imaging

US contrast agents, administered intravenously, can enhance the clarity of blood vessels and the heart. These consist of suspensions in fluid of erythrocyte-size bubbles of either air or a heavy-molecular-weight gas, stabilized with some type of shell layer, commonly of lipid, that might even be tissue targeting. The microspheres are small enough, in the 1–5 micrometer range, to traverse the capillary beds without any adverse biological effects. Yet they can produce large-amplitude echoes, since there is a leap in acoustic impedance between the gas and surrounding tissue or blood. The gas-filled bubbles are highly compressible compared to blood, and they tend to pulsate vigorously as a US wave passes by, expanding and contracting with the local pressure changes, thereby producing scattering and echoes. This can be a resonance phenomenon, with extralarge oscillations and resultant echoes, if the bubble characteristics and the US frequency are matched (typically at about 10 MHz.) If such agents are not available, one may shake or agitate normal saline and quickly inject it into the bloodstream. This also creates such microbubbles, which, while not stable for long, can still be used to diagnose and quantify shunting, for example.

A Hooke's Law spring undergoing low-amplitude oscillations is a *linear* system, in the sense that the restoring force increases linearly with displacement, $F = -\kappa x$. This combines with Newton's $F = ma$ to reveal that the resulting motion is described by a pure sine wave of constant and symmetric shape (Figure 10.25a). The same is true also of a gas-filled bubble

(a) **(b)**

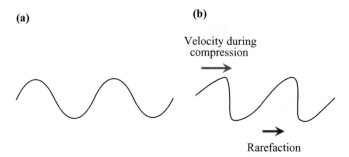

Velocity during
compression

Rarefaction

Figure 10.25 The generation of harmonics. **(a)** A spring or bubble undergoing small-amplitude oscillations obeys Hooke's law and oscillates sinusoidally. **(b)** When a material undergoes compression or extension beyond its Hooke's law limit, its properties can alter radically. In particular, the velocity of propagation of sound energy through it changes briefly under excessive compression, so that its oscillations are no longer exactly sinusoidal; the distorted pattern must now be represented as a sum of waves at multiple *harmonics* of the fundamental, as suggested in Figure 4.10.

compressing and expanding as a US wave passes by, and even for the volumetric oscillations of a small region of soft tissue.

With *high-amplitude oscillations*, however, the periodic compression of contrast bubbles, or small bits of soft tissue, can be somewhat *nonlinear*. That means that they physically distort so much that Hooke's law breaks down somewhat, and must be amended as $F = -\kappa x + \kappa' x^2 + \ldots$. Not too surprisingly, the motion becomes more complex (no longer purely sinusoidal), and its velocity changes. Equation 10.2 suggests, at first blush, that in regions of high compression where the density peaks, the speed of sound would decrease. But this is only half the picture: high compression gives rise, as well, to a change in compressibility itself, one that acts in the opposite direction – and that tends to be the dominant effect. In the crest of a very-high intensity monochromatic US wave, sound energy moves a little faster than throughout the rest of the cycle. This distorts the wave from a pure sine or, equivalently, introduces harmonics (Figure 10.25b). Fourier analysis indicates that, in analogy to the square wave of Figure 4.10b, the distorted wave comprises the fundamental sine wave plus components at a number of *harmonic* frequencies, integer multiples of the natural resonant, fundamental frequency.

There are advantages to intentionally driving the tissues or bubbles non-linear, and then creating *harmonic images* out of the echo harmonic waves only, filtering out the fundamental. Contrast agents are often used together with harmonic imaging, in which the receiver is tuned to the second (typically) harmonic of the returning echo signal. While its inherent strength is much lower than that at the fundamental frequency, the contribution of noise from clutter and some other sources may be much

less. Other techniques such as *pulse inversion* may virtually eliminate the fundamental frequency component of the echo signal, and enhance the CNR in other ways.

One early contrast agent was made by sonicating human serum albumin in the presence of air. Other agents are now available commercially, and some newer ones are currently undergoing clinical trials. While contrast agents are employed freely in Europe, so far the FDA has approved only a few agents for use in the United States to date, and these only for cardiac indications.

Doppler imaging of blood flow

Know how the whistle of an oncoming train drops in pitch as the engine rushes past you? This is an example of the Doppler effect, and the same phenomenon can be harnessed to reveal information about the flow of blood within the major arteries and veins, including the aorta, vena cava, carotid arteries, and larger vessels in the extremities. The velocity often is crucial in determining the health of the vessel itself, as well as of the organs that it feeds.

The Doppler effect is a direct consequence of the wave nature of sound. The heart of the issue is the fundamental, geometrically based relationship. $\lambda f = c$ (Equation 10.1). Suppose you are sitting in a small stationary boat, watching the ocean waves roll by you at velocity c and frequency f_0. The speed of the waves (or of US through soft tissue) is always the same relative to the shore or to the whole ocean (the body), regardless of how anyone or anything may be moving about.

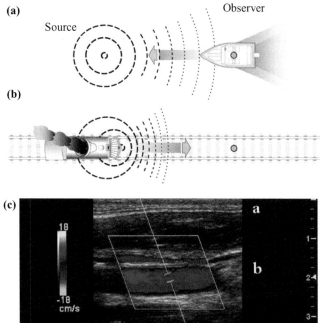

Figure 10.26 Doppler effect: someone at a source and an observer experience the same frequency when they are not moving relative to one another, but a shift occurs in the detected frequency when they are. (**a**) A frequency shift appears to the observer when she moves toward the source, and (**b**) a change in wavelength occurs when it is the source that moves. (**c**) Triplex-mode display of B-mode, color flow Doppler, spectral Doppler information at the bottom.

Now drive the boat away from the pier at speed v_{obs}, so that the speed of the waves relative to *you*, the *observer*, will be ($c + v_{obs}$). The waves will now be slapping your bow at a rate of $f_{obs} = [(c + v_{obs})/c] \times f_0$ cycles per second, which is higher than before (Figure 10.26a). This equation can easily be rearranged as $v_{obs}/c = +[(f_{obs}/f_0) - 1]$, which says that the speed at which we are traveling is directly proportional to the relative shift in the frequency that we measure. If, conversely, you are moving away from a source of waves, then the apparent frequency, f_{obs}, is shifted downward from f_0, instead, and the "+" is replaced by a minus sign.

If it is the source of the waves that moves, rather than you, the details are a little different but the result is still much the same (Figure 10.26b). A disturbance produced by a point source radiates outward, with velocity c, as a spherical wave front centered at the point, regardless of the motion of the source. But if the source moves toward you between the generation of consecutive wave crests, then the measured wavelength (i.e., the distance between the crests) will be less than what you would find if the source were stationary – and the frequency you measure would therefore have to be correspondingly higher, since the speed of sound does not differ. Once the source passes you by, the detected frequency drops *below* that actually produced by the source.

Imagine a small volume element of fluid in an artery or vein that contains cells that in effect, can reflect US. (More precisely, it is temporal variations in the numbers of erythrocytes in microscopic volumes of fluid, leading to Poisson variations in the local values of Z, that cause the reflections.) The volume element is moving at speed, v_{blood}, toward a transducer that is transmitting US of frequency, f_0. Because of their motion, the blood cells in the volume experience a source of ultrasound waves of an apparent frequency that is slightly higher than what is actually being transmitted by the transducer. That is, the blood cells, acting first like a moving "observer," encounter US wave crests at the rate of f_{obs}. Then, in reflecting this energy, the cells themselves act as an ultrasound "source" – but this new source is moving briskly along the vessel, so that the frequency of the echo signal detected back at the transducer is shifted even further upward.

The overall effect of the motion of the blood is to raise the frequency of the ultrasound echo that returns to the transducer by an amount proportional to the velocity of the fluid. By measuring the Doppler frequency shift, $\Delta f_{Doppler}$, which is technically easy to do, you can calculate the blood velocity directly:

$$v_{blood}/c = \pm^1\!/_2\, \Delta f_{Doppler}/f_0. \qquad (10.7)$$

The relative shift in frequency thus equals two times the relative (to the speed of sound in the fluid) velocity of the blood. The Doppler shift is negative if the blood is moving away from the transducer. In general, echoes are caused by blood moving through a vessel at an angle to the US beam, and from a continuum of neighboring blood volumes, both of which complicate matters.

Duplex and *color Doppler* ultrasound match high-resolution B-mode with Doppler information in ways that reveal the blood flow in a particular region. Figure 10.26c provides an example of color Doppler; blue represents blood moving in an artery or vein toward the transducer, and red blood is going the other way. The transducer produces a burst of ultrasound, similar to the transmit pulse used in B-mode imaging, but of longer duration (up to 25 cycles), hence with a narrower ultrasound frequency spectrum. Returning echo signals following a single transmit pulse are subjected to standard B-mode processing, to obtain some depth information, and also to Doppler analysis to extract the rate of blood flow. The trick here is to apply signal gating, which extracts out only those Doppler-processed echo signals originating from a well-defined depth range, discarding all other parts of the signal. Typically this "sample volume" is only 2–5 mm in thickness along the beam axis, but its location and size can be adjusted by the operator. The actual Doppler signal from blood and/or contrast agent within the sample volume is built up over several transmit-receive pulse echo sequences, where only signals from the gated region are retained.

The Doppler effect occurs with electromagnetic radiation as well as with sound. It is responsible for the red shift (i.e., downward in frequency) of the light reaching us from stars and galaxies that are speeding away from the solar system (or vice versa, depending on your point of view). Precise measurements of such red shifts are of critical impor-tance to astronomers concerned with estimating the distances of the heavenly bodies, or with assessing the size and age of the universe. Likewise, as those of us who occasionally cruise the highways a bit too exuberantly well know, police automobile Doppler RADAR can measure the speed of a gorgeous maroon Corvette with the top down on a splendid autumn afternoon in Vermont. Apparently it doesn't help much to ask the officer when and how his Doppler device was last calibrated . . . .

Elastography

Although the compressibility of a tissue may be a measure of its well being, and variations in its stiffness could be indicative of various pathological conditions, standard US provides no way to separate this out and assess it. A spin-off from US can do that, however, and recently has been finding clinical application. *Elastography*, or elastic imaging, reveals tissue elasticity parameters directly.

The basic idea is straightforward: you image an organ both before compression, and then again while it is under a known amount of acoustic or other mechanical stress to find the resultant strain. A soft object compresses, and a stiff one is displaced forward.

In a simple case, the strain occurs parallel to the stress, and is linear in it. As with Hooke's law for a spring, the more one pushes or pulls on something, the greater its deformation. *Normal* (in the sense of perpendicular to a surface) *stress*, ε, is the force per area, F/A, applied to the face of a block of tissue. *Normal strain* refers to the resulting fractional change in the length of the block, $\Delta L/L$, under compression, and is commonly represented by a sigma, σ (nothing to do with statistics!). Then $\sigma = E\varepsilon$, and the ratio of strain per unit area is called *Young's modulus*, E, also the *modulus of elasticity* – this is just Hooke's law dressed up fancy (E, here, has nothing to do with either energy or electric field strength.)

Special equipment is required both for generating precisely known stresses and for quantifying the strain. The stress can be either normal or transverse (*shear stress*), and it can be either briefly constant, or a periodic palpation, or produced through various sorts of dynamic excitation. The imaging system must be able to provide a spatial map of the types and magnitudes of the deformations taking place while the stress is being applied. While the imaging was first carried out with US, there are now systems that employ MRI, CT, optical tomography, and other means.

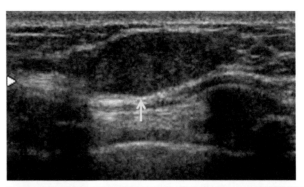

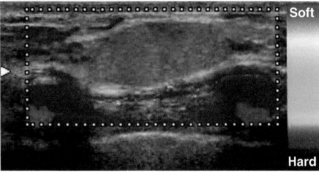

Figure 10.27 Color enhanced B-mode elastography performed on a patient presenting with a palpable breast mass of unknown etiology. The upper B-mode image demonstrates the presence of an isoechoic, oval-shaped mass with its maximal diameter parallel to the skin surface (arrow); it displays regular, well-defined contours and does not attenuate sound waves, as is typical of a benign fibroadenoma. In the lower image, color elastography confirms the diagnosis, showing that the mass is of homogeneous stiffness with a rubbery configuration.

The elasticity or stiffness of a tissue may change as a result of a pathological condition, and elastography may provide the best or only means of detecting the difference (Figure 10.27). Ductal carcinomas of the breast are much stiffer than normal glandular tissue, for example, and scirrhous carcinomas of the breast also present as hard nodules, in part due to fibrotic reactions. Cirrhotic liver tissue is considerably stiffer than normal liver. Cancers of the prostate are harder than normal prostate tissue, while prostatic hyperplasia is much less so. And uterine fibroids and a number of other abnormal tissues also have distinctive moduli. As a variation on the theme, intravascular elastography is performed where the stress is produced by the body itself, such as by varying blood pressure in vessels during the cardiac cycle, where strains are assessed with a catheter with an intravascular transducer at the tip. Recently there have been intriguing reports that the ratio of the sizes of a lesion as determined under elastography and B-mode can distinguish between benign and malignant tumors.

Areas of active technology research include improvements in resolution, signal-to-noise, and stress estimation; and also the impact of attenuation and damping on time-dependent mechanical excitation, and how to deal with it. Some predict that elastography will soon become the third leg of a stable tripod, along with B-mode and Doppler.

Safety and QA

As with all other imaging modalities (indeed, all medical activities), ultrasound images can be less than optimal because of improper performance of either the operator or the equipment. While training and management can and should ensure that the sonographers are at their best, a comprehensive quality assurance and safety program is needed to confirm that the instrument itself is behaving properly.

Quality assurance

It is important to maintain image quality and ensure patient safety with a proper ultrasound QA program, especially now that the ACR has established an accreditation program for the modality (www .acr.org/Quality-Safety/Accreditation/ultrasound.) A variety of beam, receiver, display, and other

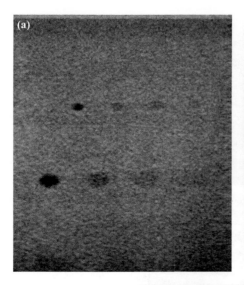
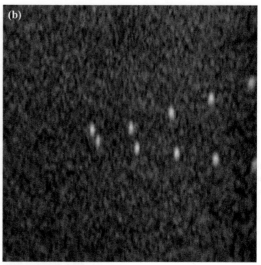
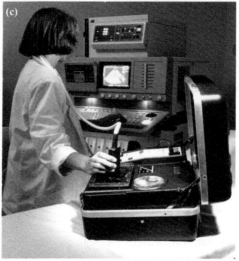

Figure 10.28 As with the other modalities, various routine and annual QA procedures range from the very simple to the complex. Checks, employing simple test devices, of **(a)** the detectability of low-contrast objects of varying contrast and size, and **(b)** axial and lateral resolution. **(c)** Doppler quality assurance phantom and fluid control system that can mimic the constant (venous) and pulsed (arterial) flow of blood through soft tissue. Courtesy of the Gammex Corporation.

characteristics should be tested with the purchase of new equipment and routinely thereafter. Routine QA should confirm that low-contrast object detectability (Figure 10.28a), axial and lateral spatial resolution (Figure 10.28b), sensitivity, depth of beam penetration, image uniformity, SNR, dynamic range, vertical and horizontal measurement, and a number of other measurable parameters exceed or at least meet stipulated criteria, with several different transducers for each system. ACR accreditation for US has special requirements for breast imaging.

Commercial QA phantoms are available in which targets ranging in size and acoustic impedance are embedded in tissue-equivalent gel, and others for Doppler (Figure 10.28c). Interpretation of the results, however, tends to be somewhat subjective and not necessarily rigorously reproductive.

Protocols of checks and measurements have been established to that end, perhaps the most widely cited of these being publications of the American Institute of Ultrasound in Medicine (AIUM) and the American College of Radiology (ACR).

Risks from properly operated diagnostic ultrasound are believed to be very low

Early in the development of SONAR, it was learned that intense bursts of sound energy can kill fish and other small animals. Since that time, the effects of ultrasound on all sorts of living organisms have been studied extensively, and at least three distinct mechanisms have been found that are capable of causing biological harm.

At the high levels of power employed in industry and some SONAR, ultrasound can cause cavitation (the creation and immediate, violent implosion of microscopic vacuum bubbles) in a fluid. It is necessary to prevent this from occurring during diagnosis, especially with patients who might be pregnant. To help the operator realize the potential risk of cavitation, modern scanners present a display of a quantity termed the *mechanical index* (*MI*), usually shown on the image monitor. The MI is computed from the estimated negative pressure amplitude, the ultrasound frequency of a transmitted pulse, and other operator-controlled settings. Cavitation is sometimes seen with MI values as low as 0.3 when stable microscopic gas bubbles happen to be naturally present in the tissue; it is believed, however, that these low values would not lead to cavitation when bubbles are absent. US power far above medical diagnostic levels is employed in *high intensity focused US* (HIFU) with the express purpose of heating or even destroying tissues.

Medium-power ultrasound does not cause cavitation, but it can raise the local temperature of tissue significantly. Indeed, this phenomenon underlies the use of US in physical therapy for various joint and soft-tissue ailments and in the hyperthermia treatment of cancer. The temperature rise is potentially dangerous if not properly controlled. Because of bone's high ultrasound absorption, considerable heat deposition and an associated rise in temperature can occur in soft tissue at bone surfaces. A second real-time output display, the *thermal index* (*TI*), is also presented to the ultrasonographer. The TI is closely related to the anticipated temperature when transmitting into tissue; a TI of 1, for exam-

ple, corresponds to an exposure that can lead to a $1\,^{\circ}\text{C}$ temperature elevation.

Ultrasound is capable, moreover, of exerting sheering and twisting forces on small objects suspended in a fluid. The spinning of intracellular particles in ultrasound fields has been observed, as has induced circulation of cellular contents. These findings (together with what some observers believe may be indications of US-induced incidences of fetal abnormalities and other effects in test mammals) suggest that there *might* be some mechanisms capable of producing some biological damage in humans even at moderate levels of exposure.

There is no single number that can serve as a comprehensive measure of beam intensity. The American Institute of Ultrasound in Medicine (AIUM) and the National Council on Radiation Protection and Measurements (NCRP) have introduced several measures that, taken together, provide useful partial information on a beam. These include the so-called *time-averaged intensity* passing through the face of the transducer, I_{TA}, where intensity is the rate of overall US energy flow across a unit area per second. The *spatial-peak, temporal-averaged intensity*, I_{SPTA}, refers to the average intensity at a point within the beam where it reaches its peak value (Figure 10.11 and Figure 10.29a), when averaged over a relatively long period of time. In practice, the pressure wave form is measured in a water tank with a small specialized piezoelectric transducer called a hydrophone, and the intensity is calculated from that.

The US energy deposited in a region of tissue is the product of the average power and the *dwell time*, which is the total time that the beam is actually on and that its focal zone covers a specific tissue volume. Combinations of I_{SPTA} and dwell time commonly employed for pulse-echo (shaded) and Doppler (hatched) systems appear in Figure 10.29b. There have been no independently confirmed significant biologic effects in mammalian tissues exposed *in vitro* with parameters in the region below the broken line, which represents recommendations by the AIUM and the NCRP.

All of that having been said, there is strong evidence that clinical diagnostic ultrasound, used properly, has no detrimental effects on patients, even fetuses. We are aware of no solid data indicating that mechanisms such as those discussed

(a)

Time-averaged intensity:
$$I_T = W / A$$

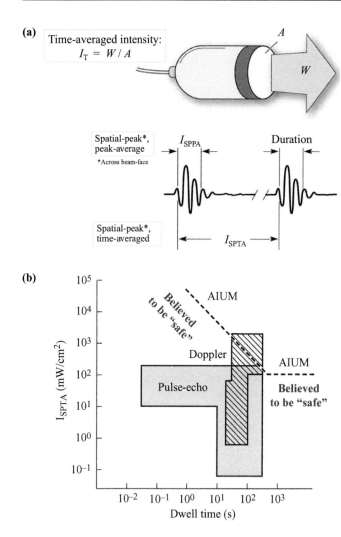

A

W

Spatial-peak*,
peak-average

*Across beam-face

I_{SPPA}

Duration

Spatial-peak*,
time-averaged

I_{SPTA}

(b)

I_{SPTA} (mW/cm²)

10^5

10^4

10^3

10^2

10^1

10^0

10^{-1}

Believed to be "safe"

AIUM

Doppler

Pulse-echo

AIUM

Believed to be "safe"

10^{-2} 10^{-1} 10^0 10^1 10^2 10^3

Dwell time (s)

Figure 10.29 US intensity and safety. **(a)** Average power, W, entering the patient from a source of area A may be related to the time-averaged intensity there I_T as $W = I_T \times A$. I_{SPPA} beam intensity, as derived from the pressure waveform, is averaged only over the pulse itself. I_{SPTA} is averaged over a long period of time. **(b)** Typical combinations of I_{SPTA} and dwell time for pulse-echo (shaded) and Doppler (hatched) systems. There have been no independently confirmed significant biologic effects in mammalian tissues exposed *in vitro* with parameters in the region below the broken line, but it is known that higher intensities can cause heating, shearing/twisting, cell streaming, and cavitation. Modified from National Council on Radiation Protection and Measurements, *Biological Effects of Ultrasound: Mechanisms and Clinical Implications*, report no. 74. Bethesda MD: NCRP1983, figs. 9.1, 9.2.

above, or others yet unknown, actually *do* cause harm in humans, even human fetuses, at the ultrasound levels used in diagnostic procedures. To the contrary, the accumulated clinical experience to date points strongly to the safety of ultrasound. Over half of all pregnant women in the United States undergo at least one ultrasound examination during pregnancy, and there have been no clear signs of adverse effects. Some ongoing, long-term follow-up epidemiological studies, in partic-

ular of the unborn, hopefully will support the general belief that ultrasound imaging poses no health risks. And there is active research on biologic effects, especially as US applications move to much higher frequencies.

But still, as with any other clinical procedure, it is prudent to employ US imaging (especially of the unborn) only if there are good medical reasons to do so – the same "justification" principle that underlies radiation safety.

CHAPTER 11

MRI in One Dimension and with No Relaxation

A Gentle Introduction to a Challenging Subject

Medical Imaging: Essentials for Physicians, First Edition. Anthony B. Wolbarst, Patrizio Capasso and Andrew R. Wyant.
© 2013 John Wiley & Sons, Inc. Published 2013 by John Wiley & Sons, Inc.

Prologue to MRI

MRI is surely the most celebrated of the newer imaging modalities. It can display high-quality slice and 3D images of the anatomy and physiology of tissues, organs, and vessels with in-plane resolution of under 1 mm, and comparable plane thicknesses. It provides contrast among radiologically similar soft tissues that is positively brilliant (Figure 11.1). And it does all of this with no exposure of patient or staff to ionizing radiation.

MRI is extraordinarily flexible, moreover, in the ways that it can generate contrast. X-ray imaging including CT is sensitive to differences in photon attenuation – as brought about by differences in tissue thickness, density, and/or atomic number – but not at all to their actual chemical or biological makeup or behavior (Box 2.1). Nuclear medicine is also a one-trick pony, indicating where the body tends to concentrate a particular pharmaceutical agent. Likewise, ultrasound locates boundaries between tissues that differ in either of two parameters, density and elasticity, or, alternatively, Doppler is sensitive to blood flow.

But MRI can create contrast in a number of radically different and unique ways, and these can provide novel kinds of information on tissue anatomy and physiology that CT and the other modalities are completely oblivious to (Figure 11.2). Imaging of proton density (PD), and of the tissue *proton spin relaxation times* known as T1 and T2, all reveal tissue anatomy and pathologies, but do so in ways so dissimilar that each is superior in only certain clinical situations; T1 and T2 are determined largely by the rotations and other motions of the water molecules involved, as modulated by their local biophysical environments within and between the cells of a voxel – and that, in turn, depends on the type of tissue and its state of health. Three more applications are MR angiography (MRA), which rivals CTA but often requires no contrast medium; diffusion tensor imaging (DTI), which indicates the diffusion of free water along the trunks of axons, and thereby brings them into view; and by distinguishing oxygenated blood from de-oxygenated, functional MRI (*f*MRI) lights up the parts of the brain that are responding to a stimulus, somewhat like PET. And there are others as well. Finally, MRI carries out all its good deeds with no ionizing radiation risk to the patient or staff – there are no X-rays and, unlike nuclear medicine, conventional MRI involves only stable, non-radioactive nuclei.

MRI may be summarized as the art and science of creating *spatial maps of the electromagnetic environments around the hydrogen nuclei of water and lipids in tissues*. Distinctions in these electromagnetic environments can be related clinically to differences in biophysical, biochemical, and

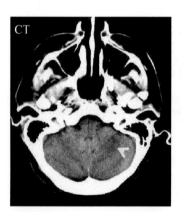
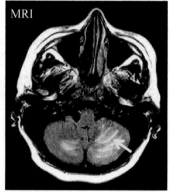

Figure 11.1 Two transverse slices of the same patient at the level of the posterior fossa, displaying the cerebellar hemispheres. The patient suffers from posterior reversible encephalopathy syndrome (PRES), which presents with edematous changes of the white matter. (**a**) Unenhanced CT axial reconstruction. The slight linear artifacts that cross the cerebellum in an arc configuration are associated with the overlying calvarium. There is a slight, ill-defined hypodensity in the white matter of the left cerebellar hemisphere (arrowhead). Recall that you are looking upward from the feet. (**b**) Unenhanced MRI FLAIR sequence axial reconstruction at the same level. Readily apparent is the hyperintensity of the cerebellar white matter representing the edema, which diffusely involves the left hemisphere (arrow), but also extends to the right side.

physiological properties and conditions of the tissues (e.g., edema, hemorrhage). Most commonly, the maps display contrast that originates from variations in tissue T1 and T2. In case the meaning of all this is not altogether clear, read on!

We begin by exploring the *nuclear magnetic resonance* (NMR) phenomenon, which underlies MRI. NMR can be introduced in either of two ways.

In the first, you can think (loosely) that a proton acts, in some ways, like a spinning charged ball, with an axis of rotation and its own minute magnetic field, like a tiny compass needle. But unlike a compass needle, the *spin axis* of a proton can

align, in the strong magnetic field of an MRI device, only "up" along or "down" against the direction of that field. This is a highly simplified version of the full *quantum mechanical* approach, but it leads to useful pictures of the NMR process occurring in a voxel. Like much of the quantum world of atoms, this may not make much sense, but it is nonetheless true. From here, it is but a short hop, skip, and jump to determining the spatial distribution of *proton density* within a one-dimensional patient, and from that, the creation of a 1D PD MR image. This will be a completely real, 100% genuine MR image that displays a physiologically essential

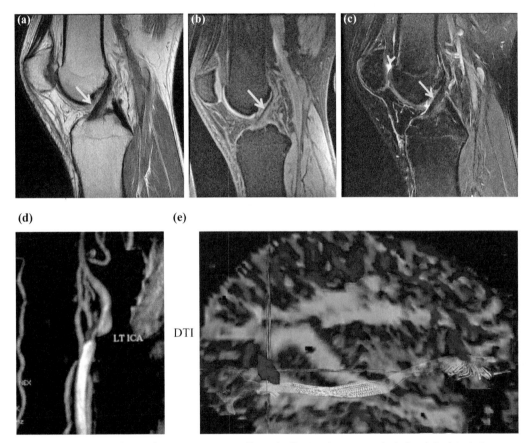

Figure 11.2 Six different forms of MRI contrast, created by and reflecting six separate physical and physiological processes, and obtained with six different sequences of RF and gradient pulses. Sagittal reconstructions of a normal left knee in (a) proton density (PD), (b) gradient-echo, and (c) T2-weighted spin-echo with saturation of fat sequences. The anterior cruciate ligament can be visualized in all sequences (arrows), as can the normal presence of a small amount of fluid within the articular space (arrowhead) in the T2-weighted spin echo image, within the suprapatellar space. (d) This gadolinium-enhanced 3D fast gradient-echo magnetic resonance angiography (MRA) study reveals a stenosis of the left interior carotid artery. (e) Diffusion tensor image (DTI) indicates the close proximity of the optic radiation to a glioma (Figure 0.6). (f) This functional MRI (fMRI) image highlights regions of the brain that respond to a flashing light.

(f)   *f* MRI

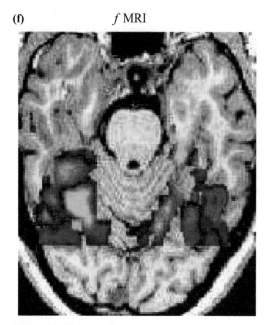

Figure 11.2 *(Continued)*

attribute – the water and/or lipid density – along the length of the patient.

The second approach to NMR and MRI, the *classical* model, focuses on the net magnetic field coming from a bunch of protons together, their *net nuclear magnetization*. Quite remarkably, the net magnetization acts in a strong magnetic field much like a gyroscope in a gravitational field. This tack is better for explaining the ubiquitous *spin-echo* and *gradient-echo* sequences of radiofrequency (RF) pulses and gradient magnetic fields that give rise to clinical MRI images.

Chapter 12 investigates the critically important issue of the two major forms of *proton-spin* relaxation, characterized by the relaxation times T1 and T2, that cause a voxel's net nuclear magnetization, $M(t)$, to decay away over time, t. We are then in a position to create clinical MR images that display the spatial variation in the values of T1 or T2 within the patient; such maps readily distinguish among separate organs, and between healthy and diseased part of the same tissue. The discussion then extends everything into two and three dimensions, and concludes with brief sketches of MRA and the remarkable techniques of DTI and *f*MRI.

You are doubtless most familiar with MRI systems with superconducting donut magnets that generate the principal field pointing along a horizontal line (Figure 11.3). Those with open magnets, on the other hand, align the principal magnetic field *vertically*, along the conventional *z*-axis; it simplifies a number of explanations to adopt the open geometry, and in this chapter and most of the next, so *the principal magnetic field, B_0, and the z-axis* will point upward, ↑.

You will recall that because a magnetic field has both magnitude and direction, it is termed a *vector* quantity; the temperature at any point in the MRI suite, by comparison, has only magnitude, and is a *scalar*.

"Quantum" approach to proton nuclear magnetic resonance

To begin, consider the up-down spin-state quantum picture of NMR. Virtually all of the relevant science was covered at the beginning of Chapter 2. Still, a brief recap of the few most salient points, plus a little good new stuff, may be helpful.

The magnetic dipole moment of a nucleus, and the two spin-orientation states of a proton in a magnetic field, *B*

A basic, defining characteristic of any magnet is that (unlike an electric charge) it always manifests with *two* "opposite" poles, and is thus a *magnetic dipole*. A compass needle is just a little magnetized bar of steel suspended at a pivot point; by convention, the "north" pole of the needle tends to point toward the Earth's *geographical* north – which is where Earth's south (!) *magnetic* pole currently resides (Figure 11.4). (Every million years or so, it flips over, and it seems that another such transition is due in perhaps 50 000 years.)

In an external magnetic field already in existence, such as *B* oriented along the positive *z*-axis in the figure, a magnetic dipole will experience a *torque*, or twisting force, trying to align it along that field. The needle would like to settle down into the orientation of lowest energy, such that its own north pole points up, toward the south pole of the external magnet. That, of course, is what enables a compass to guide your path.

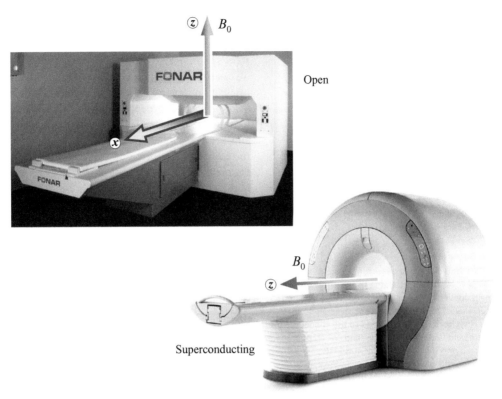

Figure 11.3 The two geometries of MRI magnets. (a) For an "open" permanent magnet or electromagnet, the principal magnetic field, B_0, is directed upward, along the $+z$-axis, and the patient table lies along the $+x$-direction. Much of the discussion in this chapter and the next will assume this configuration and coordinate system. Courtesy of the FONAR Corporation. (b) The field of a typical superconducting magnet, by contrast, is horizontal; the z-axis is, as well.

Any magnetic dipole produces its own dipole magnetic field, the lines of which, by convention, flow from its north magnetic pole to its south, also seen in Figure 11.4. It has been known for two centuries that the movement of electrically charged particles, such as an electric current in wire, gives rise to magnetic fields – indeed, that's how huge electromagnets can lift cars. It is less apparent, but also true, that nearly all atomic nuclei behave somewhat like spinning (hence moving) balls of positive charge, and generally create tiny dipole magnetic fields. A standard measure of the strength of the magnetic field produced by a dipole – that is, of the dipole's own "magnetness" – is called its *magnetic dipole moment*, and represented as the vector μ, a lower case Greek *mu*.

The only nucleus of general clinical interest in MRI is the simplest of them all, that of an atom of ordinary hydrogen – a lone proton (Figure 2.1a).

Whenever μ appears here, you can safely assume it is that of a proton, unless noted otherwise. There has been some clinical research on a few nuclei other than hydrogen-1, such as phosphorus-31 (energetics of ATP), Na-23 (stroke and cancer), and C-13 (metabolic imaging) (Table 11.1), but we shall not consider them further. It happens that $\mu = 0$ for a few biologically important nuclei, in particular for the common forms of carbon, oxygen, and calcium, which together account for about 85% of body weight. They produce no MRI signals and, indeed, cortical bone and calcifications may be most conspicuous for their absence in an image.

You can force a compass through any angle with your finger, but not so for protons: because they are subject to the sometimes counterintuitive dictates of quantum mechanics, protons in a strong external magnetic field can reside oriented either up along it, or down against it, but nowhere else.

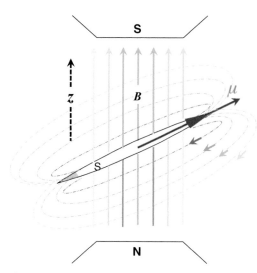

Figure 11.4 You can hold a bar magnet, such as the needle of a compass, at any angle relative to the direction of an externally applied magnetic field, *B*. But when released, the needle tends to swing around and align along that field, since its north pole is attracted to the applied field's south pole, and similarly at its other end. When pointing straight up along the positive *z*-axis, it is in its configuration of lowest potential energy. We are interested primarily in the amount of energy required to twist the needle through 180°, so that it ends up pointing in the "wrong" direction. That energy, ΔE, is proportional both to the magnitude of the external field strength, *B*, and to the magnitude of its own "magnetness," as parameterized by its *magnetic dipole moment*, μ. In the correct units, the energy needed to flip it over through 180° turns out to be simply $\Delta E = 2\mu B$.

To emphasize the point that a proton in an external magnetic field is *spatially quantized*, with its spin-axis and magnetic moment pointing *only* along or against the *z*-axis, we shall replace the symbol

μ with μ_z. The proton, moreover, has the option (totally unlike a compass needle) of remaining for a long period of time in a quasi-stable, higher-energy state, spinning and pointing the "wrong" way. So we can speak of the lower- and higher-energy spin-orientation states of a proton in a strong magnetic field, such as that produced by an MRI device; then its spin axis and its dipole magnetic moment lie anti-parallel or parallel to the external field and the *z*-direction, respectively. (*Caveat*: The upcoming *classical* picture of NMR contradicts everything said in this paragraph. But despair not – we shall explain why.)

From this simplified quantum perspective, the essentials of NMR and MRI are straightforward. Imagine a proton sitting in a strong external magnetic field in its comfortable, low-energy "ground-state" spin-orientation, with its own north pole pointing toward the external magnet's south. The trick is somehow to grab hold of the nucleus and flip or twist it over through 180°. You have to do work on it to flip it over, so it must now be in the higher-energy state. The big question is this: how much energy, ΔE, did you have to impart to it to bring about this change? (Recall that "Δ" is commonly a shorthand notation for "change in ... " or "difference in ... " whatever follows.)

You naturally (and correctly) assume that ΔE should be proportional to the strength of the external field, *B*. Likewise, it increases with the strength of the dipole's own magnetic field, $\Delta E \sim \mu_z$. In fact, with the right units, ΔE turns out to be just two times the product of these two (Figure 11.5a):

$$\Delta E = 2\mu_z B, \qquad (11.1)$$

Table 11.1 Nuclei of interest in clinical and/or research MRI. Nuclei with even numbers of protons and of neutrons, such as C-12, O-16, and Ca-40, have neither net spin nor nuclear dipole moment, and they play no active role in MRI.

Nucleus	Spin	MHz/T	Natural abundance (%)	Relative sensitivity
H-1	$\frac{1}{2}$	42.58	99.98	1
C-13	$\frac{1}{2}$	10.71	1.11	0.02
F-19	$\frac{1}{2}$	40.06	100	0.83
Na-23	$\frac{3}{2}$	11.26	100	0.09
P-31	$\frac{1}{2}$	17.24	100	0.07
C-12	0	–	–	–
O-16	0	–	–	–
Ca-40	0	–	–	–

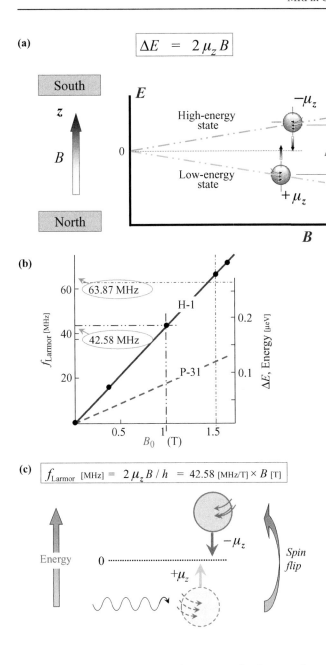

(a)

$$\Delta E = 2\mu_z B$$

South

(b)

(c)

$$f_{\text{Larmor}} \text{ [MHz]} = 2\mu_z B / h = 42.58 \text{ [MHz/T]} \times B \text{ [T]}$$

Figure 11.5 In some respects, an atomic nucleus, such as a single proton, behaves like a tiny compass needle. **(a)** It aligns in an externally magnetic field, B, but *only* along or against it and the z-axis. The strength of the weak field the proton itself produces, is its *nuclear magnetic dipole moment*, μ_z. (Every nucleus has its own value for the magnetic moment.) Unlike a compass needle, however, a proton can remain for long periods of time in a quasi-stable, higher-energy spin-orientation state, pointing the "wrong" way. The two spin states differ in energy by $\Delta E = 2\mu_z B$. The middle, horizontal, thin, solid line corresponds to the orientational energy the nucleus would have if $B = 0$. **(b)** The proton nuclear magnetic resonance (NMR) transition energy (in micro-electron volts; right-hand edge of the graph) is plotted against B (tesla) as the solid line for normal hydrogen nuclei. For a proton, the corresponding photon frequency (MHz), called its *Larmor frequency* (left-hand side), is proportional to the field strength, $f_{\text{Larmor}} = 42.58\ B$. The Larmor frequency of a free proton in a 1-T field is 42.58 MHz, 63.87 MHz at 1.5 T, and 127.7 MHz at 3 T. The second, dashed line describes the phosphorus-31 nucleus, whose nuclear magnetic moment is about $2\frac{1}{2}$ times smaller than that of the proton, and which is of some research interest in MRI. **(c)** The proton NMR phenomenon involves inducing transitions between its two spin states. Flipping it over, or twisting it through 180°, requires the transfer of the amount $\Delta E = 2\mu_z B$ of energy. The absorption of a photon of exactly that energy, $hf = \Delta E = 2\mu_z B$, can bring about such a transition.

Simple though it may seem, this is one of only a few expressions that are needed to understand clinical MRI! Apart from relaxation effects, this describes all the interesting physical science of MRI, and much of what follows involves deciding what values of B to use in it, and for how long. We'll return to this in a more useful equivalent form, known as the *Larmor equation*, in a minute – but this is, as they say, where the rubber hits the road.

The straight-line dependence of ΔE on B for protons in an adjustable magnetic field appears in Figure 11.5b, with the energy scale lying along the right-hand axis of the graph. ΔE is typically in the 0.01–0.6 micro-eV (millionth of an electron volt) range – a dozen orders of magnitude (a factor a trillion) less than the energies typically involved in X- and gamma-ray interactions! Also displayed is the corresponding dashed curve for the phosphorus-31 nucleus, the magnetic moment of which is about 40% of that of a proton.

The proton NMR resonance frequency, f_{Larmor}, is proportional to *B*

We can take this idea a huge jump forward by recalling that electromagnetic radiation displays a wave-particle dual personality. The wave and particle characteristics of an entity (whether most apparent as wave-like or particle-like) are related through $E = hf$ (Equation 2.1b and Figure 2.4). *E* stands for the energy of a (particle-like) photon, *f* is its (wave-like) frequency, and *h* is Planck's constant. This expression says that the higher the frequency of a wave of electromagnetic radiation, the greater the energy carried by each of the individual photons that comprise it.

We have talked about flipping over protons in a magnetic field, but have not explained how actually to cause these transitions. The principal mechanism for elevating a proton from the lower- to the higher-energy spin state is through its absorption of a photon of *exactly* the right energy, and frequency, indicated by the squiggle in Figure 11.5c. We can find the unique condition under which this can take place by bringing together the two fundamental ideas just discussed.

In an external magnetic field of strength *B*, the energy required to flip over a proton is $\Delta E = 2\mu_z B$. But the energy conveyed by a photon of frequency *f* is $E = hf$. Photons of energy $2\mu_z B$ are needed, and those of the *Larmor frequency* can provide it, where $hf_{Larmor} = 2\mu_z B$, or

$$f_{Larmor} = 2\mu_z B / h. \qquad (11.2a)$$

This *Larmor equation* is the basis for NMR, hence for MRI. For protons, and in the right units,

$$f_{Larmor [MHz]} = 42.58 \, [MHz/T] \times B_{[T]}. \qquad (11.2b)$$

This linear relationship between the Larmor frequency for a proton and the strength of the external magnetic field is illustrated in Figure 11.5b, again, but this time, refer to the left-hand side of the graph.

The field strength in the center of the bore of the great majority of superconducting MRI magnets is 1.5 T. The field in the vicinity of the scanner but outside the bore (the *fringe field*) is much weaker, and it is quantified in terms of a unit, the *gauss* (G), which is 10^4 times smaller: 10 000 G = 1 T.

Earth's magnetic field strength, for example, varies from place to place, but is generally on the order of 0.5 G (or 0.00005 T). Access to regions above 5 G (0.5 mT) near an MRI machine must be denied to *all* (nurses, transport personnel) except those few people known to be safe there (i.e., patients and certain family members who have been screened, and MRI-trained technologists).

The Larmor frequency for protons in a 1.0 T field is 42.58 MHz. In a 1.5 T field, it is just under 63.87 MHz. In a 3.0 T field, it is 127.7 MHz. Your National Public Radio station, by comparison, operates somewhere in the 88–108 MHz slot allotted to FM broadcasting.

A preliminary demonstration of the NMR phenomenon

This has all been a bit abstract so far – but what do you actually detect in an NMR (or MRI) study, and how do you carry out the measurements and interpret the results?

Let us design and perform (on paper, at least) the world's simplest NMR experiment (Figure 11.6a). Since the water within tissues is the molecule of major clinical interest in MRI, we shall perform our NMR experiment on a sample of water.

We begin with a standard radio transmitter that beams radiofrequency energy of a narrow band of low frequencies (like 10.00 ± 0.05 MHz, which has a *bandwidth* of 0.1 MHz = 100 kHz) into an antenna. We arrange things so that this antenna transmits a beam of RF photons, of all frequencies from 9.95 to 10.05 MHz, into an empty plastic tank. On the far side of the tank is a receiver antenna, which is attached to a power meter, and the power meter reading is noted.

Next, let's fill the tank with water. Pure water is practically transparent to 10 MHz electromagnetic energy, just as it is to visible light, so the amount of RF power reaching the meter does not change appreciably.

Then an electromagnet is turned on, and adjusted so that its magnetic field within the water sample is uniform and fixed exactly at 1 T in strength. Again, nothing interesting.

So now we slowly but steadily increase the frequency of the transmitted RF radiation, a step of 100 kHz at a time, holding the *transmitted* power level constant, and plot the *detected* power as a

Figure 11.6 A very rudimentary NMR experiment on a sample of water sitting in a uniform magnetic field that is pointing upward (as with an "open" magnet) along the z-axis, and held fixed at exactly $B_0 = 1$ tesla throughout the measurement. Radiofrequency (RF) power is absorbed precisely at, and only at, the proton Larmor frequency. **(a)** The equipment consists of a transmitter whose frequency can be slowly and continuously increased, and a receiver that leads to a power meter. **(b)** The level of detected RF power remains the same until the Larmor resonant frequency is reached (42.58 MHz for $B_0 = 1$ T), where the water absorbs power, so that less energy reaches the detector. Immediately above the Larmor frequency, the meter returns to its previous reading. For higher fixed settings of B_0, resonance occurs at correspondingly higher frequencies, in accord with the Larmor equation and Figure 11.5b.

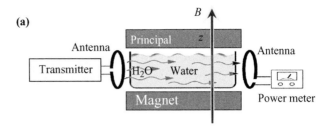

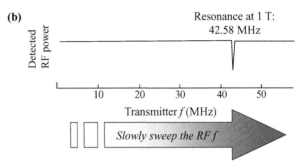

function of this frequency. The reading on the RF power meter remains unchanged up to 42.60 ± 0.05 MHz, at which point it dips sharply (Figure 11.6b). Here, and only here, some Larmor-frequency photons are being absorbed in the process of exciting some water protons into the higher-energy state – NMR occurs! – so less energy reaches the detector antenna. This is the indication we need that NMR is actually taking place, and precisely at the frequency predicted by the Larmor equation. Then, as the transmitter frequency continues to increase slowly, through and beyond the resonance condition, the detected power returns to its previous flat level. It's like being stuck in a blizzard high in North Dakota and slowly scanning up the frequency dial of your radio until suddenly, you hit a great rap station. Nothing very exciting happens until the conditions are just right, but then the signal is exactly what you wanted. (*Caveat*: When we shift to the classical picture of NMR and MRI, resonance will *not* be detected by power absorption, but rather in quite different a way.)

We name the relative magnitude of the dip in detected power the MRI *signal strength*. And for consistency with what follows, we call the dip a (negative, here) *peak*.

What we have just gone through is a simple example of a *spectral analysis*. We pump energy into the physical system over a range of frequencies, and

from the response determine how much power is absorbed (or emitted, or transmitted, etc.) at any particular frequency. Spectral analysis, sometimes called *Fourier analysis* in honor of its nineteenth-century French inventor, is a powerful mathematical tool widely used throughout the sciences, and we shall return to it soon. You saw it earlier in connection with the modulation transfer function (MTF) in Chapter 4. It's mathematically a bit complex in practice, and there is no need to explain the details of how it works, or how to carry it out – but the meaning of the resulting Fourier spectra is straightforward, and it can provide invaluable information in MRI.

If the whole experiment is repeated but with several different fixed settings of the magnetic field, this same NMR phenomenon recurs, in each case at the Larmor frequency corresponding to the current value of the field strength, as shown earlier as the distinct data points in Figure 11.5b. We have just experimentally demonstrated NMR, the main phenomenon upon which MRI is built! Hereafter, the discussion involves just filling in some interesting details.

We close this discussion of the Larmor equation by noting that it sometimes appears in an equivalent, albeit less transparent, form:

$$\omega = \gamma B. \qquad (11.2c)$$

ω is the so-called *angular frequency*, measured in radians/second. γ is the *gyromagnetic ratio*, and for protons, $\gamma = 2\pi \times 42.58$. B is still in tesla. We shall generally stick with the $f_{\text{Larmor}} = 2\mu_z B/h$ format.

Magnetic resonance imaging in one dimension

The above experiment suggests an easy way to map out water PD, the number of water hydrogen nuclei per cubic centimeter of tissue, within a body – at least a one-dimensional one. But first, this brings us to the topic of the three distinct kinds of *externally applied* magnetic fields involved in MRI.

The three distinct kinds of applied magnetic field in MRI: B_0, G_x, and B_{RF}

At any instant, the *local* field, B, felt by a proton will be comprised of one or more of three kinds of *externally applied*, superimposed components, plus fields *originating within the body itself*. It will be important to keep precise track of each of these contributions to the overall magnetic environment of the proton.

The x-, y-, z-coordinate system chosen depends on the orientation of the main magnetic field. So far, the principal field, B_0, has been aligned upward along a vertical z-axis, as is normally the case for "open" permanent and electromagnets, and we shall continue with that convention here (Figure 11.3). So imagine a patient resting on the table for a study of her leg, which lies horizontally along the x-direction. We can pretty much forget about the y-axis for now.

The three general kinds of magnetic fields will be distinguished with subscripts (Figure 11.7). The *externally applied principal field*, B_0, is very strong and *highly uniform*, or *homogeneous*, throughout the volume of the patient's body being imaged, and *constant* over time; it should never change. It is produced by the huge and very expensive principal magnet that envelops the patient.

The *gradient magnetic fields* are also always aligned entirely *along B_0*, and therefore also along the z-axis, which here is pointing upward. They are much weaker than B_0, however, and they are intentionally made to be *non*-uniform in a very predictable, controlled way; indeed, they are designed to vary regularly in *strength*, but not in *orientation*,

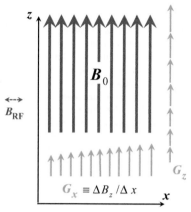

Figure 11.7 The strong (e.g., 1.5 T or 3 T), constant, and highly uniform *principal* magnetic field, B_0, is represented by the heavy, long blue vertical arrows. The *x*-gradient, G_x, in green, is produced by the separate *x*-gradient coil, and $G_x \equiv \Delta B_z/\Delta x$ represents the change in the local *z-field*, ΔB_z, that occurs when you move transversely the slight distance, Δx, in the *x*-direction; so also for G_y, not shown. Likewise, $G_z \equiv \Delta B_z/\Delta z$. For all three gradients, the field (ΔB_z) and Δz lie along the *z*-axis, parallel to B_0; that is, while the strength of each gradient field depends on position within the magnet, all involve increments in the strengths of fields aligned only along the *z*-axis. The magnetic component of the much weaker *RF* field, in red, is at or near the Larmor frequency, B_{RF}, and aligned *perpendicular* to B_0.

from place to place. For one-dimensional imaging, where the patient's leg is aligned along the *x*-axis, we write the local *x*-gradient field as $G_x \times x$. $G_x \equiv \Delta B_z/\Delta x$ reveals how much the *z*-component of the overall local field changes, ΔB_z, with a small shift, Δx, in the *x*-direction (i.e., perpendicular to B_0 and to ΔB_z). In the absence of *y*- or *z*-gradients, the local field a distance x from the center of the magnet will be $B_z(x) = B_0 + G_x \times x$. We shall later have occasion to talk about the temporarily static *z*-field at a voxel at the instant that a field gradient is being briefly (milliseconds) applied. This is just the vector sum of two entities that happen always to be pointing in the same direction, B_0 and $G_x x$, and their magnitudes simply add: $B_z(x) = B_0 + G_x x$.

Most of the time, the gradients are off; they are turned on intermittently and for a few milliseconds at a time during a real MRI study, and it is the rapid mechanical jolting of machine parts induced by the switching of these gradient fields that one hears as muffled booming.

Finally, B_{RF} is the magnetic component of a relatively weak radiofrequency field, oscillating tens of millions of times a second, at or very near the Larmor frequency. It will be turned on for short (tens or hundreds of microseconds), precisely timed periods. Produced by coil-like antennae close to the patient, it always points *perpendicular* to the alignments of B_0 and of the gradient fields. It is this RF field, made up of Larmor-frequency photons, that cause protons in tissues to undergo spin flips.

MRI is performed with the principal external field, B_0, fixed commonly at 1.5 T. For the examples that follow, however, we shall usually take B_0 to be 1.0 T, for calculational convenience, with a corresponding f_{Larmor} of 42.58 MHz; with other field strengths, in particular 1.5 T or 3.0 T, it is easy to scale things up or down with a factor of $(B_0 \text{ T})/(1 \text{ T})$.

The three kinds of magnetic fields discussed so far are all produced by an MRI machine. The other half of the MRI story, the part that deals with relaxation times T1 and T2 and related matters, involves the magnetic fields produced and sensed by protons themselves in various molecular environments in water and lipids, and by the flows of electrons within those molecules. More about that later.

Encoding of voxel *x*-position with NMR frequency, and proton density MRI of a one-dimensional patient

While MRI can display planes of tissues at any angle, suppose an orthopedic surgeon is particularly interested in transverse-slice images along a 20-cm long *field of view* (FOV) around the knee. A knee is anatomically pretty complicated, so we'll simplify matters by considering a 20-cm cylindrical plastic pseudo-leg "phantom," extending horizontally along the x-axis, instead (Figure 11.8a). The phantom consists of a number of thin-walled, pancake-shaped chambers; in this simple example, all but two of them are empty. One non-empty compartment, located at the center, is filled with pure water. The second, 5 cm to the right, contains a half-and-half mixture of water and inert filler, like Styrofoam, so that the average proton density is half that of water.

Our objective will be to determine experimentally the water content of this quasi-one-dimensional patient as a function of x-position along it. The resulting map of variations in its proton density will be a real MRI image! The process is based on *frequency encoding* of voxel position along the x-axis, in this case, with an x-gradient field on. The approach here, once again, is to sweep the RF field slowly, and keep track of the frequencies and signal amplitudes of any resonance peaks that may appear.

If the principal magnetic field were uniform at 1 T from $x = +10$ cm, above the knee, to $x = -10$ cm, below, then the water molecules in both compartments would experience the same local fields, and all would undergo resonance together at 42.58 MHz, the same value as found in Figure 11.6. Not very exciting.

But by canting the magnet pole faces a little, we can superimpose an *x-gradient* magnetic field on the principal field,

$$G_x \equiv \Delta B_z / \Delta x. \quad (11.3a)$$

(More realistically, the gradient field would come from carefully crafted electrical coils.) In the figure, B_0 is adjusted so that the total local field strength is exactly 1.0 T at the center, where $x = 0$. The added gradient field also points vertically everywhere (except in its *fringes* near the two ends), along the direction of B_0, but its *strength* now increases from left to right. Suppose that the local field strength, $B_z(x)$, runs from 0.998 T at the left side of the FOV, $x = -10$ cm, to 1.002 T at the other, $x = 10$ cm; the x-gradient is thus $G_x \equiv \Delta B_z / \Delta x = (0.004 \text{ T}/20 \text{ cm}) = 20$ mT/m, a reasonable value in practice.

At position x along the phantom, the strength of the local field there, created by combining the principal field and the gradient field is $B_z(x) = B_0 + G_x x$. Equivalently, but more usefully,

$$x = [B_z(x) - B_0] / G_x. \quad (11.3b)$$

In our example, this becomes: $x_{[meters]} = [B_z(x) - 1.0]/20$ $_{[mT/m]}$, and at the two water samples, the local fields are $B(x = 0) = 1.000$ T and $B(+5 \text{ cm}) = 1.001$ T, respectively. Conversely, by determining the local field strength at a chamber, which the instrument happens to find easy to do, this relationship leads directly its location. So how do we go about determining $B_z(x)$?

The key is the Larmor equation itself, modified slightly to account for x-position in the gradient field: measuring $f_{Larmor}(x) = 42.58 \ (B_0 + G_x x)$

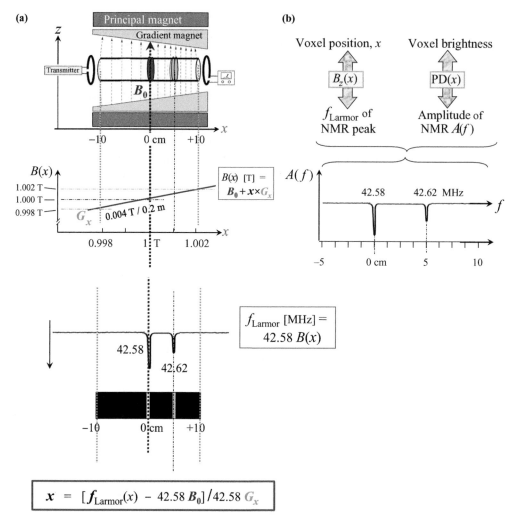

(a)

Principal magnet

Gradient magnet

Transmitter

B_0

z

x

−10   0 cm   +10

$B(x)$

1.002 T
1.000 T
0.998 T

G_x 0.004 T / 0.2 m

$B(x)$ [T] =
$B_0 + x \times G_x$

0.998   1 T   1.002

42.58

42.62

−10   0 cm   +10

f_{Larmor} [MHz] =
42.58 $B(x)$

(b)

Voxel position, x Voxel brightness

$B_z(x)$ PD(x)

f_{Larmor} of   Amplitude of
NMR peak   NMR $A(f)$

$A(f)$

42.58   42.62 MHz

f

−5   0 cm   5   10

$$x = [f_{\text{Larmor}}(x) - 42.58\, B_0]/42.58\, G_x$$

Figure 11.8 MRI in a one-dimensional patient in a *non-uniform* external field, everywhere pointing only upward along the z-axis. The patient, lying along the x-axis, is represented as a 20 cm-long cylinder that is hollow except for a thin, disk-shaped compartment in its middle filled with water, and another one 5 cm toward its upper end that conta a 50%–50% mixture of water and Styrofoam powder, somewhat like lung. **(a)** Here the magnet pole faces have been canted, superimposing a weak field gradient, G_x, on the strong uniform principal field, B_0. The composite magnetic field still points only upward, in the z-direction, but its strength increases with the x-coordinate. By our design, the field is weaker (1.000 T) at the central compartment, than at the one at $x = 5$ cm, where $B(x) = 1.001$ T. The system slowly sweeps the RF frequency through the range of anticipated resonances, and notes the frequency, f_{Larmor}, and amplitude, A(f), of any detected NMR peak. One NMR signal appears at 42.58 MHz, and another, half as tall, at 42.62 MHz. The frequency of a peak (which can be measured accurately) indicates, through the Larmor equation, the local magnetic field strength, $B_z(x)$ at any water chamber. But the field strength increases in a controlled and known (linear) manner along the length of the phantom. This rigid linkage between position, x, and local field strength, $B_z(x)$, is established through the precisely adjusted, constant linear x-gradient, $G_x = \Delta B_z/\Delta x$, and it provides the key as to where each chamber is located. **(b)** There is a direct link from NMR signal frequency, through local field strength, to position in the phantom. Also, the strength of an NMR signal at any frequency, A(f), is proportional to the proton density at the corresponding point in the phantom. One can thus relate proton density (from the NMR signal amplitude) to position along the body (from the NMR signal frequency), and thereby compute a map of water proton density throughout the phantom, PD(x); that is, an MRI image of it. The display gray scale is set so that brightness increases with signal strength (and here, with PD.)

precisely yields the local field strength, $(B_0 + G_x x)$. The argument of the preceding paragraph lets us find the location, x, where the resonance is occurring, from measurement of the resonance frequency. Combining these two expressions leads to the grand conclusion:

$$x = [\, f_{\text{Larmor}}(x) - 42.58\ B_0\,]/42.58\ G_x. \quad (11.3c)$$

To locate a slice of water, all we have to do is measure the frequency, $f_{\text{Larmor}}(x)$, of its resonance peak and plug it into Equation 11.3c. QED! As we sweep the RF frequency, the chamber at $x = 0$ will produce a peak at $42.58\ (1.00 + G_x \times 0) = 42.58$ MHz. Similarly, when we measure the resonance frequency of the upper chamber as 42.62 MHz, its location is $x = 0.05$ m, from 42.62 MHz = (42.58 MHz/T) × (1.000 T + [20 mT/m × x m]).

Equation 11.3c is just a modified form of the Larmor equation, but one that also provides an essential one-to-one correspondence that allows us to jump back and forth between voxel *x-position* within the patient and the *frequency* of the associated NMR signal. Since the PD is twice as great at the center as at $x = 5$ cm, the amplitude of the NMR peak at that frequency, $A(f)$, will be, also. By a reasonable convention, the brightness of the voxel at position x in the image is made to increase with the detected signal strength, or amplitude of the peak, $A(f)$, hence with the PD there. There is now enough information to *reconstruct* a map of water content for the phantom – a real, true, honest-to-goodness, genuine MRI image, at the bottom of Figure 11.8a. This is of the same PD MRI form as appeared earlier as Figure 11.2a.

The process is summarized in Figure 11.8b: measuring *NMR signal amplitude*, $A(f)$, as a function of *RF frequency*, allows us to generate a map of the PD as a function of *position* within the phantom. Again, this is, in effect, a spectrum, or a Fourier display, of the signal picked up by the receiver coil.

Three MRI artifacts: non-linear gradient distortion, chemical shift, and motion

MRI is technologically and computationally the most complex and flexible of the major imaging modalities; partly as a result of that, it gives rise to the greatest number and variety of artifacts. These fall into three general but somewhat overlapping categories that involve aspects related to the MRI equipment, to the patient, and to the reconstruction process, respectively. While some of these are readily apparent, others are more dangerous in that they are subtle and can be mistaken for real anatomic or physiological effects. We shall interject some examples of them throughout this chapters and the next as appropriate.

Non-linear gradient-field artifact

One MRI artifact arises from a gradient field whose strength is not perfectly proportional to position – an instrumental effect. Gradient coils are effective in producing fields that normally change linearly with position near the center of the imaging field. Toward their edges, however, it is harder to maintain these gradients, and they tend to distort, giving rise to *gradient-induced distortion artifacts* (Figure 11.9a). Software distortion-correction is usually available to compensate, as in the image to the right, so the problem is normally not evident.

Chemical shift artifact

NMR was developed independently in 1946 by Felix Bloch at Stanford and Edward Purcell at Harvard, and the two shared the 1952 Nobel Prize in Physics for this work. NMR quickly proved to be an invaluable tool for identifying organic chemical compounds and for studying their molecular structures.

The Larmor frequency of a proton in a molecule depends primarily on the field strength from the sum of the external fixed and gradient magnets. But it is exquisitely sensitive to the precise magnitude of the local magnetic field in which it resides, and slight shifts in field strength can arise from the nearby flow of all the molecule's own orbital electrons. The amount of this *chemical shift* in the local proton f_{Larmor} is determined by the details of the local molecular environment, hence of the chemical structure. This is far too small an effect, typically a few parts per million (ppm), to be apparent in normal MR images, but with MR systems of exceptional external field homogeneity and high frequency-resolution, it can be brought out with *magnetic resonance spectroscopy* (*MRS*). MRI technology can be combined with NMR spectroscopy to allow performance of *in vivo* MRS within the body, and we saw a good clinical application of this in Figure 0.4.

(a)

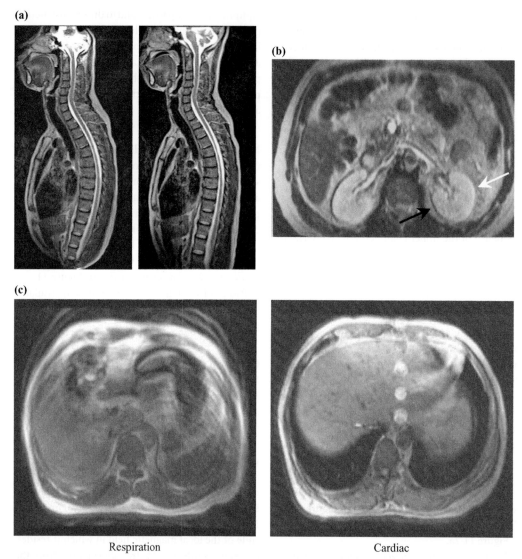

(b)

(c)

Respiration   Cardiac

Figure 11.9 Three of the numerous kinds of artifacts that can afflict MRI. (**a**) The breakdown in *linearity of the gradient field* resulted in geometric distortion of the large-FOV image of the spine, to the left. The problem vanished with application of correctional software, on the right. Courtesy of RP Gullapalli and J Zhuo. (**b**) This chemical shift artifact is apparent as the black band on one side of each kidney, and the bright line on the other; it arises from the 3.5 ppm difference between the resonant frequencies of water and fat which, in a 1.5-tesla magnetic field, translates to 220 Hz. (**c**) Effects of both respiratory and cardiac motions: breathing causes the blurring and ghosting of the thoracic image; breath-holding eliminates nearly all of that, but makes more visible cardiac pulsation effects, such as the multiple copies of the major vessels. Courtesy of J Zhou and RP Gullapalli. See also Zhou J and Gullapalli RP, Artifacts in MRI. In: Wolbarst AB, Karellas K, Krupinski EA, Hendee WR (eds), *Advances in Medical Physics*, vol. 3. Madison, WI: Medical Physics Publishing, 2010. That chapter is an expansion of Zhou J and Gullapalli RP, AAPM/RSNA physics tutorials for residents: MR artifacts, safety, and quality control. *Radiographics* 2006;**26**:275–97.

The local field at a proton can be altered either by an applied gradient magnetic field or by an inherent chemical shift, and sometimes the system confuses the two. Indeed, lipids and water in the same voxel may appear at slightly different spatial locations in an MR image for that reason, giving rise to a *chemical-shift artifact* (Figure 11.9b).

Motion artifact

Two common forms of *physiological motion*, breathing and heartbeat, may smear out an image and, because they are both somewhat periodic, they also give rise to distinct ghosts (Figure 11.9c). Of the ways to deal with the consequences of respiration, the simplest is the gated breath-hold, but this may make the effects of the cardiac cycle all the more apparent. Others that have been developed include cardiac gating, and the application of ultra-fast pulse sequences, any of which may ameliorate the problem.

"Classical" approach to NMR

We introduced NMR in terms of a single proton that acts in a magnetic field somewhat like a compass needle, but with two, and only two (higher- and lower-energy), possible spin states. With this simplified *quantum model*, we explored the imaging of the spatial distribution of proton density in a one-dimensional patient.

A completely different but complementary view of proton behavior, the *classical model*, is based on the observation that a voxel's net magnetization, *M*, produced by a sizeable cohort of the protons in it, behaves in the MRI's principal magnetic field much like an ordinary gyroscope moving about in the Earth's gravitational field. The classical picture proves helpful in discussing some of the more subtle aspects of MRI, including some relaxation phenomena.

MRI involves, in practice, the switching on and off of carefully designed and timed gradient magnetic fields, and the application of multiple, brief pulses of radiofrequency energy, each of which contains a relatively broad band of frequencies, rather than the RF energy of a single, slowly varying frequency that we have been using so far. This underlies the *spin-echo* and *gradient-echo* pulse sequences, the general methods most widely employed clinically.

And all of it can be discussed "classically" without any mention of proton quantum states or spin flips.

The magnetization, *M*, and its magnitude at thermal equilibrium, M_0

The very weak collective magnetic field that a group of hydrogen nuclei together produce per voxel (or per mm^3 or per gram) of material is called their *net nuclear magnetization*, and denoted *M*. Like a magnetic field or nuclear magnetic moment, the magnetization has both magnitude and direction, and is thus a vector. When either its magnitude or its orientation or both are changing over time, *t*, we write it as *M(t)*. Net magnetization will be the central player in the story of MRI from now on. The information provided by MRI comes from, and only from, monitoring the behavior of *M(t)* under different, carefully controlled circumstances.

We will be using *M(t)* almost entirely with the classical picture, but start out by defining it first here, just for the moment, with the quantum, spin-up, spin-down model. Suppose there are *N* protons in each voxel. In an external field of strength *B*, N_- of them happen to be in the lower-energy state, and N_+ in the higher. The total number of protons in a voxel is $(N_- + N_+) = N$, but there is a slight excess in the lower state, of magnitude $(N_- - N_+)$. Each proton contributes an amount μ_z to their composite field, so the net magnetization may be defined, within the spin-up, spin-down model, as

$$M \equiv (N_- - N_+)\mu_z. \qquad (11.4a)$$

Two big questions have surely come to mind: why should that slight excess in the lower energy state exist? And also, after everything has had time to settle down and come to rest, just how great is that difference; and, according to Equation 11.4a, is, how large is the magnetization in a sample of water or tissue when sitting in a strong magnetic field, B_0, but nothing else is going on? This *magnetization at thermal equilibrium* is so important that it has been adorned with its own special symbol: M_0.

Let's begin the discussion of M_0 with an analogy. Suppose a box contains a number of small white copper balls, and the same number of black balls of the same size but made of iron, much denser. When the box is shaken vigorously, the resulting disarray is great (Figure 11.10a). The system is constantly roiling, with balls continually bouncing about and

(a)   **(b)**   **(c)**

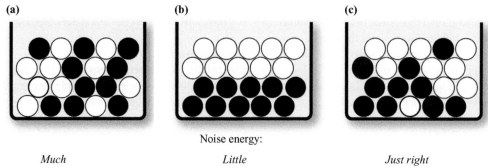

Noise energy:

Much   *Little*   *Just right*

Figure 11.10 An analogy for the battle between energy and entropy, with white and (denser) black balls in a gravitational field. **(a)** When there is much energy input through shaking, then that dominates, and the system becomes fully disordered – *high entropy* – and with the balls continually switching places with one another. **(b)** With very gentle agitation, it can end up in a state of *lowest energy*. **(c)** With some but not too much shaking, the system settles into an intermediary configuration, the nature of which depends on both the level of agitation (read: *temperature*) and the strength of the gravitational (read: *magnetic*) field.

interchanging places and, in chemistry-speak, it is seeking a condition of *maximum entropy*, of greatest disorder. If, on the other hand, the box is tapped very gently for a long while, the heavier black balls all slowly settle into the bottom rows, a state of gravitational *minimal energy* (Figure 11.10b). In between, when the disruptive forces nearly overwhelm gravity, but not completely, the result of this *battle between entropy and energy* is that there is a small excess of black balls lower down (Figure 11.10c). (Do you think the average numbers in the various rows would be the same with identical amounts of shaking if you carried out this exercise on the Moon, where gravity is only a sixth as strong?)

A similar argument describes protons in an externally applied magnetic field. If the field is initially off (i.e., $B = 0$ at $t = 0$), then the spins of the hydrogen nuclei in a glass of water or in a piece of tissue are aligned randomly in all directions (Figure 11.11a). The magnetic moments of the individual protons, each of magnitude μ, point every which way, and if you add together all their own (very small) magnetic fields, they sum to zero, and their net magnetization will also be zero, $M(t = 0) = 0$.

Place the water between the poles of a very weak, vertically aligned electromagnet, and snap the field on rapidly at $t = 0$ (Figure 11.11b). Each proton, which is subject to the sometimes counterintuitive dictates of quantum mechanics, immediately twists into alignment either along or against the external field – but with no other orientations possible. During that initial brief moment of mass confusion, at time $t = 0+$, it happens for quantum mechanical reasons that almost exactly equal numbers of them end up in the lower- and higher-energy states. We have no idea what any individual spin will do, however, so this is also a configuration of great disorder and high entropy – like black and white balls all mixed up randomly Although the situation is totally different from that before the magnet was switched on, their net magnetization will again be zero: $N_+ = N_-$, and $M(t = 0+) = 0$. With ordinary compasses, all the needles would swing rapidly into the same, lowest-energy orientation – but then again, quantum mechanics doesn't place much stock in common sense, and protons behave differently.

Now turn the magnetic field way up, so that it becomes extremely strong, far above 3 T, say. A condition of nearly complete order would arise, in which virtually all the spins drop into their lower-energy orientation, and the system into an overall state of lowest energy (Figure 11.11c). With all N protons aligned parallel to one another in the voxel, and each contributing its own magnetic field μ_z to the effort, the net magnetization will be of magnitude $M = N\mu_z$.

Finally, at body temperature and in a standard-strength MRI field, the case we're really interested in, the population of protons will settle eventually into a communal state in which *almost* (but not exactly, and that's critically important!) the same numbers of protons point up and down (Figure 11.11d). There is, in fact a slight excess of

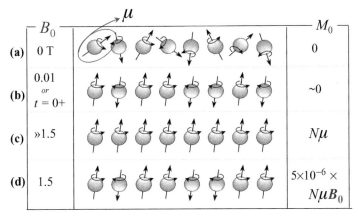

Figure 11.11 The proton spins in a voxel of water. **(a)** With no magnetic field present, the spins align every which way and the net magnetization, **M**, is zero. **(b)** Immediately after a major disruption such as that caused by abruptly turning on a strong external field, B_0, for an instant there will be equal numbers of protons aligned up and down, for reasons that can be explained with quantum mechanics. The net magnetization is zero here again, $(N_- - N_+) = 0$ briefly at $t = 0+$, but now for a very different reason. **(c)** With a high magnetic field and low temperature, on the other hand, nearly all spins do end up aligning in the orientation of lowest energy, so $(N_- - N_+) = N$, and M will be about $N \times \mu_z$. **(d)** At body temperature and clinical field strengths, the effects of thermal jostling are important again, and the outcome of this balancing act is a slight excess of protons in the lower-energy state, so that $M = (N_- - N_+) \times \mu_z$.

them in the lower-energy state. This is an especially important situation, and we shall loosely call it the condition of *thermal equilibrium*. Thermal jostling may induce individual spins to incessantly flip up and down, to some extent, but once equilibrium is achieved, as many go one way as the other. The overall balance remains quite stable, so the equilibrium magnetization does *not* have to be written as a function of time, and it is commonly designated M_0. Perhaps a better symbol would be M_∞, which suggests a very long time after any disturbance has occurred and the system has settled back down, but by convention, M_0 it is!

In short, as a result of the struggle between energy and entropy in a voxel of water or tissue, slightly more than half the protons find themselves in the lower-energy spin state at thermal equilibrium in a magnetic field suitable for imaging, with a small but definite excess of protons pointing upward, as in Figure 11.11d. This results in a net equilibrium magnetization at temperature T of magnitude

$$M_0 = \xi\, N\mu_z^2 B_0 / T, \qquad (11.4b)$$

with ξ a constant to get the units right. This follows directly from the well-known *Boltzmann equation* of chemistry and physics. No need to derive it here.

Now, many substances, when placed in an external magnetic field, will themselves create an additional field that adds to or decreases the local field within and immediately around them. That is, if such a material experiences the applied field B_0, then the strength of the field within a tiny cavity inside it, say, will be a factor of χ greater, where the lower case Greek chi symbolizes its *susceptibility*:

$$M_0 = \chi\, B_0. \qquad (11.4c)$$

For most tissues, protons rule, and chi was just seen in the previous equation to be proportional to the proton density, N; indeed, proton density MRI involves nothing more than mapping spatial variations in χ throughout the field of view. Even when mapping T1 and T2 (rather than PD), abrupt or large changes in χ may be apparent and even, in one application, be the basis for *susceptibility MRI*.

In a 1.5-tesla magnetic field and at body temperature, the relative excess of proton spins pointing north is about 5 parts per million (ppm). That may not seem to be much, until we recall that there are 70 billion billion (7×10^{19}) protons in a cubic millimeter of water. In a single voxel, there will be an excess of something like a million billion of them in the lower-energy state. This parts per million (ppm) margin may be slender, but it does give rise to a measurable communal magnetic field – the net magnetization of the water protons in the voxel – that is ultimately responsible for any MRI signal coming from it. The magnitude of the net magnetization under conditions of thermal equilibrium (i.e., M_0) is, quite simply, the ultimate determinant of the maximum possible strength of the NMR signal that gives rise to *any* kind of MR image.

As we shall see, there is a fundamental tradeoff for MRI among voxel size (and resolution), signal to noise ratio, and slice acquisition time. Raising the principal field strength increases M_0, which in turn results in a better overall balance for these three. Going from 1.5 T to 3 T, say, will double the excess number of spins in the lower energy level, and give a signal twice as great. One can adjust SNR and voxel size, for example, to create a much more revealing image (Figure 11.12a). The principal downside to more powerful magnets is the greater cost.

There is an interesting artifact sometimes encountered at 3 T. The corresponding wavelength of this RF field is of the order of about 1.2 meter, which is comparable to the dimensions of the regions of the body being imaged. This makes it possible for standing RF waves to arrive uninvited, and the subsequent wave interference effects, or *RF standing-wave MRI artifacts*, may result in false patterns of brightness and darkness, as with the breasts of Figure 11.12b. The problem does not arise at 1.5 T, where the RF wavelength is twice as great.

Normal modes of oscillation

If something is larger than a molecule (otherwise we need quantum mechanics) but smaller than a star (general relativity), and slower than greased lightning (special relativity), Newton's laws can describe its motions quite nicely.

An asteroid off in space and far from everything travels in a straight line and at constant velocity, in accord with the *law of conservation of momentum*. If it becomes subject to an applied force, however, such as that of Earth's gravity, then it will accelerate, and its state of motion will change – either its speed or its direction or both – as described by $F = ma$.

Some objects that experience certain kinds of force may undergo motion that is periodic. Consider a mass swinging at the end of a string, pulled downward by gravity and upward at an angle by the string (Figure 11.13a). High in its arc, the weight has

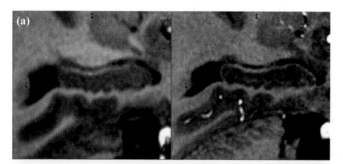

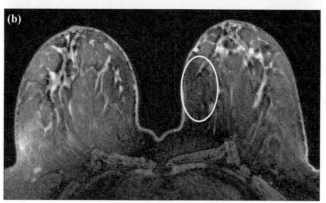

Figure 11.12 The effects of higher field strength. (a) M_0 is proportional to B_0, and MR signal strength also increases with field strength. Note the difference in image quality obtained at 1.5 T and 7 T, following i.v. contrast administration. Courtesy of Adam Anderson and John C. Gore. (b) One problem encountered occasionally at 3 T is the *RF interference artifact*. Reproduced from Zhuo J, Gullapalli RP. AAPM/RSNA physics tutorial for residents: MR artifacts, safety, and quality control. *Radiographics* 2006;**26**:275–97, with permission of the Radiological Society of North America (RSNA).

(a)

(b)

Rapid spin
about fixed axis

J

in free space

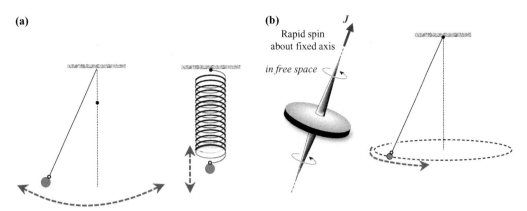

Figure 11.13 Normal modes of oscillation. (**a**) A simple pendulum and a mass on a spring both display inherent natural modes of oscillation and resonant frequencies. (**b**) A top rotating in outer space and a conical pendulum do, too.

a lot of gravitational potential energy; at the bottom, all of that has been converted to kinetic energy of motion. This simple pendulum displays a natural periodic motion, its *normal mode* of oscillation, which occurs at its own natural *resonant frequency*. Likewise for a bob bouncing on a spring.

Another kind of motion that obeys Newton's laws is the rotation of a body. A space station revolving slowly and far from the earth, say, will normally just keep on turning freely about an unchanging axis of rotation, and at a constant rate, as governed by the *law of conservation of angular momentum* (Figure 11.13b). Likewise, a conical pendulum, in which the weight travels in a circle, undergoes more complex a motion than does an ordinary swing, but it, too, experiences a normal mode of oscillation whose resonant frequency is determined by the length of the string and by the strength of the gravitational field.

What this is all leading up to is a child's gyroscope. As it spins, it feels two forces (apart from any friction): gravity pulls straight down on it, in effect at the center of the wheel, and the pedestal supporting its lower end pushes upward (Figure 11.14a). This pair of forces exerts a *torque*, or twisting force, on it that is perpendicular to the axis of rotation, and that attempts to topple the gyroscope over. But its spin, and conservation of angular momentum, resist its falling. The result is a new, and perhaps unexpected, kind of motion: the gyroscope undergoes *precession*, a swinging of its axis of rotation about the vertical (the direction of gravity's pull), at a constant rate.

The rate at which it is spinning about its axis at any instant does not change, but its overall motion does. The direction of its angular momentum, *J*, no longer remains constant, and its rate of precession is determined by the amount of torque applied. The spin-axis defines, and repeatedly slowly follows, the surface of a fixed, vertical geometrical cone. It may not be obvious why this should happen – but it is easily explained by working through Newton's math. As you might suspect, the stronger the gravitational field, the faster the rate of precession – a gyroscope on the Moon would take six times longer than on Earth to make a complete circuit around the vertical. The rate of precession also depends on the mass and shape of the flywheel, and on its rate of spin. We'll find analogous things happening with the net magnetization in a magnetic field.

"Classical" precession of the net magnetization, *M*(*t*), in a strong, fixed magnetic field, *B*₀

A proton acts somewhat like a rotating body, like the Space Station, and so it, too, possesses angular momentum, *J*, as was suggested in Figure 2.1a. It also produces (since it comprises a moving charge) its own magnetic field, parameterized by the magnetic moment, μ, the magnitude of which can be explained by your friendly neighborhood nuclear physicist or string theorist. It doesn't take so enlightened a being, however, to point out that the more rapid the spin, hence the faster the charge is moving, the greater the angular momentum, *J*, and

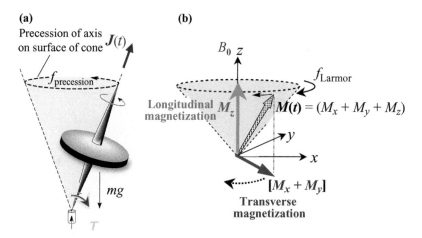

(a)

Precession of axis on surface of cone $J(t)$

$f_{precession}$

Longitudinal magnetization M_z

mg

τ

(b)

B_0 z

f_{Larmor}

$M(t) = (M_x + M_y + M_z)$

y

x

$[M_x + M_y]$

Transverse magnetization

Figure 11.14 Precessional normal modes. (**a**) A gyroscope, in which a torque is applied perpendicular to the axis of the angular momentum, J. The normal-mode behavior is *precession* of the angular momentum vector, J, and the spin axis, about the vertical. Its natural resonant frequency, or rate of precession, is determined by its mass and shape, its rate of rotation about its own axis, and the strength of the force of gravity. (**b**) The normal mode behavior of the *net magnetization* of a cohort of protons, $M(t)$, in an external magnetic field, B_0. Its precession about the field is very much like that of a top or ordinary gyroscope in gravity. As described by the Bloch equations, the precessional (Larmor) frequency is proportional to the strength of the field, $f_{Larmor} = 42.58\ B_0$, exactly what was found with the simple quantum approach! With this precession about the z-axis, it is possible to consider the z- and x-y components of $M(t)$, namely $M_z(t)$ and $M_{xy}(t)$, separately.

the stronger the proton's own field will be, so $\mu = \gamma J$. The isotope-specific constant of proportionality, γ, was introduced before, as the nucleus's *gyromagnetic ratio* in one expression of Larmor resonance (Equation 11.2c), $\omega = \gamma B$.

The rules of quantum mechanics prevent us from saying much about what any single proton does. (Indeed, some of the earlier business about spins pointing up or down was iffy, at best, and almost illegal.) But they do allow us to describe the *average* behavior of a *population* of billions of them in a voxel; and quantum mechanics says that we can even do so completely *classically*, according to old-fashioned Newtonian laws! The net magnetization, M, from a cluster of many protons is the composite field that vast numbers of them produce themselves – and quantum mechanics does allow us to discuss how M behaves in a strong, external magnetic field. All the practical physics of MRI are enshrined in a set of modifications of Newton's laws known as the *Bloch equations*. They are fully *classical* equations (although they can be derived ultimately from more advanced quantum theory), and they can describe the detailed motions of both a gyroscope in a gravitational field and a collec-

tion of protons in a magnetic field. We won't need to present or analyze the Bloch equations, but will simply discuss some of the most relevant results, which agree with what is seen in practice.

The result of experiment and also of solving the Bloch equations is that M will precess in the magnetic field, just as a gyroscope does in a gravitational field, and it should now indeed be represented as a function of time, $M(t)$. And as it precesses, it will trace out the surface of a cone aligned along the external magnetic field (Figure 11.14b). The angle of the cone; that is, the angle that $M(t)$ makes with the vertical, can assume any value at all – totally unlike the case of a spin-up or -down single proton. In a homogeneous external magnetic field of strength B_0, the frequency of proton precession turns out to be $f_{Larmor} = 42.58\ B_0$. The form of this classical equation is exactly the same as that of the corresponding quantum Equation 11.2, seen at the bottom of Figure 11.8a, but its derivation and its interpretation could not be more different! Back there, f_{Larmor} represented the frequency of an RF photon capable of flipping a proton from the lower- into the higher-energy spin-state in a strong external magnetic field. Here, it refers to the natural, normal-mode frequency of precession of a voxel's classical magnetic moment in that field. That the two should agree can be explained with the full mathematical machinery of quantum mechanics, but not with the simplified version used above.

And now for something completely different: nutation of the precessing *M(t)*

Many kinds of mechanical systems display one or more forms of normal-mode periodic behavior (Figures 11.13,11.14a). A closely related, but different, property is that of *resonance*. If applied to a system at its normal-mode frequency, even a very weak periodic external force can cause the eventual buildup of large-amplitude oscillations of the system. That is, energy is transferred to an oscillating system very efficiently through application of a periodic, resonance-frequency force.

Pushing a child on a swing offers a fine example. If you give many little pushes in very rapid succession, the swing will barely move. If you push very slowly, the swing will simply move along with your hand. But if applied at the natural frequency of the child-plus-swing system, and in phase with its motions, even modest shoves will cause the eventual buildup of large-amplitude oscillations. Resonance! So also with a circular pendulum (Figure 11.15a). If one displaces the upper end of the string slowly

in a tiny circle and at very low frequency, then the bob will simply follow along slowly, tracing out the same minute circle. If the circular "driving force" at the top is of high frequency, then the bob will not have time to follow, and it will remain nearly immobile. But if you move the string around at the circular pendulum's normal mode frequency, then the weight will move in ever higher, larger-diameter circles. The string travels on the surface of an inverted cone, and the cone opens up slowly over time, but only as long as you continue to add resonant-frequency power. You did this a thousand times as a child.

Something similar happens with a precessing gyroscope, too. Resonant transfer of energy to the gyroscope, and its response, can be demonstrated by pulling lightly on a thread attached to the top of its frame (Figure 11.15b). A very particular kind of pull is require, though: the tension in the thread should be constant, but the direction from which the pull comes must move in a circle, in phase with and parallel to the motion of the upper tip of the gyroscope at any instant. There are now *two* torques acting on the system: a strong one due to gravity, and the other caused by the thread — and these together cause the gyroscope to undergo an even more complicated kind of motion. In addition to the axis of rotation traveling on the surface of a vertical cone, *precession*, the system now *also*

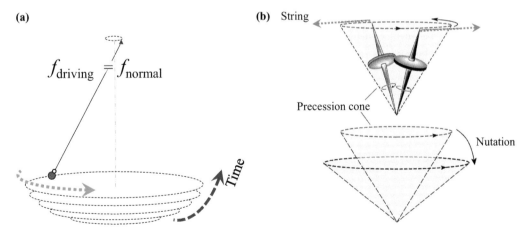

(a)

$f_{\text{driving}} = f_{\text{normal}}$

Time

(b) String

Precession cone

Nutation

Figure 11.15 Resonance. Inputting energy at a system's natural resonant frequency (**a**) can give rise to large and exaggerated oscillatory motions, the amplitudes of which depend largely on the rates at which power is being given to the system and dissipated by it. (**b**) It is possible, by way of a somewhat non-intuitive way of applying torque to a gyroscope, to provide it with in-phase, resonant-frequency power, resulting in an also non-intuitive response: *nutation*.

undergoes *nutation*: the conical surface *itself* very slowly (relative to the rate of precession) opens up, like a lotus flower unfurling in the morning sun. (Hey, this is supposed to be a work of serious literature, too). The wheel's axis of rotation now spirals gently down toward the horizontal. If the direction of the force exerted by the thread changes more slowly or rapidly than the natural precession rate, it will have little effect on the gyroscope's behavior. But applied at the resonance (Larmor) frequency – bingo!

Now back to the voxel of protons in a strong, fixed external field. Imagine a radiofrequency coil system that produces a weak radiofrequency magnetic field, B_{RF}, that lies *perpendicular* to the strong, external magnetic field and circles it in the horizontal plane. This will have the same effect on $M(t)$ as does the thread on the gyroscope. If the RF energy being generated were much above or below f_{Larmor}, then $M(t)$ would simply continue to precess in its normal-mode of motion. But RF radiation that is resonant with the natural precessional motion of the system will cause the net magnetization to undergo nutation, and the cone of precession opens up (Figure 11.16). This is the "classical picture" of the NMR phenomenon: with $M(t)$ starting out near thermal equilibrium, lying almost along B_0, the hypothetical cone on which it precesses opens up very slowly and, at some point, it actually coincides briefly with the horizontal plane. After that, it begins to fold up again, but now below the *x-y* plane. The nutation continues, until the magnetization points due south, and then it starts heading upward again, eventually returning to where it started. Then the whole process repeats itself. But this process takes place *only while the RF power is still being applied*, and that is usually only very briefly in MRI, during an RF pulse a fraction of a millisecond in duration. Indeed, nearly always, the nutation occurs only long enough for $M(t)$ to tip through either 90° or less, or through 180°.

Let's recap (Box 11.1). When experiencing only B_0, $M(t)$ is constantly precessing, and at the rate $f_{Larmor} = (\gamma/2\pi)B_0$. For a proton in a 1 T field, $f_{Larmor} = 42.58$ MHz. With application of B_{RF}, as well (which itself is oscillating also at f_{Larmor}), the system also nutates. But if we need to swing the magnetization down through 90° or 180°, say, it's necessary first to know how fast the nutation is occurring. Probably much slower than f_{Larmor}, but what? One key to the problem would be to solve the Bloch equations, but that's a little hairy and, anyway, there's an easier way, one that makes use of a cute trick.

Box 11.1   Precession versus nutation; B_0 versus B_{RF}.

Precession of $M(t)$:
  Always!
  About B_0 (fixed in the laboratory frame)
  $f_{Larmor} = 42.58$ [(MHz/T)] × B_0 [T]
Nutation of $M(t)$:
  Only when B_{RF} is *also* on!
  About B_{RF} (fixed in the rotating frame; B_0 "vanishes")
  $f_{nutation} = 42.58$ [(MHz/T)] × B_{RF} [T] = 1 kHz
  for a B_{RF} of 25 μT and for *any* B_0.
  $t_{90°} \sim {}^1/_4$ ms

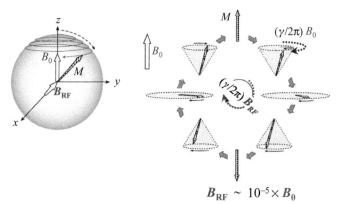

$$B_{RF} \sim 10^{-5} \times B_0$$

Figure 11.16 Two views of *M(t)* *precessing* at the Larmor frequency in a static B_0 field. While, in addition, a Larmor-frequency field, B_{RF}, is applied, *M(t)* also undergoes *nutation*, doing so with the frequency $f_{nutation} = 42.58\ B_{RF}$. This is just the Larmor equation, again, but this time the relevant magnetic field is B_{RF}, which is thousands of times less than B_0. Over the particular time interval, *t*, that B_{RF} is left on, *M(t)* nutates through the angle $\alpha = 42.58\ B_{RF}t$.

Suppose you're at Coney Island, watching the kids bob up and down on the horses of the merry-go-round. The motion is too complex for you to determine clearly who is punching whom, so you jump on board, too. The children are still oscillating vertically, but now the circular motion disappears, and each is at a fixed position on the carrousel, so the action is much simpler to untangle.

Similarly, before B_{RF} is turned on, an outside observer seated in the fixed frame of reference (also called the laboratory frame) would see $M(t)$ precessing at f_{Larmor} about the main field, B_0. The behavior of $M(t)$ over time is more readily followed, however, by someone in a frame of reference that rotates at the precessional frequency. With this perspective, $M(t)$ seems to do nothing at all, as long as $B_{RF} = 0$. The magnetization just sits there, unchanging in either magnitude or direction over time (Figure 11.17a). It's as if the act of transforming to the rotating frame has the effect of switching off the main magnetic field, B_0, just as jumping onto the carousel seems to make the horses' rotational motion go away. When viewed from the rotating frame, B_0 is really still there, of course, but when considering its influence on M from this better vantage point, you can temporarily pretend that $B_0 = 0$.

Now turn on the resonance-frequency field B_{RF} (Figure 11.17b). Seen from the laboratory frame of reference, B_{RF} is circling horizontally, in the x-y plane at the Larmor frequency. But from the rotating frame perspective, it seems to be a fixed, constant field – in fact, the only field present. So $M(t)$ will now "precess" about it (rather than around B_0,

which has "vanished") with a frequency of

$$f_{nutation} = 42.58 B_{RF}, \qquad (11.5)$$

Just as the precession rate is proportional to the strength of the main field, B_0, likewise the frequency of nutation also is linear in the RF field strength. B_{RF} is typically something like 25 μT, about five orders of magnitude weaker than B_0. So while $M(t)$ may precess at a rate of 64 MHz, in a 1.5 T field, the magnetization will nutate at only about $42.58 \times (0.000025\ \text{T}) = 1$ kHz. With this amount of B_{RF}, it will take about $t_{90°} = 250$ microseconds to cause $M(t)$ to spiral 90°, for example, from the vertical down into the x-y plane.

Apart from the occasional very brief instances when B_{RF} is turned on, of course, the system will be precessing only, and not nutating. So if M_z happens to be at equilibrium, say, and you turn on a (brief) 90° pulse, the magnetization will rapidly nutate down into the transverse plane, and then precess there indefinitely, in the absence of relaxation events. Its direction is totally different, but its magnitude has not changed.

Monitoring the NMR: the only MRI signal you ever see comes from the component of M(t) that is precessing in the x-y plane, $M_{xy}(t)$

With this classical approach, how can you tell that NMR is actually taking place? The net magnetization might be nutating like crazy, but how would anyone know?

It is possible to make the NMR process reveal itself in several ways, and the free induction decay

Figure 11.17 What you see depends on your frame of reference. (a) When you're on the carousel, too, the ponies don't advance. And as viewed from a frame rotating at the Larmor frequency, B_0 has magically vanished, in effect. When B_{RF} is off, which is nearly all the time, then $M(t)$ appears static, not precessing or doing anything else. (b) But during those brief moments that B_{RF} is turned on, there now appears to be a new fixed field, B_{RF}, and $M(t)$ nutates/precesses about it, and at the rate $42.58\ B_{RF}$ MHz. This drawing is not to scale since, in reality, $B_0 \gg B_{RF}$.

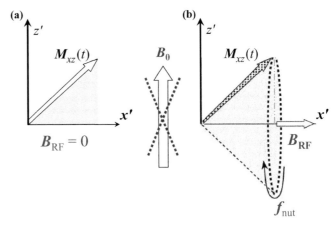

(*FID*) technique is the simplest to describe. For now, forget the "decay" or "relaxation" part – the next chapter will return to it.

Suppose, for simplicity, that a single voxel of water is sitting comfortably in a uniform magnetic field (Figure 11.18a). (We don't need to worry about gradient fields and frequency-encoding of position yet.) We're going to shake things up by applying a 90° pulse exactly at $t = 0$, and see what happens. Just before the pulse, at $t = 0-$, the z-component of the magnetization initially has magnitude, $M_z(t = 0-)$. (If the spin system has been undisturbed for a long time, then $M_z(t = 0-) = M_0$.) At this $t = 0-$, there is no component of the magnetization vector in the x-y plane: since everything is still pointing upward, $M_{xy}(0-) = 0$.

But just at $t = 0$, a pulse of Larmor-frequency power is pumped into an RF transmitter coil that is situated in the x-y plane and facing the voxel;

B_{RF} is left on exactly long enough to nutate the net magnetization from its initial vertical orientation down into the horizontal plane, and then switched off (Figure 11.18b). Just after application of this 90° *saturation* or *excitation pulse*, at $t = 0+$, $M(t)$ will be still be of magnitude $M_z(0-)$, but now precessing continuously in the x-y plane at the Larmor frequency (Figure 11.18b); it makes sense to name the x-y component of the magnetization "$M_{xy}(t)$" now, and its magnitude, right after the pulse, would be called $M_{xy}(0+)$. Since all of the magnetization is driven almost instantaneously from along the z-axis down into the x-y plane, it follows that

$$M_{xy}(0+) = M_z(0-), \qquad (11.6)$$

an expression that summarizes what just happened and that will prove conceptually useful on several occasions.

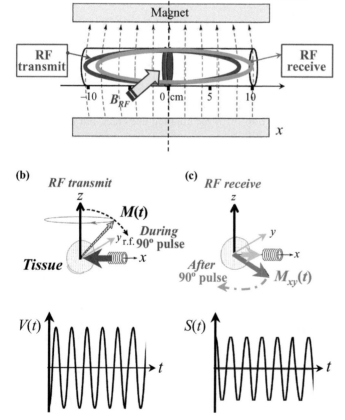

Figure 11.18 Free induction decay (FID). (a) Phantom with one water-containing voxel, in a 1-T uniform field. (b) A specially designed pulse of RF voltage, $V(t)$, is applied to the transmit coil. The corresponding 90° saturation/excitation pulse of B_{RF} causes the magnetization to nutate rapidly down into the x-y plane. With $f_{nutation} = 42.58\,B_{RF}$ and $B_{RF} = 25\,\mu T$ (about 10^5 times less than B_0), the process takes 250 μs. (c) The magnitude of the magnetization immediately after the 90° pulse, $M_{xy}(0+)$, is exactly the same as it was just before, $M_z(0-) = M_0$. By Faraday's *law of induction*, the changing magnetic field induces an f_{Larmor}-voltage signal, $S(t)$ in a nearby pickup coil. See Box 11.2.

Any changing magnetic field produces a voltage in a nearby coil, by means of Faraday induction (Figure 2.1b). That, in fact, is exactly how a generator at an electric power plant works, albeit on a somewhat grander scale. It also occurs when $M(t)$ is precessing in or near the horizontal plane, as in Figure 11.18c; its magnetic field cuts repeatedly through the pickup antenna coil that feeds the NMR system's RF receiver (Figure 11.18a), inducing a voltage in it. (When the net magnetization happens to be pointing nearly up or down, on the other hand, with almost no component in the x-y plane, then the pick-up coil is oblivious to it.) So the appearance of a Larmor frequency signal in the RF coil following application of a 90° pulse indicates the occurrence of NMR. Indeed, the *only* NMR or *MRI signal* you *ever* see comes from the *component of $M(t)$*, namely $M_{xy}(t)$, that is *precessing in the x-y plane* (Box 11.2). [Note that here, we are measuring a voltage signal, $S(t)$, induced in the pickup coil by the changing magnetic field, rather than detecting a change in power absorption, as was the case with the elementary spin-flip picture considered earlier (Figure 11.6).

Box 11.2   The *only* signal you *ever* see comes from $M_{xy}(t)$ precessing in the x-y plane!

In MRI, the *only* signal
you *ever* see comes from
$M(t)$ precessing in the x-y plane
!!!

Yes, the simple spin-state and the classical pictures are totally incompatible!

One aspect of all of this may have been troubling you a little. Or a lot. The two-state, quantum picture allows individual spins to be aligned along or against the static magnetic field, but nothing else. Yet here we find protons in a voxel whose net magnetization can be at any angle relative to the external field. $M(t)$ can even precess entirely in the horizontal plane. The two pictures are totally incompatible.

The problem is that our elementary quantum treatment, although correct enough for some purposes, is not sufficiently refined to allow us to avoid

this apparent paradox. A more advanced analysis could. The classical model of NMR can be fully presented (even including the effects of spin relaxation) by means of the Bloch equations, which describe the behavior of the net magnetization vector over time, as if it were just like a gyroscope. And the Bloch equations, in turn, can be extracted from a rigorous, comprehensive quantum mechanical treatment, which we have not pursued here. That is the only route by which the spin paradox can be resolved.

Fortunately, if you are willing to overlook this little inconsistency, you can use both pictures productively and even mix them without getting into trouble. Indeed, it's best *not* to stick with either one picture alone. As with particle-wave duality, practitioners of MRI become accustomed to living with two seemingly disparate descriptions of reality. Doesn't always make sense, but it does work well.

Free induction decay imaging (but without the decay)

We are now positioned to describe the creation of one-dimensional MRI images with RF pulses and the classical approach. One idea that does carry over completely from before, happily, is that of frequency-encoding of voxel position by way of a gradient field.

Encoding of voxel position with a gradient and a narrow-band RF pulse: a 1D FID PD MRI study

We re-introduce the phantom that consists of two thin pancake-slices of water in an x-gradient magnetic field. As before, one voxel is pure water; the other is only half filled with it (Figure 11.19a).

Two roads diverge here, and since each is well traveled, we'll take them both. The first, which can be termed the *narrow RF-band* FID approach, is somewhat similar to what we did earlier with the spin up/down picture. As described in the next chapter, it is the standard way to select individual (typically transverse) planar slices, each of which is then to be imaged in two dimensions. The other, *broad-band* road is closer to how one creates MR maps within a selected slice.

Narrow RF-band first: we begin by switching on an x-gradient that runs from 0.998 T to 1.002 T, say, over the full 20-cm length of the phantom. We

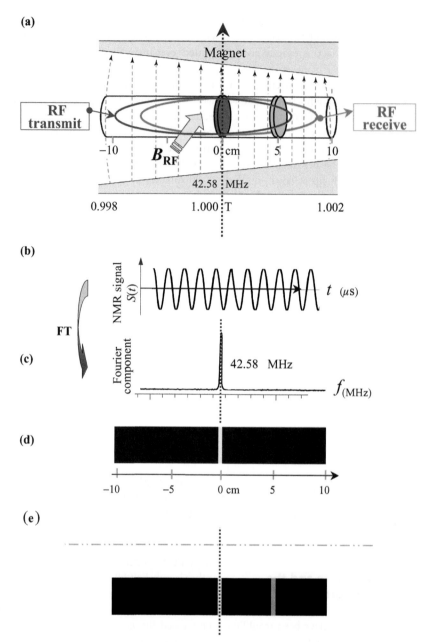

(a)

(b)

(c)

(d)

(e)

Figure 11.19 FID imaging of proton density in a 1D phantom **(a)** in an x-gradient field, with frequency-encoding of voxel x-position. There is a voxel at $x = 0$ cm containing pure water, and another at $x = 5$ cm with half the PD. The x-gradient is on during the RF pulse, as well as during readout, and adjusted so that the total field strength (principal plus gradient) is exactly 1.000 T at $x = 0$. **(b)** The system generates a sequence of separate narrow-band (0.1 MHz wide) 90° pulses of increasing center frequency, f. Nothing happens until a resonance suddenly appears. **(c)** Fourier analysis, or a Fourier transform (FT), of the resonance signal, $S(t)$, reveals that the signal is monochromatic and of a frequency 42.58 MHz. This is f_{Larmor} for water in a field of exactly 1.000 T which, with G_x on, exists only at $x = 0$ cm. **(d)** This is enough information to begin creating a PD MR image of the phantom. **(e)** This process is then repeated at increasing center frequencies, and another resonance, of half the amplitude of the first, is found at 42.62 MHz. This one occurs in a 1.001 T field, corresponding to $x = 5$ cm and half the PD. The relative amplitudes and frequencies of the signals obtained separately from the two voxels provide enough information to complete the PD MR image.

apply a 90° RF pulse made up of a mixture of all the frequencies within a *narrow band* of them, 100 kHz (0.1 MHz) wide and centered, say, at 42.00 MHz, so that the frequencies that comprise the pulse range from 41.95 to 42.05 MHz. There seems to be no water in the phantom where the resonance would occur in that frequency range, and nothing happens. We try again at 42.10 MHz and, again, nada.

After a few more uneventful steps, we finally hit pay water, with a pulse containing frequencies from 42.55 to 42.65 MHz. The pulse must have nutated the water somewhere in the phantom down into the *x-y* plane, where it proceeded to precess, because a near-sinusoidal resonance voltage signal, $S(t)$, is detected (Figure 11.19b). We shall need to find the precise value of f_{Larmor}, so we call again upon the machinery of Fourier analysis: signal in, spectrum out! This is an especially easy case, since the MR signal happens to be monochromatic, with a single spectral peak at precisely 42.58 MHz (Figure 11.19c).

The Larmor equation reveals that for this peak, the field happens to be exactly 1.000 T – and our prior knowledge of the spatial characteristics of the gradient field informs us that the relevant voxel must be at $x = 0$. And that's all that's needed to construct the MR image (Figure 11.19d). In short, this approach has *frequency-encoded* the *x*-position information about the water within the RF signal picked up by the receiver coil.

So far, we have found a resonance peak only from the water at $x = 0$. We can continue to up the frequency a few more times, and discover the other one, with a spectral peak half as tall, at 42.62 MHz. This corresponds to a voxel at $x = 5$ cm with half the PD, which makes it possible to construct the full MRI image (Figure 11.19e).

Frequency-encoding voxel *x*-position with a broad-band RF pulse: a better approach to the 1D FID PD MRI study

Back to the fork in the road.

The narrow-RF-band approach carries out separate NMR measurements at many, slightly different, nearly monochromatic frequencies, which is fine except that it would be excruciatingly slow in the clinic. The *broad-band* FID approach acts a great deal faster.

Broad-RF-band FID employs only one RF 90° pulse throughout the whole study, but that pulse is designed to contain a band of frequencies wide enough to include any and all resonances of interest, in the presence of the *x*-gradient (Figure 11.20a). To examine all the voxels in our 20-cm section of patient simultaneously, the RF pulse must contain equal amounts of all frequencies ranging from below about 42.5 MHz to 42.7 MHz, say. That way, the magnetizations of all volumes of water anywhere along the phantom will be caused, simultaneously but independently, to nutate down into the *x-y* plane, and precess there, also independently (Figure 11.20b).

In our example phantom, after the broad-band 90° RF pulse, the magnetizations of the water in the two voxels precess individually in the *x-y* plane, at 42.58 and 42.62 MHz, respectively. Each will independently attempt to induce a corresponding f_{Larmor} voltage in the pickup coil (Figure 11.20c). But what the coil actually experiences is the overall changing magnetic field, not the separate source components, and it sends to the RF receiver the composite signal generated by the two acting together. This compound signal displays a "beat" pattern characteristic of the *interference* of the two independent signals (Figure 11.20d and Figure 2.3). With more voxels containing water, the RF MR signal would be correspondingly more complex.

The remaining task is somehow to analyze this MR signal, and to determine how much water is precessing at each frequency; that is, with every local magnetic field value, hence at all positions along the gradient (and the phantom). But of course, that is exactly what Fourier analysis does best! Fourier decomposition is the converse of interference, in effect, and it quickly separates the MR signal into its constituent parts, with a peak for every voxel (Figure 11.20e). Again, every frequency is associated with a unique position along the phantom, so the positions and amplitudes of the peaks within the spectrum provide a direct anatomic map of proton density; that is, the complete PD MRI image.

First step into *k*-space

Fourier analysis is a powerful tool that is essential to image reconstruction in all the tomographic modalities, including CT, SPECT, PET, MRI, optical coherence tomography (OCT), and others. It is

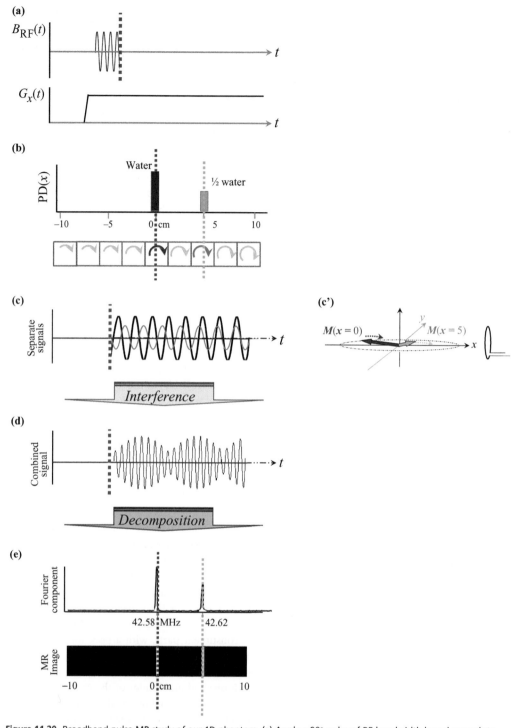

Figure 11.20 Broadband-pulse MR study of our 1D phantom. (a) Apply a 90° pulse of RF-bandwidth broad enough to simultaneously cover the Larmor frequencies of all the voxels of interest. If the *x*-gradient is on, to spread out their f_{Larmor} values, this will cause precession in the *x-y* plane of the water in any voxel. (b) The water at $x = 0$ and $x = 5$ will precess with monochromatic frequencies of 42.58 and 42.62 MHz, respectively, (c) and their magnetizations independently induce FID voltages at these frequencies in the RF pickup coil. (d) But the coil senses only the overall changing magnetic field, and it ends up sending to the receiver a compound *beat interference* pattern that arises from the two monochromatic signals, which are of slightly different wavelengths and not of the same amplitude. (e) Fortunately, the digital machinery of the *Fourier transform* (FT) can untangle the mess, working to reverse the interference process, and separate the complex signals.

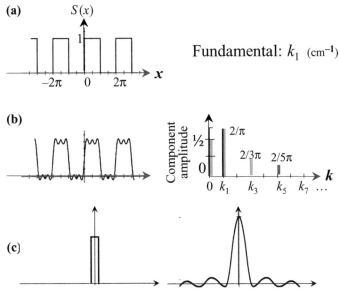

(a) $S(x)$

Fundamental: k_1 (cm^{-1})

(b)

Component amplitude

$2/\pi$

$1/2$

$2/3\pi$ $2/5\pi$

0

$0\ k_1\quad k_3\quad k_5\ k_7\ \ldots$ k

(c)

Figure 11.21 Interference of monochromatic waves and, conversely, Fourier resolution of the complex resulting wave into its constituent monochromatic components and spectrum. **(a)** A periodic spatial square wave, similar to the temporal signal seen earlier as Figure 4.10. **(b)** Such a pattern can be built up through interference among sine waves at multiples of the fundamental spatial frequency, k_1; the spectra to the right provide the appropriate amplitudes, where $k_7 = 7 \times k_1$. Conversely, *Fourier analysis* using the Fourier transform (FT) decomposes, or breaks down, a complex periodic curve into its constituent monochromatic components. The wave form and its spectrum contain equivalent information, and one form can be converted into the other with the Fourier transform. **(c)** The spectrum for a non-periodic curve, such as this single rectangle, has component frequencies so close together that their amplitudes appear to form a smooth curve

just an extension of the *Fourier sum*, which we have already talked about.

The "square wave" of Figure 11.21a is a *periodic* function of position, x (rather than of time, t, as was seen in Figure 4.10). Just as temporal frequency is typically represented as f and expressed in cycles per second, likewise, by convention, spatial frequency is shown as "k," and it comes in units of cycles per centimeter or per mm.

Recall that any periodic curve can be constructed out of the right combination of sine waves, its Fourier sum. In Figure 11.21a, specifically, the square repeats at a *fundamental spatial frequency* that we shall name k_1. Starting off with a sine wave at the fundamental frequency, one can add to it *harmonics* of the correct amplitudes (including 0) at *integer multiples* of the fundamental. For this particular function, the non-zero components have spatial frequencies $k_1, 3k_1, 5k_1, 7k_1, 9k_1, \ldots$, and amplitudes $2/\pi, 2/3\pi, 2/5\pi, \ldots$. As more such terms are added, the resulting interference patterns (which is what they really are) will grow increas-

ingly to resemble the original (Figure 11.21b). This notation is clumsy, so let's rename the fundamental and these harmonics simply as $k_1, k_3, k_5, k_7, k_9, \ldots$. They are defined to mean exactly the same thing.

The left-hand side of the diagram shows the sum pattern at an early stage of its evolution, and the Fourier spectrum is to the right. The two contain exactly the same information, just as do a number presented in digital versus binary forms, and one can jump back and forth readily between them with the mathematical tool known as the Fourier transform (FT).

Since the fundamental, k_1, corresponds to the frequency of the original pattern, there obviously can be no waves contributing to the sum that are of *longer* wavelength – the whole train of square waves does not float on a slowly undulating background wave. The harmonics, conversely, will be of progressively *shorter* wavelengths, and will be able to insert ever increasingly finer detail. That is, a high-spatial-resolution system corresponds to the ability to handle high-spatial-frequency harmonics.

Sometimes it is not obvious what spatial frequency should play the role of the "fundamental," but generally an image does not contain wavelengths longer than the entire field of view – so unless there is a clear alternative, a safe bet should be a single cycle per FOV, or $k_1 = 1/\text{FOV}$ (mm^{-1}). One could continue to add components at integer multiples of this, with shorter and shorter spatial wavelengths, up until no further improvement in the image is noticeable to the eye. If the FOV is 100 mm, for example, then you might select, say, a k_1 of 0.01 cycle/mm. Embracing harmonics up to $k_{1000} = 1000 \times k_1$ would allow inclusion of details down to the 10 cycle/mm level, or to about 0.1 mm. But the real limit in the length of the shortest useful wave is the dimension of the voxels, Δx. By Equation 6.1, this is related directly to the number of pixels and the FOV as $\mathcal{N}\Delta x = \text{FOV}$. Since $\mathcal{N}$ is typically 256 or 512 for MRI, and the FOV something like 25 cm, this would suggest that the highest-frequency, shortest-wavelength contributions to the image would be of the order of FOV/$\mathcal{N} \sim$ 0.5 mm in dimension.

With an extension of the Fourier sum, it is possible to represent a curve that is not periodic, but rather appears only once, such as a single rectangle, or something more complex. Imagine that the boxes of Figure 11.21a become narrower and spread farther apart, until only one of them appears in the FOV (Figure 11.21c, left). As this happens, the required harmonics become far more numerous and more closely spaced, and the upper tips of the spectral lines appear to blend into a smooth-seeming curve, to the right – imagine the area under the curve as being comprised of with hundreds of thin, vertical spectral lines, the upper ends of which form the curve.

So far, we have dealt with one-dimensional images. To create clinical two- or three-dimensional images, it is necessary to generalize a little. Recall that a *vector* has both magnitude and direction. The two axes of a road map can be indicated by a pair of vectors of unit length (e.g., 1 mile) and pointing along the two axes, $\underline{x}$ and $\underline{y}$. The location of the small farm of one of the authors (A.B.W.) in Clover Bottom, KY, can then be represented by two components like, say, $x = -14$ and $y = 11$ relative to an agreed-upon distance scale and an origin at the Lexington Opera House or, more simply, as $-14\underline{x} + 11\underline{y}$.

The set of all such possible map points is called a *vector space*, and this particular kind of vector space is known commonly as a two-dimensional *real space*.

In a similar fashion, one can represent a two-dimensional image out of combinations of two sets of sine curves running in perpendicular directions, so that the result has both x- and y-components. Two unit vectors are again needed, this time called $\underline{k}_x$ and $\underline{k}_y$, and they represent fundamental waves in a slightly (but not much) more abstract kind of vector space known as k-space. As in Figure 11.22a, the fundamental unit vectors are again chosen to correspond to the lowest-spatial-frequency, longest-wavelength waves that go into making up the image: if the image in real-space is simply periodic in two directions, like a chess board, then the spectral decomposition would be a 2D version of the spectrum in Figure 11.21b,c.

Consider a single black square of the chess board in real space – and let everything else be white. By the argument we have just been through, its representation in the corresponding 2D k-space is an apparently smooth, continuous 2D surface that maps out the upper ends of all the thousands of vertically-oriented spectral lines below, as to the left in Figure 11.22a. And if we are given either the k-space or the real-space representation, we can easily get to the other with a two-dimensional Fourier transform, Although we haven't demonstrated the mathematics for carrying out a FT, at least it should be clear what it is capable of doing.

A somewhat more complex entity, a widget, appears to the left in Figure 11.22b, and its Fourier/k-space representation directly above it. The center column shows what happens if one employs only a central-square section of k-space in the FT. Throwing away the higher spatial frequency components leads to a real-space image that reveals only the grosser characteristics in real space, and little fine detail. Conversely, retention only of the shorter-wavelength parts gives plenty of sharpness, but little overall sense of contrast. Obviously enough of each is needed.

What comes directly out of the MRI machine, line-by-line, happens to be the k-space representation of the MR image! This is not obvious, and you have not yet been given any reason to believe it, or see why it happens, but nonetheless it is true, and we shall discuss it in the next chapter. But

(a)

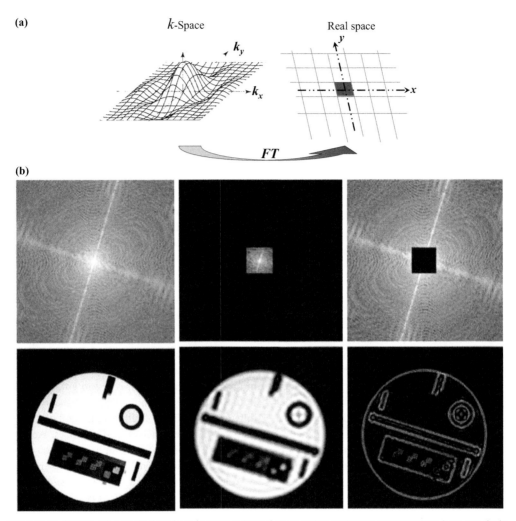

(b)

Figure 11.22 *k*-space. **(a)** A single chess-board square in 2D real-space and its 2D *k*-space representation have exactly the same information content, and can be switched back and forth by way of a 2D Fourier transform. **(b)** Fourier decomposition of the 2D real-space image of a widget (below, left) in *k*-space. If only long-wavelength components, near *k* = 0, are considered (middle), then detail is lost. Inclusion only of higher-*k*, shorter wavelength contributions (right), on the other hand, provides the spices, but not the meat. Reproduced from Zhuo J, Gullapalli RP, AAPM/RSNA physics tutorial for residents: MR artifacts, safety, and quality control. *Radiographics* 2006;**26**:275–97, with permission of the Radiological Society of North America (RSNA).

howsoever the *k*-space representation is created and then captured by the MR coil and receiver, once we have it, all that's required is to FT it back into real space to get the MR image.

Sampling and digitizing the MR signal

Nearly all clinical MRI studies employ either a *spin-echo* or a *gradient-echo* pulse sequence, to be described soon, rather than an FID. In both cases the RF signal detected and analyzed is called an *echo*

signal, and it looks something like Figure 11.23. Hereafter we shall call the MRI signal an "echo."

The patient's echo signal that is detected by the MR coil and receiver is a voltage that varies continuously over time. All the necessary calculations for image reconstruction, however, are carried out on a digital computer. That means that the input voltage must first be sampled at multiple discrete times, and then translated from the continuous to the digital form by means of an *analog-to-digital*

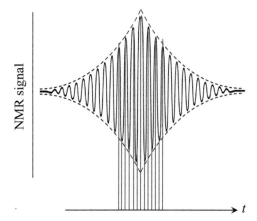

Figure 11.23 The system must sample the incoming temporal signal from the MRI pickup coils and receiver fast enough. If the highest-frequency component of importance in the signal oscillates at f_{max}, then the signal must be sampled at a rate a bit faster than $2 \times f_{max}$ to be in compliance with the Nyquist theorem.

converter (ADC). And while the initial MR signal first detected is a function of time, the final image is to be displayed in real space. On several occasions earlier (in connection with the digitized radiograph, the CCD, the active matrix flat panel imagers of DR and DSA, the nuclear medicine rectilinear scanner, B-mode, etc.), a two-dimensional spatial pattern related to properties of the body has been transformed into a (one-dimensional) function of time, and then, after processing, returned back into a 2D spatial pattern on the display – one that somehow mapped out variations in the tissue characteristics. Here it's much the same, but more complex, because of the complicated but necessary k-space middleman. We'll defer most talk of that until the next chapter.

But we can discuss here the right number of samples needed: if there are not enough, there will be insufficient information to recreate a high-quality image. But too many is wasteful of time, which, for MRI, is a highly prized commodity, and possibly also of money. Again, how many samples are needed, and how frequently must they be taken?

Although not evident from Figure 11.23, all segments of the highly complex MR signal from the coil reflect its complete frequency makeup, so you don't have to sample all of it. Fortunately, there are two simple rules that guide us in dealing with this.

The final image is generally displayed in a real-space image 512 pixels wide and, as we shall see, this requires that the temporal echo signal be sampled at least 512 times. That is, for 512 k-values, or spatial frequency components along the k_x-axis, 512 samples or more must be extracted from the MR RF signal; and

In accord with the well-known *Nyquist theorem* of signal processing, if the highest frequency contribution of interest in the echo signal is of frequency f_{max} Hz, then it is necessary but adequate to sample at the rate $2 \times f_{max}$ Hz. To make a complicated story simple: failure to sample sufficiently rapidly over time can cause problems in k-space that lead to aliasing in real space (Figure 6.9).

Spin-echo imaging (still without T1 or T2 relaxation)

FID is fine for introducing the general idea of pulse MRI, but there are two general categories of pulse sequences that are far more flexible and effective in producing images: *spin-echo* and *gradient-echo*. Both involve the creation of RF *echo signals* (totally different from those of ultrasound), and it is these that an MRI device detects and processes. We first address the more common approach, spin-echo, and sketch gradient-echo in the next chapter.

We continue to assume that no physiologically based T1- or T2-type relaxation is occurring. The next chapter will bring both into the story. Be patient.

Static field de-phasing (with characteristic time T_{SFd-P}) and the degrading effects caused by static magnetic field inhomogeneities

Spin-echo provides two immediate great benefits. One, as the name implies, is that it leads to the creation of one or more echo signals long after an FID signal would have decayed away to nothing, and these echoes can be harnessed in image creation.

The second has to do with the removal of a certain kind of image degradation that occurs naturally because of *static, time-independent* irregularities in the local magnetic field, even when the gradients are off. While nominally the principal field is uniform across a voxel and exactly of strength B_0, in fact there are slight, *fixed* spatial variation within any voxel due to several factors. The field is supposed to be homogeneous, to within 10 parts per million or so, but there is a spatial unevenness on the microscopic level caused by imperfections in magnet construction. The average variation within a voxel of the external field will be indicated ΔB_0. Another source of such irregularities is the slight gradients that arise at abrupt changes in the susceptibilities, $\Delta\chi$, of certain tissues and other materials, such as between soft tissue and cerebro-spinal fluid, or air, or bone, or any non-ferromagnetic metal at interfaces among them (Equation 11.4c). Indeed, when $\Delta\chi$ is large, as when caused by dental fillings, the resulting artifact can be quite spectacular (Figure 11.24).

After a 90° RF pulse, say, these small, static differences in field strength within a voxel bring about tiny but constant spatial differences in the precessional frequencies of separate clusters of protons in it (Figure 11.25). This causes them to de-phase from

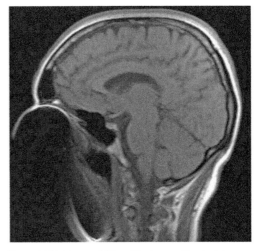

Figure 11.24 Susceptibility artifact caused by dental fillings containing magnetizable metals. Reproduced from Zhuo J, Gullapalli RP, AAPM/RSNA physics tutorial for residents: MR artifacts, safety, and quality control. *Radiographics* 2006;**26**:275–97, with permission of the Radiological Society of North America (RSNA).

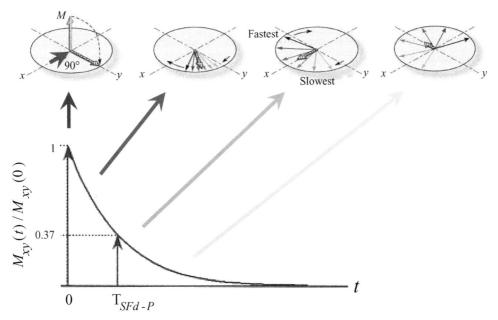

Figure 11.25 When situated in a local magnetic field that is not perfectly homogeneous, packets of spins in a voxel will spread out in the *x-y* plane after a 90° pulse, since some will precess a little faster than average, and others slower. And as this occurs, as viewed from the fixed (laboratory) frame of reference, the length of the magnetization vector, and the amplitude of the FID signal, will diminish exponentially, even in the absence of any proton spin relaxation mechanisms; the characteristic time for such static-field de-phasing and decay of $M_{xy}(t)$ to occur is $T_{SFd\text{-}P}$. As discussed in Chapter 12, T1 and T2 also, but separately, cause decay over time of the magnetization and of MR signal strength.

one another, with their individual magnetizations spreading out in the x-y plane; the magnitude of the voxel's net transverse magnetization (in the x-y plane), $M_{xy}(t)$, decreases approximately exponentially in magnitude over time as

$$M_{xy}(t)/M_{xy}(0) = e^{-t/T_{SFd-P}}, \qquad (11.7a)$$

and rather quickly vanishes. This process may be called *static-field caused de-phasing*, and the characteristic time over which it occurs, T_{SFd-P}, we shall label the Static Field *de*-Phasing time. For consistency with the convention for T1 and T2, it represents how long it takes for the static field inhomogeneities to cause $M_{xy}(t)$ to de-phase enough so as to decrease to 0.37 of its original value. (Recall that $0.37 = 1/e$.) T_{SFd-P} is also the time over which the Larmor-frequency voltage signal from the pickup coil falls to 37% of its initial value.

A short T_{SFd-P} corresponds to a fast *rate* of exponential decline, $1/T_{SFd-P}$. This overall rate for the process can be viewed as made up of two parts, parameterized by ΔB_0 and $\Delta\chi$, so that

$$1/T_{SFd-P} = \kappa\Delta B_0 + \kappa'\Delta\chi, \qquad (11.7b)$$

where κ and κ' are appropriate weighting constants. T_{SFd-P} is itself of little biological or medical interest, and we'd be better off without it. Remarkably, and fortunately, the spin-echo pulse sequence largely counteracts it and removes it from the picture – literally. But T_{SFd-P} will come up again in the next chapter in connection with the gradient-echo pulse sequence. The effect can even be put to good use in *susceptibility imaging*, which is like a clinically useful version of Figure 11.24.

Spin-echo produces readable echo signals, and it also removes field inhomogeneity and susceptibility (T_{SFd-P}) effects

Spin-echo can reverse this de-phasing effect, because, and only because, these disruptions in the local fields are *static*, not varying appreciably over time. It works just like the First (Annual) Shall Be Last Kentucky Turtle Derby (Figure 11.26a):

At $t = 0$, just before the race begins, all the competitors are aligned at the start/finish line.

(*i*) At the starting 90° pulse, the noble beasts bolt from the start/finish line in a fury of dust and thundering hooves. Some are racing faster than others, so the competitors begin to spread out.

(*ii*) At a certain pre-specified time, exactly at one-half the *echo-time* ($^1\!/_2$TE), the fleetest steed (F) will have traveled 4 meters, say, and the slowest, about $1^1\!/_2$ m, with the rest in between. In a flash, precisely at $t = {}^1\!/_2$TE, a 180° RF pulse teleports the lead turtle to a point 4 m on the far side of the start/finish line, but leaves her galloping full tilt in the original direction. At the same time, the slowest one is re-positioned $1^1\!/_2$ m from the line, and so on.

(*iii*) Over the next $^1\!/_2$TE, each turtle has exactly the right amount of time needed to reach the line, so they all cross it together exactly at $t = $ TE. Nose-to-nose photo finish!

We even can let them continue to run forward, incidentally, and apply another 180° pulse $^1\!/_2$TE later; then they'll all re-cross together at $t = $ 2TE. And again and again, *ad infinitum*, assuming they don't begin *relaxing*.

The same thing happens to the clusters of protons in a single voxel with spin-echo imaging, except that it is the spin orientation of a cohort of nuclei that is transformed at $^1\!/_2$TE, rather than its spatial location (Figure 11.26b).

Before anything happens, the magnetization is aligned completely along the z-axis, $M(t = 0) = M_z(0)$. (If, but only if, the system has been undisturbed for a good while and establishes thermal equilibrium, then $M(0) = M_0$.)

(*i*) The spin-echo sequence, 90°–$^1\!/_2$TE–180°– TE, begins with the 90° excitation at $t = 0$, with the RF field B_{RF} pointing along the y-axis. Immediately thereafter, all the spins lie along the x-axis.

(*ii*) The system is left alone for a while, during which time the spins de-phase, because of the fixed imperfections in the local magnetic field, ΔB_0 and $\Delta\chi$: any proton that happens to reside in a slightly above-average local field precesses a little faster and further than the average proton, leading to a spreading out and shortening of the net magnetization, $M(t)$.

(*iii*) At $t = {}^1\!/_2$TE, a 180° pulse is applied, either twice as strong or as long in duration as a 90° pulse. It transforms every proton spin to its mirror-image orientation relative to the x-axis, but precessing in the same direction as before.

(*iv*) Over another period of $^1\!/_2$TE, every spin precesses back to the x-axis.

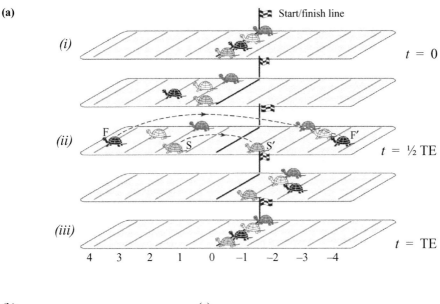

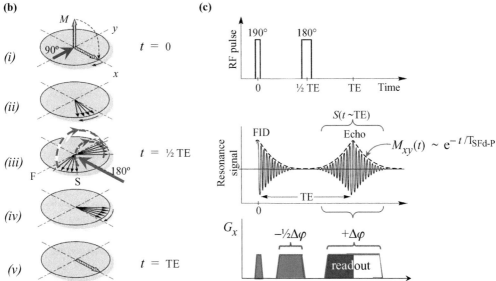

Figure 11.26 The spin-echo (S-E) process. (a) The First (Annual) Shall Be Last Kentucky Turtle Derby race begins at time $t = 0$. Exactly at $t = \frac{1}{2}TE$, each turtle is snapped to the other side of the start/finish line, facing the same direction and the same distance from it as just before the teleporting. They cross the line together at TE. (b) Spin-echo operates the same way. (i) The net magnetization of a voxel, pointing up along the z-axis, is nutated rapidly down into the x-y plane at $t = 0$ by a 90° pulse. (ii) There, $M_{xy}(t)$ precesses at the nominal Larmor frequency, but some clusters of protons in the voxel experience **static** local fields slightly higher or lower than average, because of SFd-P effects, so their orientations spread out in the x-y plane. This de-phasing causes the amplitude of $M_{xy}(t)$ to diminish over time. (iii) At $t = \frac{1}{2}TE$, a 180° Larmor frequency pulse flips all the spin packets precessing in the x-y plane back across their "starting" line. (iv) If and only if the local magnetic fields present are *static*, unchanging over time, then each packet will continue to precess in the same direction at its own fixed speed, and (v) they all recombine to form an echo at TE, and the amplitude of the echo will be the same as that of the FID signal at $t = 0$. S-E thus removes from the picture the effect of small static fields, which are generally biologically uninteresting and clinically useless anyway. (c) A more realistic spin-echo sequence consists of two RF pulses and three G_x pulses. The readout gradient is red and white. But there is also a prior anti-de-phasing pulse (blue), half as long in duration as the readout on-time. It is intended to counteract, in advance, the first half of the de-phasing caused by the readout gradient ($\Delta\varphi$) itself; that way, maximal overall re-phasing will occur at the center of the readout process, at the peak of the echo. The initial slice-selection gradient in green will be discussed in Chapter 12.

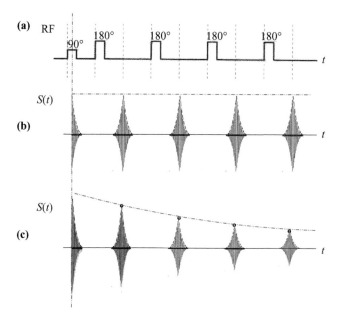

(a) RF

90°   180°   180°   180°   180°

t

(b) S(t)

t

(c) S(t)

t

Figure 11.27 Spin multiple echo. **(a)** Application of multiple 180° pulses, resulting in a train of echoes. **(b)** If all magnetic field irregularities are static, not changing in time, and there are no spin relaxation or other decay processes at play, then the amplitudes of the echoes will be the same. **(c)** Reality, when relaxation is incorporated, is far more entertaining!

(*v*) All the spins will have come back together again briefly, and will cross the *x*-axis in unison at *t* = TE, to create an echo, which is what is detected and utilized in creating an image.

One has the option of waiting another $\frac{1}{2}$TE longer, injecting a new 180° pulse, and then picking up a second echo, and so on (Figure 11.27a). In the (unrealistic) absence of relaxation mechanisms, the echoes will all have the same amplitude (Figure 11.27b). As Chapter 12 will demonstrate, however, things are much more interesting in the real world (Figure 11.27c).

Important point: since the spin de-phasing is caused entirely by static inhomogeneities in the magnetic field, which do not change over time, the amplitude of the signal from the echo magnetization at *t* = TE will be the same as that from the initial magnetization at *t* = 0. (We are still ignoring T1 and T2 relaxation effects.) For a brief instant, at exactly *t* = TE, the de-phasing caused by the static field non-uniformities is completely reversed. That is, spin-echo has completely eliminated from the echo signal (albeit only briefly, and exactly at *t* = TE) the effects of slight variations in the *static* magnetic fields from point to point within a voxel, as if no static-field de-phasing had ever occurred! Those slight static fields are biologically useless anyway, for the most part, and without spin-echo, they would just rapidly wipe out the NMR/MRI signal.

At the conclusion of the spin-echo run, the echo RF signal is detected by the pick-up coil, amplified, commonly demodulated (shifted way down in frequency, for instrumental reasons), sampled 512 or more times (Figure 11.23) and digitized, and sent to the computer for Fourier untangling.

A more complete spin-echo sequence of Figure 11.26c would include three separate *x*-gradient pulses. The brief initial one (green), turned on during the 90° RF pulse, has to do with the selection of a particular slice of tissues to be imaged, as will be discussed in the next chapter. The readout gradient following the 180° RF pulse is in red and white. There is also another, related feature that is probably surprising: an *x*-gradient (in blue) is turned on *before* the 180° pulse, and it is half as long as that used for signal readout. The reason is that whenever any gradient is activated, it will cause de-phasing of spins. This is sometimes intentional, such as in gradient-echo imaging, but usually it is not; rather, it comes along for the ride when a gradient is applied for other reasons, and it is desirable to at least partially undo such non-productive de-phasing, if possible. Because the *x*-gradient must be on during the readout process, in particular, it itself induces a cumulative phase shift of $+\frac{1}{2}\Delta\varphi$, say, as the echo signal reaches its peak, midway through reading, and another $+\frac{1}{2}\Delta\varphi$ by the time the read gradient is finally turned off. This will alter the information content of the MR signal, and can be disruptive during image reconstruction. We cannot do away with the problem altogether, but it is possible to reduce its impact by counteracting the first $+\frac{1}{2}\Delta\varphi$

with an intentional de-phasing *in the opposite direction*, by the amount $-\frac{1}{2}\Delta\varphi$. This pre-emptive blue de-phasing will cancel the red portion of the gradient near the middle of the reading process, which is a good place for that to happen. At first glance, incidentally, it may seem that the red de-phasing gradient would *add* to the blue, exacerbating the situation rather than countermanding it; that would, indeed, be so if it had been inserted after the 180° RF pulse, rather than before it.

To summarize: values of ΔB_0 or $\Delta\chi$ may well produce slight inhomogeneities within a voxel, but they remain constant over time. Spin-echo can therefore reverse and cancel out the T_{SFd-P} part (but only that part) of the spin de-phasing that is caused by these clinically uninteresting, frozen-in field irregularities, so that they have no impact on the MR signal. At the same time, it generates echoes that can be harvested to create splendid MR images.

MRI instrumentation

In 1971, the American physician and entrepreneur Raymond Damadian found that tissues surgically removed from various organs in rats may have NMR relaxation times significantly different from one another. Damadian learned, moreover, that tumors in some organs tend to have measurably longer relaxation times than do the corresponding healthy tissues. He proposed that a device be built to monitor relaxation times coming from different places within the body, but did not go far in explaining how to do it.

An American physicist, Paul Lauterbur, subsequently devised a way in which gradient fields made it possible to distinguish the NMR signals coming from different parts of the body from one another – his method builds upon and extends the 1D broadband technique described above – and in 1973 he published in *Nature* the first two-dimensional MRI image, that of a clam his daughter had found at the beach.

In 1977, after constructing the first whole-body MRI scanner, named "Indomitable" and now on permanent display at the Smithsonian Institution in Washington, DC, Damadian began producing images, too (Figure 11.28). These early efforts,

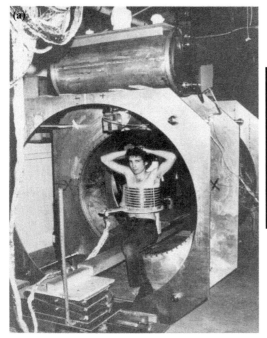
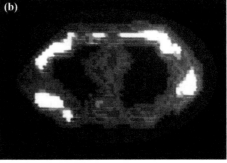

Figure 11.28 The early days of MRI. (a) The first whole-body MRI scanner, "Indomitable," built by Raymond Damadian, MD, in 1977, seen here with slender Dr. Lawrence Minkoff in the seat of honor surrounded by the electromagnet. Damadian himself served as the lead-off guinea pig, but was too large for the machine to produce an adequate signal. (b) Indomitable's first image, of Minkoff's chest, took nearly five hours to generate. Courtesy of the FONAR Corporation.

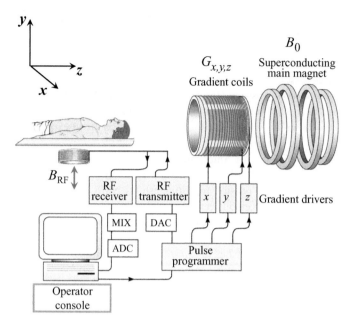

Figure 11.29 In a superconducting MRI device, the patient is bathed in the strong, static, and highly uniform field, B_0, produced by the principal magnet and pointing along the horizontal z-axis. The three gradient coils generate three independent gradient magnetic fields; for each, the field itself also points always in the z-direction, parallel to B_0, but with a strength that varies linearly along the x-, y-, or z-axis. The RF coils (radiating radiofrequency power that is produced by the RF transmitter) induce signals in the body, and the RF echo signals emerging immediately back from it are detected by these or other coils, sent to the receiver, and then analyzed by the computer. DAC, digital-to-analog converter; ADC, analog-to-digital converter; MIX, "Mixer" to shift the RF signal down to an intermediate frequency that is more manageable by the electronics.

followed by the work of hundreds of others, notably the British physicist Peter Mansfield, led to the development of MRI machines that can now map out spatial variations in T1 or T2, rapidly, in exquisitely fine detail, and with superb soft-tissue contrast – providing useful information not just about anatomy, but also on the physiology of cells, and even on their state of health. For their contributions, Lauterbur and Mansfield were awarded the 2003 Nobel Prize in Physiology or Medicine. Damadian's company, FONAR, took out full-page ads in the *New York Times* and the *Washington Post* protesting his omission, a "shameful wrong that must be righted," and some researchers in the field have been inclined to agree. It may, or may not, have been relevant that Damadian was an avowed creationist, hence not worthy, in the minds of some, of such public recognition as a scientist. Needless to say, this is not the only decision that the Nobel Committee has made over the years that has stirred up controversy.

The MRI system

A modern MRI system (Figure 11.29 and Box 11.3) consists of three major pieces of highly specialized hardware, plus a computer:

The patient is immersed in the very strong, constant, highly uniform *principal magnetic field*,

in this case generated by a horizontally aligned superconducting magnet.

Three *gradient field* electromagnet coils are energized intermittently by the gradient drivers.

The radiofrequency electronics and coils generate and radiate brief pulses of electromagnetic energy, centered at or about the Larmor frequency, that penetrate into the patient. The same coils (or others that are placed directly against the patient's body for greater sensitivity) then sense the weak resonance echo signals produced immediately by the body.

Box 11.3   Major components of a typical MRI system.

Principal magnet	*RF system*
Superconducting magnet	Transmitter
(electromagnet)	Transmit/receive RF
(permanent magnet)	coils head, body
Homogeneity correction	parallel
shim plates, coils	Quadrature
Anti-fringe shielding coils	detection
Gradient field coils	*Computer control*
Gradient drivers	Operator console
	PACS

Spatial resolution: 1 mm, 512 × 512 matrix
Slice thickness, 2D: 1 mm; 3D: 0.05 mm
FOV: 50 cm

The precise timing and shaping of the RF pulses and of the gradient fields are determined by the pulse programmer, which itself is under computer control. When not running the procedures involved in generating and acquiring the raw MRI data, the computer performs the separate tasks of analyzing the data and reconstructing and processing images for display. It normally prepares images in the DICOM format for entry into a PACS.

The principal magnetic field, B_0, and the three field gradients, G_x, G_y, and G_z

The component of a commercial machine that the patient comes into direct contact with is the *principal magnet*. This must produce a field, B_0, that is strong, most commonly 1.5 T, but in any case between 0.3 T and 3.0 T. The field must also be constant over time, and highly uniform throughout a volume of space large enough to accommodate a good portion of a body, to within a few parts per million. Passive *shim plates* usually are carefully positioned at installation to reduce field distortions, and the adjustment of low currents through active *shim coils* provides fine-tuning thereafter.

The principal magnet can be any of three, radically different types: permanent magnet, electromagnet, and superconducting magnet, in order of increasing field strength. With permanent magnets, the field is frozen into place in large, heavy blocks of ferromagnetic alloy. Electro- and superconducting magnets, on the other hand, create the principal field with electrical currents in large-diameter coils of wire. As a general rule, permanent and electromagnets are used to produce vertically aligned, lower-strength fields, while that of a supercon is generally horizontal. In any case, the direction of the principal field, B_0, is universally taken to define the z-direction of the applicable coordinate system.

The vast majority of modern MRI devices employ a superconducting magnet that produces a field typically 1.5 tesla in strength. Increasingly (and far more expensively) 3 T devices are also commercially available, with significantly improved signal-to-noise ratio. The field is created by something like 50 km of precisely wound superconducting wire that can carry hundreds of amperes of current. Niobium-titanium alloy, for example, can conduct electricity with absolutely no resistance, so that no power input is required to keep the current (hence the magnetic field) going forever. But to achieve and maintain the superconducting condition, the entire coil must be immersed in liquid helium contained within a cryostat (a highly specialized thermos/Dewar bottle) at temperature just above absolute zero (0 K; −273 °C; −460 °F) (Figure 11.30a). Intense research activity is under way to find more substances, for a wide variety of applications, that remain superconducting above liquid

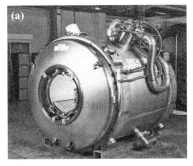
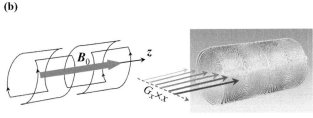

Figure 11.30 1.5 T MRI magnet. **(a)** The superconducting wires of the principal magnet are cooled by liquid helium (typically 2000 L) within a stainless steel Dewar/thermos vessel, to maintain them at an extremely low temperature, near absolute zero. Courtesy of Oxford Magnet Technology Limited, Oxford, UK. **(b)** The three independent gradient coils, which are non-superconducting, are built to fit just inside the cylindrical bore-hole of the superconducting magnet. For the G_x coil, the magnetic field everywhere points along the principal field, B_0, but its strength increases linearly with position in the x-direction. The general flow of current in an x-gradient coil is simpler in concept than in practice: design for one of multiple layers of windings. Important parameters describing the capabilities of a gradient coil are the *gradient* or slope of the field, dB_z/dx, which ranges typically from 20 to 60 mT/meter; the *rise time*, about 0.25 ms; and the *slew rate*, 50−200 mT/m/ms.

nitrogen temperatures (–77 °C), perhaps even at room temperature, but those created to date lose their superconductivity in the presence of a strong magnetic field, and they have tended to be brittle and difficult to produce in the form of wire. Three recent trends in supercon magnet design have been toward bore-holes that are shorter in length and greater in diameters, and higher in field strengths. The first two are primarily for patient comfort, but both make it harder to achieve the third.

The *x-, y-, z-gradient magnetic fields* are produced by three independent *gradient coils* (Figure 11.30b), which are intermittently energized by the *gradient drivers*, highly specialized high-power audio amplifiers. They are much weaker than the principal field, with the *gradient strength* ranging up to 50 millitesla/meter for a 1.5 T machine – so that over a 0.4 m wide FOV, the field strength varies by 0.02 T. A *rise time* (to achieve 90% of maximum gradient) of $1/4$ ms (250 μs) is typical for normal body imaging, and a gradient is pulsed "on" for only milliseconds at a time. These two measures of gradient performance are combined to give a *slew rate*, which can now approach 200 mT/m/ms (or T/m/s). Although gradient fields do not receive the attention from sales people that the main magnetic field does, gradient field strength and rise time have just as significant an effect on instrument flexibility and performance.

The RF system is like a radio transmitter/receiver pair

The transmission and reception of the radiofrequency power in MRI are very much like (but more complex than) what happens with a simple amplitude modulation (AM) radio (Figure 11.31a).

As the initial step, an AM radio transmitter, to the left, generates a nearly monochromatic RF *carrier* signal which, for commercial broadcasting in the United States, lies between 535 and 1605 kHz. Audio information of much lower frequencies is introduced by "modulating" the amplitude of the carrier (Figure 4.11a). If the carrier happens to be at 64 MHz and the information to be conveyed is, for example, a pure 4000 Hz tone, then the amplitude of the carrier is made to vary at that frequency. A spectral (Fourier) analysis of the resultant signal would reveal not only a peak at the carrier frequency, but also a pair of others, 4 kHz above and below it,

at 63.996 MHz and 64.004 MHz. It is they that are bearing the information of interest, the 4 kHz audio signal. The carrier is there just to drive the bus.

Detection of the radio signal by the antenna and receiver involves tuning to the carrier frequency, filtering out and rejecting signals and noise at all other frequencies outside a suitably narrow receiver bandwidth. The original audio signal is re-gained by "rectifying" and smoothing the RF – and becomes a pure 4 kHz tone, again, that can now be amplified and sent to the speakers. AM radio transmission thus involves producing and detecting modulated RF electromagnetic radiation that falls within a narrow band of frequencies.

A similar situation exists for MRI (Figure 11.29). Instead of audio modulation, though, a *pulse programmer* forms very brief pulses of precise and highly specialized shapes (more sophisticated than just on-off) out of the carrier RF, which is typically at about 64 MHz at 1.5 T and of power up to 30 kW – enough to energize 300 light bulbs, at least for a few milliseconds at a time. If a magnetic field gradient is also to be applied, the carrier cannot be strictly monochromatic; rather, it must contain a band of frequencies about as wide as the gradient-induced spread in Larmor frequencies. The BW of the RF generator, amplifiers, and other electronic equipment of the transmitter must be broad enough to accommodate this range of Larmor frequencies, but still narrow enough to exclude most extraneous noise.

The detection process for the NMR signal is more subtle than for a simple radio and commonly uses *quadrature detection*, with a *pair* of coils that point perpendicular to one another (and to B_0). The precessing magnetization therefore sweeps through one of them $1/4$ cycle ahead of the other; their *signals* are almost exactly identical, but 90° out of phase. The higher-frequency stochastic *noise* experienced by each, on the other hand, changes much more rapidly than f_{Larmor}, so the noise from the two will be completely uncorrelated. Quadrature detection intentionally shifts one coil signal by 90°, so that the voltages from the two are now fully in phase, and simply adds the two together. This doubles the signal strength, but largely averages and cancels out the noise, with a $\sqrt{2}$ improvement in the SNR.

The objective of transmission (the creation of an intense and uniform RF field) differs from that of

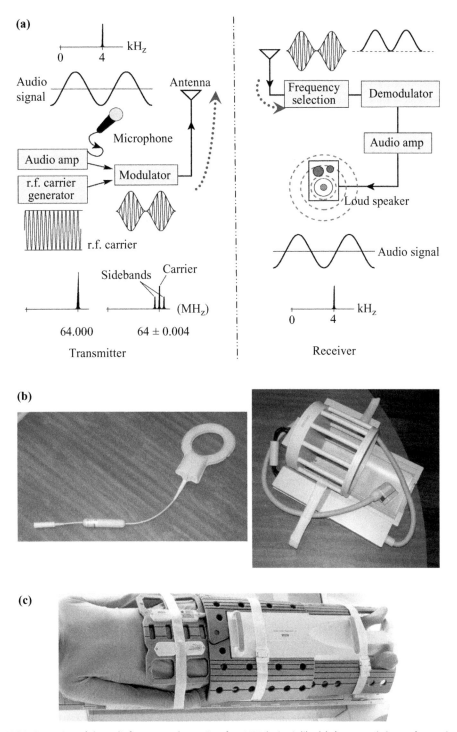

Figure 11.31 Operation of the radiofrequency electronics of an MRI device is like **(a)** the transmission and reception of an AM radio signal. **(b)** The RF receive coil(s) fit close to the patient, for greatest sensitivity. **(c)** Phased arrays of independent receiver coils have proved effective in improving both SNR and speed of data acquisition. This 16-element coil provides coverage from the pelvis to the feet. Courtesy of Nathan Yanasak, Georgia Regents University, Augusta.

reception (sensitivity to weak signals from within the patient), so separate and differently designed coils are used for some applications. In examination of the head, for example, signal-to-noise can be enhanced significantly with a so-called *birdcage* coil that surrounds it (Figure 11.31b).

The SNR improves with a smaller detection coil, but this also reduces the volume of tissue from which it can accumulate data. One solution to this dilemma is to perform MRI a number of times sequentially, moving a small coil to a new location after each study. A much faster approach is to employ *parallel* reception (pMRI). A *phased array* of multiple small coils is distributed over the region of interest (Figure 11.31c). Data acquisition speed increases with the number of independent receive coils, and currently as many as 128 of them spread out over the body simultaneously listen for the echo. Combining the separate coil signals in a meaningful manner is complicated, but the technology is becoming available. The standard measure of the increase in speed is known as the *acceleration factor*. Researchers are busy finding ways to take the next step, and synchronously transmit from more than one coil.

Quality assurance

An MRI machine is arguably the most complex and sophisticated of commercial medical imaging instruments, and initial adjustment and acceptance of a new or significantly altered machine can require a good deal of time and effort by qualified medical physicists and engineers. Also essential are periodic preventative maintenance (PM) visits by the manufacturer's or other qualified engineers, and a comprehensive program of routine QA checks by a medical physicist or so-called "MRI scientist."

Issues of concern in routine and in comprehensive annual surveys are the homogeneity of the principal magnetic field, the contrast and the SNR of the system as assessed with appropriate test phantoms within the bore, the characteristics of the detection coils, and much else. The machine tends to be quite stable, however, and its routine QA under normal conditions, including the largely automated daily check, is not very onerous. Box 11.4 lists some of the basic tests to be undertaken weekly by technologists and semi-annually by specialists. There is much QA documentation in the literature, of course, such as the AAPM's 2010 report [1]

Box 11.4 Typical QA issues for a superconducting-magnet MRI system.	
Technologist, weekly	**Physicist, semi-annual**
Visual checklist	Magnetic field homogeneity
Safety program	RF bandwidth, tuning
Center frequency and	Gradient linearity
field strength	RF coil efficiency
High-contrast	Image intensity uniformity
resolution	Low-contrast detectability
Artifact analysis	Slice thickness/position
Setup and scanning	accuracy
Geometric accuracy	Inter-slice RF interference
Table positioning	Monitors

As with mammography, CT, and ultrasound, the American College of Radiology has established a comprehensive process for ACR certification of MRI devices, like that discussed in Chapter 8 for CT. It involves examination of the training and experience of physicians, technologists, and technical staff (medical physicist or "MRI scientist"); sample images obtained both from typical patients and from the specially designed ACR MRI phantom (Figure 11.32); and the results of specific tests of machine performance. In addition, the

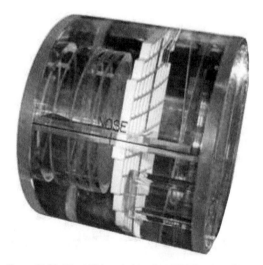

Figure 11.32 The ACR has designed an MRI phantom that allows the assessment of seven important imaging parameters: low-contrast object detectability; image intensity uniformity; high-contrast spatial resolution; slice thickness accuracy; slice position accuracy; geometric accuracy; and percent signal ghosting. With permission from the American College of Radiology.

comprehensive program for weekly and annual QA must be submitted, along with copies of representative reports.

Biological effects of the principal, gradient, and RF fields

MRI does not use ionizing radiation, and the absence of radiation dose is commonly touted as a great advantage. But an MRI machine employs extremely strong static magnetic fields, rapidly switching gradient fields, and high levels of RF power. The FDA has reported that there are about 40 MRI-related incidents per year in the USA, 10% of which involve metallic "missiles," but 70% of which are RF-induced burns. MRI is potentially very dangerous, and it must be treated with great caution, and a program to ensure the safety of patients, staff, and others is essential.

The effects on tissues of intense static magnetic fields, of rapidly switched gradient fields, and of RF power have been studied extensively. The FDA, the ACR, state Departments of Health, and other bodies publish recommendations and requirements regarding limits on the principal magnetic field strength, the rate of switching gradient fields, RF power levels, and so on, which are thought to be protective of the patient. The FDA couches its RF recommendations, for example, in terms both of *tissue temperature changes* and of the *specific absorption rate*, a measure of the rate at which RF energy (measured in watts per kilogram of tissue) is deposited within the patient: SAR = power/mass (W/kg). SAR depends on, among other things, tissue density and electrical conductivity, patient size, and the strength of the electric field of the RF pulses. It also increases with the principal magnetic field strength roughly as $B_0{}^2$, so that going from a 1.5 T field to 3.0 T may roughly double the SNR (not just increase it by $\sqrt{2}$, for several reasons), but it also quadruples the rate at which high-frequency power is pumped into tissues. The FDA provides recommendations not only on the values of SAR, but also on acceptable resulting maximum temperatures and temperature changes in various parts of the body. They also recommend that the application of the gradient fields cause no peripheral nerve stimulation, which rapidly changing, strong magnetic fields can do.

RF fields and rapidly switching gradients can induce currents and heat electrode wires or other metal objects on or within the patient, and this may lead to serious (albeit localized) burns. In addition, they can strongly disrupt the operation of most cardiac pacemakers and other electronic devices, which therefore should not be allowed near the MRI device. Methods are being developed to envelop some of these items with special materials to shield them (and the patient) from the effects of RF fields. In any case, it makes sense to exercise great caution, especially in examining pregnant women, small infants, and patients on life support systems.

An MRI machine, of course, must not be disturbed by, nor affect, the outside world. It is necessary to keep out the changing magnetic fields and RF noise produced by passing trucks and elevators and by flickering fluorescent lights. At the same time, medical electronic gear in the area, which may be very sensitive to the presence of various magnetic fields, must be protected from those of the MRI system. The necessary isolation can be achieved by means of suitable magnetic (for B_0 and B_{grad}) and electromagnetic (B_{RF}) *shielding*. The RF and, to some extent, the switching gradient problems can be solved through construction of a *Faraday cage*, a wire-mesh or solid metal panel enclosure around the patient (and RF coil) area.

Finally, and a little unrelated, a severe problem can arise from the use of gadolinium contrast agent. It has been found that associated with Gd, there is a small but serious risk of nephrogenic systemic fibrosis (NSF) in a few patients – in particular those with renal disease; severe hepatic disease; history of hypertension; history of diabetes; or age over 60. The FDA recently called for pre-screening for glomerular filtration rate (GFR) before contrast is used. It also recommends that pregnant patients *generally* avoid Gd-contrast.

Beware of aneurysm clips, pacemakers, and also flying screwdrivers, wheelchairs, and O$_2$ bottles

While the absence of ionizing radiation is one of MRI's many virtues, the machines have nonetheless been known to kill – and much more quickly and directly than any CT's X-rays ever did (Box 11.5).

The principal magnetic field is extremely strong, fills a large volume, and extends some distance beyond the bore. A screwdriver suspended in air at the center of a magnet ended up there because

Box 11.5   Eternal vigilance is the word with regard to MRI safety.
Magnetizable objects, such as some pieces of shrapnel, pins, or aneurysm clips, may reside within the body of a patient or staff member; if tugged out of place by a fringe field of the principal magnet, the damage can be fatal. Likewise, magnetizable scissors, pens, and small tool boxes flying across the room and into the magnet bore hole can also cause lethal injuries. There have been unfortunate incidents involving oxygen bottles and police guns, for example, because of lax checking of *everyone* entering the imaging suite.

in/into imaging suite	with/within patient/others
hemostat, scalpel, syringe, scissors, stethoscope, pen, mechanical pencil, phone, DPA, laptop, medical electronics, small tool, tool chest, O_2 bottle, IV pole, wheelchair, gurney, flashlight, clipboard, ax, fire extinguisher, keys, gun, handcuffs, cleaning bucket, mop. watch, credit card, . . .	aneurysm clip, shrapnel, cochlear implant, prostheses, stent, artificial heart valve, electrodes, defibrillator, pacemaker, nerve stimulator, medical infusion pump breathing apparatus, permanent denture, surgical staples, pins, drug-delivery patch, metallic IUD, tattoo

beyond the two ends of the device, where its fringe fields change rapidly with position, unavoidable gradients exert strong attractive forces on magnetizable objects. Magnetic shielding approaches have been devised that can significantly reduce the impact of fringe fields. Through *passive shielding*, the MRI magnetic fields can largely be confined and other fields excluded, with carefully sculpted steel plates either in proximity to the magnet or in the walls of the imaging room. Additional, weaker superconducting coils or electromagnets at the two ends of the bore can further reduce the fringe fields through *active shielding*. The FDA has recommended that areas where the principal

magnetic field has fallen to below 0.5 mT, about 10 times Earth's own field, are safe for the general public (Figure 11.33).

Still, the fringe fields can exert forces powerful enough to fling a wheelchair or IV pole across the room. The physician or technologist in charge must take active steps to make absolutely certain that access to the magnet room by people and all equipment is stringently restricted. Double-checking of accurate medical records of patients and *staff* can help to ensure that *nobody* comes near the high field who may have within themselves:

an aneurysm clip, surgical pin, shrapnel, plates, stent, surgical staples, metallic intrauterine device, cochlear implant, artificial heart valve, prosthesis, permanent denture, implanted drug infusion port, etc., or

a cardiac pacemaker, defibrillator, medical infusion pump, deep brain or other nerve stimulators, etc., or other potentially magnetizable or electronic items, without careful investigation to confirm that they are safe. Some items will pose no problem, of course, including pacemakers recently approved by the FDA as being MRI-compatible, but it is essential to make sure beforehand. Problems seem to arise most commonly when untrained personnel – housekeeping, maintenance, security, and transport people, police, firemen, parents, non-MRI physicians, nurses and their aids, and other medical staff, etc. – and the items they may be carrying, gain unsupervised access to areas where entry should be strictly restricted. All patients, visitors, and non-MRI staff and apparatus should be questioned, examined visually, and accompanied into the high-field area.

Flying car keys, scissors, and screwdrivers can also cause lethal damage. A firefighter was killed when the air bottle strapped to his back was dragged into the bore, and he with it. In a similar situation, a nurse's assistant placed an oxygen cylinder under a patient's gurney before they went into the scanning room; it was yanked into the bore at high velocity, fortunately before the patient had been positioned there.

Far less critical, of course, but still important is the disruption that an MRI's fields can cause to hearing aids, magnetic credit cards, watches, computer disks, and medical electronic gear. Check out www.mrisafety.com.

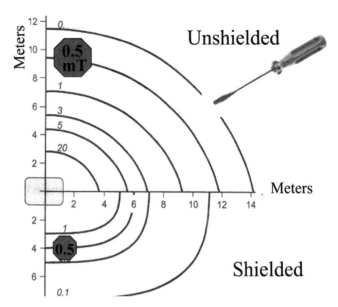

Figure 11.33 One horizontal quadrant of a contour map of the fringe fields surrounding a 1.5 T magnet, both without (upper) and with (below) passive plus active shielding. For this system, the shielding cuts to almost a quarter the area enclosed by the 0.5 mT border, within which access is normally controlled.

Some common-sense, but potentially life-saving, safety measures for medical staff and management: prevent accidents related to magnetic or RF fields or contrast agent before they can occur. Institute a multi-zone design for access to progressively more risky areas around the device, and enforce appropriate physical restrictions on admission to them. Post many, highly visible and/or audible warnings on the hazards in each zone. Institute and enforce appropriate physical restrictions on site access. Even during an emergency, scrutinize all individuals seeking to gain entry. Provide comprehensive training for those who may be coming in and out regularly or dealing with patients, including the need for especial vigilance regarding people or objects that are *not* regulars. Check staff and patient histories carefully. And always, always assume that the main magnetic field is on and potentially very hazardous.

Finally, you may someday be responsible for procuring and installing an MRI machine. First thing to do after you have settled upon a device, before anything else, go over *everything* with your vendor's installation engineers, your own facility's architect and structural engineer, and the state regulator, preferably together, until there is complete agreement. Check that sufficient electrical power, water, and HVAC are available, but that electromagnetic interference and mechanical vibrations at the site will not be excessive. Might that change in

three or five years for any foreseeable reason? There should be sufficient room for easily maneuvering of people and sensitive equipment outside the projected 0.5 mT line. And it really can be *very* cost effective, in the long run, to install a ferrous-metal-detector system for humans and equipment at the entrance to the magnet room to augment other safety procedures. Rarely, a magnet will be intentionally or otherwise *quenched*, where the wires heat and become non-superconducting and rapidly blow off vast amounts of super-cold helium gas; there must be plans to evacuate the gas and the patient immediately, to avoid freezing and asphyxiation. Last but not least, make sure beforehand that the magnet can pass readily into and through *all* the doors, corridors, elevators, *etc.*, and temporary holes in walls, roofs, and floors to and at its final destination, and that *all* the floors can support its multi-ton weight. Yes, there have been little miscalculations . . . . And do bear in mind also that you may eventually choose to remove the machine, or even upgrade it with a larger one.

Reference

1 AAPM. *Acceptance Testing and Quality Assurance Procedures for Magnetic Resonance Imaging Facilities*, report no. 100. College Park, MD: American Association of Physicists in Medicine.

CHAPTER 12

Mapping T1 and T2 Relaxation in Three Dimensions

The "classical" picture of NMR and MRI centers on the net magnetization, $M(t)$, of a cohort of protons in a tissue voxel in a strong magnetic field. So far, it has discussed the special state of thermal equilibrium, $M(t) = M_0$, and also the gyroscope-like precession of $M(t)$ in the x-y plane following a 90° pulse. There has been no consideration, however, of possible *proton spin relaxation* mechanisms. Time now to move on from that simplistic ideal to harsh reality.

Two preliminary comments: in much of this chapter, we shall assume the spin-echo pulse (SE) sequence, so that we can mostly ignore the *Static*

Field spin *de-Phasing* caused by fixed, unchanging magnet field imperfections and susceptibility effects, with associate characteristic time, $T_{\text{SFd-P}}$. They are unrelated to biology, for the most part, and of little clinical value, and with S-E we can generally forget that they exist.

Also, the *rates* at which relaxation processes occur and the associated *relaxation times* are inverses of one another: the faster the rate, the less time the process takes. Physicians tend to discuss the relaxations times that parameterize clinically interesting properties of a tissue, and researchers into the underlying biophysical processes may be more inclined to speak

Medical Imaging: Essentials for Physicians, First Edition. Anthony B. Wolbarst, Patrizio Capasso and Andrew R. Wyant.
© 2013 John Wiley & Sons, Inc. Published 2013 by John Wiley & Sons, Inc.

of the rates at which they take place. Two sides of the same coin.

Longitudinal spin relaxation and T1

The longitudinal spin-relaxation time T1, and the exponential re-growth of $M_z(t)$ toward M_0

The previous chapter concluded the discussion of precessing spins giving rise to a sequence of echo signals, the amplitudes of which were expected to remain constant – but that, when recorded, actually declined over time (Figure 11.27c). Nothing discussed up to that point could explain it.

To do so, indeed, it is now necessary to introduce a radically different concept, that of *relaxation* of a spin system. Relaxation is a common enough everyday physical phenomenon, whether it be the fading away of a church bell, or the settling down of a swinging pendulum or a bobbing mass on a spring. Likewise, after a spin system is disturbed, it undergoes a number of spin-relaxation processes, all on the atomic level. Two of these are particularly important. One is the spontaneously occurring *longitudinal spin-relaxation* of the protons, trying to nudge $M(t)$ back toward M_0. The second is *transverse relaxation*, in which cohorts of protons precessing in the x-y plane lose their mutual phase coherence.

Longitudinal relaxation is simpler to describe, so we shall tackle it first. Let's place a voxel of water in a powerful magnet and switch it on rapidly. Over the next few milliseconds, every proton starts out pointing either up or down, but nowhere else (Figure 11.11b, reproduced in modified form as Figure 12.1a). Initially there are equal numbers of spins pointing up and down, but over time some individual spins spontaneously flip over (we'll see why in a minute). At first, $M(t)$ increases from an initial value of zero linearly with time as, on average, 0, 2μ, 4μ, 6μ, ... (Figure 12.1a,b,c). Some may flip the other way, as well, but since they are moving toward equilibrium, there is a greater tendency to evolve in this direction.

Graphing this phenomenon experimentally over longer times, it becomes apparent that what we have seen is just the early part of an exponential curve that describes the spin system's approach to its final, equilibrium-state magnetization value, M_0, which

has a small but highly significant excess of spins pointing along the external magnetic field (Figure 12.1d). As $M(t)$ moves from $M = 0$ toward that end condition, its sense of urgency to do so diminishes, as does its rate of approach. The shape of the curve describing the process is of the form

$$M_z(t)/M_0 = (1 - e^{-t/\text{T1}}), \qquad (12.1)$$

by an argument similar to those leading to Equations 3.1 and 9.2 and Figure 9.8a. The parameter that characterizes how long this process takes, designated T1, is called the *longitudinal nuclear spin relaxation time* (or sometimes the *spin-lattice relaxation time*, for historical reasons).

From Equation 12.1, T1 can be defined as the time required by the system to go $(1 - e^{-\text{T1}/\text{T1}}) = (1 - e^{-1}) = 0.63$ of the way from a configuration of zero net magnetization to thermal equilibrium. In the figure, the tissue under examination has a T1 = 0.5 seconds. At $t = 2 \times$ T1, $M_z(t)$ reaches 0.86 M_0, and so on. Re-growth/relaxation curves for three different materials and T1-values appear in Figure 12.1e.

Biophysical mechanisms of T1 relaxation: random f_{Larmor} fluctuations in $B_{\text{local}}(t)$ cause proton spin-state transitions

After being disturbed, a system of proton spins evolves unaided toward thermal equilibrium. This presumably involves spin flips – but, after the RF is turned off, what is making them take place?

Analysis of the relevant physics reveals that the NMR interaction is different, in a fundamental way, from the photon-*electron* interactions that play central roles in gamma- and X-ray imaging. With photoelectric and Compton interactions, it is primarily the *electric field* of the photon that exerts a force on a (charged) atomic electron, resulting in a change in its orbital quantum state, along with absorption or scattering of the photon. With NMR, by contrast, it is the rapidly oscillating *magnetic field* component of the incident Larmor-frequency electromagnetic radiation that interacts with the magnetic moment of the nucleus and brings about a change in the nuclear spin orientation quantum state.

This suggests that *any* magnetic field that happens to be varying at the Larmor frequency (not just one from an RF photon pumped in by an RF transmitter and coil) could couple with a proton

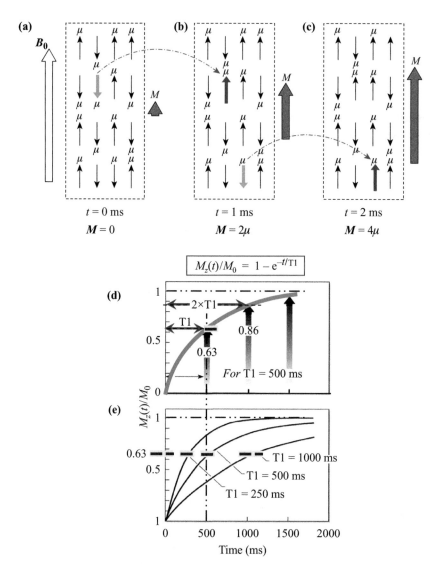

Figure 12.1 A magnetic field, B_0, is switched on abruptly, and the net magnetization, M, of a voxel of water protons relaxes exponentially toward its thermal equilibrium value, M_0, with characteristic time T1, that is, at the rate 1/T1. **(a)** Immediately after the field is switched on, at time $t = 0+$, equal numbers of protons point up and down, and $M(0+) = 0$. **(b,c)** But individual spins will flip over, both up and down, independently of one another; more will flip into the lower-energy state, however, than the other way, at first. And initially, until about the time 0.1 T1, the net magnetization will tend to move toward M_0, on average, linearly in time. Early on, that is, the number that do so is nearly linearly proportional to the time. **(d)** Over a longer period of time, the net longitudinal magnetization curve is of the form $M_z(t)/M_0 = (1 - e^{-t/T1})$ (which does start off, for small t, as a straight line). At the particular time $t = T1$, $M_z (T1)/M_0 = 0.63$ which provides the quantitative definition of T1. Much later, after the passage of 10 T1 or so, say, protons will be flipping up and down at the same rate; that is, the magnitude of the net magnetization will hold steady at M_0, but the state of equilibrium is a dynamic one. **(e)** T1 spin relaxation for three materials with T1 of 500 milliseconds, 1000 ms, and 1500 ms, respectively.

to elevate it from its lower- into its higher-energy spin state. Just as likely, for reasons explained by quantum mechanics, it can tickle a proton sitting in its higher-energy state down into the lower one. That is, if there happen to be naturally occurring magnetic fields present with a component fluctuating at the Larmor frequency, then those fields are perfectly capable of stimulating a proton flip, either up or down. And if the system is not sitting at thermal equilibrium, then the Larmor-frequency component of the naturally fluctuating local magnetic field that the protons experience will drive it over time, for the most part, preferentially toward that condition.

Once again, because this is such an important idea: Larmor-frequency magnetic fields, whether coming from an RF pulse or arising spontaneously in a material, not only can excite a ground-state proton into its excited spin-state, but also can tickle it out of the higher state back down to the ground state, with the release of an RF photon or of some vibrational energy that dissipates as a tiny amount of heat. So the population dynamics of protons in a strong field are generally not static, but rather they are churning away with protons everywhere continually flopping up and down like mad. But during all this, there is an overwhelming tendency to drive the magnetization of a voxel, over a period of the order of T1, relentlessly toward M_0.

There are a number of ways that protons can themselves produce and be subjected to spontaneous, random fluctuations in the local magnetic field. The most important involves the magnetic interaction between the two hydrogen nuclei of the same water molecule as it rotates and collides with other molecules. The spin axis of each proton, and the magnetic field it produces, remains pointing along or against the external magnetic field, so the strength of the weak field from one proton overlapping its partner is determined, at any moment, by their instantaneous relative positions in the external field (Figure 12.2a). As a water molecule rotates, the amount of proton-proton field overlap will also change, at the molecular rotation frequency. And whenever a water molecule happens to be tumbling at the Larmor frequency, in particular, then the local magnetic dipole fields at each of the two protons will also cycle at that rate – and it is such naturally occurring Larmor-frequency fields that stimulate

proton spin-state transitions. The larger the fraction of water molecules in a sample for which this is occurring, the faster that T1-type relaxation occurs, and the shorter T1.

The above discussion drives straight to the heart of the matter: the only thing a proton is ever aware of, or reacts to, is the local magnetic field, $B_{local}(t)$, that it experiences (Box 12.1). So we can rephrase this as: how many water protons are experiencing f_{Larmor} magnetic fields? Or, almost equivalently, how many of a cell's water molecules will be rotating, at any instant, at the Larmor frequency?

Box 12.1   In MRI, the *only* thing a proton is *ever* aware of, or reacts to, is the *local magnetic field*, $B_{local}(t)$.

!!!

The motions of the water molecules within a voxel of tissue are strongly influenced by how tightly they are interacting with various ions or biomolecules in solution or with the cellular membranes. It simplifies matters to think of a tissue as comprising three distinct and separate sub-populations of water molecules (Figure 12.2b): those that are essentially free water; those bound tightly to membranes or to massive molecules; and those in between, that are attached moderately loosely (so that they can come and go fairly easily) to intermediate-sized biomolecules.

Consider first a "free" H_2O molecule surrounded only by pure water, the lowest curve in Figure 12.3a. It will rotate briefly about some axis in space, bang into another water molecule, rotate at a different rate about another axis, collide again, and so on. Because they are small and light, many free water molecules will be off far to the right in the figure, rotating at rates much higher than the Larmor frequency. It may be surprising, but there will also be a wide range of other motions that the waters are undergoing. Some will even be moving at frequencies down near zero, to the left in the figure. The spectrum of local magnetic "noise" frequencies for the free water sample as a whole is flat and broad, so the relative number causing magnetic field fluctuation at the Larmor frequency, in particular, will be small. For those free water molecules that *do* happen

(a)

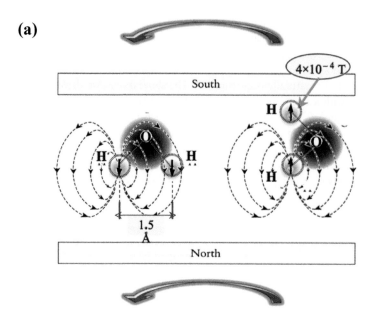

(b)   **Bound**   **Hydration**   **Free**

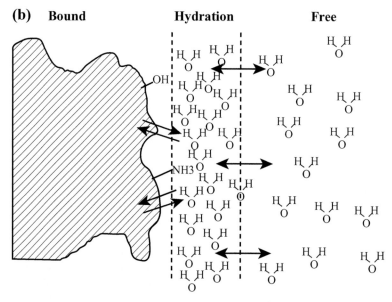

Figure 12.2 The principal T1 relaxation mechanism for water: inter-proton magnetic dipole-dipole interactions within the same molecule. **(a)** Each hydrogen nucleus of the water molecule aligns either along or against the strong external magnetic field, and generally stays that way. But a proton experiences also the small magnetic dipole field created by its partner proton. (The separation of the protons in water is about 1.5 angstroms, where $1\,\text{Å} = 10^{-10}$ m, and the maximum field generated this way, 4×10^{-4} T, is greater than that of the RF typically produced by the system's transmitter and coil.) If the molecule happens to be tumbling naturally at the Larmor frequency, then the resulting f_{Larmor}-field can induce spin transitions either up or down in energy. **(b)** T1 depends on the tightness of the bonds between water molecules and the various cellular biomolecules, and on the viscosity of the cellular fluid. Both affect the rate at which the water molecules move about, and the likelihood that they will experience naturally occurring Larmor-frequency fields. One can view the behavior of water molecules as if they exist in three different local environments: free water, in which most (but not all) molecules rotate much faster than f_{Larmor}; water bound tightly to large, slow-moving macromolecules and membranes; and water in between these extremes, such as in a layer of hydration, which is of greatest interest for T1. In reality, of course, these three zones form a continuum.

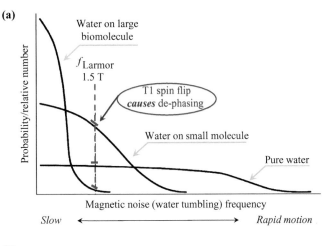

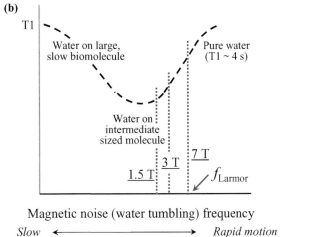

Figure 12.3 The rate of longitudinal relaxation, 1/T1, is proportional to the number of protons that are tumbling at about the rate f_{Larmor} and therefore experiencing magnetic "noise" with a significant component at that frequency. That, in turn, depends largely on how many are in "free" water, on the sizes of the biomolecules to which others tend to attach, and on the strength of those attachments. (a) The rotational spectrum for pure water is wide and flat, giving rise to only a small amount of Larmor-frequency magnetic noise. Likewise, few water molecules that are bound to the large, slowly moving macromolecules will experience Larmor-frequency fields. The greatest contribution to relaxation comes from water held loosely to large molecules or membranes, or adhering to those of mid-size. (b) For that reason, it is the waters on intermediate-size molecules that are most responsible for the rate 1/T1, and for the relaxation time T1. As f_{Larmor} moves from that at $B_0 = 1.5$ T to 3.0 T and 7.0 T and perhaps higher, T1 values tend to lengthen, roughly as $B_0^{1/3}$. Probably more important is the improvement in SNR (See Figure 11.12a).

to be moving about near f_{Larmor}, and thereby generating magnetic "noise" for each partner proton at that frequency, protons may undergo spin-state relaxation transitions. Relatively few protons will be doing this, however, and if that were the whole story, T1 would be long (Figure 12.3b).

Likewise, for water connected firmly to membranes or to large macromolecules that tumble very slowly, each proton again would experience an overlap field from its partner that varies at the tumble frequencies. But those tend to be much *lower* than the proton Larmor frequency at 1.5 T. There will be relatively few of them able to undergo relaxation, so again T1 is long.

That leaves the third category, water bound loosely and intermittently in the hydration layers of macromolecules, or held to mid-sized biomolecules

that are themselves rotating much more slowly than free water because of their greater mass and friction-like forces dragging on them. The tightness of the binding and the extent to which that will hinder rotation depend on the macromolecule's chemical makeup and three-dimensional structure, and on its tendency to hold onto water of hydration. A fair amount of such water may end up rotating at rates close to the Larmor frequency – and protons in this sub-population, unlike those in the other two groups, may undergo relaxation at a fast rate, causing the tissue to display relatively *short* T1.

Numerous normal and abnormal physiologic processes affect the amounts of water residing within and between cells, the concentrations of certain specific molecules or organelle parts, the binding of water to the cellular contents, the viscosity and ionicity of the solution, and other factors. The type and status of health of a tissue determine how much water is in its cells, where it is located, what is dissolved or suspended in it, and what it has latched onto, all of which is reflected in the measured values of relaxation times. This is why spatial variations in the values of T1 are of such interest: because water proton spin relaxation times depend on cell-type, T1-MRI can distinguish one tissue or organ from another. Because they also reflect the physiological status of a tissue, MRI may even reveal pathological conditions. The story for T2 is similar but different, and we shall turn to it soon.

We have focused attention, so far, on the protons of water molecules. Protons on other kinds of molecules produce their own NMR signals, at Larmor frequencies very close to that of water protons, and this is particularly significant in cells with high aliphatic lipid content. Such molecules undergo motions that are somewhat unlike those of water, and display correspondingly dissimilar relaxation behavior. Proton relaxation times for cerebral white matter, for example, tend to be shorter than those for gray matter, because of the relatively greater number of fast-relaxing lipid protons (Table 12.1).

The protons in any voxel of tissue inhabit a broad range of environmental conditions, and may take part in a wide variety of spin relaxation processes, only one of which has been described above, and each has its own characteristic times. It is possible, however, to correlate much of this with the single pair of gross relaxation parameters, T1 and T2. This is plausible when relaxation is at least nearly exponential, as would be appropriate for so-called "one-compartment" kinetic models of the processes involved. Fortunately, the two relaxation times, crude though they be, are still sufficiently tissue-sensitive and -specific that T1- and T2-weighted MRI maps are clinically highly useful.

Quantitative T1 FID study of the 1D patient

The previous chapter explored several ways in which frequency-mediated spatial-encoding, by way of an applied field gradient, allowed determination of proton density along a 1D phantom. Now we shall go through a similar exercise to generate MRI maps of T1 values, instead. The geometry is the same, with two exceptions. The pancake chambers at $x = 0$ and $x = 5$ cm now contain lipid and cerebral spinal fluid, respectively, rather than water (Figure 12.4). The voxels have been filled so as to have about the same number of protons, which implies that their separate values of M_0 will be the same, as well. Lipid has relatively fast T1 ($^1/_4$ s), while that of CSF is close to 1 s, and the difference should be clearly visible in the phantom's image. Second, the RF transmit and receive coils now lie along the region of interest, rather than at its ends, which is more realistic; much more significantly, the receive coil now feeds into an RF receiver, rather than into a power meter.

Table 12.1 For various tissues, typical values of proton density, of T1 at 1.0 T, 1.5 T, and 3.0 T, and of T2, which is largely independent of field strength. T1 tends to increase with field strength (Figure 12.3b). Values of T2 in tissues are in the tens and hundreds of milliseconds, typically an order of magnitude shorter than those of T1, which are mostly in tenths of seconds. Numbers for relaxation times vary considerably among tabulated sources largely because of the use of dissimilar data acquisition techniques; those listed here are typical.

Tissue	PD p+/mm³, rel.	T1, 1 T (ms)	T1, 1.5 T (ms)	T1, 3 T (ms)	T2 (ms)
Pure H₂0	1	4000		4000	4000
Brain					
CSF	0.95	2500	2500	2500	200
White matter	0.6	700	800	850	90
Gray matter	0.7	800	900	1300	100
Edema			1100		110
Glioma		930	1000		110
Liver			500		40
Hepatoma			1100		85
Muscle	0.9	700	900	1800	45
Adipose	0.95	240	260		60

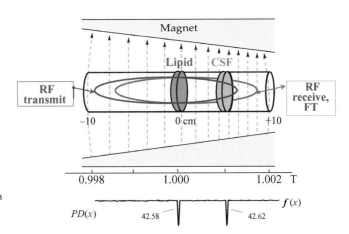

Figure 12.4 Phantom for mapping T1 values. The proton-density phantom has been replaced with another in which the two pancake chambers contain lipid in the center and CSF at 5 cm, respectively. These are arranged to have the same PD, but they will display different T1 values. (In a simple proton-density study, Fourier transform of the temporal signal arriving at the receiver would result in a spectrum of two equally tall peaks at the two (different) resonant frequencies.)

To simplify matters at first, let's consider only the lipid voxel, and drain out the CSF. Alternatively, we can use a narrow-bandwidth pulse that covers only the lipid voxel – since it is at $x = 0$ cm, we can even forget about the x-gradient.

The approach is to disturb the system at $t = 0$, then follow the exponential re-growth of the longitudinal magnetization, $M_z(t)$, over time, and fit the data points to $M_z(t)/M_0 = (1 - e^{-t/T1})$ (Equation 12.1 and Figure 12.1d). Let's start off at thermal equilibrium, where $M_z(0) = M_0$. At $t = 0$, we apply an f_{Larmor} 90° pulse. A *first* FID signal appears immediately, and its strength at its leading edge $S(t = 0+)$ comes from the full magnetization now precessing in the x-y plane: $S(0+) = M_{xy}(0+)/M_0 = M_z(0-)/M_0 = 1$ (Equation 11.6). The signal decays away over time from its initial maximum of 1, while the magnetization precesses in the x-y plane, as the magnetization begins to recover along z. We then wait a short period TR and then apply another 90° pulse. Over the period of duration TR, the magnetization has been re-growing along the z-axis, but it does not even come close to reaching M_0. Then exactly at $t = $ TR, a *second* 90° pulse swings whatever amount has recovered, $M_z(TR)$, back down into the x-y plane, where it generates a *second* FID signal, which starts out with amplitude $S(TR+) = M_z(TR+)/M_0$ (Figure 12.5a). The longer the TR delay, the more the re-growth along the z-axis occurs, and the closer $M_z(TR)/M_0$ and $S(TR)$ will be to 1.

We now leave the spins alone long enough to re-equilibrate to M_0, and repeat this "saturation-recovery" pulse sequence and measurement. Doing this for several different choices of TR (Fig-

ure 12.5b,c) allows a fit of the initial amplitudes of the second FID signal, in each case, to $(1 - e^{-TR/T1})$, thereby yielding an estimate of T1 (Figure 12.5d).

It will shortly prove advantageous to take the Fourier transform of each second-FID signal, to the right in Figure 12.5a–c. The signal from a voxel will be quite narrow in frequency, and centered on the local f_{Larmor} there, and its FT will provide a direct measure of its amplitude. So the set of amplitudes of the peaks in $\mathbf{FT}[S(TR)]$ for all the TR settings will also indicate magnetization recovery (Figure 12.5d, again). Statistically based curve fitting to $(1 - e^{-TR/T1})$ leads to an estimated T1 value of 250 ms. Because T1-relaxation for a lipid is characteristically quite fast, the corresponding region of the MR T1 image is bright. This is a matter of *convention*, and does not come from any fundamental law of nature.

To finish off, we could re-fill the CSF voxel at $x = 5$ cm, and go through this entire business again with the x-gradient on and a Larmor frequency appropriate for $x = 5$ cm, $f_{Larmor} = 42.62$ MHz. A much faster method, however, is to drive *all* the voxel-magnetizations in the entire phantom down through 90° simultaneously, using a broad-bandwidth 90° RF pulse, and repeating after TR with the read x-gradient on. The Fourier transform can untangle the second-FID signals, yielding one peak for each voxel (Figure 12.6a). Repeats at a few TRs would provide all the data needed to find the separate re-growth curves (Figure 12.6b), and provide the desired T1 values to create the entire MR image.

The above approach is known as *quantitative MRI*, where the objective is to obtain an anatomic

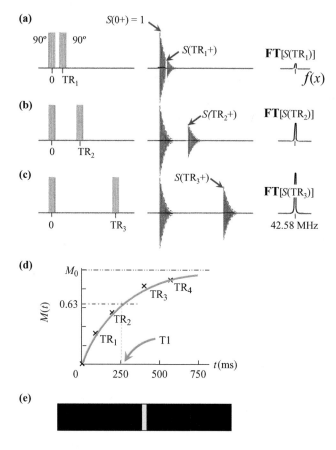

Figure 12.5 "Quantitative T1 mapping" of 1D phantom, with lipid in the voxel at $x = 0$ cm, but no CSF, at $x = 5$ cm for the time being. (a) At $t = 0$, a 90° RF pulse centered at 42.58 MHz kHz is applied, and a signal appears immediately, caused by the magnetization of amplitude M_0 precessing in the x-y plane. During a subsequent (very brief) recovery period of duration TR_1, $M_z(t)$ re-grows (a very small amount) along the z-axis, reaching the (very small) magnitude $M_z(TR_1+)$. A second 90° pulse then drives this back down into the x-y plane, where it precesses and gives rise to a (very weak) MR signal, $S(TR_1+)$. For future use, we sample the signal and find its spectrum, that is, take its Fourier transform, **FT**, shown to the right. That's the end of round 1. (b) Now the spins are allowed to re-equilibrate for a long while, and they settle back to M_0. The procedure is repeated, but with a longer value for TR, namely TR_2, and the detected signal $S(TR_2+)$ is found to be stronger, since there was more time for magnetization to re-grow along the z-axis. (c) After doing this several more times, each with a new value of TR_i, (d) the resulting data points are fitted to $S(TR_i) = (1 - e^{-TR_i/T1})$ to estimate T1, and (e) a T1 MRI image is created. By convention, the shorter the T1 of the material, the lighter the pixels in the image.

map of precise values of T1, T2, or proton density, and it has some clinical and research applications. But it is relatively slow, and does not lend itself to the efficient generation of large numbers of routine images in the clinic. It is possible, however, to produce, much faster, a map of something that reflects T1 (or T2 or proton density) indirectly – namely, the relative magnitudes of local magnetization in each of the voxels all at the same single, particular instant of time after a 90° pulse. Fortunately, such a *weighted* magnetic resonance image turns out to be clinically adequate and much faster, and it is the kind produced in practice.

T1-weighted FID study of the 1D patient

What is normally sought clinically is a rapidly created image that somehow indicates, in a significant way, the differences in relaxation times among the various healthy and pathologic tissues. Things can be speeded up significantly from the quantitative

approach just described by assessing the magnitude of the MR signal only once (Figure 12.7a). This gives only one magnetization amplitude per voxel, but that measurement will depend strongly on T1 relaxation in tissue there, and the same is true for all the other voxels as well. This results in a T1-*weighted* (T1-*w*) image; it is not exactly the same thing as a map of precise T1 values, but which, for nearly all clinical tasks, it is just as good at discriminating among tissues (Figure 12.7b). Normally this is done with a spin-echo or gradient-echo pulse sequence, but for simplicity, we have introduced it via FID.

This is pretty basic and important, so let's go through it briefly again in different words. The spins in a set of tissue voxels are allowed to stand undisturbed long enough for their magnetizations to be close to their equilibrium configurations, pointing along B_0. (The values of M_0 may differ among them, depending on their proton densities.) A broadband 90° "saturation" pulse is applied, driving the

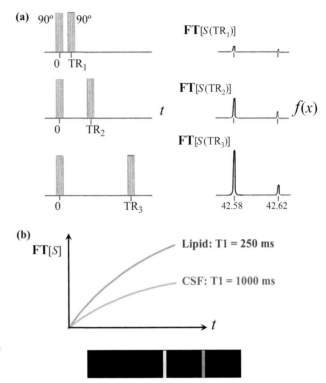

Figure 12.6 The same as the previous figure, but with CSF in the voxel at $x = 5$ cm, as well, and the x-gradient being applied. (**a**) The signals from the two voxels overlap, but can be separated with a Fourier transform. (**b**) Again, exponential curves are fitted from the data, yielding their respective T1 values and the T1 MR image.

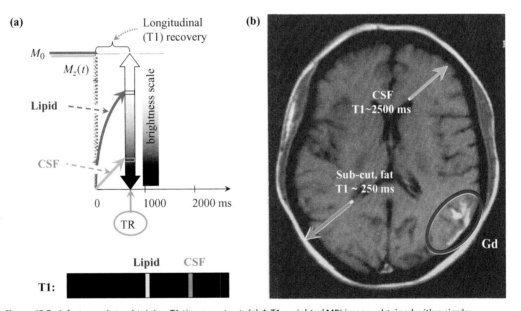

Figure 12.7 A faster path to obtaining T1 tissue contrast. (**a**) A T1-*weighted* MRI image, obtained with a single broad-band 90–90° saturation-recovery sequence, with the second pulse at a value of TR selected carefully for optimal contrast, and with G_x on. (How might one go about choosing a good value for TR?) (**b**) 1.5 T T1-*w* study displaying adipose tissue, CSF, and Gd contrast agent taken up by a neoplasm. With T1 imaging, tissues with short T1 show up bright.

magnetizations for all voxels separately down into the x-y plane, after which the $M_z(t)$ begins to re-grow along the external field, each at its own 1/T1 rate. A second 90° pulse is then applied at a single, pre-selected $t = $ TR, and the signal from *it* is obtained immediately, with the readout gradient being G_x applied. FT of the composite signal effects a separation of the contributions from all the voxels, which have been spatially encoded (spread apart in frequency) by G_x according to their positions, and this provides a measure (but not a precise value) of T1 for each. It reveals the *relative* amount of proton NMR signal that originates in each voxel at that instant, and from this alone one can create a T1-w map: the greater the re-grown magnetization in a voxel at the time of signal detection, the stronger the NMR signal coming from it, and the brighter the pixel in the corresponding MRI image.

After introducing T2 imaging, we shall return to this issue and see how this works (to great advantage) with a spin-echo pulse sequence (90−180°), rather than this FID saturation-recovery (90−90°).

Imaging at 3 and 7 Tesla

There is a fundamental tradeoff in MRI among contrast/SNR, spatial resolution, and imaging time (Figure 12.8a). Any of these can be made better, but only to the detriment of one of the other two.

One way to improve this balance is to increase the principal magnetic field strength. The magnitude of M_0 is proportional to B_0, and you might suspect that the strength, $S(t)$, of the MR signal coming from the patient goes up linearly with field strength. For reasons not pursued here, it actually increases more closely with the square of the field strength, as B_0^2. Because there is more $S(t)$, and the SNR increases accordingly, so a new and significantly better trade-off is possible among tissue contrast, imaging time, and resolution. Indeed, microvasculature that is not even suggested at 1.5 T can appear clearly in 7 T images (Figure 11.12a).

Thus greater field strengths enable higher SNR and/or smaller voxel size, thereby increasing resolution and decreasing the partial volume effect and generally improving anatomical imaging, such as in MR microscopy (Figure 12.8b). In addition, both functional MRI (*f*MRI) and diffusion-weighted MRI (DWI) tend to do better at 3 T or 7 T than at 1.5 T, also in part because some intrinsic properties

(a)

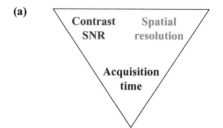

(b)

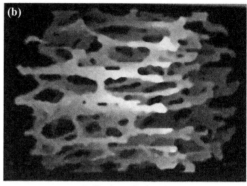

$5\ \text{mm} \times 5\ \text{mm}$

Figure 12.8 A fundamental tradeoff for any MRI device. (a) Specific sequences of RF pulses and gradients optimize this balance for various studies in different ways. Adjustable parameters include TE and TR, slice thickness, flip angle (90° is not necessarily best), matrix size, field of view, number of acquisitions, etc. But it is possible to make the whole pie bigger, or float all the boats higher, by switching to a machine with greater B_0. (b) Improved resolution, together with especially strong gradients, makes possible microscopic MRI, such as of this $5 \times 5 \times 5$ mm³ bone marrow sample. Courtesy of Scott Huang, Felix Wherli, John Williams, and the journal *Medical Physics*.

of the tissues themselves are field-dependent in ways that can affect contrast. Finally, since it would lead to greater chemical shifts, a high field can separate overlapping resonance peaks, enhancing magnetic resonance spectroscopy studies.

There are, of course, ~~significant challenges~~ great opportunities that come along with higher fields, and most of these have something to do with the higher Larmor frequencies.

T1 lengthens with field strength approximately as $T1 \sim B_0^{1/3}$. (T2 appears much less sensitive to B_0.) An increase in B_0 and resulting shift of f_{Larmor} to the right in Figure 12.3, for example, means that water attached to an intermediated-sized molecule would experience a reduction in the strength of the Larmor-frequency magnetic noise, hence slower relaxation, and an increase in T1. So it is not enough to state T1; one must know the field strength at which the measurement was made, as indicated by the different T1 columns in Table 12.1. Indeed, people familiar with reading T1 images at 1.5 T may have to re-adjust their thinking a little at 3 T and 7 T, and they will find that a 1.5-T T1-*w* protocol is not necessarily optimal for higher field strength imaging.

In addition, motion, blood flow, and chemical shift artifacts tend to worsen as field strength increases, along with geometrical distortions associated with external field inhomogeneities and patient susceptibility effects.

As mentioned in the previous chapter, the specific absorption rate (SAR) increases roughly as the square of the field strength, so the issue of tissue heating may become more problematic. Also, the wavelength of the RF approaches the dimensions of the anatomic entities being viewed, which may introduce various wave interference effects not encountered at lower fields (Figure 11.12b).

Finally, there are new biological interactions and effects that can occur above 3T, including photophosphenes (patients may experience flashes in the eye), altered cardiac electrophysiology (pulse sequences that gate with the heart may require new methodologies), and hazards from stronger static field gradients near the ends of the magnet bore. The amount of development work ongoing, however, indicates that these and other obstacles may well be surmountable.

A research area where the experimental complications are much less severe, and the biophysics possibilities unlimited, is in small animal studies. These are currently ongoing at fields typically from 7 T to near 20 T, with accompanying resolution of down to 10 microns. There are numerous reports of the imaging of amyloid plaques in transgenic mice that display Alzheimer's disease, for example, and of the movement of individual cells in real time. This is stimulating the development of new contrast agents specific to particular cell-types and individual proteins involved in gene expression, and the behavior of intra-cellular structures. And that's just the beginning.

While machines that operate at 1.5 T are still the norm, largely because of their lower purchase cost, sales of 3-T devices are increasing briskly. And as of 2012, moreover, there are already about 50 whole-body devices in the world that operate at 7 T; there is even talk of developing clinical machines with fields twice as strong as that.

Contrast agents and counter-indications

Unlike the situation in radiography, where iodine or barium atoms are particularly effective at absorbing X-ray photons, MRI contrast agents work indirectly, by altering the local magnetic environments of certain water protons (such as those that have crossed the blood-brain barrier) thereby affecting their relaxation rates and their values of T1 and T2.

Electrons orbiting an atom are normally spin-paired, in the sense that the magnetic field generated by one is effectively canceled out by that from another oriented in the opposite direction. As a result, water, many organic compounds, soft tissues, oxyhemoglobin, and other materials are slightly *diamagnetic* – that is, they reduce an applied magnetic field within them a little, below what it would be in free space, and for them, $\chi < 0$ in Equation 11.4c.

A few atoms, however, find it energetically favorable for one (or more) of their electrons to go against the grain, and remain unpaired. The magnetic moment of an unpaired orbital electron is 657 times that of a proton, so the field it produces at a nearby water proton will be far stronger than even that of its own partner. While some such *paramagnetic* materials occur naturally in the body, such as deoxyhemoglobin, others are introduced as MR contrast agents. In the extreme case, gadolinium carries seven unpaired electrons (in inner orbitals, so that it does not act as a chemically reactive free radical.) This gives rise to a fluctuating magnetic field thousands of times stronger than that of any proton, and, again, this can radically affect the local environment of nearby water protons.

As with the radionuclide and carrier/agent of a nuclear medicine radiopharmaceutical, a paramagnetic contrast agent must be tissue-specific and safe at concentrations that are high enough for it to have an appreciable effect. Unfortunately many of the strong paramagnetic elements are transition metals or rare earth elements, which are frequently quite toxic in raw form. Hence, most common contrast agents consist of a paramagnetic ion within a large chelate molecule, where the effectiveness of the agent depends on whether it is hydrophilic or hydrophobic, etc. Chelating also helps with purging the paramagnetic ion from the patient's system (e.g., via the kidneys), as the lifetime for many chelate complexes in the body is fairly short, easily less than 24 hours. The most widely explored agents contain chelated ions of iron, manganese, dysprosium, and especially gadolinium, commonly complexed with diethelenetriaminepenta-acetic acid (Gd-DTPA). Non-chelated materials, such as manganese chloride, have higher levels of toxicity and do not evacuate the body rapidly; they can probe some internal cellular properties more readily, however, due to the small size and properties of the free ion.

The overall relaxation rate, 1/T1, depends on the tissue T1 and on the concentration of agent, [Gd], and because the two phenomena are independent, $1/T1 = 1/T1_{tissue} + \kappa[Gd]$ with constant κ. This suggests the involvement of two quite distinct populations: water molecules in tissue away from the chelated ions, and those in the contrast agent hydration layers, which exchange rapidly with the pool of tissue water (Figure 12.9). Clinical trials have already demonstrated the efficacy and general safety of Gd-DTPA, for example, in imaging breakdown of the blood-brain barrier (Figure 12.7b), renal lesions, myocardial infarctions, and other pathologic conditions. But as noted before in the discussion of MRI safety, there are risks associated with gadolinium-based contrast agents for some patients, in particular with the possible causation of nephrogenic systemic fibrosis (NSF).

Nanoparticles of ferric oxide and a few other *superparamagnetics* have magnetic susceptibilities hundreds or thousands of times stronger even than those of paramagnetic materials, and find some limited use as MR contrast agents.

Dynamic contrast enhanced (DCE) is a perfusion modality that employs rapid sequential acquisition of multiple MR images to follow the flow and diffusion of contrast agents into certain tissues, and the subsequent washout. It has shown itself to be effective in the detection, classification, and prognosis of cancer, in the evaluation of synovial activity in patients with rheumatoid arthritis, and elsewhere. It involves the analysis of the shape of the enhancement curve over time, and the kinetics (e.g., www.imageanalysis.org.uk).

Transverse spin relaxation and T2-*w* images

As was seen in the study of gray matter (Figure 11.27), there is no need to be satisfied with a single spin-echo. Multiple repetitions of the 180° pulse of the spin-echo sequence will lead to a train of multiple echoes. Figure 12.10 reproduces the interesting part of the signal, in which echoes appear regularly every TE. Those are the only times at which we can determine the echo amplitude – so that's what we do. The envelope of the train seems to decline exponentially, with some characteristic time that we shall call T for now – but the earlier discussion would suggest that field inhomogeneities and susceptibility effects should *not* be causing it to happen, since we are using spin-echo. So what's going on?

Ah-ha!, you exclaim in a moment of characteristic extreme lucidity, it's that T1 business that we were just talking about. Sure, in the previous chapter we ignored T1 when playing with the quantum and classical pictures. But in a realistic situation, longitudinal relaxation spin-flips are doubtless ongoing, and that could cause recurring echoes to diminish in amplitude over time. Certainly we can mix the spin-up/spin-down and the gyroscope-like pictures together enough to explain the signal reduction in terms of longitudinal relaxation.

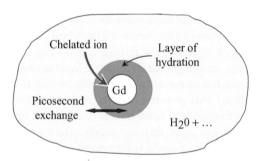

Figure 12.9 Most MRI contrast agents are paramagnetic (gadolinium, dysprosium, manganese) or superparamagnetic (iron oxide) nanoparticles; their fields can be thousands of times stronger than those from a proton, since the magnetic moment of an unpaired electron is hundreds of times greater than that of a proton. Interactions between contrast agents and protons can speed up proton relaxation rates 1/T1 considerably and (to a lesser extent) 1/T2, and thereby shorten T1 and T2.

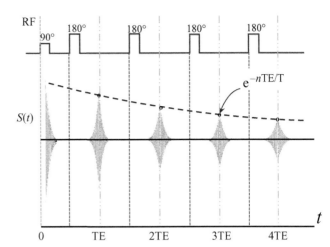

Figure 12.10 Relaxation. In this pulse, multi-echo sequence, echoes appear at times $t = n$ TE for integer n. The echo amplitude is decreasing with time exponentially as $e^{-n\text{TE}/\text{T}}$, for some value of T.

As we explore the situation a bit more fully, we recall that many decay/survival phenomena of all sorts occur exponentially over time or distance (radionuclide decay, decay of a flash of scintillation light, X-ray and ultrasound attenuation, and much else.) So we try and succeed in fitting the amplitudes in Figure 12.10 for this study to a general trial term

$$M_{xy}(t)/M_{xy}(0) = e^{-t/\text{T}}. \quad (12.2a)$$

(Note that t, and this equation, are meaningful only at the center of an echo.) From the peak-echo data points, we get a very good fit to the exponential form, and the measured numerical value of T turns out to be 100 ms. No doubt this "T" is just T1 with a different name, right? So far so good.

The transverse relaxation time, T2, and spin de-phasing in the *x-y* plane: the much faster exponential decay of $M_{xy}(t)$

Until, that is, you examine a table of T1 relaxation times, and discover, to your shock and dismay, that T1 for gray matter is not 100 ms, which we just measured, but rather much longer, something like 900 ms at 1.5 T, (Table 12.1). Puzzled but undeterred by this hopefully minor setback, you study liver tissue next, and again the data seem to fit your trial exponential curve nicely, with T = 45 ms. But T1 for liver has been measured independently and reported to be 490 ms. And so on and on for other tissues. In each case, the relaxation time you measure, as in Figure 12.10, is between about 0.1 and 0.3 of the corresponding tabulated value of T1. In

other words, something else is going on, above and beyond T1 relaxation, and it's even a good deal faster.

This new phenomenon is known as *transverse-* or *spin-spin-relaxation*, and it is parameterized by a new characteristic time called T2. So our T = T2, and not T1, and we can re-write Equation 12.2a as

$$M_{xy}(t)/M_{xy}(0) = e^{-t/\text{T}2}. \quad (12.2a')$$

You are right in thinking that T1 relaxation events contribute to the fall-off in echo signal amplitude over time. But that seems to be only a part of the story, and a fairly small part, at that. The above comparison of T2 with T1 values indicates that something *else* must be taking place, in addition, a quite different spin process, one with a much bigger impact. That something else is, indeed, a distinct form of relaxation known as the *secular component* in the T2 process. So two distinct atomic-scale mechanisms, the T1 and the secular contributions, together are responsible for overall T2 relaxation (Figure 12.11a). The relaxation rate 1/T2 can therefore be expressed as the sum of the two independent parts:

$$1/\text{T}2 = \tfrac{1}{2}/\text{T}1 + 1/\text{T}2_{\text{secular}}. \quad (12.2b)$$

(The $\frac{1}{2}$ is there because $\text{T}2_{\text{secular}}$ events occur in the two-dimensional *x-y* plane, while T1 relaxation occurs only along one axis.) That is, both 1/T1 and $1/\text{T}2_{\text{secular}}$ events contribute to the proton spin de-phasing within the *x-y* plane that determines the rate 1/T2.

(a)

$$1/T2 = \tfrac{1}{2}\,/\,T1 + 1/T2_{secular}$$

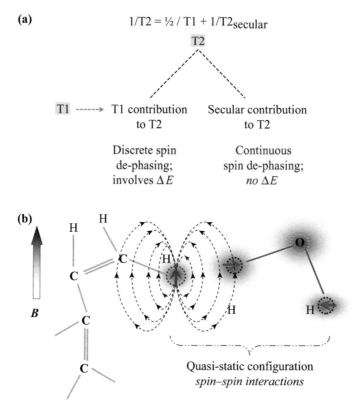

T2

T1 - - - - → T1 contribution   Secular contribution
              to T2   to T2

        Discrete spin   Continuous
        de-phasing;   spin de-phasing;
        involves ΔE *no ΔE*

(b)

B

H   H
H
C   C
C
C
C

Quasi-static configuration
spin–spin interactions

Figure 12.11 T2 is the measure of the rate at which spin packets lose spin phase coherence in the *x-y* plane following a 90° pulse. **(a)** The decay rate 1/T2 consists of two parts. One is simply attributable to T1-type events, caused by Larmor-frequency field fluctuations. Spin flips along the *z*-axis cause loss of phase in the *x-y* plane. (No, it may not really make any sense, but live with it.) The *secular* part, on the other hand, comes from relatively slow field variations, between which the phase packets have time to de-phase and spread apart as they precess, somewhat like the case of T$_{SFd-P}$. But because the magnetic fields underlying both contributions to 1/T2 vary randomly over time, unlike those of T$_{SFd-P}$, they cannot be reversed or eliminated with S-E, so that decay similar to that of Figures 11.25 and 12.10 is unavoidable. **(b)** An example of how de-phasing might occur, mixing the quantum and classical pictures: a water molecule lingers for a short time near a proton aligned along B_0 that is part of an organic macromolecule. The two water protons happen to be precessing in the *x-y* plane but, because one is closer to the hydrogen of the slowly moving macromolecule, their local fields differ a little, as do their precession rates, and they lose phase coherence at a rate parameterized by T2$_{secular}$.

The T1 portion is just the longitudinal transitions that flip spins from the spin-down state to spin-up, and vice versa. It may seem odd that changes of orientation along or against the *z*-direction can have an impact on (the same!) spins seemingly precessing in the *x-y* plane, but you may as well just take that leap of faith, and blame the illogic of it on quantum weirdness. The bottom line is that T1-type relaxations do, indeed, help to disrupt $M_{xy}(t)$ and expedite its decline.

The secular contribution to 1/T2 involves *slowly* and *randomly* varying local magnetic fields that arise from sluggish molecular motions. Imagine a group of protons immediately after a 90° pulse at $t = 0$, with their spin axes all aligned parallel and giving rise to a transverse magnetization, $M_{xy}(t)$. They start out precessing in the *x-y* plane in phase, but 1/T2$_{secular}$ changes that phase coherence quickly. Suppose that, for some biophysical and clinically relevant reason, the motions of water molecules are very leisurely compared to the Larmor frequency. Each proton will be subject to (among other things) vertically aligned nuclear magnetic dipole fields, from its partner proton or from others nearby. At some times they will add locally a slight amount to B_0; at others they will reduce it (Figure 12.11b).

Each proton will therefore be precessing, just after a 90° pulse, a little faster or slower than average, and the individual spins in a voxel lose their mutual phase coherence, in a manner similar to that of Figure 11.25. Since these $B_{local}(t)$ fields fluctuate randomly, this spin de-phasing cannot be undone by spin-echo, and they just continuously and irreversibly add to the overall spin de-phasing over time. As their orientations become more evenly spread out in the transverse plane, the fields from their magnetic moments will increasingly cancel one another out, leading to a transverse magnetization, $M_{xy}(t)$, that falls off as $e^{-t/T2_{secular}}$. $T2_{secular}$ can be defined as the time it takes, in a spin multi-echo study (Figure 12.10), for the echo signal amplitudes to decrease by a factor of $0.37 = 1/e$ because of the *secular component* of T2-relaxation. This secular

de-phasing phenomenon is the principal mechanism by means of which T2 relaxation occurs (Figure 12.11a). Together with the *T1 component*, it determines T2 (Equation 12.2b and Figure 12.10).

The amounts of either Larmor-frequency or low-frequency magnetic fields arising spontaneously and experienced by a proton in a water molecule depend, of course, on the molecule's motions (Figure 12.12, which is an extension of Figure 12.3). The effect of molecular motions on the relaxation times may be illustrated with this fact: when water freezes, its T2 drops from a few seconds to 10^{-5} s. In solids, there is relatively little motion of the nuclei, so that the slowly changing local fields give the spins ample time to de-phase. The secular relaxation mechanism is therefore very fast, and the transverse relaxation time is much shorter than T1 alone. Protons

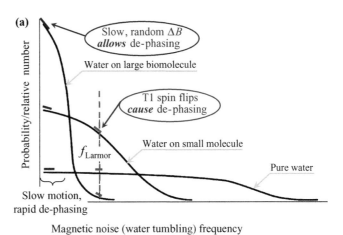

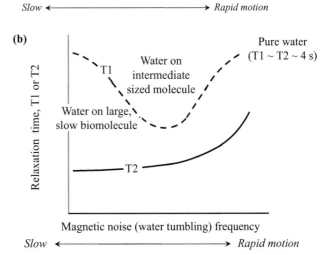

Figure 12.12 The explanation of T2 relaxation is similar to that for T1 (Figure 12.3), differing only in the details. (a) One of the two contributions to the rate 1/T2 is T1 relaxation itself (Equation 12.2b); every time a spin flips up or down along the z-axis, triggered by an f_{Larmor} local field fluctuation, the affected proton loses whatever precessional coherence it had in the x-y plane with the others in the voxel. The second *secular* mechanism involves slow but irregular molecular motions of water molecules; these do not involve spin flips, nor the expenditure of energy, but they do afford each proton time to de-phase from other protons in the voxel. (b) As a result, water molecules in cellular environments that tend to provide plenty of low-frequency fields undergo rapid T2 decay.

in solid-like environments undergo T2$_{secular}$ relaxation that is so fast, in fact, that their transverse magnetization may decay away even before it can be detected for the construction of an image.

In non-viscous liquids such as water, at the other extreme, the molecular motions and the resulting fluctuations in the local fields are far too rapid to be effective in causing secular spin de-phasing. In this special case, T2 is nearly all attributable to T1-type transitions (spin flips), so T2 ∼ T1. Soft tissues lie somewhere in between: 1/T2 for a tissue is usually three to ten or so times faster than 1/T1, and T1 is correspondingly longer. This means that the transverse magnetization is normally long gone by the time that the longitudinal magnetization has re-grown significantly.

Pharmacological and molecular biological MRI

MRI reflects primarily upon the interactions of water with the biomolecules that happen to be present within and between the cells of tissues. T1- and T2-imaging are powerful because they provide forms of image contrast, based on those interactions, that are altogether different from those of other modalities – these ones are sensitive, in particular, to differences in soft tissue types and correlate with specific pathologies. As medical physicists, computer scientists, and others continue to provide technical improvements at a rapid clip, the transfer of these evolving developments to the clinic will open new areas of medical research and, thereafter, widespread application.

One area of significant clinical growth potential in MRI is in the prediction and monitoring of response to treatment, whether radiation therapy, chemotherapy, local heat ablation with US, gene therapy, whatever. In cancer therapy, for example, ionizing radiation and certain tumoricidal drugs are relatively ineffective on tumor cells that are poorly oxygenated. Indeed, the most resistant cells are commonly those inhabiting a barely viable hypoxic rind between active tumor, on the outside, and necrotic tumor cells within that have died from anoxia. MRI might be able to reveal whether a pharmaceutical intended to promote angiogenesis in that rind, or to facilitate the perfusion or diffusion of water or oxygen into it, will be successful on a specific patient. And following the adminis-

tration of a drug or dose of radiation, MRI and perhaps MR spectroscopy can assess the degree to which the opening or proliferation of blood vessels has increased the oxygen level in hypoxic regions, hence the likelihood of destruction of the tumor. These are but two out of countless examples of *image-guided therapy* (involving MRI alone or in collaboration with other modalities, e.g., PET) that either already exist or are soon to be forthcoming.

In the long run, perhaps the most extraordinary (from our current perspective) advances will arise from ongoing efforts to establish strong linkages between physiologic imaging, especially MRI, nuclear medicine, and optical imaging, with genomics, proteomics, molecular biology, and nanotechnology. These fields are just beginning to unify, yet already have yielded the creation of novel families of biologically derived *imaging biomarkers* as measures of biological processes. It is easy to suppose that this is still just the lowest hanging fruit, and that eventual results could be far beyond our imaginings at present.

Optimizing the contrast in T1-*w*, T2-*w*, and PD-*w* spin-echo images

Figure 12.5 and Figure 12.6 indicated how to measure T1 values throughout a 1D body simply, with a saturate-recovery, 90−90° pulse sequence. The objective in MRI normally is not so ambitious as to attempt to produce an accurate map of T1; rather, it is to create images in which visual contrast indirectly reflects, but in a clinically significant and rapid fashion, the *differences* in the various relaxation times among the tissues. For this reason, it is generally adequate to generate a *relative* T1-*w*, T2-*w*, PD-*w*, or other MR image. While Figure 12.7a explored a simple FID means of carrying that out, an extension of the standard 90−180° spin-echo sequence is especially adept at the task.

As we have seen, multiple repetitions of the spin-echo pulse sequence will give rise to a train of echoes. The sequences for two such repetitions are labeled *i* and *ii* in Figure 12.13a. Each of them contains both a 90° and a 180° pulse, both broadband, and each produces an echo. Figure 12.13b displays the behavior over time of the longitudinal and transverse components of the magnetization, $M_z(t)$ and $M_{xy}(t)$, for two tissues, adipose (amber)

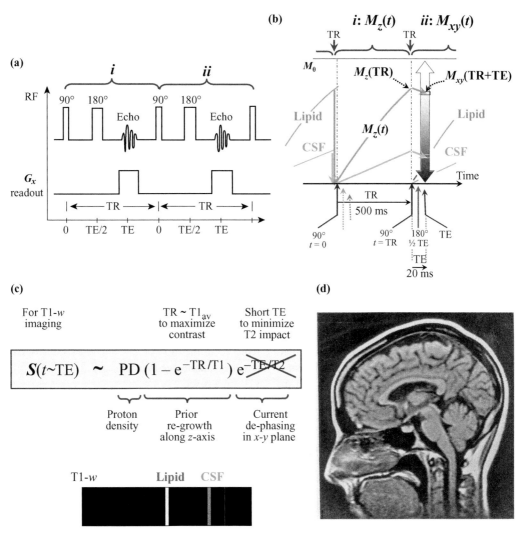

Figure 12.13 Weighted imaging of our phantom that consists of a pair of voxels; the one at the center of the phantom contains lipid, and that at 5 cm holds CSF, with equal proton densities. **(a)** Two of many repetitions in a multi-spin-echo train, labeled *i* and *ii*, and small parts of two others on either side. **(b)** To the left, a broadband 90° pulse, with the *x*-gradient on, initiates repetition *i*, and the magnetizations of the lipid and CSF voxels are driven down into the *x-y* plane. The *longitudinal* components, $M_z(t)$, of the magnetizations of both materials re-grow for as long as they are given time, and they achieve their peak magnitudes (generally a good deal less than M_0) of M_z(TR) just before the next sequence is begun, at $t =$ TR. At the beginning of *ii*, the two magnetization vectors are once again swung down through 90°, at TR. Just after that instant, at $t =$ TR+, the new *transverse* magnetization for each is its respective M_{xy}(TR+) (which is equal to its M_z(TR−) by Equation 11.6). A re-phasing 180° pulse applied at $t = \frac{1}{2}$TE produces in an echo at TE of amplitude M_{xy}(TR + TE) from each voxel, and the signal picked up by the receiver coil is a mixture of those from both of them. Then the compound signal will be disentangled and related to voxel position by means of a Fourier transform. **(c)** T1-weighted imaging is accomplished with a TR near the average T1 values of the tissues of interest, to maximize subject contrast between them (even though this does not necessarily maximize signal strength.) Also, by Equation 12.3, a short TE will force $e^{-TE/T2}$ to a value of about unity, minimizing the effects of T2-type spin de-phasing in the *x-y* plane, and leaving T1 relaxation with the dominant influence. Just after TE, the lipid signal will be far stronger than the CSF, because of its much shorter T1, and by convention, strong signal tissues are made to appear bright. **(d)** T1-*w* image of a lipoma at the pituitary, which, because lipids have short T1 values, appears bright. The CSF has a relatively long T1, and is darker.

and cerebro-spinal fluid (green), in a pair of nearby voxels.

Segment i of the diagram focuses on the z-component of the magnetization over time, $M_z(t)$, and for a less confusing diagram, we leave out the 180° pulse and echo. The segment begins with a 90° pulse to the far left at $t = 0$. $M_z(t)$ for each material thereafter recovers separately according to $M(0)$ $(1 - e^{-t/T1})$, but that for lipid occurs much faster, hence further, than that of CSF because its T1 (250 ms at 1.5 T) is much shorter than that of CSF (2500 ms). There is not, however, enough time between 90° pulses for either material to re-grow fully to its M_0; the increase in $M_z(t)$ is cut off from further growth, rather, when the next repetition is initiated at the *repetition time*. $t = $ TR by the next 90° pulse. Just before that instant, at $t = $ TR–, $M_z(t)/M(0)$ has reached $(1 - e^{-TR/T1})$. This is like Equation 12.1, but it is meaningful *only* at the particular moment $t = $ TR.

The action in part ii is exactly the same as in the previous one, but this time we pay particular attention to what is going on with the x-y *component* of the magnetization, $M_{xy}(t)$, instead, and only during the brief period from $t = $ TR+ to TR+TE. (TR+TE) is virtually the same as [TR+]+TE, of course, just expressed a little more simply.) At the instant of the second 90° pulse, at $t = $ TR, the $M_z(t)$ of each material is again driven down into the x-y plane. The *longitudinal* magnetization, M_z(TR–) is reincarnated as a new *transverse* magnetization vector, M_{xy}(TR+), of the *same magnitude*: M_{xy}(TR+) = M_z(TR–), again Equation 11.6. This magnitude is determined by the choice, the *selection* by the device operator, of the duration of TR relative to the natural value of the T1s for the substance (lipid or CSF) in the voxel. The magnetization, $M_{xy}(t)$, is now entirely transverse and precessing in the x-y plane, and it begins decaying at the rate 1/T2 (Equation 12.2a). For T1-imaging, TE is chosen by the operator to be short, and the spin-echo sequence now quickly fires a 180° pulse, a short time ½ TE after the $t = $ TR excitation 90° pulse. The echo materializes (with the readout gradient G_x turned on) another ½ TE after that. Between the initiation of the echo at $t = $ TR and its appearance at $t = $ TR + TE, its peak amplitude will have diminished by only the small factor of M_{xy}(TR + TE)/M_{xy}(TR+) = $e^{-TE/T2}$, as indicated by the short arrows falling off to the right

in Figure 12.13b. (Note that this is equivalent to M_{xy}(TE)/M_{xy}(0) = $e^{-TE/T2}$.) This decline will last only a brief time (because TE is short!), so that during echo readout, M_{xy}(TE) will be hardly different from M_z(TR), and $e^{-TE/T2}$ is practically 1, which removes all information about the impact of TE.

Putting this all together: the strength of the contribution of a voxel to the echo signal depends primarily on the three biologically determined parameters T1, T2, and PD, and also on the two operator settings TR and TE. The important, unifying expression

$$S(TR, \ TE) \sim PD(1 - e^{-TR/T1})e^{-TE/T2}, \quad (12.3)$$

which comes from Equations 12.1 and 12.2', fully describes and codifies one of the central ideas of standard MRI. It suggests, moreover, how to produce T1-w, T2-w, and PD-w images (Figure 12.14 and Table 12.2).

For T1-w imaging with a short TE, in particular, $S(t)$ describes the effect of T1 relaxation, but removes all mention of TE (Figure 12.13c). What remains is an image that reflects only the T1 (and PD) for a voxel.

The normal objective is to create an optimal T1-w image for our phantom, and in people (Figure 12.13d). To achieve high contrast, we need strong signals from both the CSF and lipid voxels and, just as essential, a large difference in their amplitudes: A good T1 strategy to make this happen consists of two decisions, one for each part of Figure 12.13b:

(i) Select a TR value (500 ms, here) that lies midway between the T1 values for the materials in the two voxels. This TR setting is long enough for $M_z(t)$ in both lipid and CSF to have re-grown far above $M_z(0) = 0$, but not yet to have come close together – that is, near their equilibrium values, M_0 – in agreement with the $(1 - e^{-TR/T1})$ term in Equation 12.3. There should be a significant difference in the strengths of the signals they generate in the pickup coils, hopefully, giving rise to strong T1 contrast between the two voxels. Meanwhile,

(ii) Set TE to a value (e.g., 20 ms) that is very short relative to the T2 values of both lipid (T2 = 60 ms) and CSF (200 ms), so that neither voxel will have sufficient time to undergo much T2 relaxation (Figure 12.13c). The term $(e^{-TE/T2})$ in Equation 12.3 remains near unity since TE/T2 is small, and

Figure 12.14 Representative Gd-enhanced (**a**) T1-*w*, (**b**) T2-*w*, and (**c**) PD-*w* spin-echo images showing slices through a glioma.

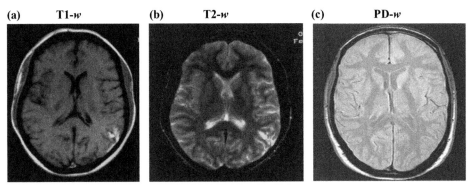

(a)   **T1-*w***   (b)   **T2-*w***   (c)   **PD-*w***

	T1-w	*T2-w*	*PD-w*
TR	~Long (~T1$_{av}$)	Long	Long
(ms)	(300–700)	(1500–3500)	(1500–3500)
TE	Short	~Short (~T2$_{av}$)	Short
(ms)	(10–25)	(60–150)	(10–25)
Bright	Short T1	Long T2	High PD
SNR	Good	Lower	Best

Table 12.2 Typical operational parameter settings, TR and TE, to produce spin-echo T1-*w*, T2-*w*, and PD-*w* studies.

the effect of T2 is thereby largely removed from the picture.

This combination of TR and TE settings yields an image that is heavily weighted toward T1 spatial variations, with some unavoidable PD influence, and with still a little admixture of T2 effects (Figure 12.13d). As with carving *David*, to produce a T1-*w* image, we try to remove signs of those processes (i.e., T2 relaxation) that don't look like T1.

The argument is much the same for T2-*w* images, just turned around a little (Figure 12.15a). To remove T1 effects, we set TR *long* relative to the T1s of the two voxel materials; their signals reach a maximum near their respective M_0 values (which we shall no longer assume to be the same.) That is, the $(1 - e^{-TR/T1})$ term in Equation 12.3 is near 1 for both, and this eliminates the T1 presence. The right-hand side of the diagram indicates that as one lengthens TE, on the other hand, two counterbalancing important processes occur. Contrast is enhanced, up to a point, because of the difference in T2s and the $e^{-TE/T2}$ for each; but at the same time, signal strength decreases over time

for both, again because of the $e^{-TE/T2}$ terms, as does the SNR. Selecting an optimal TE once again presents a tradeoff decision. Here, too, it is commonly best to choose TE midway between the two T2 times. This time, *long* T2 materials like CSF keep their signals high longer, and show up brighter.

Finally, a long TR and short TE produce images that reveal little about either T1 or T2 processes (Figure 12.15b). What is left is primarily proton density, and PD-*w* does have few specialized applications. Since they involve a TR similar to that for T2-*w*, PD-*w* images are readily collected from sequences that acquire two echoes during the same excitation: one at short TE to provide a PD-*w* image, and another with long TE for the T2-*w*. That's twice the bang for the buck at little more time, so why not obtain both?

Hiding distracting water and lipids with FLAIR and STIR

The *inversion-recovery* (IR) pulse sequence is an alternative to simple spin-echo that was originally employed to generate images with strong

(a)

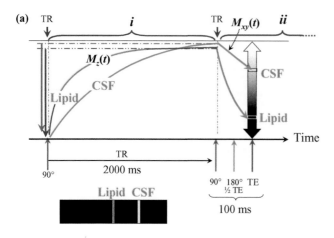

(b)

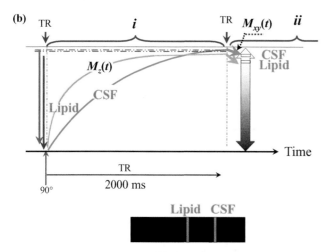

Figure 12.15 T2-*w* and PD-*w* spin-echo MR images. To make these examples more realistic the two voxels no longer have the same PDs. **(a)** For T2-*w*: after the 90° excitation pulse, $M_z(t)$ for the CSF and lipid spin packets are allowed to recover over a good period, to eliminate T1 effects from the image. After the next excitation pulse, the $M_{xy}(t)$ for each, newly created from its respective $M_z(t)$, precesses in the *x-y* plane over a TE span comparable to the average value of T2 among the tissues. **(b)** For PD-*w*: long TR and short TE remove both T1- and T2-effects, leaving only PD.

T1 weighting. More important applications now involve the suppression of unwanted signals that obscure others of greater interest.

Damaged brain tissues may locally take up excess fluid, but the extent of this edema may be obscured by cerebrospinal fluid at nearby CSF interfaces. The FLAIR (*FL*uid *A*ttenuated *I*nversion *R*ecovery) sequence largely nulls out materials with long-T1, like CSF, and this may render an edematous region more clearly delineated, as in Figure 12.16a, which is contrasted to a T2-*w* fast S-E. FLAIR also helps to reveal periventricular lesions like multiple sclerosis plaques.

Likewise, STIR (*S*hort *TI I*nversion *R*ecovery) sequences find use in musculoskeletal studies by attenuating the signal from lipids, such as in marrow (Figure 12.16b). STIR, which can be either T1-

or T2-weighted, can also counteract the presence of metal within a patient. A T1-*w* fast S-E echo is to the right for comparison.A

T2* and the gradient-echo (G-E) pulse sequence

We have been extolling the virtues of spin-echo, among the most impressive of which is its elimination of the $T_{SFd\text{-}P}$-type effects of imperfections in the principal magnetic field and of susceptibility discontinuities within the body. Neither of these is normally of any clinical value, and both disrupt the estimation of T2, which *is*. Spin-echo rids us of these problems, and a chain of echoes decays with characteristic time T2.

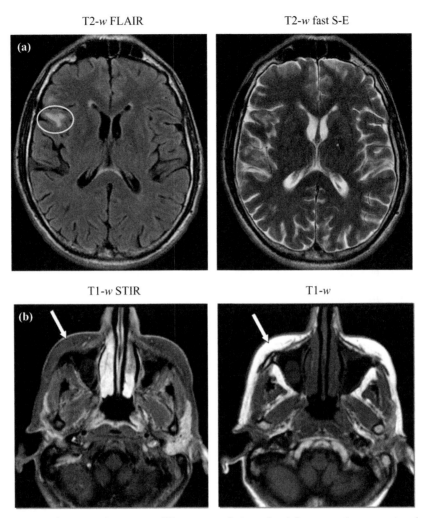

T2-*w* FLAIR

T2-*w* fast S-E

T1-*w* STIR

T1-*w*

Figure 12.16 FLAIR and STIR inversion recovery (IR) sequences eliminate signals from some tissues so as to enhance the appearance of others. (**a**) CSF suppression with FLAIR. (**b**) One type of fat suppression ("fat-sat"). STIR nulls the fat signal, which renders the bone marrow edema more visible than does the T1-*w* fast S-E to the right.

1/T2* is 1/T2 speeded up by static field inhomogeneities, 1/T$_{SFd-P}$

With free induction decay, a single $90°$ pulse drives the magnetization down into the transverse plane, where it undergoes free precession. It does *not* include, in particular, a phase-reversal $180°$ pulse that counteracts the biologically irrelevant T$_{SFd-P}$ de-phasing caused by the static fields associated with ΔB_0 and $\Delta \chi$ of Equation 11.7b As a consequence, an FID signal decays at a characteristic rate $1/T2^* = 1/T2 + 1/T_{SFd-P} = 1/T2 + [\kappa \Delta B_0 + \kappa' \Delta \chi]$. T2* is called "tee two star" and, as suggested by Figure 12.17, it has the most effects contribut-

ing to it, and is therefore the fastest member of the relaxation family.

Gradient-echo

Most magnetic resonance imaging employs variations on the spin-echo sequence because signal strength is relatively high and T$_{SFd-P}$ effects are minimized. But other approaches have also been developed, in particular the category of *gradient-echo* (G-E), also known as *gradient-recalled echo* (GRE) (Box 12.2). The gradient-echo family generate maps of T1, and of T2* rather than of T2. This is tolerable because while such T2* MRI images are only

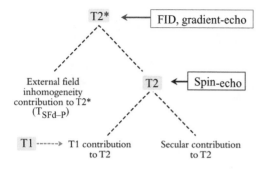

Figure 12.17 The complete spin-relaxation family tree. T1 spin-state transitions are caused by random, Larmor-frequency fluctuations occurring naturally in tissue. T2 de-phasing arises not only from T1 events, but also from random, but slow, variations in the local magnetic field, as some proton packets precess faster than average and others slower. De-phasing from either T1 or T2 events cannot be undone. On the other hand, T_{SFd-P} de-phasing, which contributes to 1/T2* signal decay in gradient-echo, can be reversed and removed with spin-echo.

partially biologically based, and clinically less revealing than those of the spatial distribution of T2, they are still of some use, and the gradient-echo sequence has the great benefit that it can be much faster than most spin-echo.

Box 12.2   Some of the general categories of spin-echo and gradient-echo sequences.

Spin-echo: T1 and T2
Standard spin-echo
Fast/turbo spin-echo
Inversion-recovery (STIR, FLAIR

Gradient-echo: T1 and T2*
(*aka* gradient-recalled echo, GRE)
Fast gradient-echo
Echo-planar imaging (EPI)
Coherent gradient-echo
Incoherent gradient-echo
Balanced gradient-echo
Steady-state free precession

A GRE sequence creates an echo signal by first *intentionally de-phasing* the spins with a briefly applied gradient field, such as $+G_x$, then *re-phasing*

them with a subsequent, oppositely polarized gradient, $-G_x$, where this second gradient is on during readout (Figure 12.18a). That is, a while after a 90° (or, more commonly, a smaller angle α°) pulse brings about FID, you intentionally apply a gradient to eliminate prematurely, but in a controlled fashion, the phase coherence that exists among the spins precessing in the *x-y* plane. You then bring about re-phasing with a second, equal but opposite gradient and, as a result, create an echo at $t = $ TE, which serves as the MRI signal. A short time (TR) later (10–100 ms), the process starts anew.

Unlike SE, GRE does not eliminate T_{SFd-P} effects, and it suffers the partial downside of yielding T2*-*w* rather than T2-*w*, images. But T2*-*w* studies are still of some clinical usefulness. Indeed, revealing a susceptibility effect with a T2* examination can at times elucidate diagnosis, such as for old bleeds, slow leaks, and vascular malformations (Figure 11.18b). And partly because there is no 180° pulse and associated delay of duration $2 \times \frac{1}{2}$TE, it has the virtue of being generally a good deal faster than spin-echo.

Gradient-echo sequence trains are of two general categories, known as *steady-state* and *spoiled*. For the first of these, after the initial few GRE sequences, during which the process stabilizes, $M_z(t)$ is tipped consistently through the same flip angle of α° by subsequent excitation pulses. Spoiled GE applies a *spoiler gradient* after readout to remove any residual transverse magnetization, so that only the *z*-component remains at the time of the next excitation. These topics get pretty involved, and will not be pursued here.

Into two and three dimensions

Much of the excitement and success of the CT revolution stemmed from the ability to isolate and represent thin transverse slices of tissue that are unobscured by over- and underlying layers. This is even more so for MRI as well, which has long been displaying planes with *any* orientation.

Choosing the *x-y* plane to image: slice selection

Up until now, with 1D MR phantoms and images, the magnetic field pointed vertically, as in an open-magnet system, and the position of a voxel was

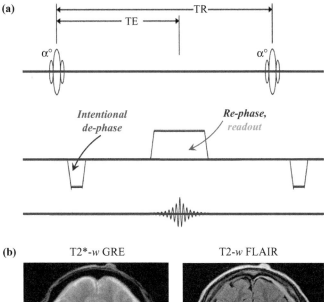

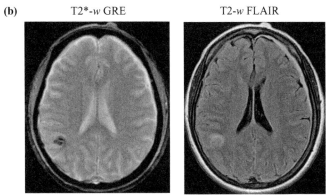

Figure 12.18 Gradient-echo (G-E), also known as gradient-recalled echo (GRE). (a) Typical GRE pulse sequences involve an echo signal produced by intentionally de-phasing, then re-phasing, spins with a sequence of oppositely-polarized gradients, such as $\pm G_x$, rather than with spontaneously occurring de-phasing and a 180° re-phasing RF pulse. For a multiple-echo sequence, the echo amplitude falls off over time with characteristic time T2*, rather than T2. (b) T2*-*w* GRE and T2-*w* FLAIR images of a hemorrhage. The contrast from GRE is enhanced by the shortening of T2* because of the susceptibility effect caused by the hemoglobin and its byproducts; that effect is largely absent in the FLAIR.

expressed as its *x*-value (Figure 12.19a). In moving on to two and three dimensions, it simplifies matters to adopt another geometry – that of a standard superconducting magnet, with B_0, the *z*-axis, and the patient all lying horizontally and co-linear (Figure 12.19b). We then select only a single thin transverse (for simplicity here) slice of tissue at some specific value of *z* to work with, and then map out PD, T1, T2, or whatever else throughout the *x*-*y* plane crossing the *z*-axis there.

Selection of a thin transverse slice of protons at a particular *z*-position entails applying a

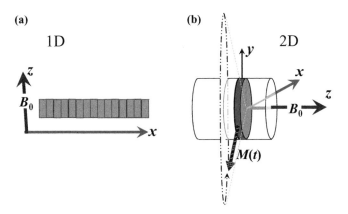

Figure 12.19 Coordinate systems and field geometries for (a) an "open" magnet with a vertical field and *z*-direction, which we have used up until now with our ID patient; and (b) a standard superconducting magnet, with horizontal field and *z*-axis, and 2D transverse slice of patient.

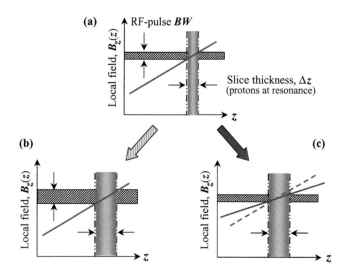

Figure 12.20 Slice thickness, RF bandwidth, and gradient strength. **(a)** Keep an eye on the thickness of the horizontal and vertical "bars," and on the slope of the diagonal line. One can produce a thicker (in the z-direction) tissue slice either by **(b)** increasing the bandwidth of the RF transmitter, or by **(c)** reducing the strength of the gradient, G_x. A third approach, familiar from multi-slice CT, is to combine the data from several adjacent tissue slices. However accomplished, acquiring thicker slices will improve signal-to-noise, but perhaps at the expense of reduced contrast and spatial resolution because of more overlapping of tissues and greater partial volume effects.

narrow-band 90° pulse, at the system's fixed B_0 (typically 1.5 T) and f_{Larmor} (63.87 ± Δf MHz) and with the z-gradient on. The bandwidth of the RF pulse and the gradient ($G_z = dB_z/dz$) together determine the *thickness* of the slice, and the z-gradient coil current is adjusted to set its *location* along the z-axis (Figure 12.20). The 90° pulse then drives the spins in the slice at the currently selected z-position, and *only* them, over into the x-y plane, where they precess at the local f_{Larmor}. Again, of all the protons in the phantom, it is only these in this single slice that will be imaged at present.

Since we want only the protons within one slice, of small but finite thickness Δz, to resonate at any time, then the narrow range of frequencies in the RF pulse should be no more than its shift over one voxel-length: $\Delta f_z = 42.58 \, G_z \Delta z$ [MHz], from Equation 11.3c. For our above example, this amounts to about 1 kHz per 1-mm thickness of slice. Here, the electronics must be adjusted to handle an *RF bandwidth* (BW) of only a few kHz. *Caveat*: The term "bandwidth" has several different applications and meanings in MRI, of which this is but one, and the numbers in Hz can differ considerably among them.

Phase encoding of voxel y-position

Up until now, we have been dealing with frequency encoding of voxel position along the x-axis. With a broadband spin-echo or gradient-echo pulse sequence, an echo signal, $S(t)$, appears over

a brief time interval centered on TE; it is comprised of contributions at $\mathcal{N}_x$ slightly different frequencies, $f(x)$, one for each voxel position, x (Figure 6.6 and Figure 12.19a). Fourier analysis then provides the frequency spectrum of the signal, with the amplitude of each spectral peak proportional to the signal strength from the corresponding voxel (Figure 12.21). This has been fine for imaging one-dimensional patients, but it cannot be simply extended into 2D or 3D.

Fortunately, there is a second, and independent, way to track a voxel's position. It involves modulating and detecting the *phases* of various components that make up the RF echo signal, rather than their frequencies, and it serves nicely in introducing the y-axis, perpendicular to the other two, into the story. So it is necessary here to say a word or two about the *phase* of a wave. For 2D MR imaging, it is 100% as important as its frequency.

Phase doesn't get much respect. We routinely adjust the frequency setting and amplitude of the radio, thinking not at all of the phase. But it can be just as significant as frequency in, for example, trying to excite a resonant system, such as a child on a swing: if the impulses are applied at the right frequency but 180° out of phase with the motion, the oscillations will be suppressed, rather than enhanced – and this is true in MRI as well.

The two dashed sine curves in Figure 12.22a are of the same frequency and amplitude, but differ

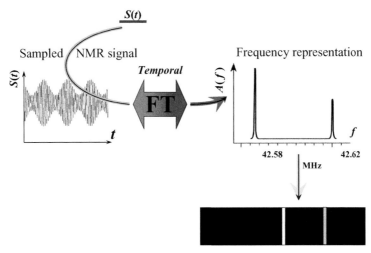

Figure 12.21 Summary of the image reconstruction process in one dimension. This works nicely because x-position, magnetic field strength, and MR signal frequency are all functions of only one variable, namely x, and can therefore be linked directly with each another. This same tactic is not viable when voxels are distributed in two dimensions, but it is possible to generalize it: voxel position in the second (y) direction will be represented by the *phase* of an RF echo signal, rather than by its *frequency*, and a more complex, two-dimensional Fourier transform is required.

in phase by 90°, or $\pi/2$. When each is separately added to the solid sine wave, which is one third the frequency but three times the amplitude of the others, the two resulting composite signals are notably dissimilar (Figure 12.22b). So the relative phases of waves (which can range between −180° and 180° or, equivalently, $-\pi$ and π) have an obvious importance when they are superimposed. A sophisticated Fourier analysis program can tell the difference, and even determine the relative magnitudes of the phases. That is central to how phase-encoding works in voxel y-localization.

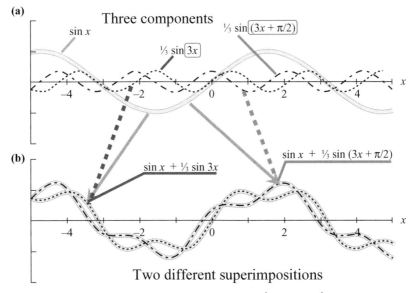

Figure 12.22 The importance of phase. The two higher-frequency waves, $\frac{1}{3} \sin 3x$ and $\frac{1}{3} \sin (3x + \pi/2)$, are the same except for a 90° difference in phase. When each is separately added to sin x, the results, [sin x + $\frac{1}{3}$ sin 3x] and [sin x + $\frac{1}{3}$ sin (3x + $\pi/2$)], appear completely distinct, and the difference can be quantified as part of Fourier analysis.

Spin-echo/spin-warp with a 2 × 2 voxel patient

As with CT earlier, we'll work through the image reconstruction process with a 2 × 2, four-voxel transverse slice (Figure 12.23a). The voxels contain different water densities, but are otherwise the same, and our mission, should we choose to accept it, is to estimate the PD of each. We can achieve this by finding the magnitude of the net magnetization in each, $M(i)$, for $i = 1$ through 4. And

we'll accomplish *that* by detecting (with the pickup coil and receiver) the signal, S, from the entire slice, from the four voxels acting together, while applying several different combinations of G_x and G_y at various times. We then untangle all the signal data with FTs to extract the part contributed by each voxel individually.

Assume that an x-y plane has just been selected during the 90° pulse of a spin-echo sequence, and is now sitting facing a uniform external field. The

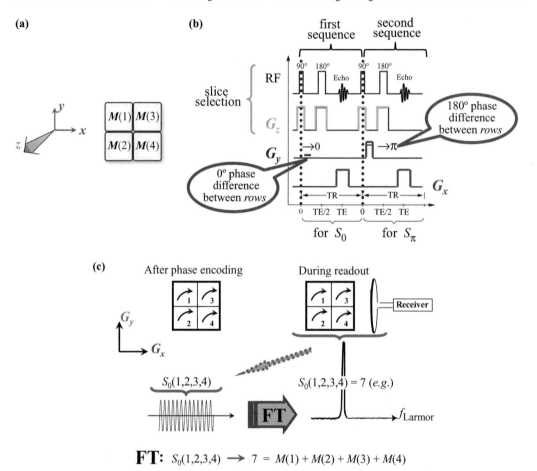

$$\textbf{FT:}\quad S_0(1,2,3,4) \longrightarrow 7 = M(1) + M(2) + M(3) + M(4)$$

Figure 12.23 Our patient **(a)** consists of four voxels lying in the plane to which B_0 and the z-axis are normal (perpendicular). **(b)** Spin-echo, spin-warp for this 2 × 2 matrix consists of two "repetitions." Each invokes the simple 90–180° S-E sequence, but the y-gradient is applied only in the second; the signal from the two are labeled S_0 and S_π, to indicate the amount of phase shift that the y-gradient, G_y, introduces. **(c)** When no gradients of either type (x- or y-) are ever applied, the four magnetizations precess in phase and at the same resonant frequency. This gives rise to a simple, monochromatic sinusoidal signal, $S_0(1,2,3,4)$. Its spectrum, obtained by Fourier analysis, consists of a single peak, which, in this example, is 7 units tall; the subscript 0 indicates that there is zero phase difference introduced between the spins in the first and second rows. **(d)** For our four-voxel patient, the first pulse/gradient repetition sequence is straightforward spin-echo with the x-gradient on during read-out, while **(e)** in the second, a 180° G_y pulse introduces that amount of phase shift between the spins of the lower row and those of the upper before readout (during which the x-gradient is again on.).

(d) **First S-E sequence**

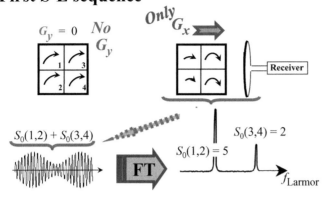

$$FT: S_0(1,2) + S_0(3,4) \begin{cases} S_0(1,2) = 5 = M(1) + M(2) \\ S_0(3,4) = 2 = M(3) + M(4) \end{cases}$$

(e) **Second S-E sequence**

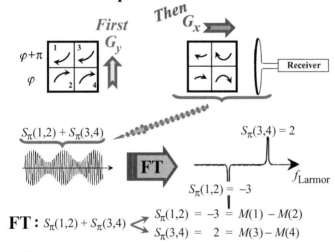

$$FT: S_\pi(1,2) + S_\pi(3,4) \begin{cases} S_\pi(1,2) = -3 = M(1) - M(2) \\ S_\pi(3,4) = 2 = M(3) - M(4) \end{cases}$$

Figure 12.23 (*Continued*)

basic idea underlying what follows is that the contribution to the overall detected signal, $S(t)$, that comes from the ith voxel alone, namely $S(i)$, is proportional to $M(i)$, which is itself linear in PD(i).

Spin-echo, spin-warp for a 2×2 voxel patient consists of two separate, independent standard S-E sequences (Figure 12.23b). The first sequence consists of a straightforward 90–180° pulse pair, with the x-gradient turned on during readout but the y-gradient always left off, $G_y = 0$. Nothing new here. But for the second, the y-gradient is activated long enough, *before* the readout, for the spins in the

upper row to gain π in phase relative to those in the lower row; thereafter, G_x is again turned on as the signal comes in. In the current four-voxel example, since G_y is made to induced phase shifts of only two possible values 0° (first sequence) and π (second), the corresponding signals will be labeled S_0 and S_π, to distinguish RF pulses (0° and 180°) from phase shifts (0 and π).

This may have been a little mind-messing the first time around, so let's go through it again more slowly, and begin with the simplest possible situation.

Preliminary sequence: $G_y = G_y = 0$

If there is neither an x-gradient nor a y-gradient *ever* present, then the four voxel magnetizations evolve over time in complete synchrony (Figure 12.23c). Following the initial 90° pulse, they precess in a uniform magnetic field all at the same frequency, and there are no phase differences among them. So their magnetization vectors just add together, $M = M(1) + M(2) + M(3) + M(4)$; and, after the 180° re-phasing RF pulse, the strength of each of their contributions to the overall RF echo signal sensed by the pickup coil is still proportional to its own PD.

To simplify notation, let's choose units such that $S(i) = M(i)$. The signal strength from any voxel, $S(i)$, is proportional to the magnetization there, so the detected signal from the four together produces a monochromatic sine wave voltage in the pickup coil of amplitude $S_0(1,2,3,4) = S_0(1) + S_0(2) + S_0(3) + S_0(4)$. Suppose the signal is measured, in this example, to have an amplitude/strength of 7: $S_0(1,2,3,4) = 7$. The subscript "0" on $S_0(1,2,3,4)$ indicates that indeed, there are no phase unit shifts brought about by G_y. We can pass the signal through a Fourier analysis program and it indicates, as expected, that the signal is monochromatic, and 7 units in strength.

Things become more interesting, however, with the two-part spin-warp, spin-echo pulse train of Figure 12.23d. Now, G_x is turned on for readout of each of the two echoes; this aspect of the process is commonly called *frequency-encoding*.

There is a fundamental difference, however, between the pulse sequences of Figure 12.23d and e: the first keeps the phase-encoding y-gradient off throughout, but in the second, G_y is turned on with exactly the right strength and span of time, the *phase-encoding period*, to cause the two magnetizations in the *upper row* of the matrix to precess exactly π (180°) farther than those in the lower row (hence the subscript on S_π.) Fleshing this out a little . . .

First S-E repetition sequence: $G_y = 0$; G_x on during readout

For the *first* of the two S-E sequences (Figure 12.23d), no y-gradient is applied at any point. Just before readout begins, the four magnetizations are in phase, as they were in Figure 12.23c. But G_x is turned on during readout/frequency encoding,

and so the two magnetizations in the right-hand column precess a little faster than those to the left, as indicated by the longer curved arrows. Part of the echo signal from the patient is generated by the pair of left-column voxels, and the other part and at slightly higher frequency, by the ones on the right. The pickup coil senses a single beat interference signal created by two independent sources, namely $[M(1) + M(2)]$ and $[M(3) + M(4)]$. These two pairs of voxels produce separate contributions, at two slightly different values of f_{Larmor}, to the overall RF signal. The pickup coil receives a composite signal, S_0, that contains components proportional to each of these sources. After sampling and digitizing, a Fourier analysis reveals that the amplitudes of the components at the two frequencies separately can be expressed, for our example, as the two equations $S_0(1,2) = M(1) + M(2) = 5$ and $S_0(3,4) = M(3) + M(4) = 2$, where the 5 and the 2, say, are the signal strengths that were measured. This is exactly the kind of thing that went on when we were dealing earlier with the 1D phantom.

These measurements comprise a system of two equations with four unknowns, $M(i)$. But to learn the values of the four unknowns, we need a total of four independent relationships among them. What to do now?

Second S-E repetition sequence: $G_y \to \pi$ before readout; G_x on during readout

Spin-warp uses a clever trick to salvage the situation: after completion of the pulses and gradients that gave us S_0, we now perform the second spin-echo measurement (Figure 12.23e) – but this time with a twist, literally. In the second set of S-E pulses of the pulse train, G_y is applied briefly, at some time *before* readout, in such a manner that, by our design, the upper row magnetizations both twist through exactly one extra half-turn, a shift by the amount π, relative to those in the bottom row. After G_y is switched off, the four magnetization vectors again precess all at the same original rate, but there is a new phase relationship among them – in particular, the upper row is now 180° out of phase with the lower. $M(1)$ and $M(3)$ of the top row are still pointing parallel to one another as they go around, that is, but they are now aligned *opposite* to those of voxels 2 and 4. We cannot measure and use the *sum* of $M(1)$ and $M(2)$ again, but rather they now exactly

$$\text{FT}: \quad S_0(1,2) + S_0(3,4) \quad \left\{ \begin{array}{l} S_0(1,2) = 5 = M(1) + M(2) \\ S_0(3,4) = 2 = M(3) + M(4) \end{array} \right.$$

$$\text{FT}: \quad S_\pi(1,2) + S_\pi(3,4) \quad \left\{ \begin{array}{l} S_\pi(1,2) = -3 = M(1) - M(2) \\ S_\pi(3,4) = 2 = M(3) - M(4) \end{array} \right.$$

$$\begin{array}{|c|c|} \hline 1_{\ 1} & 2_{\ 3} \\ \hline 4_{\ 2} & 0_{\ 4} \\ \hline \end{array}$$

Figure 12.24 Four equations in four unknowns, $M(i)$, makes it possible to solve for all of them.

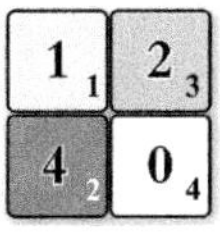

Check:

$$\text{FT}: \quad S_0(1,2,3,4) \rightarrow 7 = M(1) + M(2) + M(3) + M(4)$$

counteract one another (because of the phase shift of exactly π); the combined field from the two of them is now their *difference*, $[M(1) - M(2)]$. Likewise for $[M(3) - M(4)]$. We apply the x-gradient during readout; G_x, and Fourier analysis of this second echo signal indicates $S_\pi(1,2) = M(1) - M(2) = -3$, say, and $S_\pi(3,4) = M(3) + M(4) = 2$.

Now we *can* solve the set of four equations in four unknowns (Figure 12.24), and a little algebra reveals the values of the $M(i)$, hence of the corresponding relative proton densities. Adding the first and the third together, $[M(1) + M(2) = 5] + [M(1) - M(2) = -3]$ leads immediately to $M(1) = 1$, while subtracting them yields $M(2) = 4$. So, too, for the other two equations. These results, incidentally, are in agreement with the results of the preliminary no-gradient study of Figure 11.23c.

It's a heady jump to a 512×512 spatial matrix, involving 512 settings of G_y, and 512 different phase angles rather than only 2, but at heart the approach is much the same – just a good deal more complicated.

Fast imaging with EPI, FISP, FLASH, GRASS, RARE, *et al.*

As with any other imaging modalities, the selection of operating parameters involves tradeoffs. For MRI, the principal ones influence contrast and noise level (i.e., SNR), resolution, and image acquisition time (Figure 12.8a). What perhaps most distinguishes the operation of an MRI machine, from the physician's and radiographer's perspectives, is the number of possible combinations of parameters, and the extent to which the nature of the information revealed is sensitive to the particular set chosen. Parameter selection is a complicated (and

still evolving) business, and it is determined by the clinical objective, the methods chosen to enhance the contrast-to-noise ratio or resolution, the need for contrast agent, aspects of patient anatomy, etc.

While some parameters are difficult or impossible to alter, such as the strength of the principal magnetic field, others are under the immediate control of the operator and subject to well-known general guidelines. These include the type of sequence (spin-echo, inversion-recovery, gradient-echo) and the timing (TE, TR) of RF pulses and briefly applied gradient fields; the slice thickness and inter-slice separation; the dimensions of the voxel matrix and of the field of view (which together determine voxel size and a limit on possible resolution); the use of contrast agent or of physiologic (such as electrocardiogram) gating; parallel surface coils to detect the echo RF pulses; and other factors.

A major objective of MR researchers and manufacturers has been to reduce image-acquisition time without loss of image quality. Some are designing special radiofrequency and gradient pulse sequences that are now fast enough even to capture the beating of a heart in cine form. Many techniques have been devised to increase the speed at which images are produced, and these come under the heading of *fast MRI imaging*.

Fast (or *turbo*, or *rapid*) *spin-echo* (*FSE*) imaging techniques such as RARE (Rapid Acquisition with Relaxation Enhancement) and its derivatives produce images in much less time than standard spin-echo. They may employ trains of multiple 180° pulses to generate corresponding sequences of multiple echoes (Figure 12.10), each created with a separate phase encode. The overall scan time for a slice is reduced by the number of echoes, or *echo train length*, picked up in each sequence. Typically the ETL = 4 to 16 for FSE sequences – although by the time you read this, that number may be greater. The data acquisition time for the FSE can thereby be reduced from something like 12 minutes to just 2 or 3.

The first fast-MRI method to become widely accepted was a form of gradient-echo imaging, rather than spin-echo. Manufacturers offer a variety of GRE sequences on commercial machines that do much the same thing, or not, and that go by acronyms like GRASS, spoiled GRASS, fast multi-planar spoiled GRASS, FISP, FLASH, TurboFLASH, MP-RAGE, SSFP, Balanced SSFP, FIESTA. . . . And the list goes on.

The fastest acquisition methods currently in regular clinical use are variations on the GRE *echo planar imaging* (*EPI*) theme. The phase is not set fully anew after each echo, like normal spin-echo and GRE, but rather is incremented slightly from its previous value with a little phase-encoding G_y nudge, by an amount that corresponds to the row's y-position. An entire slice can be obtained in 50 ms, but it will have more noise and lower spatial resolution than typical anatomical images, along with possible artifacts. EPI is used commonly in functional imaging, such as for contrast-enhanced perfusion imaging and for diffusion imaging.

Other recent advances in hardware and software have also been reducing imaging times. Perhaps most significant has been the advent of *parallel imaging* (pMRI) methods such as SMASH, SENSE, and GRAPPA. Multiple small RF pickup coils are spread out over the region being examined, and the signal from each is recorded separately and sent to its own, independent receiver (Figure 11.31c). This can greatly enhance the speed of data acquisition when a good part of the body is being examined, and provide improved resolution, and it is likely to find increasing application at higher field strengths (3 T). There is a need to integrate the various images obtained, one from each coil, into a single overall picture; since each coil has a relatively small FOV, each requires far fewer phase-encoding lines in *k*-space; the ratio of the number of lines in full *k*-space to the number of lines for one coil is known as the *acceleration factor*, R. *Parallel imaging artifacts* may arise if too large an acceleration factor is selected, or too small an FOV.

As with multi-gated (MUGA) nuclear medicine and CT angiography (CTA), an electrocardiogram (ECG) signal can be harnessed to gate highly specialized, extremely fast pulses of RF energy and gradient fields to image the heart throughout the cardiac cycle. Cardiac MRI can distinguish patients with severe coronary artery disease from others presenting with chest pain – and it may do so more effectively than can ECG, blood enzyme levels, and other measures.

MR imaging of fluid movement/motion

There are many variations on the general MRI theme, some of which explore MR-related time-dependent biophysical processes. As in a number of other modalities, the detection of something *changing* gives rise to novel forms of contrast among different tissues.

Factors that can radically alter the apparent relaxation time for a voxel of tissue are the perfusion of blood or the diffusion of water or other materials through it. Specialized pulse sequences can reveal such movements, and make it possible to devise various kinds of contrast that are clinically relevant. Three that have found significant application are *magnetic resonance angiography* (*MRA*) of flow of blood through vessels (a form of change); *diffusion tensor imaging* (*DTI*) of diffusion of water along neural tracts; and *functional MRI* (*fMRI*) which monitors local changes in blood flow in the brain induced by certain stimuli.

MR angiography and cardiac MRI

Spin relaxation times of protons in fluids will be affected by the bulk flow of their water molecules within spatially or temporally varying magnetic fields. As a consequence, MRI can be exploited in several ways to image the movement of blood within the arteries and veins, providing approaches to angiography. MRA is different from fluoroscopic or CT angiography, however, in that it is non-invasive, involves no ionizing radiation exposure, and does not lead to the kinds of complications that may arise with intra-arterial contrast angiography, such as vascular injury, reactions to iodine-based contrast agent, or stroke. (Some forms of MRA, however, do involve Gd contrast agent.) As with

Doppler ultrasound, MRA can assess the rate of blood flow in the vessels, but with much greater ability to localize that flow; and it can then go on to display the vasculature in three dimensions.

Flow can alter the measured magnitude and phase of the NMR signal from blood, and the flowing blood itself acts the part, in effect, of a contrast agent. With *time-of-flight* (*TOF*) angiography, a blood vessel is oriented perpendicular to and passes through a hypothetical thin slice of voxels (Figure 1.23a). Suppose that nearly all the voxels are filled with static tissue, but a single voxel at the vessel contains blood flowing across the plane, instead. We saturate all the voxels in the plane with a 90° pulse, for example, and monitor the return toward equilibrium of each of them separately. Nearly all will recover at a rate determined by the local tissue T1 value, but not the one containing moving blood: for it, the change will occur much more rapidly, as its saturated blood is rapidly replaced with fresh, unsaturated blood from upstream. Indeed, the parameter characterizing its $M_z(t)$ curve will be determined primarily by the

blood's velocity, not by its T1; and the shorter the *apparent* time constant is, the brighter the blood will appear on what is essentially a T1-weighted image. For this reason, TOF is called a form of *bright blood* angiography; for *dark blood* techniques, voxels corresponding to areas of blood flow yield low NMR signal.

Another form of MR angiography, *phase contrast* (*PC*) MRA, has the advantage of indicating not only the speed of flow, but also its direction (Figure 1.23b). PC-MRA is a relative of diffusion-weighted imaging, described next. Its downside is that it may take considerably more time than TOF.

Diffusion tensor imaging

The brief, enticing scent of a garlic-calamari pizza wafts off all too quickly as it passes by and, likewise, a drop of color dye in a glass of water slowly spreads out in an expanding gradient of paleness (Figure 12.25a). The dye does this because whenever one of its molecules bangs into a tumbling water molecule, it is equally likely to end up moving away

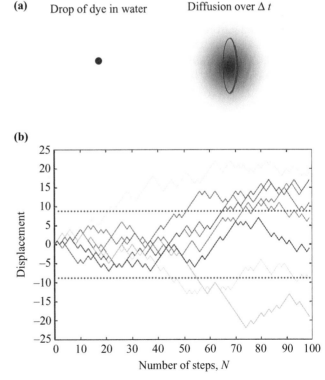

(a)   Drop of dye in water   Diffusion over Δt

(b)

Figure 12.25 Diffusion tensor imaging (DTI). (**a**) Diffusion of a drop of dye in water. Dye slowly diffuses outward from the initially high-concentration point, and as the entropy (degree of disorder) increases. The ring on the right indicates the average distance that dye molecules have traveled by a certain time. (**b**) A complementary explanation employs a branch of probability theory that deals with "random walks."

Displacement

Number of steps, N

(a)   Conventional T2   **(b)**   DWI

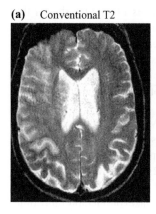 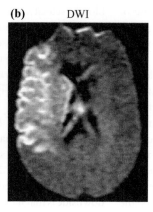

Figure 12.26 For a patient with an acute stroke, comparison of **(a)** conventional T2 and **(b)** diffusion-weighted images. Contrast is created by identifying voxels through which water is self-diffusing rapidly, in particular through failing cells or along nerve tracts. Courtesy of David K. Powell, University of Kentucky MRISC.

from the original center of the spot as back toward it. Over time, this sort of thing causes a broadening and thinning of the spherically symmetric, near-Gaussian cloud about its center. Likewise within tissue, unconstrained intercellular water itself drifts continuously from place to place. For these, the principal driver is the process of *diffusion*. Diffusion is a molecular-scale, non-equilibrium process that takes place when there is a concentration gradient of a substance (dye) between regions (the center of the original drop and the surrounding pure water), and a channel along which the substance can slowly wend its way. This is a loose definition of Fick's law, which is the starting point for a quantitative analysis.

There is a different, interesting way to look at this. Recall the legendary late-night reveler trying to get home after an evening at his favorite establishments. He staggers up the street to the nearest lamppost and rests there awhile. But when beginning the next leg of his journey, he forgets which way he was headed, and flips a coin to decide which way to go this time. And so on, again and again. Figure 12.25b follows his route for all the evenings in a week. It happens in this probabilistic 1D *random walk* exercise that, on *average*, he will end up $0.8\,N^{\frac{1}{2}}$ from the starting point after N steps – but there's no telling which side of the starting point he will be on. The same happens when a proton's water molecule undergoes collisions with others, ends up spinning at a different rate about a new axis of rotation and drifting in a new direction, accumulating a bit more de-phasing – but whether it acquires a positive or negative increment of phase angle is anybody's guess.

The propensity of water to diffuse, parameterized by the *diffusion constant*, D, depends on its local environment. In the case of early acute stroke, for example, *diffusion-weighted imaging* can detect early on that the sodium-potassium pump has failed, and that water is not moving properly inward and out of the afflicted cells. While this may be noticeable on a conventional T2 image (Figure 12.26a), it is quite unmistakable with DWI (Figure 12.26b). Later, the cells will burst, and the stroke area gets very dark.

The diffusion of intracellular water is generally more restricted than that of extracellular water – a special case of that being diffusion along an axon. Structures such as cell membranes and myelin layers form powerful barriers that restrict diffusion out of the cells, so anisotropic diffusion along the long lengths of axon fascicles is generally much quicker than radially across the cell membrane and myelin. The form of the technique known as *diffusion tensor imaging* (*DTI*) is valuable, and visually striking, in delineating the paths of trunks of axons in the brain, as in Figure 0.6 and on the front cover. DTI can examine such directional differences in diffusion that arise from characteristics like organized cellular structure. When pathology of structured organs changes, such as demyelination of white matter in multiple sclerosis, diffusion out of cells becomes much faster.

While originally applied to brain studies, DTI has extended its range, and now finds application in the study of carpal tunnel syndrome, compressed lumbar nerves, cervical spondylotic myelopathy, neural tumors, and other pathologies affecting the nervous and musculoskeletal systems.

Functional MRI with blood oxygenation level-dependent (BOLD) MRI

*f*MRI and PET have been bringing about a revolution in the neurosciences. Research and clinical psychologists and psychiatrists are employing them to correlate neural metabolism and the activities of local cranial microvasculature with normal and abnormal mental function, including sensation, emotional responses, cognitive tasks, and a broad range of neurological diseases. *f*MRI is similar to PET in some regards, but it differs from it in its fundamental mechanism: while PET commonly reveals changes in cellular *glucose metabolism* in various parts of the brain in response to stimuli, *f*MRI monitors the response of the microvasculature and variations in the local *flow of oxygenated blood* needed for that metabolism. So the two are complementary and often correlated, but they are not the same.

*f*MRI, and in particular *blood oxygen level-dependent* (*BOLD*) imaging, is built upon the difference in magnetic properties (as parameterized by the susceptibility, χ, Equation 11.4c) between oxygenated and non-oxygenated blood. Deoxyhemoglobin is *paramagnetic* — it contains an unpaired electron on the iron ion, which produces a magnetic field three orders of magnitude greater than that of a proton, somewhat like gadolinium contrast agent. Oxyhemoglobin, on the other hand, is diamagnetic, and the magnetic field produced by its cloud of (spin-paired) electrons is extremely weak. Under "resting" conditions, the brain maintains a balance of the two, but during neural activity, there is local increased need and utilization of oxygen. This causes the conversion of some of the oxyhemoglobin present to deoxyhemoglobin, disturbing the former balance and altering the local magnetic fields near capillary beds and veins.

The BOLD process involves some stimulus that gives rise to neural activation, followed by an alteration in the hemodynamic balance in a small region of the brain, and an altered BOLD *f*MRI signal (Figure 0.5). Suppose a subject is receiving regularly spaced stimuli, such as periodic touches to the right middle toe, or regular flashing images of Sarah Palin doing something curious with a moose. Alternatively, the subject herself might be intermittently bending and straightening the left thumb. Either way, there will be an associated activity in some part of the sensory or motor regions of the brain, which will therefore consume a little more oxygen than normal, thereby increase the level of deoxyhemoglobin.

Changing the concentrations of the two forms of hemoglobin will create variations and gradients in the local magnetic fields. We have already seen that addition of a paramagnetic material can shorten T1 relaxation times, and T2 and T2* times as well. BOLD images are usually T2*-*w*, and areas of the brain with signal variations that correlate well with the cyclical task pattern can be displayed as an overlay on top of an anatomical MRI image.

To monitor rapid changes in the brain that are associated with these stimuli, one must collect multiple images within short periods of time. Achieving adequate SNR requires repeating the stimulus periodically a number of times, and the use of high-powered statistics to separate information from noise. For the same reason, *f*MRI is one technology that performs significantly better at higher B_0. Typically, one would obtain a set of 20–30 images, covering the whole brain, every 2–4 seconds. For an *f*MRI experiment lasting four minutes, say, that would correspond to more than a thousand images.

Deoxyhemoglobin is paramagnetic, acting like a contrast agent; you would therefore naturally expect relaxation processes to speed up, with shorter T2* or T2 coming from the faster de-phasing of $M_{xy}(t)$ (Figure 12.27a). A shorter T2* gives rise to a weaker MR signal, and you should find a darker region in an image. Makes perfect sense, but it's the opposite of what actually happens. Because of the need for more oxygen, rather, there occurs a local vasodilation and increase in blood flow that overcompensates, removing deoxyhemoglobin from the region so fast that its concentration *falls* below what it is in the resting condition (Figure 12.27b). Turning that around: a slower 1/T2* rate gives rise to a decrease in the signal strength, which indicates where in the brain the instantaneous flow of oxygenated blood is unusually high, and where the neurons are unusually busy. In other words, your brain is smart enough not only to think deep thoughts, but also to keep track of what part of it needs special attention to make the deep thoughts happen!

BOLD thus is a powerful research tool that makes it possible to track precisely what parts of the brain

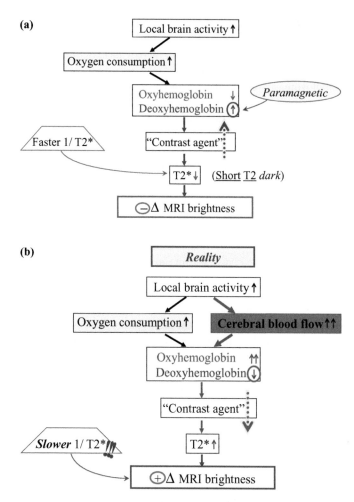

(a)

Local brain activity ↑

Oxygen consumption ↑

Oxyhemoglobin ↓
Deoxyhemoglobin ↑   *Paramagnetic*

Faster 1/ T2*   "Contrast agent"

T2* ↓   (Short T2 *dark*)

⊖Δ MRI brightness

(b)

Reality

Local brain activity ↑

Oxygen consumption ↑   **Cerebral blood flow ↑↑**

Oxyhemoglobin ↑↑
Deoxyhemoglobin ↓

"Contrast agent"

Slower 1/ T2*   T2* ↑

⊕Δ MRI brightness

Figure 12.27 Oxyhemoglobin, which is diamagnetic, and deoxyhemoglobin (paramagnetic) have magnetic properties sufficiently dissimilar that they have different impacts on the relaxation times of protons in nearby water. When a patient receives a stimulus, certain parts of the brain will respond, consuming oxygen, and this will indirectly modify the local balance of oxygenated to oxygen-depleted blood. That, in turn, will alter the local blood flow, and that also affects the proton relaxation times, hence the MRI signal. (**a**) The obvious, but incorrect, mechanism of BOLD. (**b**) What really happens.

are responding to various specific external or self-initiated stimuli. But *f*MRI has clinical applications, as well. Enhancing standard MRI with *f*MRI, for example, can assist in the planning of delicate operations; not only can a neurosurgeon see exactly where an astrocytoma is, but she can also take more fully into account potential losses of cognitive, sensory, or motor abilities that might be caused by damage to nearby healthy tissues from various surgical or radiation treatment strategies. She might even be able to see if the corresponding region in the contra-lateral hemisphere is unexpectedly active, indicating some compensation that the brain is performing to circumvent loss of function from the tumor.

Other modalities, such as electroencephalography (EEG) and magnetoencephalography (MEG), are also being utilized for mapping brain function, as discussed in Chapter 13. Establishing connections between their results and those of (much higher spatial resolution) *f*MRI and PET will be essential for their progress.

CHAPTER 13

Evolving and Experimental Modalities

Researchers have been exploring the clinical potentials of a number of imaging modalities other than the principal ones already described. Some are familiar and others are fresh, and any of them may, or may not, eventually find wide use in the clinic.

The newer ones include optical and molecular imaging, nanotechnology, and bioinformatics, perhaps in combination with new forms of computational hardware and software, and may well lead to novel approaches to medical imaging.

Among the ones that have been around for a while, thermography, electroencephalography, and magnetocardiography create images from extremely faint electromagnetic signals that the body itself produces and emits naturally, rather like nuclear medicine but without need for the radio-pharmaceutical contrast agent. Tissue impedance tomography and diaphanography, conversely, operate like X-rays and ultrasound, observing how probes passing through the body interact with it.

The catchword *du jour*, the area that is receiving a noticeable increase in attention and funding, is *translational research* from lab to clinic. Meanwhile, biomedical research is becoming ever more interdisciplinary, as it depends increasingly on cross-fertilization between the physical sciences and engineering on the one hand and biology and clinical medicine on the other. The recent trend in importing ideas, devices, and software from elsewhere will surely continue to grow. The National Security Agency (NSA), the Defense Advanced Research Projects Agency (DARPA), and the National Aeronautics and Space Administration (NASA), for example, have developed highly sophisticated imaging techniques to sharpen the eyes of spy satellites, to keep cruise missiles on track, and to search the heavens back to the beginnings of time. These agencies are constantly looking for civilian applications of some of their technologies, and they have already transferred numerous ideas and equipment designs to medicine. Similarly, much of the technology that makes modern imaging so vibrant and flexible was produced first by the entertainment and communications industries for games, special effects for

Medical Imaging: Essentials for Physicians, First Edition. Anthony B. Wolbarst, Patrizio Capasso and Andrew R. Wyant.
© 2013 John Wiley & Sons, Inc. Published 2013 by John Wiley & Sons, Inc.

films, etc. – and they, too, clearly have much more to share.

This chapter provides very brief comments on (rather than explanations of) a small sample of the innovations and changes that may have the potential for clinical adoption. Some are obvious, and others just happen to interest the authors. It draws largely from a review article [1] Bear in mind that there are thousands of other approaches out there, and one of them might come from nowhere and become the next MRI.

Optical and near-infrared imaging

Gamma-rays and X-rays reside at the top of the useable electromagnetic spectrum (Figure 2.2b), and those fields are well plowed. Heading southward in energy, after meandering through the ultraviolet region (where currently there are few applications), one comes to visible and near-infrared light.

The intensity, $L(x)$, of monochromatic light in a homogeneous medium is attenuated approximately exponentially, with penetration distance,

$$L(x)/L(0) = e^{-\mu_{opt}x}. \qquad (13.1)$$

This is essentially the same as the corresponding attenuation laws for high-energy photons and ultrasound (Equations 3.1 and 10.2), and as with them, the attenuation process can be partitioned into absorption and scatter parts. The *optical attenuation coefficient*, μ_{opt}, and closely related entities go also by other names like "molar extinction factor," "absorption/scattering cross-sections," "opacity," and "optical density," depending on the context.

Our eyes evolved to respond to visible light largely because the atmospheric gases happen to be nearly transparent to electromagnetic energy in that range. Fortunately for us, on the other hand, they do rapidly attenuate ionizing gamma-rays from outer space and ultraviolet light; they also absorb most of the infrared spectrum, down to the microwave and radiofrequency range, where communications and radio-astronomy again become feasible. Water and some cellular materials and tissues, such as those of glass fish, are also nearly transparent to visible and infrared light.

Nearly all soft tissues, on the other hand, are rather opaque throughout most of the infrared, visible, and ultraviolet parts of the electromagnetic spectrum, and behave optically much like milk. When you shine light onto them, it will penetrate centimeters, more or less, over which it is both absorbed and scattered, and the attenuation coefficient varies strongly with the photon energy for reasons that have largely to do with the vibrational modes of the molecules involved.

The clinical utility of optical methods depends largely on the ability to extract image information about objects embedded in turbid media, so there have been serious efforts to reduce the level of scattered radiation reaching the image receptor. Improvements in time-resolved spectroscopy techniques and in the theory of photon transport in tissues have both contributed to recent advances in scatter suppression.

Endoscopy and laparoscopy

One of the simplest ways to look within the body is, well, just to look. Physicians long used rigid tubes, mirrors, and candles or sunlight to peer down the throat and along other bodily passageways, but it was the introduction of fiber optics in the 1950s that transformed *endoscopy* and *laparoscopy* into major clinical modalities.

Light (typically incandescent) entering the tip of a flexible glass fiber, a tenth of a millimeter or so across, will reflect again and again off its interior surface, like a stone skipping on water, and can travel great distances with little loss of intensity. Whether inserted through a natural orifice or through a small surgical incision, a bundle of thousands of fibers, commonly with lenses at the two ends, can carry a clear and sharp optical image. A modern endoscope consists of such a bundle, along with another bunch of fibers that bring in bright light to illuminate the region being viewed. It may also have channels to convey gases or liquids in or out, or perhaps even a mechanical device such as a biopsy forceps at its business end. Alternatively, a high-power laser beam carried by a fiber optic bundle may be used to burn away diseased tissues.

Traditional laparoscopy involves making three small incisions into the patient and directly manipulating the optical camera and the mechanical arms that perform the cutting and suturing. With some recent devices, only a single small (1.5 cm) incision is required (such as through the navel), and the surgeon controls all the action of robot arms from a computer console. While this leads to faster healing and less scarring, the jury is still out on which procedures warrant the extra cost.

A fairly recent variation on this theme is doubtless a harbinger of things to come. Gastroscopy and CT are sometimes unable to image the small intestine adequately, requiring exploratory surgery. But a camera and radio-transmitter combination the size of a large pill has been developed that can be swallowed, sending images throughout its transit of the gastrointestinal tract. Shades of *Fantastic Voyage* but, alas, without Raquel Welch.

These devices provide photographic views of tissue coverings only, directly revealing little of what lies below the exterior. For that, one has to turn to the less direct modalities.

Diaphanography of the breast

Diaphanography, also termed *transillumination*, is a form of *transmission* imaging that is similar to radiography or fluoroscopy, except that it employs visible-light photons, rather than X-rays, as its probes – as when you shine a bright flashlight through your hand. It is sensitive to the differential absorption and scatter of high-intensity laser light as it scans through relatively thin blocks of tissues, and records images with an electronic optical camera such as a CCD.

Transillumination of the breast can sometimes distinguish between benign and malignant masses, but mammography and ultrasound produce fewer erroneous positive and negative results. It is of some clinical interest, however, the more so now that researchers are finding ways to prevent light scattered within the tissues from reaching the detector, but it has not been accepted as a standard clinical tool.

Infrared-guided biopsy

Each year, 1 million women undergo core-needle breast biopsy in the United States. While considerably easier on the patient than excisional biopsy, the core-needle technique suffers too high a rate of false-negatives, despite needle guidance with X-ray fluoroscopy or US. A more sophisticated type of probe currently under development may reduce the false-negative rate substantially. After the probe has been guided to the tumor site within the breast, its tip transmits near-infrared (NIR) laser light into the breast tissue and then senses the light coming back from the tissue. The light returning from a tumor may differ from that coming back from normal tissue because of irregularities in the degree of oxygenation, fluorescence characteristics, or other properties. In cases where no abnormality is detected, the tip of the probe is advanced in further search for disease. On finding tissue that yields an irregularity in the returning light, the probe acquires a core biopsy specimen. Unlike mammograms, the NIR probe works well in the dense breast tissue of many young women, and may find applications in other organ systems, as well.

Optical tomography

Laser optical tomography or *optical coherence tomography (OCT)* yields cross-sectional images by irradiating tissue with laser beams and capturing the relatively small amount of light that is *reflected* coherently (not scattered randomly) from subsurface features; scattered light, which contributes only optical noise, is filtered out and rejected. The technique normally employs NIR radiation, to which tissues are relatively transmissive, and it can provide resolution of 0.01 mm or better, but it works only at a surface or to a depth of several millimeters. The images are useful in studies of blood perfusion, tissue oxygenation, and neovascularity in the brain, breast, and extremities (Figure 13.1).

Diffuse optical tomography is a related but different NIR-based technology that provides measurements of hemodynamics and neural activation at depths of several centimeters in tissue.

With a somewhat different approach, *confocal scanning laser tomography* can non-invasively acquire three-dimensional images of the posterior surface of the eye, creating a quantitative description of the head of the optic nerve and the surrounding retinal surface (Figure 13.2). A laser beam is focused to some depth within the eye and scans a two-dimensional plane. Only light from that focal plane is allowed to reach the detector. A sequence of such two-dimensional optical planar views is acquired for increasing depths of the focal plane, and the result can be displayed as a three-dimensional topographic image of the nerve head and peripapillary retinal nerve fiber layer. With expert interpretation, the power of the technique as an aid in the diagnosis and management of

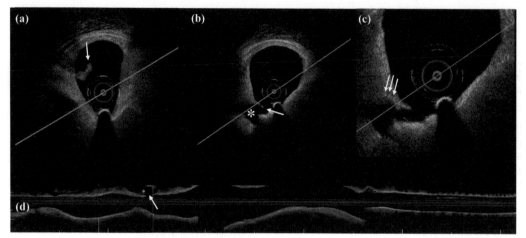

Figure 13.1 Optical coherence tomography (OCT) findings in acute ST elevation myocardial infarction following mechanical thrombectomy. (**a**) Cross-sectional image of highly reflective intraluminal structure with shadowing (arrow) representing residual red thrombus. (**b**) Large superficial lipid pool (asterisk) with a recently ruptured thin-cap fibroatheroma (arrow). (**c**) Adjacent residual fibrous cap with spotty reflective areas (arrows), consistent with macrophage infiltration in the recently ruptured vulnerable plaque. (**d**) Longitudinal view. Images obtained with a 2.7 French C7 Dragonfly™ intravascular imaging catheter. Image and interpretation courtesy of Michael Jones, Curtis Given, Central Baptist Hospital, Lexington, KY.

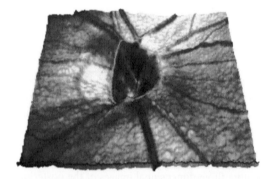

Figure 13.2 Confocal scanning laser tomographic image of the posterior surface of the eye shows the topography of the optic nerve head and of the surrounding retinal surface in three dimensions. In less than 2 seconds, the 670-nm laser performed a sequence of 64 scans of the retina over a 15° × 15° field, creating sixty-four 386 × 386-pixel planar images out of light reflected from different depths. The shape of the indentation edge, emphasized by the drawn green line, indicates a nerve fiber layer defect at the rim of the optic nerve head. Courtesy of Heidelberg Engineering, Dossenheim, Germany. Reproduced from [1], fig. 11, with permission of the Radiological Society of North America (RSNA).

glaucoma may be comparable to that of the accepted standard of stereofundus photography.

Finally, *non-linear microscopy* employs non-linear optical methods, such as multi-photon molecular excitation, optical harmonic generation, and depletion of stimulated emission. It can image subcellular morphology and trace molecular dynamics at sub-nanometer resolution at depths of up to a fraction of a millimeter in living tissue.

Molecular imaging and nanotechnology

Cellular and molecular fluorescence imaging

"Molecular imaging" describes the minimally invasive *in vivo* sensing, depiction, and characterization of spatially localized biologic processes at the cellular and molecular levels. It has evolved largely out of conventional nuclear medicine and optical fluorescence imaging, and its studies of image-based surrogate markers and biomarkers and of biosensors are in their infancy. Perhaps what most distinguishes it from its precursors is its focus on *in vivo* pathology at the microscopic level, rather than on detecting sizeable regions where disease is occurring. It generally refers to work that is still largely in

Figure 13.3 Biomolecular imaging. (a) Optical bioluminescence imaging of cardiac gene delivery for three rats injected directly into the lateral wall with: (left) control adenovirus (*Ad*), indicating the low background activity; (middle) adenovirus carrying firefly luciferase (*Fluc*) driven by cytomegalovirus (*CMV*) promoter, revealing the expression in the myocardium and liver due to leakage of adenovirus into the bloodstream from the injection site; (right) adenovirus carrying luciferase driven by myosin light chain (*MLC*) promoter. The image shows only cardiac expression of luciferase due to use of myosin light chain promoter, which is not markedly active in hepatocytes. In all three cases, the bioluminescence image, in relative light units (*RLU*) per minute, is superimposed on a normal photograph of the rat. Courtesy of Sanjiv Gambhir, Stanford University. (b) Serial transverse microPET images of reporter gene expression in a rat as a function of time in days after dose injection: (top) the animal was injected with ^{13}N-labeled ammonia; (bottom) the injected agent is ^{18}F-labeled *HBG* gene. Courtesy of Heinrich Schelbert, David Geffen School of Medicine, UCLA. (c) Dependence on particle size of the emission spectra of quantum dots comprised of various semiconducting materials. Courtesy of Xavier Michalet. Reproduced from [1], fig. 16ab, with permission of the Radiological Society of North America (RSNA) (parts a and b). See Michalet X, Bentolila LA, Weiss S, Molecular imaging: physics and bioapplications of quantum dots. In: Wolbarst AB, Mossman KL, Hendee WR (eds), *Advances in Medical Physics*, vol. 2. Madison, WI: Medical Physics Publishing, 2008 (part c).

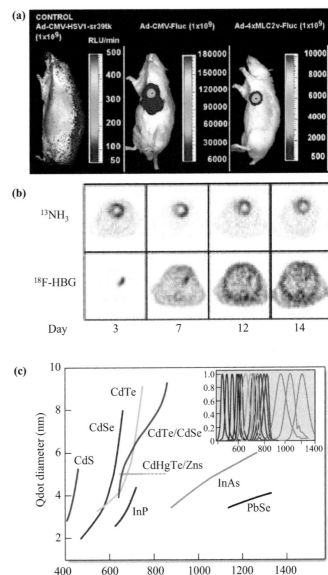

an active preclinical stage, and involves "the convergence of multiple image-capture techniques, basic cell/molecular biology, chemistry, medicine, pharmacology, medical physics, biomathematics, and bioinformatics into a new imaging paradigm" [2].

The development of molecular imaging is attributable, in part, to the synthesis of novel molecular agents that attach with high specificity to genes, proteins, or other biomolecular targets and that can then be sensed with various imaging technologies.

Among these are substances that are activated in response to particular changes in the local biochemical environment, such as specific gene expression or enzyme activity (Figure 13.3a).

Considerable numbers and varieties of molecular imaging systems are being investigated and, as with any new field, they are undergoing rapid growth. This is being driven in part by the design of micro-CT, micro-MR, micro-PET, optical bioluminescence, fluorescence molecular tomography, and other devices for the study of small (approximately 70 g) laboratory animals (Figure 13.3b). The corresponding clinical machines built for 70 kg humans are scaled down – often with improved image quality and almost always at substantially reduced cost. The image receptor for micro-CT, for example, can be built around commercially available off-the-shelf charge-coupled devices.

Molecular imaging technology – indeed, the whole field of *biophotonics* – is undergoing leaps in sophistication. In addition to new pharmaceuticals, imaging techniques, and methods for therapeutic monitoring, there are numerous recent reports on the monitoring or imaging of exogenous gene delivery and expression, protein-protein interactions, apoptosis as a predictor of therapeutic response, tumor growth, dopamine and serotonin neurotransmission, and much else. Also being studied are the absorption, scatter, and fluorescence of various wavelengths of light by tissues, and dependences of their kinetics (e.g., fluorescent lifetime imaging microscopy) on the water, lipid, deoxyhemoglobin, and other biochemical contents, which, in turn, are influenced by the state of health of the cells, matrix materials, and vasculature – all of which may depend on the patient's age, sex, and other characteristics.

Mini- and nanotechnology

Nano-scale technology offers exciting possibilities for medical imaging. Truly microscopic sensors, motors, and other electromechanical devices (which might contain biologic components) could be injected into the bloodstream or bowel, say, and directed to an area of concern. Once there, they might obtain and transmit images, perform chemical tests or biopsies, or even carry out small-scale surgery. While some might find all of this to be just a little too sci-fi, others would argue that it's already happening.

At the finest level, *nanoparticles* display specific physical or chemical characteristics (such as paramagnetism or stimulated fluorescence) that can be quite at variance with the properties of the bulk material, as may objects coated with nanoparticles. *Quantum dots*, or *qdots*, are single fluorescent semiconductor or other nanocrystals only nanometers in diameter. At such sizes, a nanosystem begins to act somewhat like a large molecule or a set of interacting large molecules, with quantum mechanical properties quite different from those of a bulk piece of the same crystalline or amorphous material. Because of quantum confinement effects, the narrow laser-stimulated emission spectra of quantum dots, in particular, depend on the size of the dots, which can be precisely controlled during synthesis (Figure 13.3c). When quantum dots emitting various colors are conjugated to antibodies, antibiotics, or other recognition molecules and are then injected intravenously, they can help detect and map out a number of specific cellular markers of diseased tissues simultaneously – a form of multiplexed, *in vivo* optical biopsy. Also, MR, PET, and CT contrast agents can be grafted to their surface so that they, too, can provide molecular imaging diagnostics. It might even be possible to attach therapeutic agents to quantum dots, moreover, which could be activated once in proper position.

Thermography

In contrast to the modalities discussed so far, thermography, electrocardiography, electroencephalography, magnetoencephalography, and magnetocardiography all involve extraction of information from the electromagnetic radiation that the body itself produces and emits naturally.

The warmer and bigger something is, the more infrared (heat) electromagnetic radiation it emits, at a rate that is approximately proportional to the fourth power of the absolute temperature, as T^4. (Another reason anodes don't all fry is that the hotter they get, the ever more rapidly they radiate off energy – a kind of protective negative feedback effect.) Like some night-vision techniques, medical emission thermography is able to sense infrared radiation (of lower frequency than visible light) emitted through the skin as a result of heat brought to the surface by blood flowing up from deeper regions. Irregularities that affect blood flow in the outermost few millimeters of the skin or that influence its temperature directly (e.g., angiogenesis and neovascularity that accompany breast disease) can be detected by means of an infrared camera (Figure 13.4).

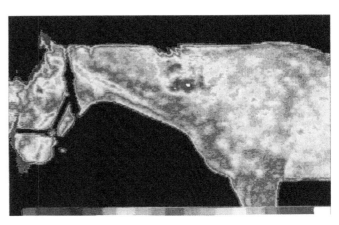

Figure 13.4 Thermogram of Stewball, who recently received an intramuscular injection in his neck. Skin in the region of the injection is about 2 °C warmer than elsewhere, and it shows up as a red area of increased brightness. Courtesy of Martin Furr, Virginia-Maryland Regional College of Veterinary Medicine. Reproduced from [1], fig. 14, with permission of the Radiological Society of North America (RSNA).

The FDA has warned women not to substitute breast thermography for mammography in screening for breast cancer (www.fda.gov/MedicalDevices/Safety/AlertsandNotices/ucm257259.htm), but it is useful in monitoring inflammatory conditions, such as rheumatic disease, injured muscles, damaged nerve enervation of muscles, burns, and frostbite.

Terahertz (T-ray) imaging of epithelial tissues

The terahertz portion of the electromagnetic spectrum lies between 300 and 100 μm in wavelength. So-called terahertz rays, or T-rays, do not penetrate water or tissue well, so they would be of little use in the examination of deep-seated tissues. A substantial fraction of cancers lie in the epithelium, however, and while many of these are readily apparent to the trained eye, some that are small and flat can be overlooked, inaccessible, or are simply not visible. Standard modalities are not adept at depicting or characterizing epithelial tumors – but terahertz imaging can recognize the spectral fingerprints of surface proteins that are markers for certain cancers, and is capable of demonstrating them at an early stage when they can still be treated effectively (Figure 13.5). Terahertz rays are non-ionizing and offer imaging resolution of less than a millimeter; the equipment is safe and portable. Terahertz sensing and imaging devices are inefficient and still costly, but recently created so-called photonic band-gap materials may change that situation.

Microwave and electron spin resonance imaging

Microwave imaging is particularly sensitive to differences in absorption between fat and other soft tissues. The wavelength is too long normally to allow the degree of spatial resolution normally required for diagnostic imaging, but microwave devices may

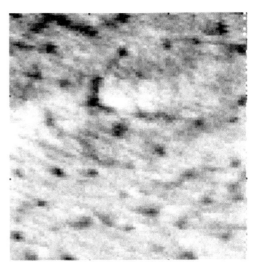

Figure 13.5 *In vivo* terahertz image of a 15 × 15-mm² region of a volunteer's forearm, with a scar running upward from left to right in the upper half. The image was generated by plotting the electric field value reflected from beneath the skin surface; small dark circular regions are hair follicles of normal skin, which are not present at the scar. Courtesy of Vincent Wallace, TeraView, Cambridge, UK. Reproduced from [1], fig. 12, with permission of the Radiological Society of North America (RSNA).

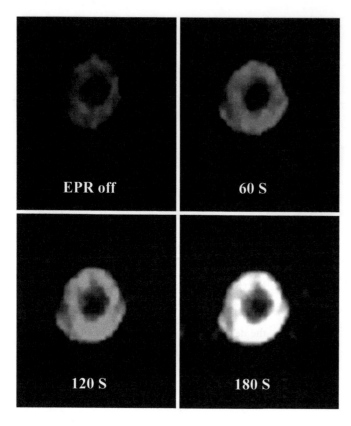

Figure 13.6 Proton electron double resonance imaging (PEDRI; also known as Overhauser imaging). Time course of PEDRI study of myocardial uptake of free radical probe TEMPONE (4-oxo-2,2,6,6-tetramethylpiperidine-1-oxyl) by isolated perfused rat heart. Two-dimensional PEDRI sections were then sequentially acquired every 30 seconds, with each scan taking 27 seconds. At the low field strength of 0.02 T (201 G), the electron-spin resonance and nuclear MR frequencies are 567 and 0.856 MHz, respectively. Courtesy of Haihong Li, Jay Zweier, Ohio State University. Reproduced from [1], fig. 13, with permission of the Radiological Society of North America (RSNA).

find other applications. For example, promising preliminary clinical studies have been reported on a small device called a tissue resonance interferometer. This device generates low levels of 400–1350 MHz radiation (less than that of a cell phone), and the returning signal is altered by tissue irregularities, including tumors.

Electron-spin resonance (ESR) imaging, also known as electron paramagnetic resonance (EPR) imaging, is analogous to the process underlying MRI, but it involves spin transitions of unpaired atomic orbital *electrons* (found typically on *free radicals*, Chapter 5) rather than of hydrogen nuclei. Since an electron has the same magnitude of charge as a proton but is three orders of magnitude lighter (and therefore seems to spin much faster), it has a considerably greater magnetic moment and a correspondingly higher Larmor frequency. At 1 T, an electron's magnetic resonance occurs at 28 GHz, rather than at 42 MHz for a proton (1 GHz = 1000 MHz). As with MRI, ESR imaging involves both the absorption of microwave-energy photons and the subsequent relaxation of electrons between their spin states. In a variation on the theme, known as proton-electron double-resonance imaging (PEDRI), electron-spin resonance and nuclear MR imaging take place simultaneously (Figure 13.6).

Electroencephalography, magnetocardiography, and impedance imaging

The normal flows of ionic currents in cardiac muscle cells and within and among the neurons in the brain give rise to weak, low-frequency, transient *electric* and *magnetic* fields. General approaches have been devised to detect and examine these fields with devices positioned external to the body.

Electroencephalography and electrocardiography

Electrocardiography (ECG or EKG), the method of detecting and quantifying electric fields resulting from the activity of the heart, is ubiquitous, and increasing numbers of laboratories are investigating potential clinical applications of its cousin, *electroencephalography* (EEG) of the brain, as well. Either way, electrodes are attached to the skin surface of the chest or along the scalp to record the faint voltages produced when the heart fires or when the brain does whatever it does. The studies are sensitive, and the shapes and temporal patterns of the voltage pulses can yield medically critical information.

With the traditional approach, a few electrodes attached to the skin surface record the faint voltages produced when the heart pulses or an area of the brain is activated. At present, it is the shapes of the voltage pulses changing over time that are diagnostic. Arrays of many electrodes spread over an area of the patient may eventually succeed in generating spatial information in image form, as well. One problem is the rapid attenuation of electric signals in the body, so that those that do reach the electrodes are very weak and difficult to extract from background electrophysiologic noise. Another is that electrical currents in the body do not travel in straight lines, exacerbating the problem of source location. Computer and electrical engineers have made great strides forward, though, in filtering out the junk while leaving the principal signals intact.

Magnetoencephalography and magnetocardiography

Electric currents within tissues generate weak, time-varying magnetic fields. Magnetoencephalography (MEG) measures them with detectors positioned around the head, and back-calculates the locations and strengths of the neural currents that gave rise to them. The fields are about one billionth as strong as the earth's, so near-perfect magnetic shielding and an exceedingly responsive detector are required to map their variations in time and space around the head. Fortunately, the exquisitely sensitive Superconducting QUantum Interference Device (SQUID) fills the latter bill nicely (Figure 13.7). In breast studies, moreover, iron oxide nanoparticles bound to antibodies serve as a MEG contrast agent; attached to HER-2 receptors, the approach can reveal a breast tumor one thousand times smaller than what mammography can find.

MEG and EEG have already proven to be clinically of value in non-invasive studies of epilepsy, migraine headache, diabetic coma, and post-traumatic stress disorder. Like PET and functional

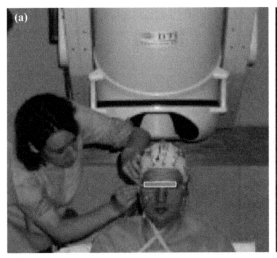 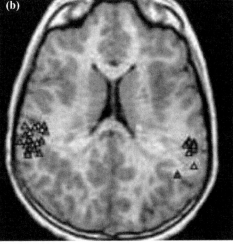

Figure 13.7 Magnetoencephalography. (a) A MEG device, based on a Superconducting QUantum Interference Device (SQUID) is hypersensitive to weak magnetic fields. Courtesy of Yang Jiang, University of Kentucky. (b) MEG spatial information superimposed on a transverse T1-weighted MR section. Spike activity (△) in a 10-year-old patient with Landau-Kleffner syndrome. Courtesy of M Funke, University of Utah. Reproduced from [1], fig. 15, with permission of the Radiological Society of North America (RSNA).

MRI, moreover, they can also follow the brain's response to stimuli. And they can demonstrate subtle abnormalities in a region of brain that appears to be structurally and physiologically normal when viewed by other modalities.

Magnetocardiography (MCG) tracks the much stronger magnetic field changes that accompany the cardiac cycle. While MEG and MCG, together known as magnetic source imaging, are not yet employed widely, a number of researchers consider them well worth vigorous pursuit. Also being investigated, as an alternative to electroshock therapy, is the converse process of magnetic nerve stimulation, in which a pulse of electric current flow is generated in a well-localized region of the brain by rapidly changing the field from a powerful external magnet.

With millimeter and millisecond spatial and temporal resolutions, MEG and EEG assess neural activity directly, as it takes place. Functional MRI and PET, by contrast, provide indirect assessments of brain function, and can display only relatively slow variations in metabolic and oxygenation activity. Still, it is clearly apparent that these modalities are complementary, and ripe for further fusion.

Tissue electric impedance tomography

Biological materials contain electrons and ions that can move about, to a greater or lesser extent, in response to an applied electric field. The measure of their responsiveness to externally applied electric pushes and pulls is called their *electrical impedance* (or, which is practically the same thing for most purposes, their *resistance*). Tissue impedance imaging assesses the resistance between numerous pairs of electrodes attached to the skin of a region of the body. It does this by applying a low voltage between any two of them, and gauging the current produced everywhere; it then employs CT-like reconstruction calculations to generate maps of tissue impedance throughout the region. Like MRI, tissue impedance imaging is sensitive to changes in the water content of tissues; indeed, it is being developed by the military to monitor blood loss from the wounded. Other reported applications include studies of gastric emptying, pulmonary ventilation, cardiac output, blood flow, and intracranial hemorrhaging in infants. Since malignant tumor tissue may be an

order of magnitude or so more conductive than surrounding normal tissue, instruments have been built to explore the assessment of ambiguous breast masses.

Electric impedance tomography is safe, can be used at the bedside, allows for long-term data acquisition, costs little, and images a new physiologic function that may turn out to be uniquely revealing for some disorders.

Photo-acoustic imaging

Photo-acoustic tomographic (*PAT*) imaging displays strong contrast and the fine resolution obtainable from ultrasound. While this hybrid modality is still far from routine clinical use, it could well have a big impact.

A typical simple PAT system might start off with a microsecond-long pulse from a laser, spread out with an optics assembly so as to form a thin beam of parallel rays of intense, monochromatic light (Figure 13.8a). When directed into a portion of compressed breast, say, much of the light passes through, but that which strikes a blood vessel is strongly absorbed by the hemoglobin (Figure 13.8b). (Oxygenated and deoxygenated hemoglobin both absorb optical radiation well, incidentally, but they have spectra that differ enough to allow distinction between the two species.) The energy is absorbed over a period of microseconds, and the heat causes a burst of thermal expansion so rapid that it causes a pulse of ultrasound to radiate from the vessel. Finally, this ultrasound energy is detected by a 2D array of small and extremely sensitive transducer elements. Obviously, untangling the mess of signals and making sense of them is a remarkably nasty reconstruction job, but filtered back-projection appears somewhat able to handle it.

Photo-acoustic imaging is still in the exploratory phase, but its ability to find and display breast lesions, in particular, is impressive. Applications are constrained, at present, by the power of penetration of the laser light and by the sensitivity of the transducers, to blocks of tissue, test animals, etc., less than 1 cm or so thick, but researchers are searching for possible ways around that limit.

Thermo-acoustic (TAT) imaging is similar, but employs pulses of microwave energy, rather than light, to deliver high power to a region.

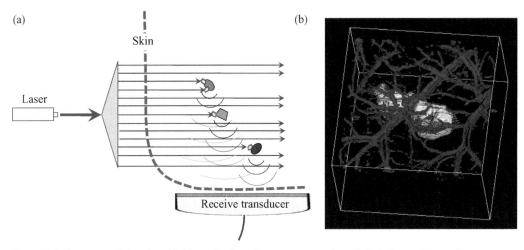

Figure 13.8 Photo-acoustic imaging. **(a)** Schematic of a rudimentary system. Laser light is dispersed into a fan or continuous band of parallel rays, and enters tissue. When striking a highly absorbing entity, such as a blood vessel, the optical energy is transformed into heat, which brings about a burst of thermal expansion. This generates MHz acoustic waves, and these are picked up by a transducer and untangled by a computer to create an image. **(b)** Frame from a 3D movie of a melanoma (http://upload.wikimedia.org/wikipedia/commons/1/17/Melanoma3DMovie.gif).

Computer technology: the constant revolution

"She suffered a stroke at the age of 42, and for nearly a decade after, she was unable to move or communicate beyond shaking her head . . . . but today, thanks to a neural implant that links her brain to a computer, she has used her mind to control a keyboard and move a robotic arm."

Science 2011;**333**:1108

What is perhaps most amazing about this report is not only the extraordinary power of connecting brain-implanted electrodes to computers to create the beginnings of cyborg-like minds, but also that this sort of thing has been going on for two decades. Current brain-machine interfaces (BMI) can even allow paralyzed patients to manipulate their own or bionic hands with their thoughts and experience tactile feedback.

It is only recently, however, that researchers and patients are able to do this non-invasively, with electrodes sitting on the scalp rather than passing through it. Like *f*MRI, and PET, electroencephalography has for some while been capturing electrical wave forms diagnostic of various diseases of the brain non-invasively. But here we enter a whole new domain, and the possibilities are literally mind-boggling in many areas, including medicine. The prospects of genuine computer-based thinking caps assisting severely disabled individuals appear limitless but so, too, does the notion of criminals, many politicians, and other expert liars having actually to tell the truth. Meanwhile, a number of companies are marketing a variety of EEG-related computer games and other apps, and no doubt the technology will develop rapidly and in unanticipated directions. Meanwhile . . .

First appearing in the clinic in the 1970s, computers have enabled novel computation-intensive imaging (CT, MRI, PET); provided image processing and analysis tools ranging from windowing and noise reduction to CAD for all modalities; and allowed the instantaneous storage, retrieval, display, and transmission of images and other information with PACS, electronic notepads, and so on. In so doing, they have altogether changed how medicine is practiced. The deployment of digital imaging systems; high-bandwidth, fast networks to transport images between acquisition, interpretation, consultation, and storage sites; and algorithms for computer recognition of image features for computer-aided detection and diagnosis are ushering in a whole new approach to medical imaging. The only certainty is that what we see today is just the beginning. Tomorrow – perhaps the one-stop digital diagnostician in a box? And after that?

Computers themselves will keep on getting faster, smarter, and less costly. The CPU of a typical PC is now made up of some 10^9 transistors, separated apart by 30 nanometers. A fast new desktop personal computer may be able to manage ten billion operations in a second. The most advanced supercomputers operate more than 10^5 times faster, at a thousand trillion operations per second, and draw on a quintillion (a million trillion) bytes of local mass storage in doing so.

In 1965, Gordon Moore, co-founder of Intel, predicted that that the number of individual transistors that could be fitted onto a small chip of silicon, hence its speed, would double every year or so, and that the cost per chip would decline accordingly. A half century later, some assert that Moore's law has run its course, and that it is finally bumping up against ultimate size limitations raised by inter-transistor electron leakage, or the need to dissipate ever-increasing amounts of heat. That may or may not be true. Certain innovations, including carbon and silicon nanowires and nanotubes, the discovery of the remarkable electronic properties of graphene (a carbon film one atom thick) and of spintronics (which affect the spin orientations of electrons in a magnetic field, rather than their responses to electric fields), building arrays of transistors in three dimensions instead of two, and other developments, show promise in keeping Moore's law valid. And cloud and grid technologies, by means of which computation and memory tasks are distributed over wide networks of facilities, are coming to the fore, and promise virtually unlimited amounts of computer power and memory.

The boundary between computation and communication is blurring. In the second decade of the new millennium, something like a billion cell phones are filling the airwaves with chatter. More than 10% of them are smart cell phone–computer hybrids that cruise the Web, support complex games, and send and receive email, text messages, and images. This wireless technology is already nosing its way into the clinic in the form of systems for computerized physician order entry and real-time verbal updating of patient charts by way of tablet personal computers that incorporate dictation, transcription, and error-prevention software.

Beyond producing ever bigger and faster computers, some researchers at the cutting edge are taking the first tentative steps toward creating computing machines that are different in kind, not just in degree. Rather than sending currents of electrons along routes determined by the settings of silicon-based switches, a DNA computer, for example, would operate by snipping and joining segments of DNA in solution. Such a computer would consume a billion times less energy than its solid-state siblings, require a trillionth of the space, and perform some kinds of computations that are otherwise impossible now.

At the same time, preliminary *quantum computers* are being explored that operate according to the counterintuitive quirky rules of quantum mechanics, rather than the linear, "if-this-then-that" Boolean logic of everyday life. While digital computers operate, ultimately, with electronic switches that can be in either the "on" or the "off" bit state, quantum devices would manipulate "qubits," or states that comprise a range of combinations of the two. Like practical DNA devices, they would provide calculational powers currently undreamed of but – also like DNA computers – probably not for decades, if ever.

DNA and quantum computers will act somewhat like massively parallel conventional computers – in effect, performing gargantuan numbers of relatively simple computations with blinding speed. They will be able to crack certain mathematic problems in minutes that would give today's computers centuries-long nightmares, such as separating a thousand-digit number into its two prime-number factors – a task that is of critical importance in making and breaking secret codes. But they may also be relatively inflexible and, as with supercomputers, challenging to provide software for and to program. Still, all it might take is one good idea to change all that.

Another species of biological computer, the neuron computer, might be relatively slow, but it could open up a limitless universe of possibilities. Perhaps grown as clusters of human nerve cells and self-assembling according to building plans contained within a genetically modified DNA set, a neuron computer might interface with the outside world by way of a solid-state substrate – at the confluence of semiconductor, information, nano-, and biotechnologies. Or perhaps it could talk directly with the neurons of a human brain through attached electrodes or other means. Conceivably, a neuron computer could be made to mimic the structure or function of some of our own neural complexes. And that might be just the start.

The most advanced computers play increasingly central roles in circuit design, and Darwinian (i.e., "genetic" programming) methods encourage their rapid, and sometimes non-obvious, paths of "evolution." New machines may come into being that function in desirable ways but that will conceivably be far, far too complicated for humans to understand. And these machines will, in turn, design future generations of computers, and so on, and so on – an interesting prospect, and no longer the stuff of science fiction.

Imaging with a crystal ball

Much of optical and molecular imaging, thermography, electrocardiography and electroencephalography, magnetocardiography and magnetoencephalography, terahertz imaging, tissue impedance imaging, and electron-spin resonance imaging is still largely experimental, and some of the potential applications have achieved only limited clinical success so far. It is quite possible, however, that one or more of these technologies may burst without warning onto the clinical scene. High-technology companies are expending considerable resources to push MRI, CT, SPECT, PET, EEG, and other established modalities farther along – and on the way, they may well find exactly what is needed to bring magnetoencephalography or tissue impedance or electron spin resonance imaging to the fore. Just as likely, methods that combine modalities, such as happened with PET plus CT, and perhaps optical plus US imaging, will continue to break new ground. And then there are all those wild ideas not yet even imagined …

So maybe the clinic of 2050 will be as astonishing to us as MRI would be to Roentgen. You just never know!

> "Everything that can be invented has been invented."
> Charles H. Duell, Commissioner,
> US Patent Office, 1899

References

1 Wolbarst AB, Hendee WR. Evolving and experimental technologies in medical imaging. *Radiology* 2006;**238**:16–39.

2 Massoud TF, Gambhir SS. Molecular imaging in living subjects: seeing fundamental biological processes in a new light. *Genes Dev* 2003;**17**(5):545–80.

Suggested Further Reading

General imaging

Clinical and technical

The Essential Physics of Medical Imaging, 3rd edn. Jerrold T Bushberg, J Anthony Seibert, Edwin M Leidholdt, Jr., John M Boone. Wolters Kluwer | Lippincott Williams & Wilkins, Philadelphia (2012). Recommended to follow *Medical Imaging – Essentials for Physicians*. Very wide (1000 pages), up-to-date coverage of many topics.

Physics of Radiology, 2nd edn. Anthony B Wolbarst. Medical Physics Publishing, Madison (2005). Like the technical parts of *Medical Imaging – Essentials for Physicians*, but more of it.

Medical Imaging Physics, 4th edn. William R Hendee, E Russell Ritenour. Wiley-Liss, New York (2002). Nice problem sets with solutions.

Advances in Medical Physics series (volumes 1–4). Anthony B Wolbarst, William R Hendee, *et al.*, eds. Medical Physics Publishing, Madison (2006, 2008, 2010, 2012). Some chapters suitable for physicians, others for medical physicists, etc., and some for both.

Clinical

Essentials of Radiology, 2nd edn. FA Mettler, Jr. Elsevier Saunders, Philadelphia (2005).

Squire's Fundamentals of Radiology, 6th edn. RA Novelline. Harvard University Press, Cambridge (2004).

Bontrager's Handbook of Radiographic Positioning and Techniques, 7th edn. KL Bontrager, J Lampignano. Mosby, Maryland Heights (2009).

Grainger & Allison's Diagnostic Radiology: A Textbook of Medical Imaging, 4th edn. RG Grainger, DJ Allison, AK Dixon, eds. Churchill Livingstone, London (2001).

Comprehensive Radiographic Pathology, 4th edn. R Eisenberg, N Johnson. Mosby, Marryland Heights, MO (2007).

Technical

Webb's Physics of Medical Imaging, 2nd edn. MA Flower, ed. CRC Press, Boca Raton (2012).

Foundations of Image Science. Harrison H Barrett, Kyle J Myers. Wiley, Hoboken (2004). Massive, mathematical, and deep.

Digital radiology and fluoroscopy

Clinical and technical

Radiography in the Digital Age: *Physics-Exposure-Radiation Biology*, 1st edn. QB Carroll. Charles C Thomas, Springfield (2011).

"Mammography and other breast imaging techniques." Libby Brateman, Andrew Karellas. In: *Advances in Medical Physics*, vol. 1. Anthony B Wolbarst, Robert G Zamenhof, William R Hendee, eds. Medical Physics Publishing, Madison, pp 25–58 (2006).

PACS: *A Guide to the Digital Revolution*, 2nd edn. KJ Dreyer, DS Hirschorn, JH Thrall, eds. Springer, New York (2010).

Clinical

Digital Mammography, 1st edn. ED Pisano, MJ Yaffe, CM Kuzmiak. Lippincott Williams & Wilkins, Philadelphia (2003).

Abram's Angiography: Interventional Radiology, 2nd edn. S Baum, MJ Pentecost, eds. Lippincott Williams & Wilkins, Philadelphia (2006).

Technical

"Digital radiology and fluoroscopy." Wei Zhao, Katherine P Andriole, Ehsan Samei. In: *Advances in Medical Physics*, vol. 1. Anthony B Wolbarst, Robert G Zamenhof, William R Hendee, eds. Medical Physics Publishing, Madison, pp 1–24 (2006).

"Recent developments in fluoroscopic imaging systems in interventional procedures." Barry Belanger. In: *Advances in Medical Physics*, vol. 4. Anthony B Wolbarst, Patrizio Capasso, Devon J Godfrey, *et al.*, eds. Medical Physics Publishing, Madison, pp 23–58 (2012).

Medical Imaging: Essentials for Physicians, First Edition. Anthony B. Wolbarst, Patrizio Capasso and Andrew R. Wyant.
© 2013 John Wiley & Sons, Inc. Published 2013 by John Wiley & Sons, Inc.

Computed tomography

Clinical and technical

Computed Tomography, 2nd edn. Willi A Kalender. Publicis Corporate Publishing, Erlangen (2005).

Computed Tomography: Physical Principles, Clinical Applications, and Quality Control, 3rd edn. E Seeram. Saunders, Philadelphia (2008).

"CT dose index and patient dose: they are not the same thing." CH McCollough, S Leng, L Yu, DD Cody, JM Boone, MF McNitt-Gray. *Radiology* 2011;259:311–16.

Clinical

Computed Body Tomography with MRI Correlation, 4th edn. JKT Lee, SS Sagel, RJ Stanley, JP Heiken, eds. Lippincott Williams & Wilkins, Philadelphia (2003).

CT and MRI of the Whole Body, 5th edn. JR Haaga, D Boll (authors), VS Dogra, M Forsting, RC Gilkeson, *et al.*, eds. Mosby, Philadelphia (2008).

CT and MR Angiography: Comprehensive Vascular Assessment, 1st edn. GD Rubin, NM Rofsky, eds. Lippincott Williams & Wilkins, Philadelphia (2008).

Technical

"Principles of computer assisted tomography (CAT) in radiographic and radioisotope imaging." Rodney A Brooks, Giovanni di Chiro. *Physics in Medicine and Biology*, 1976;21:689–732.

"Computerized tomography." Thomas G Flohr, Dianna D Cody, Cynthia H McCollough. In: *Advances in Medical Physics*, vol. 1. Anthony B Wolbarst, Robert G Zamenhof, William R Hendee, eds. Medical Physics Publishing, Madison, pp 59–100 (2006).

"Advances in CT." Thomas G Flohr, Bernhard T Schmidt. In: *Advances in Medical Physics*, vol. 4. Anthony B Wolbarst, Patrizio Capasso, Devon J Godfrey, *et al.*, eds. Medical Physics Publishing, Madison, pp 75–110 (2012).

"CT, PET, and SPECT reconstruction algorithms." David S Lalush. In: *Advances in Medical Physics*, vol. 2. Anthony B Wolbarst, Kenneth L Mossman, eds. Medical Physics Publishing, Madison, pp 1–24 (2008).

Nuclear Medicine

Clinical and technical

Nuclear Medicine Physics: The Basics, 6th edn. Ramesh Chandra. Lippincott Williams & Wilkins, Philadelphia (2004).

Physics in Nuclear Medicine, 3rd edn. Simon R Cherry, James A Sorenson, Michael E Phelps. Saunders, Philadelphia (2003).

Clinical

Nuclear Medicine Technology: Procedures and Quick Reference, 2nd edn. P Shackett. Lippincott-Raven, Philadelphia (2008).

Clinical Nuclear Medicine, 4th edn. GJR Cook, MN Maisey, KE Britton, V Chengazi. Hodder Arnold, London (2007).

Technical

Recent Developments in Nuclear Medicine. Frederic H Fahey. In: *Advances in Medical Physics*, vol. 3. Anthony B Wolbarst, Andrew Karellas, Elizabeth A Krupinski, William R Hendee, eds. Medical Physics Publishing, Madison, pp 19–36 (2010).

Molecular imaging

Clinical and technical

"Quantitative imaging biomarkers of cancer." John C Gore, H Charles Manning, Todd E Peterson, *et al.* In: *Advances in Medical Physics*, vol. 3. Anthony B Wolbarst, Andrew Karellas, Elizabeth A Krupinski, William R Hendee, eds. Medical Physics Publishing, Madison, pp 89–112 (2010).

"Molecular imaging and tomography with near-infrared fluorescence." Eva M Sevick-Muraca. In: *Advances in Medical Physics*, vol. 4. Anthony B Wolbarst, Patrizio Capasso, Devon J Godfrey, *et al.*, eds. Medical Physics Publishing, Madison, pp 155–72 (2012).

"Molecular imaging." X Michalet, LA Bentolila, S Weiss. In *Advances in Medical Physics*, vol 1. Anthony B Wolbarst, Robert G Zamenhof, William R Hendee, eds. Medical Physics Publishing, Madison (2006).

"Molecular imaging: physics and bioapplications of quantum dots." X Michalet, LA Bentolila, S Weiss. In *Advances in Medical Physics*, vol. 2. Anthony B Wolbarst, Kenneth L Mossman, eds. Medical Physics Publishing, Madison (2008).

Clinical

Molecular Imaging, 1st edn. R Weissleder, BD Ross, SS Gambhir. People's Medical Publishing House USA, Beijing (2010).

Molecular Imaging: Radiopharmaceuticals for PET and SPECT, 1st edn. S Vallabhajosula. Springer, New York (2009).

Ultrasound

Clinical and technical

Ultrasound Physics and Instrumentation, 4th edn. Wayne R Hedrick, David L Hykes, Dale E Starchman. Elsevier/Mosby, St. Louis (2005).

Basic Doppler Physics. Hans-Jorgen Smith, James A Zagzebski. Medical Physics Publishing, Madison (1991).

Clinical

Diagnostic Ultrasound, 4th edn. CM Rumack, SR Wilson, JW Charboneau, D Levine. Mosby, Philadelphia (2011).
Ultrasound: The Requisites, 2nd edn. WD Middleton, AB Kurtz. Mosby, Philadelphia (2003).
Sonography Principles and Instruments, 8th edn. FW Kremkau. Saunders, Philadelphia (2010).

Technical

"Recent advances in ultrasonic imaging and ultrasound imaging technology." Jeremy J Dahl, Gregg E Trahey. In: *Advances in Medical Physics,* vol. 4. Anthony B Wolbarst, Patrizio Capasso, Devon J Godfrey, *et al.*, eds. Medical Physics Publishing, Madison, pp 219–234 (2012).
"2D and 3D data acquisition in ultrasound." James A Zagzebski. In: *Advances in Medical Physics,* vol. 4. Anthony B Wolbarst, Patrizio Capasso, Devon J Godfrey, *et al.*, eds. Medical Physics Publishing, Madison, pp 235–52 (2012).
Quality Assurance Manual for Gray Scale Ultrasound Scanners (Stage 2), E Madsen, ed. American Institute of Ultrasound in Medicine, Laurel, (1995).
"Real-time B-mode ultrasound quality control test procedures. Report of AAPM Ultrasound Task Group No. 1." MM Goodsitt, PL Carson, S Witt, *et al. Medical Physics* 1998;**25**(8):1385–1406.

Magnetic resonance imaging

Clinical and technical

A Non-Mathematical Approach to Basic MRI. Hans-J Smith, Frank N Ranallo. Medical Physics Publishing, Madison (1989). Recommended next step.
Questions and Answers in Magnetic Resonance Imaging, 2nd edn. Allen D Elster, Jonathan H Burdette. Mosby, St. Louis (2001).
"Artifacts in MRI." Jiachen Zhou, Rao Gullapalli. In: *Advances in Medical Physics,* vol. 3. Anthony B Wolbarst, Andrew Karellas, Elizabeth A Krupinski, William R Hendee, eds. Medical Physics Publishing, Madison, pp 55–72 (2010).

Clinical

MRI in Practice, 4th edn. C Westbrook, CK Roth, J Talbot. Wiley-Blackwell, Chichester (2011).

Technical

"Physical foundations of proton NMR: parts 1 & 2." In: *NMR in Medicine: Instrumentation and Clinical Applications.* Stephen R Thomas, Robert L Dixon, eds. AAPM Medical Physics Monograph no. 14, American Institute of Physics, New York, pp 1–58 (1986). An old but classic technical overview.
Handbook of MRI Pulse Sequences. Matt A Bernstein, Kevin E King, Xiaohong Joe Zhou. Elsevier, Amsterdam (2004).
"Developments in ultra-high-field MRI." Adam M Anderson, John C Gore. In: *Advances in Medical Physics,* vol. 4. Anthony B Wolbarst, Patrizio Capasso, Devon J Godfrey, *et al.*, eds. Medical Physics Publishing, Madison, pp 75–110 (2012).

Radiobiology

Clinical and technical

Radiobiology for the Radiologist, 6th edn. Eric J Hall, Amato J Giaccia. Lippincott Williams & Wilkins, Philadelphia (2006). The standard.
"The 2007 Recommendations of the International Commission on Radiological Protection." *Annals of the ICRP,* publication 103. J Valentin, ed. Elsevier, Orlando (2007).
Health Risks from Exposure to Low Levels of Ionizing Radiation: BEIR VII Phase 2. National Research Council. National Academies Press, Washington (2006).
Biological Effects of Low Doses of Ionizing Radiation. Antone L Brooks, Mathew A Coleman, Evan B Douple, *et al.* In: *Advances in Medical Physics,* vol. 1. Anthony B Wolbarst, Robert G Zamenhof, William R Hendee, eds. Medical Physics Publishing, Madison, pp 255–86 (2006).
"Medical response to a major radiologic emergency: a primer for medical and public health practitioners." Anthony B Wolbarst, Albert L Wiley, Jeffrey B Nemhauser, *et al. Radiology* 2010;**254**:660–77.
Basic Clinical Radiobiology, 4th edn. A Van der Kogel, M Joiner. Hodder-Arnold, London (2009).

Index

Page numbers in **bold** represent tables, those in *italics* represent figures.

Medical Imaging: Essentials for Physicians, First Edition. Anthony B. Wolbarst, Patrizio Capasso and Andrew R. Wyant.
© 2013 John Wiley & Sons, Inc. Published 2013 by John Wiley & Sons, Inc.

Printed and bound by CPI Group (UK) Ltd, Croydon, CR0 4YY

16/04/2025

14658537-0002

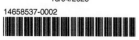